Pharmacology **Success**

A Course Review Applying Critical Thinking to Test Taking

Pharmacology **Success**

A Course Review Applying Critical Thinking to Test Taking

Ray A. Hargrove-Huttel RN, PhD

Trinity Valley Community College

Kaufman, Texas

Kathryn Cadenhead Colgrove RN, MS, CNS, OCN

Trinity Valley Community College

Kaufman, Texas

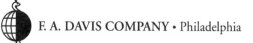 F. A. DAVIS COMPANY • Philadelphia

F. A. Davis Company
1915 Arch Street
Philadelphia, PA 19103
www.fadavis.com

Printed in the United States of America

Last digit indicates print number: 10 9 8 7 6 5 4 3 2 1

Publisher, Nursing: Robert G. Martone
Director of Content Development: Darlene D. Pedersen
Project Editor: Padraic J. Maroney
Art and Design Manager: Carolyn O'Brien

As new scientific information becomes available through basic and clinical research, recommended treatments and drug therapies undergo changes. The author(s) and publisher have done everything possible to make this book accurate, up to date, and in accord with accepted standards at the time of publication. The author(s), editors, and publisher are not responsible for errors or omissions or for consequences from application of the book, and make no warranty, expressed or implied, in regard to the contents of the book. Any practice described in this book should be applied by the reader in accordance with professional standards of care used in regard to the unique circumstances that may apply in each situation. The reader is advised always to check product information (package inserts) for changes and new information regarding dose and contraindications before administering any drug. Caution is especially urged when using new or infrequently ordered drugs.

Contributors

Leslie Prater, RN, MS, CNS, CDE
Clinical Diabetes Educator
Associate Degree Nursing Instructor
Trinity Valley Community College
Kaufman, Texas

Helen Reid, RN, PhD
Dean, Health Occupations
Trinity Valley Community College
Kaufman, Texas

Reviewers

Sue Bond, RN, BSN, MSN
Interim Advanced Project Coordinator, Nursing Instructor
Prima Community College Center for Training and Development
Practical Nurse Program
Tucson, Arizona

M. Joyce Dienger, DNSc, RN
Assistant Professor
University of Cincinnati
Cincinnati, Ohio

Pamela Fifer, MS, RN
Nursing Faculty
Chemeketa Community College
Salem, Oregon

Lois Griffin, MSN, FNP
Instructor
Shelton State Community College
Tuscaloosa, Alabama

Lori A. Hart, MS, APRN
Assistant Professor
Weber State University
Sitka, Arkansas

Carol Masker
Senior Analyst
Hoffman-La Roche Labs
Nutley, New Jersey

Maureen McDonald, MS, RN
Professor
Massasoit Community College
Brockton, Massachusetts

Karen Mitchell, RN, MSN
Course Coordinator, Clinical Instructor
The Christ Hospital School of Nursing,
The Christ College of Nursing and Health Sciences
Cincinnati, Ohio

Janice Palese, BS, MS, PhD, RN
Professor
John A. Logan College
Carterville, Illinois

Elizabeth A. Palmer, PhD, MS, BS
Associate Professor
Indiana University of Pennsylvania
Indiana, Pennsylvania

Acknowledgments

The authors are dedicating this book to the Trinity Valley Community College Associate Degree nursing students, faculty, and staff. Without the support and encouragement of the faculty and staff this book would not be possible. The nursing students' enquiring minds and thirst for knowledge challenge us daily to continue our own learning. We would like to thank Rob Martone for giving us the opportunity for our second book in the series and our appreciation goes to Barbara Tchabovsky for her editorial assistance. Our sincere thanks go to Glada Norris for sharing her incredible computer skills in the process of preparing the book for the publisher.

I would like to dedicate this book to Ruth, Ann, and Jan, Sue and Marvin and all the members of my family who have been by my side throughout the years. Always in my heart is the memory of my husband, Bill, and my parents, T/Sgt. Leo and Nancy Hargrove, who are the rocks on which my life is built. I also thank and acknowledge my sisters, Gail and Debbie, my nephew Benjamin, and Paula for their support and encouragement. My children, Teresa and Aaron, continue to amaze me as they enter their adulthood and remain the most important people in my life. Congratulations Aaron on your graduation.

RAY ANN HARGROVE-HUTTEL

I would like to thank my extended family for the love and support they showed to a small child and have never ceased to be there for me; Evelyn and Joe Young, Carolyn Wood, Charles Wood, George Rogers, Evelyn Davis, Roger Cadenhead, Jodi Greenbaum, and Stacy Shudak. I would like to dedicate this book to my husband, Larry, daughter Laurie and son-in-law Todd, and son Larry Jr. and daughter-in-law Mai, and grandchildren Chris, Ashley, Justin C., Justin A., Connor, and Sawyer without their support and patience the book would not have been possible.

KATHRYN COLGROVE

Table of Contents

1 **Basic Concepts in Medication Administration** 1

2 **Neurological System** 7
PRACTICE QUESTIONS 7
A Client with Head Injury 7
A Client with Seizures 8
A Client with Cerebrovascular Accident 10
A Client with Brain Tumor 11
A Client with Parkinson's Disease 12
A Client Diagnosed with Alzheimer's Disease 14
A Client with a Migraine Headache 15
PRACTICE QUESTIONS ANSWERS AND RATIONALES 17
COMPREHENSIVE EXAMINATION 29
COMPREHENSIVE EXAMINATION ANSWERS AND RATIONALES 32

3 **Cardiovascular System** 37
PRACTICE QUESTIONS 37
A Client with Angina/Myocardial Infarction 37
A Client with Coronary Artery Disease 39
A Client with Congestive Heart Failure 41
A Client with Dysrhythmias and Conduction Problems 42
A Client with Inflammatory Cardiac Disorders 45
A Client with Arterial Occlusive Disease 46
A Client with Arterial Hypertension 47
A Client with Deep Vein Thrombosis 49
A Client with Anemia 51
PRACTICE QUESTIONS ANSWERS AND RATIONALES 53
COMPREHENSIVE EXAMINATION 69
COMPREHENSIVE EXAMINATION ANSWERS AND RATIONALES 72

4 **Pulmonary System** 77
PRACTICE QUESTIONS 77
A Client with Upper Respiratory Infection 77
A Client with Lower Respiratory Infection 78
A Client with Reactive Airway Disease 79
A Child with Reactive Airway Disease 81
A Client with Pulmonary Embolus 82
PRACTICE QUESTIONS ANSWERS AND RATIONALES 85
COMPREHENSIVE EXAMINATION 94
COMPREHENSIVE EXAMINATION ANSWERS AND RATIONALES 97

5 **Gastrointestinal System** 101
PRACTICE QUESTIONS 101
A Client with Gastroesophageal Reflux 101
A Client with Inflammatory Bowel Disease 102
A Client with Peptic Ulcer Disease 104

An Elderly Client with Diverticulosis/Diverticulitis 105
A Client with Liver Failure 106
A Client with Hepatitis 108
A Child with Gastroenteritides 109
A Client Who Is Obese 110
A Client Experiencing Constipation or Diarrhea 112
A Client Undergoing Abdominal Surgery with General Anesthesia 113
PRACTICE QUESTIONS ANSWERS AND RATIONALES 115
COMPREHENSIVE EXAMINATION 133
COMPREHENSIVE EXAMINATION ANSWERS AND RATIONALES 137

6   Endocrine System **141**
PRACTICE QUESTIONS 141
A Client with Type 1 Diabetes 141
A Client with Type 2 Diabetes 142
A Client with Pancreatitis 144
A Client with Adrenal Disorders 145
A Client with Pituitary Disorders 146
A Client with Thyroid Disorders 148
PRACTICE QUESTIONS ANSWERS AND RATIONALES 150
COMPREHENSIVE EXAMINATION 162
COMPREHENSIVE EXAMINATION ANSWERS AND RATIONALES 165

7   Genitourinary System **169**
PRACTICE QUESTIONS 169
A Client with Chronic Renal Failure 169
A Client with a Urinary Tract Infection 170
A Client with Benign Prostatic Hypertrophy and Spinal Anesthesia 172
A Client with Renal Calculi 173
An Adolescent with a Sexually Transmitted Disease 175
A Client Experiencing Pregnancy 176
A Client Experiencing Infertility 177
A Client Using Birth Control 179
PRACTICE QUESTIONS ANSWERS AND RATIONALES 181
COMPREHENSIVE EXAMINATION 195
COMPREHENSIVE EXAMINATION ANSWERS AND RATIONALES 198

8   Musculoskeletal System **203**
PRACTICE QUESTIONS 203
A Client with Low Back Pain 203
A Client with Osteoarthritis 204
A Client with Osteoporosis 206
A Client Undergoing an Orthopedic Surgery 207
PRACTICE QUESTIONS ANSWERS AND RATIONALES 209
COMPREHENSIVE EXAMINATION 217
COMPREHENSIVE EXAMINATION ANSWERS AND RATIONALES 220

9   Integumentary System **225**
PRACTICE QUESTIONS 225
A Client with Burns 225
A Client with Pressure Ulcers 226
A Client with a Skin Disorder 228
PRACTICE QUESTIONS ANSWERS AND RATIONALES 230
COMPREHENSIVE EXAMINATION 235
COMPREHENSIVE EXAMINATION ANSWERS AND RATIONALES 238

10   Immune Inflammatory System **241**
PRACTICE QUESTIONS 241
A Client with an Autoimmune Disease 241

A Client with Acquired Immunodeficiency Syndrome 242
A Client with Allergies 244
A Client with Rheumatoid Arthritis 245
A Child Receiving Immunizations 247
PRACTICE QUESTIONS ANSWERS AND RATIONALES 249
COMPREHENSIVE EXAMINATION 258
COMPREHENSIVE EXAMINATION ANSWERS AND RATIONALES 261

11 Cancer Treatments 265
PRACTICE QUESTIONS 265
A Client Receiving Chemotherapy 265
A Client Receiving a Biologic Response Modifier 268
A Client Receiving Hormone Therapy 269
A Client Receiving an Investigational Protocol 270
A Client Undergoing Surgery for Cancer 272
A Client with Chronic Pain 273
PRACTICE QUESTIONS ANSWERS AND RATIONALES 276
COMPREHENSIVE EXAMINATION 287
COMPREHENSIVE EXAMINATION ANSWERS AND RATIONALES 291

12 Mental Health Disorders 295
PRACTICE QUESTIONS 295
A Client with a Major Depressive Disorder 295
A Client with Bipolar Disorder 296
A Client with Schizophrenia 298
A Client with an Anxiety Disorder 299
A Child with Attention Deficit–Hyperactivity Disorder 301
A Client with a Sleep Disorder 302
A Client with Substance Abuse 304
PRACTICE QUESTIONS ANSWERS AND RATIONALES 306
COMPREHENSIVE EXAMINATION 319
COMPREHENSIVE EXAMINATION ANSWERS AND RATIONALES 323

13 Sensory Deficits 327
PRACTICE QUESTIONS 327
A Client with an Eye Disorder 327
A Child with an Ear Infection 328
PRACTICE QUESTIONS ANSWERS AND RATIONALES 331
COMPREHENSIVE EXAMINATION 335
COMPREHENSIVE EXAMINATION ANSWERS AND RATIONALES 338

14 Emergency Nursing 341
PRACTICE QUESTIONS 341
A Client Experiencing Shock 341
A Community Facing Bioterrorism 342
A Client Experiencing a Code 344
A Child Experiencing Poisoning 345
PRACTICE QUESTIONS ANSWERS AND RATIONALES 347
COMPREHENSIVE EXAMINATION 354
COMPREHENSIVE EXAMINATION ANSWERS AND RATIONALES 357

15 Nonprescribed Medications 361
PRACTICE QUESTIONS 361
A Client Taking Herbs 361
A Client Taking Vitamins/Minerals 362
A Client Self-Prescribing Medications 364
PRACTICE QUESTIONS ANSWERS AND RATIONALES 366
COMPREHENSIVE EXAMINATION 371
COMPREHENSIVE EXAMINATION ANSWERS AND RATIONALES 374

16 Administration of Medications **379**
    PRACTICE QUESTIONS 379
        The Nurse Administering Medications 379
        The Nurse Computing Math to Administer Medications 380
    PRACTICE QUESTIONS ANSWERS AND RATIONALES 383
    COMPREHENSIVE EXAMINATION 387
    COMPREHENSIVE EXAMINATION ANSWERS AND RATIONALES 390

17 Comprehensive Examination **395**
    COMPREHENSIVE EXAMINATION ANSWERS AND RATIONALES 410

Index **425**

Basic Concepts in Medication Administration

The nurse should never put a medication in any client's orifice, manmade or natural, if the nurse does not know what the medication is, how it acts in the body, and what the safe administration guidelines for that medication are.

—Ray A. Hargrove-Huttel

PHARMACOLOGY TEST-TAKING HINTS

The test taker must know medications, and memorization is part of administering medications safely. This chapter contains some tips to assist the test taker in learning about medications; they apply to all the questions in this book.

First, learn the specific classification of the medication, including the actions, side effects, and adverse effects of the medications in that classification. Also learn how to safely administer a medication in the classification. Generally speaking, medications in a classification share characteristics. However, be sure not to be too broad in the classification. For example, do not combine all medications administered for hypertension in the same category. Angiotensin converting enzyme (ACE) inhibitors, beta blockers, and calcium channel blockers do not work in the same manner and are not in the same classification—even though they may all be used to treat hypertension. Similarly, oral medications for diabetes mellitus and diuretics fall into several classification groups; the facts about each specific classification must be learned. Each classification has its own effects on the body, its own side effects, and its own adverse effects; in addition, the nurse must take specific steps before administering a medication in a specific classification category.

When administering medications for a group of clients, the test taker must realize that time is a realistic problem. It is not feasible for the nurse to look up 50 to 60 medications and administer them all within the dosing time frame, so it is imperative that the nurse learn about the most common medications.

One tip for learning about medications is for the test taker to complete handmade drug cards. This is better than buying ready-made cards because in completing the drug cards the test taker uses more than one method of learning—reading, deciding which information to put on the card, and writing the pertinent information on the card. All of this assists the test taker in memorizing the information.

When the test taker is deciding which information is the most important to write on a drug card, the following five questions can be used as a guide. The test taker should always ask "why" an intervention is being implemented. That is the key to critical thinking.

1. *What classification is the medication that the nurse is administering to the client in, and why specifically is this client receiving this medication? Many medications are categorized in one classification group, but the client is receiving the medication for a different reason. For example, the anticonvulsant valproic acid (Depakote), commonly used to treat seizures, is also administered as an antimania medication. What action does the medication have on the body? This is known as the scientific rationale for administering the medication.*

Example #1:

Digoxin (Lanoxin) 0.25 mg po

- The classification of this medication is a cardiac glycoside.
- The medication is administered to clients diagnosed with congestive heart failure or rapid atrial fibrillation.
- Cardiac glycosides increase the contractility of the heart and decrease the heart rate. (In heart failure, the medication is administered to increase the contractility of the heart, but in atrial fibrillation, the medication is administered to slow the heart rate.)

Example #2:

Furosemide (Lasix) 40 mg intravenous push (IVP)

- The classification of the medication is a loop diuretic.
- The medication is administered to clients with essential hypertension or congestive heart failure or with any other condition in which there is excess fluid in the body.
- This medication helps remove excess fluid from the body.
- Loop diuretics remove water from the kidneys along with potassium.

2. *When should the nurse question administering this medication? Does the medication have a therapeutic serum level? Which vital signs must be monitored? Which physiological parameters should be monitored when the medication is being administered?*

Example #1:

Digoxin (Lanoxin)

- Is the apical pulse (AP) less than 60 beats per minute (bpm)?
- Is the digoxin level within the therapeutic range?
- Is the potassium level within normal range?

Example #2:

Furosemide (Lasix)

- Is the potassium level within normal range?
- Does the client have signs/symptoms of dehydration?
- Is the client's blood pressure below 90/60?

3. *What interventions must be taught to the client to ensure the medication is administered safely in the hospital setting? What interventions must be taught for taking the medication safely at home?*

Example #1:

Digoxin (Lanoxin)

- Explain the importance of getting serum levels checked regularly.
- Teach the client to take his or her radial pulse and not to take the medication if the pulse is less than 60.
- Inform the client to take the medication daily and notify the health-care provider (HCP) if not taking the medication.

Example #2:

Furosemide (Lasix)

- Teach about orthostatic hypotension.
- Instruct the client to drink water to replace insensible fluid loss.
- If the medication is IVP, inform the client about how many minutes the medication should be pushed, what primary IV is hanging, and whether it is compatible with Lasix.

4. *What are the side effects and potential adverse reactions? Side effects are undesired effects of the medication, but they do not warrant discontinuing or changing the medication. Adverse reactions involve any situation that would require notifying the health-care provider or discontinuing the medication.*

Example #1:
Digoxin (Lanoxin)
- Decrease in heart rate to below 60 bpm.
- Signs of toxicity—nausea, vomiting, anorexia, and yellow haze.

Example #2:
Furosemide (Lasix)
- Side effects—dizziness, lightheadedness.
- Adverse effects—hypokalemia; tinnitus if administered too quickly by IVP.

5. *How does the nurse know the medication is effective?*

Example #1:
Digoxin (Lanoxin)
- Have the signs/symptoms of congestive heart failure improved?
- Is the client able to breathe easier? How many pillows does the client have to sleep on when lying down? Is the client able to perform activities of daily living (ADL) without shortness of breath? What do the lung fields sound like?

Example #2:
Furosemide (Lasix)
- Is the client's urinary output greater than the intake?
- Has the client lost any weight?
- Does the client have sacral or peripheral edema?
- Does the client have jugular vein distention?
- Has the client's blood pressure decreased?

SAMPLE DRUG CARDS

Front of Card

Classification of Drug	Route
Action of drug	
Uses	
Nursing implications (When would I question giving the medication?)	
How will I monitor to see if it is working?	

Back of Card

Side Effects
Teaching needs
Drug names

It is suggested that the test taker complete these cards from a pharmacology textbook and not a drug handbook because most test questions come from a pharmacology book.

Sample Card for Digoxin

Digoxin Cardiac Glycosides		PO/IV
Action:	Positive inotropic action, increases force of ventricular contraction and thereby increases cardiac output; slows the heart, allowing for increased filling time.	
Uses:	Congestive heart failure and rapid atrial cardiac dysrhythmias	
Nursing Implications:	Check apical pulse for 1 full minute; hold if <60. Check digoxin level (0.5–2.0 normal, >2.5 = toxic). Check K+ level (hypokalemia is most common cause of dysrhythmias in clients receiving dig [3.5–5.0 mEq/L]). Monitor for S/S of CHF, crackles in lungs, I > O, edema. Question if the AP <60 or abnormal lab values. IVP—over 5 minutes: maintenance dose 0.125–0.25 mg q day	
Effectiveness:	S/S of CHF improve, output > intake, weight decreases, breathing improves, activity tolerance improves, atrial rate decreases	
Side Effects:	Toxic = yellow haze or nausea and vomiting; ventricular rate decreases. If given along with a diuretic, increased risk of hypokalemia.	
Teaching Needs:	To take radial pulse and hold if <60 and notify HCP. K+ replacement—eat food high in K+ or may need supplemental K+. Report weight gain of 3 lbs or more.	
Drug Names:	Digoxin (Generic) Lanoxin Lanoxicap	

Sample Card for Furosemide

Furosemide Loop Diuretic		PO/IVP/IM
Actions:	Blocks reabsorption of sodium and chloride in the loop of Henle = prevents the passive reabsorption of water = diuresis	
Uses:	CHF, fluid volume overload, pulmonary edema, HTN	
Nursing Implications:	I & O, monitor K+ level, check skin turgor, monitor for leg cramps, provide K+-rich foods or supplements, give early in the day to prevent nocturia. If giving IVP, give at prescribed rate (Lasix 20 mg/minute); ototoxic if given faster	
Effectiveness:	Decrease in weight, output > intake, less edema, lung sounds clear	
Side Effects:	Hypokalemia, muscle cramps, hyponatremia, dehydration	
Teaching Needs:	Take early in the day Eat foods high in K+	
Drug Names:	Furosemide (Lasix) Bumetanide (Bumex) Torsemide (Demadex) Ethacrynic acid (Edecrin)	

The test taker is encouraged to use these guidelines/test-taking hints when answering the questions about medications in the following chapters. The questions cover medications prescribed for many different disease processes. The book is intended to cover the most commonly occurring health-care problems, but it is not all-inclusive. New medications are approved for use every month.

In each chapter there are medication questions for specific disease processes and a comprehensive test that may have some questions regarding less common disease processes and the medications prescribed to treat these problems.

POPULATION-SPECIFIC INFORMATION

Pediatric Clients

The nurse must be aware that pediatric clients have specific prescribing and drug administration needs. The weight of the child's body directly affects the amount of medication that can safely be administered. In addition, possible effects on the liver and brain, which are not fully mature in pediatric clients, must be considered. Pediatric dosing is frequently prescribed in mg/kg. The nurse must have the mathematical ability to convert pounds to kilograms and grams to milligrams. A kilogram is equal to 2.2 pounds.

Elderly Clients

The nurse must be aware that as the body ages, the body processes slow and do not function as they once did. The liver and kidneys are responsible for processing medications and eliminating the excess from the body. These organs are two of the most important organs to monitor when administering medications. The client's reaction to the medications prescribed, laboratory studies, and potential toxicities must all be carefully monitored. In the elderly, doses may need to be decreased to account for the body's decreased ability to process and detoxify medications.

Females of Childbearing Age

Any time a female client is mentioned in a question and an age is given that indicates the client is of childbearing age and could be pregnant, the test taker must determine if the medication is safe to administer to two clients—the female client and a potential fetus.

IMPORTANT DATA TO REMEMBER

The test taker must know commonly used abbreviations and their meanings. Examples include PRN, an abbreviation for *pro re nata*, a Latin term meaning "as needed" or "as circumstances require," and b.i.d., an abbreviation for *bis in die*, a Latin term meaning "twice a day." Many such abbreviations are used in medical prescribing, and the nurse must be knowledgeable about them.

This book and the NCLEX-RN examination assume the test taker knows common terminology such as "efficacy," which means "effectiveness," and "teratogenic," which means "causing developmental malformations."

Different medications affect different body organs and may affect different laboratory values. The nurse should be aware of which body organs and laboratory values may be affected by a specific problem or by a specific medication and monitor accordingly. For example, if there is a problem with the pancreas, the nurse might monitor blood glucose levels or lipase and amylase levels. As stated earlier, the two major organs of the body responsible for detoxifying and eliminating excess substances from the body are the liver and the kidney; therefore the nurse must monitor liver function tests, blood urea nitrogen (BUN), and creatinine levels. The nurse must know what normal laboratory values are, including normal electrolyte values, because many medications can alter the homeostatic balance of the body. The nurse should also know which laboratory values indicate a potential threat to the life or the health status of the client.

The nurse must always be aware of the effects of medications on the body to determine if a medication is effective. The medication is effective if the signs and symptoms of the disease process for which the medication is being administered are improving. For example, if an antibiotic is being administered to a client with an infection caused by an agent sensitive to that antibiotic, the white blood count should decrease; similarly, if furosemide or digoxin is given to a client with heart failure, the lung fields should be clear if the medication is effective.

All medications have side effects. A side effect is an untoward reaction to the medication. Side effects are not uncommon and are not necessarily a reason for discontinuing the medication. Frequently the nurse must teach the client how to manage a side effect. For example, anticholinergic medications have the side effect of drying secretions. The client is taught to chew sugarless gum or hard candies to alleviate this problem.

Adverse effects of medications, however, could be life threatening, and the health-care provider should be notified of the problem. For example, an adverse effect of many medications is agranulocytosis, bone marrow suppression, that results in a decreased production of white blood cells and increased susceptibility to infections and often manifests itself by flulike symptoms.

When reading a question in this book or on the NCLEX-RN examination, the test taker can assume that if the option is in the question, the nurse has a health-care provider's order for that option. The test taker should not eliminate an option because he/she does not think there is a health-care provider order for the intervention.

Medication Memory Jogger

In each chapter there are comments that apply to some of the questions and some that are basic medication administration guidelines. These memory joggers are designed to "jog" the test taker's critical thinking ability. Pay particular attention when one of these comments appears in a chapter.

Neurological System

A prudent question is one half of wisdom.

—Frances Bacon

PRACTICE QUESTIONS

A Client with a Head Injury

1. The client with a head injury is experiencing increased intracranial pressure. The neurosurgeon prescribes the osmotic diuretic mannitol (Osmitrol). Which intervention should the nurse implement when administering this medication?
   1. Monitor the client's arterial blood gases during administration.
   2. Do not administer if the client's blood pressure is less than 90/60.
   3. Ensure that the client's cardiac status is monitored by telemetry.
   4. Use a filter needle when administering the medication.

2. The client with increased intracranial pressure is receiving the osmotic diuretic mannitol (Osmitrol). Which data would cause the nurse to hold the administration of this medication?
   1. The serum osmolality is 330 mOsm/kg.
   2. The urine osmolality is 550 mOsm/kg.
   3. The acetone level is 1.5 mg/dL.
   4. The creatinine level is 1.8 mg/dL.

3. Which discharge instruction should the emergency room nurse discuss with the client that has sustained a concussion and is being discharged home?
   1. Do not take any type of medication for at least 48 hours.
   2. Take two acetaminophen (Tylenol) up to every 4 hours for a headache.
   3. If experiencing a headache, take one hydrocodone (Vicodin) every 8 hours.
   4. It is all right to take a couple of aspirin if experiencing a headache.

4. All the following clients have a head injury. Which client would the nurse question administering the osmotic diuretic mannitol (Osmitrol)?
   1. The 34-year-old client who is HIV positive.
   2. The 84-year-old client who has glaucoma.
   3. The 68-year-old client who has cor pulmonale.
   4. The 16-year-old client who has cystic fibrosis.

5. The client has an open laceration on the right temporal lobe secondary to being hit on the head with a baseball bat. The emergency department physician sutures the laceration and the CT scan is negative. Which instruction should the nurse discuss with the client?
   1. Do not put anything on the laceration for 72 hours.
   2. Use hydrocortisone cream 0.5% on the laceration.
   3. Cleanse the area with alcohol three times a day.
   4. Apply Neosporin ointment to the sutured area.

6. The client with a head injury is ordered a CT scan of the head with contrast dye. Which statement by the client would warrant immediate intervention?
    1. "I take medication for my hypertension."
    2. "I am allergic to many types of fish."
    3. "I get nauseated whenever I take aspirin."
    4. "I had about three beers before I fell and hit my head."

7. The nurse is preparing to administer medications to the following clients. Which medication would the nurse question administering?
    1. The loop diuretic furosemide (Lasix) to a client with a serum potassium level of 4.2 mEq/L.
    2. The osmotic diuretic mannitol (Osmitrol) to a client with a serum osmolality of 280 mOsm/kg.
    3. The cardiac glycoside digoxin (Lanoxin) to a client with a digoxin level of 2.4 mg/dL.
    4. The anticonvulsant phenytoin (Dilantin) to a client with a Dilantin level of 14 μg/mL.

8. The client with a head injury is admitted into the intensive care unit (ICU). Which health-care provider medication order would the ICU nurse question?
    1. Osmitrol (Mannitol), an osmotic diuretic.
    2. Methylprednisolone (Solu-Medrol), a corticosteroid.
    3. Phenytoin (Dilantin), an anticonvulsant.
    4. Oxygen, 6 L via nasal cannula.

9. The client with increased intracranial pressure is receiving the osmotic diuretic mannitol (Osmitrol). Which intervention should the nurse implement to evaluate the effectiveness of the medication?
    1. Monitor the client's vital signs.
    2. Maintain strict intake and output.
    3. Assess the client's neurological status.
    4. Check the client's serum osmolality level.

10. The client has increased intracranial pressure and the health-care provider orders a bolus of 0.5 g/kg IV of 25% osmotic diuretic solution. The client weighs 165 pounds. How much medication will the nurse administer to the client?

    Answer _____

A Client with Seizures

11. The client with a seizure disorder is prescribed the anticonvulsant phenytoin (Dilantin). Which statement indicates the client understands the medication teaching?
    1. "If my urine turns a reddish-brown color, I should call my doctor."
    2. "I should take my medication on an empty stomach."
    3. "I will use a soft-bristled toothbrush to brush my teeth."
    4. "I may get a sore throat when taking this medication."

12. The client with a seizure disorder who is taking carbamazepine (Tegretol) tells the clinic nurse, "I am taking evening primrose oil for my premenstrual cramps and it is really working." Which statement would be the nurse's best response?
    1. "You should inform your health-care provider about taking this herb."
    2. "It is very dangerous to take both the herb and Tegretol."
    3. "Herbs are natural substances and I am glad it is helping your PMS."
    4. "Are you sure you should be taking herbs along with Tegretol?"

13. Which data should the nurse assess for the client with a seizure disorder who is taking valproate (Depakote)?
    1. Creatinine and BUN.
    2. White blood cell count.
    3. Liver enzymes.
    4. Red blood cell count.

14. The nurse is preparing to administer the following anticonvulsant medications. Which medication would the nurse question administering?
    1. Carbamazepine (Tegretol) to the client who has a Tegretol serum level of 8 μg/mL.
    2. Clonazepam (Klonopin) to the client who has a Klonopin serum level of 60 ng/mL.
    3. Phenytoin (Dilantin) to the client who has a Dilantin serum level of 26 μg/mL.
    4. Ethosuximide (Zarontin) to the client who has a Zarontin serum level of 45 μg/mL.

15. The client with a seizure disorder is prescribed the anticonvulsant fosphenytoin (Cerebyx). Which interventions should the nurse discuss with the client? Select all that apply.
    1. Instruct the client to wear a MedicAlert bracelet and carry identification.
    2. Tell the client to not self-medicate with over-the-counter medications.
    3. Encourage the client to decrease drinking of any type of alcohol.
    4. Discuss the importance of maintaining good oral hygiene.
    5. Explain the importance of maintaining adequate nutritional intake.

16. The client is having status epilepticus and is prescribed intravenous diazepam (Valium). The client has an IV of D_5W 75 mL/hr in the right arm and a saline lock in the left arm. Which intervention should the nurse implement?
    1. Dilute the Valium and administer over 5 minutes via the existing IV.
    2. Do not dilute the medication and administer at the port closest to the client.
    3. Question the order because Valium cannot be administered with D_5W.
    4. Inject 3 mL of normal saline in the saline lock and administer Valium undiluted.

17. The client newly diagnosed with a seizure disorder also has Type 2 diabetes. The health-care provider prescribes phenytoin (Dilantin) for the client. Which intervention should the nurse implement?
    1. Instruct the client to monitor his or her blood glucose more closely.
    2. Explain that the Dilantin will not affect the client's antidiabetic medication.
    3. Discuss the need to discontinue oral hypoglycemic medication and take insulin.
    4. Call the health-care provider to discuss prescribing the Dilantin.

18. The female client diagnosed with epilepsy tells the nurse, "I am very scared to get pregnant since I am taking medication for my epilepsy." Which statement is the nurse's best response?
    1. "You are scared because you take medication for your epilepsy."
    2. "Many women with epilepsy give birth to normal infants."
    3. "You should not get pregnant when you are taking anticonvulsants."
    4. "Have you discussed your concerns with your health-care provider?"

19. The client newly diagnosed with epilepsy is prescribed an anticonvulsant medication. Which information should the nurse tell the client?
    1. The medication dosage will start low and gradually increase over a few weeks.
    2. The dosage prescribed initially will be the dosage prescribed for the rest of your life.
    3. The health-care provider will prescribe a loading dose and decrease dosage gradually.
    4. The dose of medication will be adjusted monthly until a serum drug level is obtained.

20. The nurse is preparing to administer phenytoin (Dilantin) intravenous push. The client has an IV of D_5W 0.45 NS at 50 mL/hr. Which action should the nurse implement?
    1. Administer the Dilantin undiluted over 5 minutes via the port closest to the client.
    2. Dilute the medication with normal saline and administer over 2 minutes.
    3. Flush tubing with normal saline (NS), administer diluted Dilantin, and then flush with NS.
    4. Insert a saline lock in the other arm and administer the medication undiluted.

A Client with Cerebrovascular Accident

21. The 55-year-old African American male client presents to the emergency department with blurred vision, slurred speech, and left-sided weakness. The client has a history of hypertension (HTN) and benign prostatic hypertrophy (BPH). Which statement regarding the client's medications should the nurse ask at this time?
    1. "Have you been taking over-the-counter herbs to treat the BPH?"
    2. "Do you take an aspirin every day to prevent heart attacks and strokes?"
    3. "Do you eat green, leafy vegetables frequently?"
    4. "Have you been taking medications routinely to control the HTN?"

22. The nurse in the emergency department is preparing to administer the thrombolytic medication alteplase (Activase) to a client whose initial symptoms of a stroke began 2 hours ago. Which intervention should the nurse implement first?
    1. Check the client's armband for allergies.
    2. Hang the medication via IVPB and infuse over 90 minutes.
    3. Check the results of the client's CT scan of the brain.
    4. Teach the client that this medication dissolves clots.

23. The long-term-care facility nurse is caring for a client diagnosed with a cerebrovascular accident (CVA) 6 months ago who has residual cognitive deficits. The HCP has ordered alprazolam (Xanax), an antianxiety medication, to be administered at bedtime. Which intervention should the nurse initiate for this client?
    1. Offer toileting every 2 hours.
    2. Move the client to the end of the hall for less noise.
    3. Administer the medication at 1800.
    4. Give the medication with a full glass of water.

24. The client diagnosed with a stroke has been prescribed phenytoin (Dilantin), an anticonvulsant. Which statement explains the scientific rationale for prescribing this medication?
    1. The client's stroke was caused by some damage to cerebral tissue.
    2. The stroke caused damage to the brain tissue that could result in seizures.
    3. Hemorrhagic strokes leave residual blood in the brain that causes seizures.
    4. This medication can help the client with cognitive deficits think more clearly.

25. The female client presents to the emergency department diagnosed with a stroke. Which of the client's current medication regimen is a risk factor for developing a stroke?
    1. Propranolol (Inderal), a beta blocker.
    2. Furosemide (Lasix), a loop diuretic.
    3. Estradiol/norgestimate (Ortho-Cyclen), a combination hormone.
    4. Metformin (Glucophage), a biguanide.

26. The client diagnosed with chronic hypertension is prescribed furosemide (Lasix), a loop diuretic, and enalapril (Vasotec), an ACE inhibitor. The client's blood pressures for the last 3 weeks have averaged 178/95, and the HCP has added atenolol (Tenormin), a beta blocker, to the client's current medication regimen. Which statement is the scientific rationale for including this medication in the client's regimen?
    1. Achieving a lower average blood pressure will help to prevent a stroke.
    2. The other medications are not effective without the addition of atenolol.
    3. The atenolol will potentiate the effects of loop diuretics.
    4. The HCP will taper off the ACE inhibitor and eventually discontinue it.

27. The elderly client diagnosed with a stroke is being discharged. When preparing the discharge instructions, the nurse notes many medications that are ordered to be taken at different times of the day. Which intervention should the nurse implement first?
    1. Complete a comprehensive chart for the client to use.
    2. Refer the client to a home health care agency for follow up.
    3. Teach the client to return to the HCP office for follow up.
    4. Discuss the multiple medications and times with the HCP.

28. The nurse is caring for a client diagnosed with a hemorrhagic stroke. Which medication should the nurse question administering?
    1. Clopidogrel (Plavix), an antiplatelet.
    2. Osmitrol (Mannitol), an osmotic diuretic.
    3. Nifedipine (Procardia), a calcium channel blocker.
    4. Dexamethasone (Decadron), a glucocorticoid.

29. The nurse is preparing to administer an oral medication to a client diagnosed with a stroke. Which intervention should the nurse implement first?
    1. Crush all oral medications and place them in pudding.
    2. Elevate the head 60 degrees.
    3. Ask the client to swallow a drink of water.
    4. Have suction equipment at the bedside.

30. The nurse in the intensive care unit is caring for a client diagnosed with a left cerebral artery thrombotic stroke who received a thrombolytic medication in the emergency department. Which intervention should be implemented?
    1. Administer the antiplatelet medication ticlopidine (Ticlid) po.
    2. Place the client in the Trendelenburg position.
    3. Keep the client turned to the right side and high Fowler's position.
    4. Monitor the anticoagulant heparin infusion.

A Client with Brain Tumor

31. The nurse is caring for a client with a malignant brain tumor. Which medication would the nurse anticipate the health-care provider ordering?
    1. Cyclophosphamide (Cytoxan), an alkylating agent, IVPB.
    2. Octreotide (Sandostatin), a pituitary suppressant.
    3. Erythropoietin (Epogen), a biologic response modifier.
    4. Phenytoin (Dilantin), an anticonvulsant.

32. The client diagnosed with a pituitary tumor has the pituitary hormone vasopressin (DDAVP) ordered. Which statement by the client indicates that the medication is effective?
    1. "My headaches are much better since I have been on this medication."
    2. "My nasal drainage was initially worse, but now I don't have any."
    3. "I am not so thirsty when I take this medication."
    4. "My seizures have been eliminated."

33. The client diagnosed with a brain tumor is being admitted to the medical oncology unit at 2000. Which health-care provider's order should be implemented first?
    1. Regular soft diet with between-meal snacks.
    2. Dexamethasone (Decadron), a steroid, every 6 hours IVP.
    3. Prochlorperazine (Compazine), an antiemetic, ac.
    4. CBC and chemistry panel laboratory tests.

34. The client diagnosed with a brain tumor is ordered the osmotic diuretic mannitol (Osmitrol) to be given intravenously. Which interventions for this medication should the nurse implement? Select all that apply.
    1. Inspect the bottle for crystals.
    2. Record intake and output every 8 hours.
    3. Auscultate the client's lung fields.
    4. Perform a neurological examination.
    5. Have calcium gluconate at the bedside.

35. The 6-year-old client diagnosed with a brain tumor has returned from the postanesthesia care unit to intensive care. Which medication should the nurse question?
    1. Meperidine (Demerol), a narcotic analgesic, IVP every 2 hours.
    2. Methylprednisolone (Solu-Medrol), a steroid, IVPB every 8 hours.
    3. Acetaminophen (Tylenol), an antipyretic, po or rectal PRN.
    4. Promethazine (Phenergan), an antiemetic, IVP PRN.

36. The client diagnosed with a brain tumor has been placed on narcotical analgesic medications to control the associated headaches. Which intervention should the nurse implement?
    1. Instruct the client to limit fluids after taking the medication.
    2. Talk to the client about taking bulk laxatives.
    3. Teach the significant other to perform a neurological assessment.
    4. Discuss limiting the amount of medication allowed per day.

37. The client diagnosed with a brain tumor is undergoing radiation therapy. Which medication should the home health nurse suggest the health-care provider order to assist the client in managing the side effects of the radiation therapy?
    1. An antiemetic to be taken before meals and as needed.
    2. An increase in the narcotic pain medication.
    3. A topical medicated lotion for the scalp.
    4. An antianxiety medication to control anxiety during treatments.

38. The client diagnosed with a pituitary tumor has acromegaly. The health-care provider has prescribed the hormone suppressant octreotide (Sandostatin). Which interventions should the nurse implement regarding this medication?
    1. Implement fall precautions.
    2. Administer calcium tablets to replace the lost calcium.
    3. Have the client discuss acnelike skin problems with a dermatologist.
    4. Contact the client's insurance provider to determine if the medication is covered.

39. The 8-year-old male client has been determined to have a benign tumor in the anterior pituitary gland. Surgery has resulted in an inadequate production of growth hormone (GH). The nurse is teaching the parents about growth hormone therapy. Which statement indicates the parent understands the medication?
    1. "If I give too much, then my child will grow to be a giant."
    2. "After a few months I can taper my child off the growth hormone."
    3. "If I don't give the hormone, my child will become retarded."
    4. "I should monitor my child's blood glucose levels."

40. The male client diagnosed with a brain tumor tells the clinic nurse that he has been having seizures more frequently. The client is taking the anticonvulsant phenytoin (Dilantin), the narcotic morphine sulfate (Roxanol), the analgesic acetaminophen (Tylenol), and the antianxiety medication alprazolam (Xanax). Which question about the client's medications should the nurse ask next?
    1. "How often do you need to take the Xanax?"
    2. "Do you take any vitamins that might cause the seizures?"
    3. "What was your last Dilantin level?"
    4. "Have you had any x-rays to determine the cause of the seizures?"

A Client with Parkinson's Disease

41. The elderly client diagnosed with Parkinson's disease (PD) has been prescribed carbidopa/levodopa (Sinemet). Which data indicates the medication has been effective?
    1. The client has cogwheel motion when swinging the arms.
    2. The client does not display emotions when discussing the illness.
    3. The client is able to walk upright without stumbling.
    4. The client eats 30%–40% of meals within 1 hour.

42. Which statement made by the wife of a client diagnosed with Parkinson's disease (PD) indicates that teaching about the medication regimen has been effective?
    1. "The medications will control all the symptoms of the PD if they are taken correctly."
    2. "The medications provide symptom management, but the effects may not last."
    3. "The medications will have to be taken for about 6 months and then stopped."
    4. "The medications must be tapered off when he is better or he will have a relapse."

43. Which statement indicates the scientific rationale for the combination drug carbidopa/levodopa (Sinemet) prescribed for Parkinson's disease?
    1. The carbidopa delays the breakdown of the levodopa in the periphery so more dopamine gets to the brain.
    2. The medication is less expensive when combined, so it is more affordable to clients on a fixed income.
    3. The carbidopa breaks down in the periphery and causes vasoconstriction of the blood vessels.
    4. Carbidopa increases the action of levodopa on the renal arteries, increasing renal perfusion.

44. The client diagnosed with Parkinson's disease has been on long-term levodopa (L-dopa), an anti-Parkinson's disease drug. Which data supports the reason for placing the client on a "drug holiday"?
    1. The medication is expensive and difficult to afford for clients on a fixed income.
    2. The therapeutic effects of the drug have diminished and the adverse effects have increased.
    3. The client has developed hypertension that is uncontrolled by medication.
    4. An overdose is being taken and the medication needs to clear the system.

45. The client diagnosed with early-stage Parkinson's disease has been prescribed pramipexole (Mirapex), a dopamine agonist medication. Which side effect of this medication should the nurse teach the client?
    1. Daytime somnolence.
    2. On–off effect.
    3. Excessive salivation.
    4. Pill rolling motion.

46. Which statement is an advantage of administering the catechol-O-methyltransferase (COMT) inhibitor entacapone (Comtan) to a client diagnosed with Parkinson's disease?
    1. Comtan increases the vasodilating effect of levodopa.
    2. Levodopa can be discontinued while the client is taking Comtan.
    3. There are no side effects of the drug to interfere with treatment.
    4. Comtan causes blood levels of levodopa to be smoother and more sustained.

47. The client diagnosed with Parkinson's disease is prescribed the antiviral drug amantadine (Symmetrel). Which information should the nurse teach the client?
    1. Do not get the flu vaccine because there may be interactions.
    2. If the symptoms return, the client should notify the HCP.
    3. The dose should be decreased if taking other PD medications.
    4. If a dry mouth develops, discontinue the medication immediately.

48. Which client diagnosed with Parkinson's disease should the nurse question administering the anticholinergic medication benztropine (Cogentin)?
    1. The client diagnosed with congestive heart failure.
    2. The client who has had a myocardial infarction.
    3. The client diagnosed with glaucoma.
    4. The client who is undergoing hip replacement surgery.

49. The nurse is caring for a client newly diagnosed with Parkinson's disease who is receiving the anti-Parkinson's disease medication levodopa (L-dopa). Which interventions should the nurse implement? Select all that apply.
    1. Instruct the client to rise slowly from a seated or lying position.
    2. Teach about on–off effects of the medication.
    3. Discuss taking the medication with meals or snacks.
    4. Tell the client that the sweat and urine may become darker.
    5. Inform the client about having routine blood levels drawn.

50. The nurse is preparing a care plan for a client diagnosed with Parkinson's disease. Which statement is the goal of medication therapy for the client diagnosed with Parkinson's disease?
    1. The medication will cure the client of Parkinson's disease.
    2. The client will maintain functional ability.
    3. The client will be able to take the medications as ordered.
    4. The medication will control all symptoms of Parkinson's disease.

A Client Diagnosed with Alzheimer's Disease

51. The family member of a client diagnosed with early-stage Alzheimer's disease (AD) who was prescribed the cholinesterase inhibitor donepezil (Aricept) without improvement asks the nurse, "Can anything be done to slow the disease since this medication does not work?" Which statement is the nurse's best response?
    1. "I am sorry that the medication did not help. Would you like to talk about it?"
    2. "You need to prepare for long-term care because confusion is inevitable now."
    3. "Your loved one may respond to a different medication of the same type."
    4. "No, nothing is going to slow the disease now. Have the client make a will."

52. Which statement is the scientific rationale for prescribing and administering donepezil (Aricept), a cholinesterase inhibitor?
    1. Aricept works to bind the dopamine at neuron receptor sites to increase ability.
    2. Aricept increases the availability of acetylcholine at cholinergic synapses.
    3. Aricept decreases acetylcholine in the periphery to increase movement.
    4. Aricept delays transmission of acetylcholine at the neuronal junction.

53. The client diagnosed with Alzheimer's disease (AD) is prescribed rivastigmine (Exelon), a cholinesterase inhibitor. Which medication should the nurse question administering to the client?
    1. Amitriptyline (Elavil), a tricyclic antidepressant.
    2. Warfarin (Coumadin), an anticoagulant.
    3. Phenytoin (Dilantin), an anticonvulsant.
    4. Prochlorperazine (Compazine), an antiemetic.

54. The nurse caring for clients on a medical psychiatric unit has received the morning shift report. To whom should the nurse administer medications first?
    1. The client diagnosed with Alzheimer's disease who has a po cardiac glycoside daily.
    2. The client diagnosed with Alzheimer's disease who needs a PRN for nausea.
    3. The client diagnosed with Alzheimer's disease who has a cholinesterase inhibitor ordered t.i.d.
    4. The client diagnosed with Alzheimer's disease who is angry and disoriented and has an antipsychotic PRN.

55. The nurse is completing an admission assessment on a client being admitted to a medical unit diagnosed with pneumonia. The client's list of home medications includes Lasix, a loop diuretic; Metamucil, a bulk laxative; and Reminyl, a cholinesterase inhibitor. Which intervention should the nurse implement first?
    1. Make sure the client has a room near the nursing station.
    2. Check the client's white blood cell count and potassium level.
    3. Have the unlicensed assistant get ice chips for the client to suck on.
    4. Determine the client's usual bowel elimination pattern.

56. The home health care nurse is caring for a client taking donepezil (Aricept), a cholinesterase inhibitor. Which finding would indicate the medication is effective?
    1. The client is unable to relate his or her name or birth date.
    2. The client is discussing an upcoming event with the family.
    3. The client is wearing underwear on the outside of the clothes.
    4. The client is talking on the telephone that is signaling a dial tone.

57. The daughter of an elderly client diagnosed with Alzheimer's disease asks the nurse, "Is there anything I can do to prevent getting this disease?" Which statement is the nurse's best response?
    1. "Not if you are genetically programmed to get Alzheimer's disease."
    2. "Yearly brain scans may determine if you are susceptible to getting Alzheimer's."
    3. "There are some medications, but research has not proved that they work."
    4. "Hormone replacement therapy may prevent the development of Alzheimer's."

58. The client diagnosed with Alzheimer's disease is taking vitamin E and *Ginkgo biloba*. Which information should the nurse teach the client?
    1. Take the medications on an empty stomach.
    2. Have regular blood tests to assess for toxic levels.
    3. The medications only slow the progression of the disease.
    4. Use a sunscreen of SPF 15 or greater when in the sun.

59. Which statement is the advantage of prescribing donepezil (Aricept) over the other cholinesterase inhibitors?
    1. The dosing schedule for Aricept is only once a day.
    2. Aricept is the only one that can be given with an NSAID.
    3. Aricept enhances the cognitive protective effects of vitamin E.
    4. There are no side effects of Aricept.

60. The client diagnosed with Alzheimer's disease is prescribed galantamine (Reminyl), a cholinesterase inhibitor. Which interventions should the nurse implement? Select all that apply.
    1. Inform the client to take the medication with food.
    2. Check the client's BUN and creatinine levels.
    3. Teach the client to wear a MedicAlert bracelet with information about the medication.
    4. Assess the client's other routine medications.
    5. Discuss not abruptly discontinuing the medication.

A Client with a Migraine Headache

61. The client presents to the emergency department complaining of a migraine headache and is prescribed medication. Which scientific rationale is most appropriate for administering the medication by the parenteral route?
    1. The client requests the medication be given IVP.
    2. Migraine headaches do not respond to oral medications.
    3. Migraine headaches can cause nausea, vomiting, and gastric stasis.
    4. The client is not as likely to develop an addiction to the medications.

62. The 29-year-old female client is taking feverfew, an over-the-counter herb, for chronic migraine headaches. Which information should the nurse teach the client?
    1. Decrease the dose of prescription NSAIDs while taking this herb.
    2. Do not breast-feed and avoid getting pregnant while taking feverfew.
    3. The medication will immediately relieve a migraine headache.
    4. Menstrual problems will become worse while taking this medication.

63. The male client diagnosed with chronic migraine headaches, who has taken medications daily for years to prevent a migraine from occurring, tells the clinic nurse that now he has a headache "all the time, no matter what I take." Which situation would the nurse suspect is occurring?
    1. The client has developed a resistance to pain medication.
    2. The client is addicted and wants to get an increase in narcotics prescribed.
    3. The client has developed medication overuse headaches.
    4. The client may have a complication of therapy and has a brain tumor.

64. The client diagnosed with a migraine headache rates the pain at a 4 on a 1–10 scale. Which medication would the nurse administer?
    1. Ibuprofen (Motrin) po, a nonsteroidal anti-inflammatory drug.
    2. Butorphanol (Stadol) IM, an opioid analgesic.
    3. Dihydroergotamine (D.H.E. 45), an ergot alkaloid, intranasally.
    4. Sumatriptan (Imitrex), subcutaneous, a selective serotonin receptor agonist.

65. The nurse is caring for a client diagnosed with migraine headaches. Which information should the nurse teach regarding abortive medication therapy?
    1. Use the medication every day even if no headache.
    2. Take the radial pulse for 1 minute prior to taking the medication.
    3. The medications can cause severe hypertension.
    4. Limit use of the medication to 1 or 2 days a week.

66. The client is prescribed sumatriptan (Imitrex), 6 mg subcutaneously, for a migraine headache. The medication comes 12 mg/mL. How many milliliters should the nurse administer?

    Answer _____

67. The client diagnosed with migraine headaches that occur every 2 to 3 days is placed on preventive therapy with the beta blocker propranolol (Inderal). Which data indicates the medication is effective?
    1. The client has had only one headache in the past week.
    2. The client's apical pulse is 78 beats per minute.
    3. The client has developed orthostatic hypotension.
    4. The client supplemented Inderal with Imitrex four times.

68. The male client presents to the outpatient clinic complaining of headaches that occur suddenly with throbbing in the right orbital area and on the right side of the forehead that last for an hour or longer and that have been occurring regularly for the past 2 weeks. Which medications would the nurse anticipate being prescribed?
    1. Propranolol (Inderal), a beta blocker, and almotriptan (Axert), a triptan.
    2. Prednisone, a glucocorticoid, and lithium (Lithobid), a psychotherapeutic agent.
    3. Amitriptyline (Elavil), a tricyclic antidepressant, and the estrogen patch Climara.
    4. Ibuprofen (Motrin), an NSAID, and metoclopramide (Reglan), an antiemetic.

69. The nurse in an HCP's office is assessing a female client with a tension headache. Which question should the nurse ask the client?
    1. "Have you been sunbathing recently?"
    2. "Do you eat shellfish or other iodine-containing foods?"
    3. "Is there a chance you might be pregnant?"
    4. "What over-the-counter medications have you tried?"

70. The nurse is administering 1600 medications. Which medication should the nurse administer first?
    1. Humalog insulin for a client with a blood glucose level of 200 mg/dL.
    2. Meperidine (Demerol), a narcotic analgesic, for a client with a headache rated an 8.
    3. Divalproex (Depakote ER) for a client diagnosed with migraine headaches.
    4. Metoclopramide (Reglan), an antiemetic, for a client with gastric stasis.

The correct answer number and rationale for why it is the correct answer are given in **boldface blue type**. Rationales for why the other possible answer options are not correct are also given, but they are not in boldface type.

A Client with a Head Injury

1. 1. The client's ABGs are not affected by the administration of mannitol; therefore, there is no need to monitor them.
   2. The client's blood pressure does not affect the administration of mannitol.
   3. The client with a head injury would be in the intensive care unit receiving telemetry, but mannitol does not affect cardiac status.
   4. **The nurse must use a filter needle when administering mannitol because crystals may form in the solution and syringe and be inadvertently injected into the client if a filter needle is not used.**

2. 1. **The normal serum osmolality is 275–300 mOsm/kg. Mannitol is held if the serum osmolality exceeds 310–320 mOsm/kg.**
   2. The normal urine osmolality is 250–900 mOsm/kg; therefore, the data is within normal limits. However, urine osmolality is not usually monitored when administering mannitol.
   3. The normal acetone level is 0.3–2.0 mg/dL; therefore, the data is within normal limits. However, acetone is not monitored when administering mannitol.
   4. The normal creatinine level is 0.7–1.4 mg/dL; therefore, the data indicates an elevated level. However, the creatinine level is not affected by the administration of mannitol; there must be another reason for the elevated creatinine level.

   MEDICATION MEMORY JOGGER: The nurse must be knowledgeable about accepted standards of practice for medication administration, including which client assessment data and laboratory data should be monitored prior to administering the medication.

3. 1. The client can take nonnarcotic analgesics if experiencing a headache.
   2. **Tylenol can be taken for a headache in a patient who has sustained a concussion. If the Tylenol does not relieve the headache, the client should contact the health-care provider.**
   3. Narcotic analgesics should not be taken after a head injury because such medications may further depress neurological status.
   4. Aspirin could lead to bleeding, and a client with a concussion does not need a chance of increased bleeding.

4. 1. Mannitol would not be contraindicated in a client who is HIV positive.
   2. Mannitol would not be contraindicated in a client who has glaucoma.
   3. **Cor pulmonale is right-sided heart failure, often secondary to chronic obstructive pulmonary disease (COPD). Because mannitol pulls fluid off the brain, it may lead to a circulatory overload, which the heart with right-sided failure could not handle. This client would need an order for a loop diuretic to prevent serious cardiac complications.**
   4. The client is 16 years old, and, even with cystic fibrosis, the client's heart should be able to handle the fluid volume overload.

5. 1. The sutured area may get infected; therefore, the client should keep the wound clean and apply antibiotic ointment.
   2. Hydrocortisone cream is an anti-inflammatory medication and would not be applied to a laceration.
   3. Alcohol would be very painful and should not be used to clean the laceration.
   4. **The sutured area must be cleansed with soap and water and patted dry, and an antibiotic ointment, such as Neosporin, should be applied to prevent infection.**

6. 1. Antihypertensive medication would not interfere with the contrast dye that is used when performing a CT scan.
   2. **The contrast dye used in a CT scan is iodine based, and an allergy to shellfish suggests an allergy to iodine and would warrant the nurse notifying the HCP to cancel the contrast part of the CT scan. Further assessment would be needed.**
   3. Aspirin would not interfere with the contrast dye that is used when performing a CT scan.
   4. Alcohol is not contraindicated when performing a CT scan.

   MEDICATION MEMORY JOGGER: The nurse must be knowledgeable about accepted standards of practice for disease processes and conditions. If the nurse administers a medication the health-care provider has prescribed and it harms the client, the nurse could be held accountable. Remember the nurse is a client advocate.

7. 1. The normal serum potassium level is 3.5–4.5 mEq/L. Because the client's potassium level is within normal range, the nurse has no reason to question this medication order.
   2. The normal serum osmolality is 275–300 mOsm/kg. Because the client's level is within this range, the nurse would have no reason to question administering this medication.
   3. The normal digoxin level is 0.8–2.0 mg/dL. A digoxin level of 2.4 mg/dL would warrant the nurse questioning the administration of this medication.
   4. The therapeutic serum level of Dilantin is 10–20 µg/mL. Because the client's level is within this range, the nurse should not question administering this medication.

8. 1. An osmotic diuretic is the treatment of choice to help decrease intracranial pressure that occurs with a head injury.
   2. Research supports the finding that clients with head injuries who are treated with anti-inflammatory corticosteroids are 20% more likely to die within 2 weeks after the head injury than those who aren't so treated. The nurse should question this medication.
   3. Seizures are a common complication of head injuries; therefore, an order for an anticonvulsant medication would be appropriate.
   4. There is no reason for the nurse to question an order for oxygen—which is considered a medication—for a client with a head injury.

9. 1. The client's vital signs should be evaluated, but these readings are not the best indicators of the effectiveness of an osmotic diuretic.
   2. Monitoring the client's intake and output evaluates the client's hydration status, but it does not determine the effectiveness of the medication.
   3. Mannitol is administered to decrease intracranial pressure. Changes in intracranial pressure affect neurological status; therefore, the client's neurological status should be evaluated to determine the effectiveness of the medication.
   4. The client's osmolality serum level is assessed when administering mannitol, but this level does not evaluate the effectiveness of the medication.

MEDICATION MEMORY JOGGER: The nurse determines the effectiveness of a medication by assessing for the symptoms, or lack thereof, for which the medication was prescribed.

10. **Answer: 37.5 g**
To determine this, first find the client's weight in kilograms (165 pounds ÷ 2.2 = 75 kg). Then, multiply 0.5 g by weight in kilograms (0.5 × 75 kg = 37.5 kg).

A Client with Seizures

11. 1. Dilantin may cause the client's urine to turn a harmless pinkish-red or reddish-brown; therefore, the client does not need to call the health-care provider.
    2. The client should take Dilantin at the same time every day with food or milk to prevent gastric upset.
    3. The client should use a soft-bristled toothbrush to prevent gum irritation and bleeding. Gingival hyperplasia (overgrowth of gums) is a side effect of this medication.
    4. A sore throat, bruising, or nosebleeds should be reported to the health-care provider because this may indicate a blood dyscrasia.

12. 1. Evening primrose oil may lower the seizure threshold, and the Tegretol dose may need to be modified. Therefore, the client should notify the health-care provider.
    2. Evening primrose oil is not dangerous, and the nurse should not scare the client.
    3. Although the evening primrose oil may help the client's PMS, the nurse should inform the client that because she is also taking Tegretol, she should inform her HCP because the dose of Tegretol may need to be adjusted.
    4. The nurse needs to give factual information to the client— not ask the client a question.

13. 1. Depakote does not cause nephrotoxicity.
    2. Depakote does not cause blood dyscrasia.
    3. Hepatotoxicity is one of the possible adverse reactions to Depakote; therefore, the liver enzymes should be monitored.
    4. Depakote does not affect the RBC count.

MEDICATION MEMORY JOGGER: The nurse must be knowledgeable about accepted standards of practice for medication administration, including which client assessment data and laboratory data should be monitored prior to administering the medication.

14. 1. The therapeutic serum level of Tegretol is 5–12 μg/mL. Because the client's level is within that range, the nurse has no reason to question administering the drug.
 2. The therapeutic serum level of Klonopin is 20–80 ng/m. Because the client's level is within that range, the nurse has no reason to question administering the drug.
 3. **The therapeutic serum level of Dilantin is 10–20 μg/mL. Because the client's level is above that range, the nurse should question administering this medication.**
 4. The therapeutic serum level of Zarontin is 40–100 μg/mL. Because the client's level is within that range, the nurse has no reason to question administering the drug.

15. 1. **The client should wear a MedicAlert bracelet and carry identification so that a health-care provider and others possibly providing care know that the client has a seizure disorder.**
 2. **The client should not take any over-the-counter medications without first consulting with the HCP or pharmacist because many medications interact with Cerebyx.**
 3. Alcohol and other central nerve depressants can cause an added depressive effect on the body and should be avoided, not just decreased.
 4. Gingival hyperplasia (overgrowth of gums) is a side effect of Dilantin, not of Cerebyx.
 5. **Dilantin may cause anorexia, nausea, and vomiting; therefore, the client should maintain an adequate nutritional intake.**

16. 1. Valium is oil based and should not be diluted.
 2. Valium is oil based and should not be administered in an existing intravenous line if another option is available.
 3. Valium should not be administered in an existing intravenous line, but the nurse does not need to question the order because there is an existing saline lock.
 4. The nurse should administer the Valium undiluted through the saline lock.

17. 1. Serum glucose must be monitored more closely because phenytoin may inhibit insulin release, thus causing an increase in glucose level.
 2. This is not a true statement. Dilantin may affect the client's antidiabetic medication.
 3. This is not a true statement. The client can still take oral hypoglycemic medications.
 4. The nurse should call and discuss any questionable medication with the HCP, but there is no reason to discuss Dilantin being prescribed for a client with Type 2 diabetes.

18. 1. This is a therapeutic response that is used to encourage the client to ventilate feelings, but the nurse should provide factual information to this client.
 2. **Many anticonvulsant medications have teratogenic properties that increase the risk for fetal malformations, but many women with epilepsy give birth to normal infants. The nurse should provide the client with facts.**
 3. A female client with epilepsy can give birth to a normal infant.
 4. The client should discuss a potential pregnancy with the significant other, but this is not addressing the client's concerns.

19. 1. **Anticonvulsant dosages usually start low and gradually increase over a period of weeks until the serum drug level is within therapeutic range or the seizures stop.**
 2. It is incorrect to state that the dosage prescribed will be the dosage for the rest of the client's life, but it is correct to state that the client will most likely be on the medication for the rest of his or her life.
 3. This is incorrect information. The medication is started in low dosages and gradually increased.
 4. The dose of medication will be adjusted until a serum drug level is reached but it will be more frequently than monthly.

20. 1. Dilantin cannot be administered with dextrose because it will cause precipitation.
 2. Dextrose solutions should be avoided because of drug precipitation.
 3. **Dilantin should be diluted in a saline solution and the IV tubing should be flushed before and after administration because a dextrose solution will cause drug precipitation.**

4. There is no reason for the nurse to cause more pain to the client by starting a saline lock because the IV tubing is already in place and can be flushed before and after the administration of Dilantin.

MEDICATION MEMORY JOGGER: Any time a nurse administers an intravenous push medication the nurse should dilute the medication. This causes less pain for the client, helps prevent infiltration of the vein, and allows the nurse to administer the medication over the correct amount of time if it is diluted to a 10-mL bolus.

A Client with Cerebrovascular Accident

21. 1. The nurse should ask all clients about taking over-the-counter preparations when being admitted, but this question would have no bearing on the client's presenting symptoms of a stroke.
    2. The client has symptoms of a stroke. Whether he was taking an aspirin to prevent a potential problem is irrelevant. The client has a problem at this time.
    3. Green, leafy vegetables are high in vitamin K, the antidote for Coumadin. The client has no reason to be taking an anticoagulant at this time.
    4. **Many medications for HTN have the adverse effect of causing erectile dysfunction, which many men are hesitant to discuss with their HCP, and the man may simply stop taking the medication to avoid this side effect. The nurse should assess how the client has been controlling his HTN and ask specifically about erectile dysfunction related to hypertensive medication. HTN is a risk factor for developing other cardiovascular diseases, including stroke. This client has two risk factors for developing a stroke: HTN and his racial background.**

22. 1. This is an important intervention, but it is not the first.
    2. This is the correct procedure when hanging the medication, but it is not the first intervention.
    3. **There are three types of strokes: thrombotic, embolic, and hemorrhagic. The nurse must know that the client has not had a hemorrhagic stroke before hanging a medication that** destroys clots. Administering a thrombolytic to a client who has had a hemorrhagic stroke can result in the client's death. In this question the steps in order would be three, one, two, and four.
    4. Teaching the client can be done after the medication has been administered.

23. 1. **This medication has a side effect of drowsiness, which is why the HCP chose this medication for the client—to help the client rest at night. The client has cognitive deficits and should be on fall precautions, so it is hoped that assisting the client to the bathroom every 2 hours will prevent the client from falling while trying to get to the bathroom.**
    2. The client at risk for falling should be as near the nursing station as possible. This allows the staff to keep a closer watch on the client.
    3. The medication is ordered for bedtime, usually 2100, in most health-care facilities.
    4. Giving the medication with a full glass of water would increase the client's need to get up during the night to use the bathroom, increasing the risk of falling.

24. 1. Strokes cause damage to the cerebral tissue; the brain does not cause the damage to itself.
    2. **Stroke-caused loss of function in areas of the brain leads to a problem with nerve impulse transmission; this blocked transmission can initiate a seizure.**
    3. If the client survives a hemorrhagic stroke, the body will reabsorb the blood. There should not be any residual blood.
    4. Anticonvulsants do not increase cognitive ability.

25. 1. Inderal is administered for cardiac dysrhythmias and hypertension and for migraine headache prophylaxis. The medication could help prevent a stroke by lowering the blood pressure.
    2. Loop diuretics have an indirect ability to lower the blood pressure by decreasing the volume of fluid in the body. This would decrease the risk of a stroke.
    3. **Combination oral contraceptives have been associated with venous and arterial thromboembolism, pulmonary embolism, myocardial infarction, and thrombotic stroke.**

4. Adverse reaction to Glucophage is lactic acid buildup, not stroke.

26. 1. **Hypertension is a risk factor for developing a stroke. Some clients require multiple medications to control their hypertension.**
    2. If this were true, then atenolol would be the only medication the client needs. Beta blockers are frequently used in combination with other antihypertensive medications to control a client's blood pressure.
    3. Atenolol does not potentiate the effectiveness of loop diuretics.
    4. Beta blockers, not ACE inhibitors, must be tapered off when discontinuing them to prevent rebound cardiac dysrhythmias. The HCP is adding the beta blocker to the current medications.

    MEDICATION MEMORY JOGGER: Typically medications ending in "ol" or "al" are in the beta blocker classification. Typically medications ending in "il" are ACE inhibitors; verapamil, a calcium-channel blocker, is an exception to the rule.

27. 1. This could be done if the nurse and HCP cannot simplify the medication routine.
    2. This may need to be done based on the nurse's evaluation of the client's situation, but it is not the first intervention.
    3. This should be done, but it is not the first intervention and does not address the problem of many medications and multiple administration times.
    4. **The client has had a stroke and may have difficulty complying with multiple medications and different administration times. Research (for all clients) indicates that the fewer medication administration times during the day, the better the compliance with taking the medication as ordered. The nurse should discuss simplifying the medication regimen with the HCP.**

28. 1. **The client has experienced a bleed into the cranium. Plavix interferes with the client's clotting ability. This medication should be held and discussed with the HCP.**
    2. There is no reason to question giving a medication that will decrease intracranial pressure. Mannitol is the diuretic of choice for this client.
    3. Procardia will decrease the client's blood pressure, which is elevated in clients with increased intracranial pressure.

4. Decadron will decrease edema, resulting in decreased intracranial pressure.

29. 1. Some medications can be crushed and administered in pudding if the client has difficulty swallowing; however, enteric-coated or timed-release medications should not be crushed. The possibility of difficulty in swallowing must be determined first, before an oral medication is given.
    2. The head of the bed should be elevated to 90 degrees when the client is swallowing food or medications.
    3. **The client's ability to swallow must be assessed before attempting to administer any oral medication. Water is the best fluid to use because it will not damage the lungs if aspirated.**
    4. Equipment is usually charged to the client. The nurse should first determine if suction equipment is needed prior to setting it up.

30. 1. Ticlid may be ordered in the future once the cause of the thrombus is determined, but this would not be ordered in the intensive care unit.
    2. The Trendelenburg position is head down and would increase intracranial pressure.
    3. There is no reason to restrict the client to lying on the right side, and high Fowler's is sitting upright. This would be a difficult position for the client to maintain. The client should have the head of the bed elevated approximately 30 degrees to decrease intracranial pressure by gravity drainage.
    4. **The anticoagulant heparin is administered to prevent clot reformation after lysis of the clot by the thrombolytic, and its infusion should be monitored.**

A Client with Brain Tumor

31. 1. Most drugs do not cross the blood–brain barrier, so most antineoplastic agents are not effective against cancers in the brain.
    2. Octreotide is a growth hormone suppressant and is useful in the treatment of acromegaly, not malignant tumors of the brain.
    3. Brain tumors rarely metastasize outside of the skull cavity to cause systemic manifestations of disease such as anemia, for which erythropoietin would be prescribed. Brain tumors, malignant or benign, kill by

occupying space and causing increased intracranial pressure.

4. A brain tumor has the potential to cause erratic stimulation of the neurons in the brain, resulting in seizures. The nurse should expect the HCP to order an anticonvulsant to prevent or control seizures.

32. 1. Vasopressin is the antidiuretic hormone produced by the pituitary gland that is instrumental in the body's ability to conserve water. It does not affect headaches or any other type of pain. Diabetes insipidus is caused by a lack of vasopressin.
   2. DDAVP is given intranasally, and the nurse should be alert to symptoms of rhinitis, but lack of nasal drainage does not indicate that the medication is effective.
   3. DDAVP is a synthetic form of the antidiuretic hormone vasopressin. Without vasopressin, the body does not conserve water and a large amount of very dilute urine is excreted. The body will attempt to have the client replace the fluid by producing the symptom of extreme thirst. Lack of thirst indicates the medication is effective.
   4. DDAVP will not affect seizure activity.

MEDICATION MEMORY JOGGER: The nurse determines the effectiveness of a medication by assessing for the symptoms, or lack thereof, for which the medication was prescribed.

33. 1. The diet is not a priority over preventing increased intracranial pressure resulting from the tumor. It is 2000, or 8 P.M., and meals are usually served in hospitals around 0800, 1200, and 1700. The next meal will be served at 0800.
   2. Dexamethasone is the glucocorticoid of choice for brain swelling. The client is at risk for increased intracranial pressure as a result of the tumor and edema caused by the tumor. The nurse should administer the steroid first to initiate the positive effects of the medication.
   3. This medication is ordered ac, which means before meals. The next dose of this medication is not until 0730 in the morning.
   4. These are routine laboratory tests and will not be drawn until the next morning.

34. 1. Mannitol can crystallize in the containers in which it is packaged, and the

crystals must not be infused into the client. The nurse should inspect the bottle for crystals before beginning the administration.
   2. Any client receiving a diuretic should be monitored for intake and output to determine if the client is excreting more than the intake.
   3. Mannitol is an osmotic diuretic and works by pulling fluid from the tissues into the blood vessels. Clients diagnosed with heart failure or who may be at risk for heart failure may develop fluid volume overload. Therefore, the nurse should assess lung sounds before administering this medication.
   4. The nurse does not have to perform a neurological examination for this medication. The nurse should do this for the disease diagnosis.
   5. Calcium gluconate will not affect this medication, nor is it an antidote.

35. 1. Meperidine metabolizes into normeperidine in the body, and accumulation of this substance in the body can cause seizures. It is not recommended to give Demerol to children, and the schedule may be excessive. The nurse should not automatically administer narcotics to a client who is neurologically impaired. The nurse should determine the neurological status of the client before administering a medication that can mask symptoms.
   2. There is no reason to question prescription of a steroid.
   3. The client may need this medication to control mild pain or fever until the body has a chance to readjust its thermoregulatory mechanism.
   4. An antiemetic can prevent the child from vomiting and increasing intracranial pressure during that activity. The vomiting center is in the brain and can become irritated as a result of increased intracranial pressure.

36. 1. The client is at risk for constipation because of the effects of narcotics on the gastrointestinal tract. The client should be encouraged to increase the amount of fluid intake.
   2. The client is at risk for constipation. A bowel regimen should be instituted, including bulk laxatives as part of the regimen.

3. The significant other does not need to be taught to perform a neurological assessment for this medication. He or she should be told that if the client becomes excessively drowsy, hold the next dose and notify the HCP. It may be necessary to allow the drowsiness to control the pain.
4. The medication may need to be increased, not limited, to control the pain. The amount of pain medication needed should be provided.

37. 1. **Radiation therapy may cause nausea. An antiemetic should be ordered so the client can maintain nutritional status and comfort.**
2. As the tumor shrinks from the radiation, the pain associated with the tumor should decrease, not increase, so an increase in the medication is not needed.
3. The skin in the radiation field should be cleaned with mild soap and water, being careful not to obliterate the markings. Medicated lotions can irritate the skin.
4. The therapy sessions take from 5 to 10 minutes and do require the client to lie still, but usually antianxiety medications are not needed.

38. 1. Octreotide does not increase the risk of falls.
2. Octreotide does not cause bone resorption, so calcium replacement is not needed.
3. Octreotide does not cause acne or acnelike problems.
4. **Octreotide can cost thousands of dollars a year (about $8,000). Before beginning the treatment, the nurse and HCP must know that the client can afford the medication.**

39. 1. **The HCP will regulate the dose to achieve a normal growth rate for the child. Heights and weights are determined on a monthly basis to determine the effectiveness of the medication. This therapy is continued until the epiphyseal closure occurs or to about age 20–24 years.**
2. Tapering is not needed.
3. Lack of growth hormone can result in dwarfism but will not cause mental retardation.
4. **Human growth hormone is diabetogenic and can cause hyperglycemia.**

40. 1. Xanax does not cause seizures; the client has a brain tumor that is the most likely cause of the seizures.

2. The client would not know if a vitamin were causing a seizure. The most probable cause of the seizure is the brain tumor.
3. **Therapeutic levels of Dilantin are needed to control aberrant brain activity. The therapeutic level is 10–20 mg/dL.**
4. The client may need a CT scan or MRI to determine if tumor growth is causing the increase in frequency of seizures, but the nurse should determine if a therapeutic level of Dilantin is being maintained first.

A Client with Parkinson's Disease

41. 1. Cogwheel motion is a symptom of PD. Displaying cogwheel motion does not indicate the medication is effective.
2. Sinemet is a combination medication designed to delay the breakdown of levodopa (dopamine) in the periphery. A flat affect or no emotions would not indicate the medication is effective.
3. **One of the symptoms of PD is a forward shuffling gait, so being able to walk upright without stumbling would indicate that the medication is effective.**
4. The client should be encouraged to consume at least 50% of the meals provided. Meal times that last 1 hour are not encouraged because the client becomes fatigued and the food temperature changes. Hot foods become cold and cold foods become lukewarm. The client should be served frequent small meals each day.

42. 1. All the symptoms may not be controlled even if the client adheres to a strict medication regimen.
2. **PD is treated with medications and surgery. The medications have side effects and adverse effects, and the effectiveness of the medications may be reduced over time.**
3. The client diagnosed with PD will need to take the medications for life unless surgery is performed and a significant improvement is achieved.
4. The medications do not have to be tapered when discontinued.

43. 1. **In Parkinson's disease there is a decreased amount of dopamine in the brain. Carbidopa delays the breakdown of levodopa (dopamine) in the periphery so that more of the levodopa**

crosses the blood–brain barrier and reaches the brain.

2. The expense of the medication is not the reason for the combination of the drugs. Sinemet comes in only one strength combination, which is a disadvantage of the medication.

3. Levodopa breaking down in the periphery is the reason that the medications are combined.

4. Carbidopa does not increase the action of levodopa; it delays the breakdown of the compound in the periphery.

44. 1. The medication is not interrupted for this reason.

2. **With long-term use of levodopa, the adverse effects tend to increase and the client may develop a drug tolerance where the therapeutic effects decrease. A short hiatus from the medication (10 days) may result in beneficial effects being achieved with lower doses.**

3. Early in the treatment of PD with levodopa the client may have postural hypotension, but hypertension is not associated with levodopa.

4. An overdose is not being taken; the client's tolerance to the medication has changed.

45. 1. **Daytime somnolence is seen in about 22% of clients taking Mirapex. A few clients experience an overwhelming and irresistible sleepiness that comes on without warning.**

2. The on–off effect with levodopa occurs when the therapeutic effects of the medication wear off.

3. Salivation is not a side effect of Mirapex.

4. Pill rolling motion is a symptom of PD, not a side effect of a medication.

46. 1. Increased vasodilatation causes hypotension. This is not a reason to administer this drug.

2. Comtan is given in conjunction with levodopa to inhibit metabolism of levodopa in the intestines and peripheral tissues. There is no substitute for dopamine. Medications can increase the relative availability of the dopamine present in the body or can be a form of dopamine itself.

3. Many side effects may interfere with treatment, including hallucinations, postural hypotension, dyskinesias, and sleep disturbances.

4. **Comtan increases the half-life of levodopa by 50–75%, thereby causing**

levodopa blood levels to be smoother and more sustained. This delays the "off" effects and prolongs the "on" effects of levodopa.

47. 1. Clients diagnosed with chronic illnesses should receive the flu vaccination. There is no reason not to get the flu vaccine when receiving amantadine.

2. **The effectiveness of amantadine may diminish in 3–6 months. If signs and symptoms of Parkinson's disease reoccur, the client should notify the HCP.**

3. Amantadine can enhance the response of the other PD medications and is given in the same dosage as if given alone.

4. A dry mouth is a side effect, not an adverse effect. The client should be taught to chew sugarless gum or hard candies to relieve the dry mouth.

48. 1. Anticholinergic medications are not contraindicated in clients diagnosed with heart failure.

2. Anticholinergic medications are not contraindicated in clients who have had a myocardial infarction.

3. **Anticholinergic medications block cholinergic receptors in the eye and may precipitate or aggravate glaucoma.**

4. Anticholinergic medications are not contraindicated in clients undergoing surgery.

MEDICATION MEMORY JOGGER: Glaucoma is affected by any medication that has the effect of drying secretions.

49. 1. Initially levodopa can cause orthostatic hypotension. The client should be taught to rise slowly to prevent falls.

2. **The client may experience an "on" effect of symptom control when the medication is effective and an "off" effect near the time for the next dose of medication.**

3. Food can decrease the absorption of levodopa; administration with meals should be avoided, if possible.

4. **Clients should be warned that darkening of the urine and sweat is a harmless side effect of this medication.**

5. Routine blood levels of levodopa are not drawn.

50. 1. There is currently no cure for Parkinson's disease.

2. **The goal for most clients diagnosed with a chronic disease is to maintain functional ability as long as possible.**

3. Taking the medications as ordered does not guarantee a positive response by the client's body to the medication and thus is not a goal of the medication therapy.
4. All the symptoms may not be controlled; in fact, the medications may exacerbate the symptoms or create new symptoms.

MEDICATION MEMORY JOGGER: All medications have some type of side effects.

A Client Diagnosed with Alzheimer's Disease

51. 1. There are three other medications in the classification of cholinesterase inhibitors that may be tried because the medications are not identical. Additionally, vitamin E in large doses, selegiline, and *Gingko biloba* have been shown to slow progression of AD. This answer on the part of the nurse is not providing information and is not directly answering the family member's question.
2. The progression of AD is inevitable at some point. Cholinesterase inhibitors are prescribed for clients with mild to moderate symptoms of AD, and they can delay the progression of AD. This is not the time to discuss long-term care.
3. **If the client does not respond to one of the cholinesterase inhibitors, then another may be tried because the drugs are not identical. The client may be responsive to a different medication in the same classification.**
4. There are more options to discuss regarding treatment of AD at this time.

52. 1. Aricept does not bind dopamine.
2. **Cholinesterase inhibitors increase the availability of acetylcholine at cholinergic synapses, resulting in increased transmission of acetylcholine by cholinergic neurons that have not been destroyed by the Alzheimer's disease.**
3. Aricept does not decrease acetylcholine in the periphery.
4. Aricept enhances the availability of acetylcholine at the receptor sites.

53. 1. Tricyclic antidepressants, first-generation antihistamines, and antipsychotics can reduce the client's response to cholinesterase inhibitors. Antipsychotics are useful for clients whose behavior is erratic and uncontrollable in the end stage of the disease. The cholinesterase inhibitor Exelon would not be useful in end-stage disease.
2. Coumadin interacts with several medications but not with cholinesterase inhibitors.
3. Cholinesterase inhibitors do not interact with Dilantin.
4. Compazine may be used to control the nausea produced by Exelon; there is no reason to question administering this medication.

54. 1. This is a daily medication and could be administered at any time.
2. This client is nauseated and should be given medication after protecting the client at risk for injury.
3. This medication can be administered after the client's nausea medication in option #2, but it is not a priority at this time.
4. **This client is at risk of harming self or others. Antipsychotic medications are used to control this type of behavior.**

55. 1. **Reminyl is prescribed for mild to moderate AD, and the safety of the client should be the nurse's first concern. Moving the client to a room that can be observed more closely is one of the first steps in a falls prevention protocol.**
2. This should be done, but it is not a priority over client safety.
3. The medications do not cause dry mouth. The unlicensed assistive personnel (UAP) can provide water for the client, providing that there is no reason not to. Clients taking bulk laxatives should increase the fluid intake, but this is not the first intervention.
4. The nurse should assess for effectiveness of all medications, including laxatives, but this is not the first concern.

56. 1. This may not indicate a decrease in abilities, but it definitely does not indicate an improvement in cognitive abilities, which is what the question is asking.
2. **Cholinesterase inhibitors are prescribed to increase cognitive ability for clients diagnosed with AD. Discussing an upcoming event indicates the client is able to focus on a topic and remember that something will happen in the future.**

3. This may not indicate a decrease in abilities, but it definitely does not indicate an improvement in cognitive abilities, which is what the question is asking.

4. This may not indicate a decrease in abilities, but it definitely does not indicate an improvement in cognitive abilities, which is what the question is asking.

57. 1. There are medications that can be taken to reduce the risk of developing Alzheimer's disease (AD). There is a genetic link to developing AD.
    2. Brain scans are not recommended to determine if neuronal damage is occurring leading to the development of AD.
    3. Research has proved the efficacy of HRT and NSAIDs in prevention of AD.
    4. **Hormone replacement therapy has been proved to reduce the risk of developing AD by 30–40% in postmenopausal women. Other medications that have been proven to aid in prevention of AD are nonsteroidal anti-inflammatory drugs (NSAIDs).**

58. 1. The medications may be taken at any time.
    2. There is no reason for routine blood tests to determine toxicity.
    3. **Medications used to treat AD only slow the progression of AD. Currently no medications, prescribed or over the counter, have been proven to reverse or permanently prevent progression of neuronal destruction.**
    4. The medications do not produce photosensitivity. The client should use sunscreen but not because of the medications.

59. 1. **An advantage of Aricept is once-a-day dosing. Research has proved that the more doses required to be taken each day, the less the actual compliance with the medication regimen. Additionally, Aricept is not hepatotoxic and is better tolerated than some of the cholinesterase inhibitors.**
    2. There is no contraindication to administering NSAIDs and cholinesterase inhibitors simultaneously.
    3. Aricept does not enhance vitamin E.
    4. There are side effects with any medications. The common side effects of Aricept are nausea, diarrhea, and bradycardia.

60. 1. **Reminyl's most common side effect is gastrointestinal disturbance. This can**

be minimized if the medication is taken with food.

2. **Reminyl is excreted by the kidneys. The dose is limited for clients with renal or liver impairment and used with caution in clients with severe impairment.**

3. There is no reason to require the client to wear a MedicAlert bracelet. All clients should keep a list of current medications with them in case of an emergency.

4. **The effects of cholinesterase inhibitors may be reduced by first-generation antihistamine medications, tricyclic antidepressants, and antipsychotics, and the client should not take these medications simultaneously. The nurse should ask the client about other medications taken.**

5. The medication does not have to be tapered off to avoid adverse effects.

MEDICATION MEMORY JOGGER: Because the hepatic and renal systems are responsible for metabolizing and excreting all medications, monitoring the liver and kidney laboratory values is a pertinent nursing action.

A Client with a Migraine Headache

61. 1. The client request is not a scientific rationale for prescribing the route of a medication.
    2. Migraine headaches respond to oral medication when administered prophylactically, but the client is less likely to respond to oral medication after the attack has begun.
    3. **Because migraine headaches often cause nausea, vomiting, and gastric stasis, oral medications may not be tolerated or may not be effective once an attack has begun.**
    4. Addiction to medications depends on many factors. The parenteral, intramuscular, intravenous, or oral route may all be addicting, depending on the medication in question.

62. 1. **Feverfew decreases the effectiveness of prescription NSAIDs. The HCP should be notified when a client is taking both medications simultaneously so dosage adjustments can be made. The dose of**

NSAIDs would have to be increased to achieve the same effectiveness.

2. **The client is of childbearing age and should be warned that feverfew crosses the placental barrier and may cause problems with the fetus. The nurse should teach the client to avoid pregnancy and not to breastfeed while taking feverfew.**

3. The client may not see results for 4–6 weeks when taking feverfew. The best results are achieved when the medication is taken continuously for prophylaxis of migraine headaches.

4. Feverfew is also given to relieve menstrual problems; it should not increase menstrual difficulties.

MEDICATION MEMORY JOGGER: Any time the female client is of childbearing age, the nurse must be concerned with possible pregnancy when administering medications. Many medications are teratogenic.

63. 1. These symptoms indicate the client is responding to the long-term use of headache medication, not developing a resistance to the medications.

2. Pain is whatever the client says it is and occurs whenever the client says it does. The client is reporting a subjective symptom and seeking help, not judgment.

3. **Medication overuse headaches occur when clients take headache medication every day. These headaches are also known as rebound headaches or drug-induced headaches. The headache will persist for days to weeks after the medication has been discontinued.**

4. The use of medications for migraine headaches does not cause brain tumors.

64. 1. **The client rates the pain as a 4. NSAIDs are given for mild to moderate migraine pain.**

2. An opioid analgesic should be given only if ergot alkaloids or selective serotonin receptor agonist medications (migraine-specific medications) are not effective in treating the pain.

3. The patient reports mild to moderate pain. A migraine-specific drug, such as an ergot alkaloid, should be given for moderate to severe pain.

4. The patient reports mild to moderate pain. A migraine-specific drug, such as a selective serotonin receptor agonist, should be given for moderate to severe pain.

65. 1. Abortive therapy is used to treat an actual migraine headache in an effort to limit the intensity and duration of the headache. Using the medication more than 1–2 days per week can cause medication overuse headaches (MOH).

2. The client should take his or her radial pulse if receiving preventive therapy with a beta blocker medication—not for the medications used to abort a headache.

3. The common side effects of abortive medications are nausea, vomiting, and diarrhea. The development of hypertension is not associated with these medications. Care should be taken to ensure the patient is experiencing a migraine because a headache can also be caused by severe hypertension.

4. **Use of abortive medications more than 1–2 days per week frequently results in a drug-induced headache, called medication overuse headache (MOH).**

66. **0.5 mL.** To set this problem up algebraically

The first step is:	$6 : X = 12 : 1$
Then cross-multiply to get:	$12\,X = 6$
The next step is to get the X by itself:	$X = \dfrac{6}{12}$
Simplify:	$X = 1/2$ or 0.5 mL

67. 1. **This indicates an improvement in the number of headaches the client normally experiences and is the only option that indicates an improvement in a condition.**

2. This client should be taught to take the radial pulse for 1 minute and to hold the Inderal if the pulse is less than 60 because beta blockers slow the heart rate. This does not indicate the medication is effective.

3. This may be a side effect of the medication because beta blockers are frequently prescribed for hypertension, but this effect does not indicate the medication's effectiveness in preventing migraine.

4. Supplementing the Inderal with an abortive medication four times indicates that the Inderal has not been effective in preventing the occurrence of the headaches.

68. 1. Inderal is used to prevent and Axert is used to treat migraine headaches. The client's symptoms support the diagnosis of cluster headaches, not migraines.
2. **The client's symptoms support the diagnosis of cluster headaches, which are related to migraines but differ in several ways. Cluster headaches are less common than migraines and occur in males 5:1. Cluster headaches do not cause nausea and vomiting; they can be more debilitating than migraines; they do not have an aura; and they are not linked to genetics. The drugs of choice to treat cluster headaches are prednisone and lithium. High-dose prednisone can reduce symptoms within 48 hours, and lithium can prevent the headaches altogether. Lithium takes 1–2 weeks before relief is noted.**
3. Elavil is useful in preventing migraine headaches, not cluster headaches, and Climara is useful in preventing menstrual migraine headaches.
4. Motrin is used to treat mild to moderate migraine headaches, and Reglan is the antiemetic of choice to treat the nausea and vomiting and relieve the gastric stasis of migraine headaches.

69. 1. Sunbathing does not affect a tension headache. Clients with migraine headaches may be sensitive to light.
2. Iodine will not affect a tension headache. Caffeine intake may prevent a headache for some clients.
3. This would be a good question if the client were suffering from a migraine headache because a drug commonly used to treat migraine—ergotamine—should not be taken by a pregnant woman because it may cause uterine contractions. However, this client has a tension headache, not a migraine.
4. **Clients will attempt to self-treat with over-the-counter medications prior to seeking medical attention. The nurse should assess what the client has already tried for relief of the headache.**

70. 1. The meal trays are usually served between 1630 and 1700 on most nursing units. Humalog has an onset of action of 5–7 minutes. The nurse should not administer this insulin until closer to the time for the meal to be served.
2. **Demerol is used to treat severe migraine headaches when other measures have not been effective. This client needs the medication as soon as possible (pain is rated as 8), and this should be the first medication administered.**
3. Depakote ER is used to prevent migraine headaches in the extended-release form. This medication would not be administered prior to treating a headache that is occurring.
4. Reglan is given for nausea and vomiting and to relieve gastric stasis in clients with a migraine headache. The option did not say that the client was vomiting at this time. A headache of an "8" would be priority.

MEDICATION MEMORY JOGGER: Pain is a priority, and pain of an "8" indicates severe pain. The test taker should look at the times and know the actions of the medications administered; this eliminates option "1" as a possible answer.

1. The male client diagnosed with urinary retention is receiving bethanechol (Urecholine), a muscarinic agonist, medication. Which intervention should the nurse implement?
   1. Limit the client's fluid intake to 1000 mL daily.
   2. Have the client's urinal readily available.
   3. Maintain hourly intake and output for the client.
   4. Monitor the client's serum creatinine level.

2. Which client would the nurse question administering the muscarinic antagonist atropine?
   1. The 69-year-old client diagnosed with glaucoma.
   2. The 60-year-old client diagnosed with symptomatic sinus bradycardia.
   3. The 55-year-old client being prepped for an abdominal surgery.
   4. The 28-year-old client with severe diarrhea.

3. The 28-year-old client who is obese is complaining of nervousness, irritability, insomnia, and heart palpitations. Which question should the clinic nurse ask the client first?
   1. "How much weight have you gained or lost within the last 12 months?"
   2. "Do you make yourself vomit after eating large meals?"
   3. "Is there any history of you taking illegal drugs such as amphetamines?"
   4. "Have you been taking any over-the-counter appetite suppressants?"

4. The client is undergoing electroconvulsive therapy (ECT) for major depression and is receiving tubocurarine, a nondepolarizing neuromuscular blocker. Which data would warrant immediate intervention by the nurse?
   1. The client's apical pulse is 58.
   2. The client's oral temperature is 99.8°F.
   3. The client's respiratory rate is 10.
   4. The client's blood pressure is 110/70.

5. The client prescribed phenytoin (Dilantin) for epilepsy calls the clinic and reports a measles-like rash. Which action should the nurse implement?
   1. Instruct the client to come to the clinic immediately.
   2. Determine if the client is drinking grapefruit juice.
   3. Encourage the client to apply a hydrocortisone cream to the rash.
   4. Explain that this is a common side effect of this medication.

6. The client diagnosed with Parkinson's disease has been taking amantadine (Symmetrel), an antiparkinsonian drug. The home health nurse notes a new finding of mottled discoloration of the skin. Which action should the nurse take?
   1. Ask the client if he or she has changed soap products.
   2. Prepare the significant other for the client's imminent death.
   3. Notify the health-care provider to discontinue the medication.
   4. Explain that this is expected and document the finding.

7. The daughter of a client diagnosed with Alzheimer's disease tells the home health nurse that she has been giving her mother *Ginkgo biloba*, an herbal medication. Which action should the nurse take?
   1. Tell her to stop giving her mother the herb because it will not help.
   2. Teach her that herbs have many life-threatening adverse effects.
   3. Explain that the effects may only last for 6–12 months.
   4. Ask the HCP to prescribe tacrine (Cognex) instead of the herb.

8. The client diagnosed with late-stage Alzheimer's disease is agitated and having delusions. Which medication should the nurse anticipate the health-care provider prescribing?
   1. The cholinesterase inhibitor donepezil (Aricept).
   2. The antipsychotic medication haloperidol (Haldol).
   3. The selective serotonin reuptake inhibitor fluoxetine (Prozac).
   4. The tricyclic antidepressant amitriptyline (Elavil).

9. The client diagnosed with Parkinson's disease who is taking selegiline (Eldepryl) has had hip surgery and is being admitted to the orthopedic department. The nurse is transcribing the postoperative orders. Which postoperative order would the nurse question?
   1. The low molecular weight heparin enoxaparin (Lovenox).
   2. The narcotic analgesic meperidine (Demerol).
   3. The MAO-B inhibitor selegiline (Eldepryl).
   4. The prophylactic broad-spectrum antibiotic cefazolin (Ancef).

10. The client diagnosed with epilepsy has undergone a spontaneous remission of the epilepsy, a rare but occasional occurrence. What information should the nurse discuss with the client when discontinuing antiepileptic drugs?
    1. Discuss the need to slowly taper off the antiepileptic drugs.
    2. Explain the importance of getting routine serum levels.
    3. Teach the client to continue taking the antiepileptic drugs.
    4. Instruct the client to use a soft-bristled toothbrush.

11. The client diagnosed with history of a gastric ulcer is having transient ischemic attacks (TIA) and is prescribed a daily 325-mg aspirin. Which information is most important for the nurse to discuss with the client?
    1. Encourage the client to take the aspirin with food.
    2. Notify the health-care provider if ringing in the ears occurs.
    3. Instruct the client to take an enteric-coated brand of aspirin.
    4. Explain that the client may experience black, tarry stools.

12. The client with a severe head injury was exhibiting decorticate posturing during the nurse's assessment 2 hours ago. The client is receiving mannitol (Osmitrol), an osmotic diuretic. Which data indicates the medication is not effective?
    1. The client pushes the nurse's hand away in response to pain.
    2. The client's Glasgow Coma score is a 13.
    3. The client is not able to state the day of the week.
    4. The client exhibits flaccid paralysis to painful stimuli.

13. The client presents to the emergency department complaining of a migraine headache. The health-care provider prescribes sumatriptan (Imitrex), a serotonin receptor agonist. When the nurse enters the room to administer the medication, the client is laughing with his or her significant other. Which action should the nurse take?
    1. Notify the health-care provider of the client's drug-seeking behavior.
    2. Ask the client how bad is the headache if he or she is able to laugh.
    3. Administer the medication after checking for allergies and the ID bracelet.
    4. Discharge the client and recommend taking over-the-counter medication.

14. The client is admitted into the emergency department complaining of profuse salivation, excessive tearing, and diarrhea. The client tells the nurse he had been camping and living off the land. Which medication would the nurse anticipate administering?
    1. Atropine, a muscarinic antagonist.
    2. Diphenhydramine (Benadryl), an antihistamine.
    3. Magnesium/aluminum hydroxide (Maalox), an antacid.
    4. Pantoprazole (Protonix), a proton-pump inhibitor.

15. The client with epilepsy is seen in the clinic and has a serum Dilantin level of 5.4 mg/dL. Which action should the nurse implement first?
    1. Request that the laboratory verify the results of the test.
    2. Ask the client when the dose was taken last.
    3. Instruct the client to not take the Dilantin for 2 days.
    4. Discuss the need to increase the dose of the medication.

16. The client diagnosed with cerebrovascular accident (CVA) is complaining of a headache. Which interventions should the rehabilitation nurse implement? List in the order of performance.
    1. Assess the client's neurological status.
    2. Administer oral acetaminophen (Tylenol).
    3. Have the client swallow a drink of water.
    4. Ask the client to give his or her date of birth.
    5. Ask the client to rate pain on a scale of 1 to 10.

17. The client is going on a cruise and asks the clinic nurse, "I am worried about getting seasick. What should I do?" Which statement would be the nurse's best response?
    1. "You are worried about getting seasick. Let's sit down and talk about it."
    2. "Take the motion sickness medication when you start getting nauseated."
    3. "If you get seasick, you should take an antacid to help with the nausea."
    4. "I would recommend taking Dramamine 30 minutes before your departure."

18. The client is prescribed meclizine (Antivert), an antihistamine, for vertigo. Which statement by the client would warrant intervention by the nurse?
    1. "I have had someone drive my car because I have been getting dizzy."
    2. "I will tell my health-care providers about taking this medication."
    3. "I usually have one or two glasses of wine with my evening meal."
    4. "I will chew sugarless gum or suck on hard candy if my mouth is dry."

19. The client with a brain tumor is complaining of headache that is a "5" on a scale of 1–10. The client's Medication Administration Record (MAR) has acetaminophen (Tylenol) 2 po PRN pain, hydrocodone (Vicodin) 2 po PRN pain, morphine 4 mg IVP PRN pain, and lorazepam (Ativan) 1 mg IVP PRN. Which medication should the nurse prepare to administer?
    1. Tylenol 2 tablets.
    2. Vicodin 2 tablets.
    3. Morphine 4 mg IVP.
    4. Ativan 1 mg IVP.

20. The nurse is administering mannitol (Osmitrol) to the client with a head injury. The order reads 1000 mL intravenous piggyback over 6 hours. At which rate should the nurse administer the medication via a pump?

    Answer _____

1. 1. If the nurse decreases the client's fluid intake, the client could become dehydrated as a result of the increase of urine output caused by the Urecholine as well as sweating, salivation, bronchial secretions, and increased secretions of gastric acid.
   2. **This medication relaxes the urinary sphincters and increases voiding pressure by contracting the detrusor muscle of the bladder; therefore, the client will need to have a urinal available for frequent urination.**
   3. An every-shift intake and output would be sufficient to determine the effectiveness of this medication; an hourly intake and output is not needed.
   4. The client's kidney function does not need to be evaluated prior to administering this medication.

2. 1. **Atropine is contraindicated in a client with glaucoma because atropine causes mydriasis and paralysis of the ciliary muscle, which would increase intraocular pressure and may cause blindness.**
   2. Atropine is the medication of choice for the client with lightheadedness and dizziness from sinus bradycardia manifested by low apical pulse rate; therefore, the nurse would not question administering this medication.
   3. Preoperative treatment with atropine can prevent a dangerous reduction in heart rate, and it dries secretions, which is needed during surgery. The nurse should not question administering this medication.
   4. By blocking the muscarinic receptors in the intestine, atropine can decrease both the tone and motility of intestinal smooth muscle, which will decrease episodes of diarrhea.

   MEDICATION MEMORY JOGGER: Glaucoma is affected by any medication that has the effect of drying secretions.

3. 1. Asking about weight loss and weight gain is an appropriate question for a client who is obese, but this client's physiological signs/symptoms require a more specific question.
   2. This is a question the nurse would ask a client who is suspected of having bulimia, which is not apparent with this client.
   3. Asking the client about illegal drug use may be appropriate, but the nurse should first ask about prescribed or self-medications from over the counter. This question likely will cause the client to become defensive.

   4. **These physiological signs/symptoms could indicate long-term use of anorexiants (appetite suppressants); therefore, the nurse should discuss this question with the client.**

4. 1. This medication does not affect the apical heart rate.
   2. This medication does not affect the client's temperature.
   3. **The primary effect of tubocurarine is relaxation of skeletal muscles, producing a state of flaccid paralysis. Paralysis of the respiratory muscles can cause respiratory arrest. Therefore, a respiratory rate of 10 would warrant immediate intervention by the nurse.**
   4. This blood pressure is within normal limits and therefore would not warrant intervention by the nurse.

5. 1. **This morbilliform (measles-like) rash may progress to a more serious reaction; therefore, the client should come to the clinic immediately and the medication should be stopped immediately.**
   2. Grapefruit does not cause a measles-like rash; therefore, the nurse should not ask this question.
   3. This rash has potential life-threatening consequences, and hydrocortisone cream will not help the client.
   4. This is not a normal side effect of the medication.

   MEDICATION MEMORY JOGGER: Grapefruit juice interacts with many medications and causes problems with absorption, but the interaction with medications does not cause a rash.

6. 1. This change in status would not result from soaps. A rash or skin irritation would be expected with soap products.
   2. Mottling of the skin is a sign of imminent death in some clients, but the nurse must be aware of potential side effects of medications. This client is not dying.
   3. This side effect is not life threatening, and as long as the medication is effective, there is no reason to discontinue the medication.
   4. **Clients taking amantadine for 1 month or longer often develop a mottled discoloration of the skin called livedo reticularis, a benign condition that will gradually disappear following discontinuation of the drug. This condition is not**

a reason to discontinue the medication as long as it is effective. The effectiveness of this medication begins to diminish within 3–6 months.

7. 1. This herb is able to stabilize or improve cognitive performance and social behavior for 6–12 months; therefore, it does help the symptoms of uncomplicated Alzheimer's.

   2. Most herbs do not have life-threatening adverse effects. *Ginkgo biloba* should be taken with caution when taking antiplatelets or anticoagulants because it will increase the risk of bleeding.

   3. **Research has determined that *Ginkgo biloba* has biologic activity in treating uncomplicated Alzheimer's disease for up to 12 months. At this time, medications for Alzheimer's disease result in temporary improvement of the symptoms.**

   4. *Ginkgo biloba* extract has proved to be as effective as tacrine, so there is no reason to change to this medication. Tacrine has a significant risk of liver damage and is avoided in favor of the other cholinesterase inhibitors.

8. 1. Aricept is prescribed in the early stages of Alzheimer's disease but would not be effective in the late stages.

   2. **Delusions and agitation respond to antipsychotic medications. Haldol has been used and has proven to be effective in treating these symptoms, so the nurse should anticipate this prescription.**

   3. SSRIs are useful in treating the depression of Alzheimer's, but these symptoms do not indicate depression.

   4. Tricyclic antidepressants have significant anticholinergic actions and may intensify the symptoms of Alzheimer's disease; therefore, the nurse would not anticipate this being prescribed.

9. 1. The nurse would expect the client to be taking a prophylactic anticoagulant to prevent deep-vein thrombosis secondary to bed rest.

   2. **Meperidine can cause a dangerous interaction with selegiline (Eldepryl), resulting in stupor, rigidity, agitation, and hyperthermia. The nurse would question administering meperidine because the client is receiving selegi-**

line for the Parkinson's disease and it cannot be discontinued abruptly.

   3. This is a medication routinely prescribed for the treatment of Parkinson's disease and the nurse should not question administering it because it cannot be discontinued abruptly.

   4. Prophylactic antibiotics should be prescribed for a client undergoing surgery; therefore, the nurse would not question this medication.

MEDICATION MEMORY JOGGER:
Meperidine (Demerol) metabolizes into normeperidine, which is not readily eliminated from the body and results in the accumulation of toxic substances. The use of Demerol is questioned in many situations and is currently not being used as the first-line medication for pain.

10. 1. **The most important rule in discontinuing antiepileptic drugs (AED) is that they be withdrawn over a period of 6 weeks to several months to avoid side effects. If the client is taking two AEDs, the drugs should be discontinued sequentially, not simultaneously.**

    2. There is no need to obtain serum levels when the medication is being discontinued.

    3. When the epilepsy is in remission, the client should stop taking the AED because a client should not take medication if it is not necessary.

    4. Soft-bristled toothbrushes are recommended for clients taking phenytoin (Dilantin) because of gingival hyperplasia, but this client will stop taking an AED because of being in remission.

11. 1. The client should take the aspirin with food, but because the client has a history of a gastric ulcer, it is more important that the medication not dissolve until after it has passed through the stomach.

    2. Tinnitus, ringing in the ears, is a sign of aspirin toxicity, but if the client takes the medication only once a day, this is a very low risk; thus, this is not a priority intervention.

    3. **Because the client has a history of a gastric ulcer, the client should take an enteric-coated aspirin to ensure that the medication will not dissolve in the stomach and potentially cause gastric irritation leading to bleeding.**

4. If the client has black, tarry stools the health-care provider should be notified because this is a sign of gastric bleeding. One aspirin a day should not cause bleeding; therefore, this is not the most important information to teach the client.

12. 1. This behavior indicates the client's neurological status is improving; therefore, the medication is effective.
   2. The highest possible score on the Glasgow Coma Scale is 15. Therefore, a 13 indicates the client is getting better and the medication is effective.
   3. If the client is alert, even if unable to identify the day of the week, this indicates the client is getting better and the medication is effective.
   4. **Flaccid paralysis is the client's worst response to painful stimuli, equivalent to a 3 on the Glasgow Coma Scale. Decorticate posturing would receive a 5 on the Glasgow Coma Scale. Therefore, flaccid paralysis indicates the medication is not effective.**

13. 1. Clients experiencing chronic pain must adjust to living with the pain and do not always act as the nurse assumes they should. Imitrex is not a narcotic. Therefore, this is not drug-seeking behavior.
   2. Laughing may be the client's way of dealing with the pain, and the nurse should not be judgmental.
   3. **The nurse must check two forms of identification and allergies prior to administering any medication. The nurse should not be judgmental when caring for any client. Pain is what the client states it is.**
   4. Over-the-counter medications are not effective in treating severe vasospasm headaches, which is what a migraine headache is.

14. 1. **The client reports living off the land, and the symptoms reported are clinical manifestations of muscarinic poisoning from eating wild mushrooms. Therefore, the nurse should anticipate administering the antidote, which is atropine.**
   2. An antihistamine would be prescribed for an allergic reaction, not for muscarinic poisoning.
   3. Maalox neutralizes gastric acid and would not be used for mushroom poisoning.

4. A proton-pump inhibitor decreases gastric acidity and would not be prescribed for muscarinic poisoning.

15. 1. There is no indication of a reason for verifying the serum Dilantin level.
   2. **This level is below the therapeutic range of 10–20 mg/dL; therefore, the nurse should determine if the client is taking the medication as directed.**
   3. This is below the therapeutic range; therefore, the medication should not be omitted.
   4. Because this level is below therapeutic range, the nurse must determine how the medication is being taken before discussing the need to increase the dose.

16.   **1, 5, 4, 3, 2**
   1. **The nurse should apply the nursing process and always assess the client unless the client is in distress. The nurse must determine if this is routine pain for which the HCP has prescribed acetaminophen or if it is a complication that warrants medical intervention.**
   5. **The nurse must then determine how much pain the client is in to determine which medication would be most appropriate. The pain scale will also help evaluate the effectiveness of the medication.**
   4. **The nurse must identify the client prior to administering the medication.**
   3. **Because the client has had a CVA, the nurse must determine if the client can swallow prior to administering medication. If the client has problems swallowing water, then the nurse should thicken liquids to help prevent aspiration.**
   2. **The nurse should administer the medication after all the previous steps are completed.**

17. 1. This is a therapeutic response and the patient needs information. Therefore, it is not the nurse's best response.
   2. Antivertigo or anti–motion-sickness medications are most effective when administered prophylactically, rather than after symptoms have begun.
   3. Antacids neutralize the gastric acid and will not help the nausea experienced with motion sickness.
   4. **Dimenhydrinate (Dramamine) is the over-the-counter drug of choice for motion sickness. It should be taken**

30–60 minutes before departure and 30 minutes before meals thereafter.

18. 1. Because of the illness and its drug treatment, the client should not be driving a car; therefore, this statement does not warrant immediate intervention by the nurse.
    2. This client should make sure all the HCPs know about this medication; therefore, this statement does not warrant intervention by the nurse.
    3. **The client should avoid other central nervous system depressants, including alcohol. Therefore, this statement requires intervention and further teaching by the nurse.**
    4. This medication may cause dryness of the mouth and chewing sugarless gum or sucking hard candy would be appropriate; therefore, this statement does not warrant intervention.

MEDICATION MEMORY JOGGER: Usually if there is a question regarding alcohol consumption and medication interaction, the recommendation is to avoid alcohol altogether, not limit the intake.

19. 1. Tylenol, a nonnarcotic analgesic, is useful in the relief of mild to moderate pain, 1–3 on the pain scale.
    2. **Vicodin, a narcotic analgesic, is equivalent to codeine. It is useful for the relief of moderate to severe pain, 4–6 on the pain scale. This client has a brain tumor, which would include increasing intracranial pressure and pain. Therefore, this would be the most appropriate medication at this time.**
    3. Morphine, a narcotic analgesic, intravenous push (IVP), is a potent analgesic and used to treat severe pain, 7–10 on the pain scale.
    4. Ativan, an antianxiety medication, is not used to treat pain.

20. **167 mL/hr** The nurse should divide the volume (1000 mL) by the number of hours (6); this equals 166.6666. The nurse should round up if the number is greater than 5; therefore, the nurse should set the pump at 167 mL/hr.

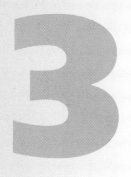

Cardiovascular System

A love affair with knowledge will never end in heartbreak.

—Michael Garrett Marino

PRACTICE QUESTIONS

A Client with Angina/Myocardial Infarction

1. The nurse is teaching the client diagnosed with angina about sublingual nitroglycerin (NTG), a coronary vasodilator. Which statement indicates the client needs more medication teaching?
   1. "I will always carry my nitroglycerin in a dark-colored bottle."
   2. "If I have chest pain, I will put a tablet underneath my tongue."
   3. "If my pain is not relieved with one tablet, I will get medical help."
   4. "I should expect to get a headache after taking my nitroglycerin."

2. The nurse is preparing to administer nitroglycerin, a coronary vasodilator transdermal patch, to the client diagnosed with a myocardial infarction. Which intervention should the nurse implement?
   1. Question applying the patch if the client's B/P is less than 110/70.
   2. Use nonsterile gloves when applying the transdermal patch.
   3. Date and time transdermal patch prior to applying to client's skin.
   4. Place the transdermal patch on the site where the old patch was removed.

3. The client is complaining of severe chest pain radiating down the left arm and is nauseated and diaphoretic. The HCP suspects the client is having a myocardial infarction (MI) and has ordered morphine sulfate (MS), a narcotic analgesic, for the pain. Which intervention should the nurse implement?
   1. Administer the morphine intramuscularly in the ventral gluteal muscle.
   2. Dilute the MS to a 10-mL bolus with normal saline and administer intravenous push.
   3. Question the order because MS should not be administered to a client with an MI.
   4. Assess the client's pain prior to administering the medication orally.

4. The nurse is administering 0900 medications to the following clients. To which client would the nurse question administering the medication?
   1. The client receiving a calcium channel blocker who drank a glass of grapefruit juice.
   2. The client receiving a beta blocker who has an apical pulse of 62 beats per minute.
   3. The client receiving a nitroglycerin patch who has a blood pressure of 148/92.
   4. The client receiving an antiplatelet medication who has a platelet count of 150,000.

5. The client diagnosed with angina is prescribed nitroglycerin (Nitrobid) and tells the nurse, "I don't understand why I can't take my Viagra. I need to take it so that I can make love to my wife." Which statement is the nurse's best response?
   1. "If you take the medications together, you may get very low blood pressure."
   2. "You are worried your wife will be concerned if you cannot make love."
   3. "If you wait at least 8 hours after taking your NTG, you can take your Viagra."
   4. "You should get clarification with your HCP about your taking Viagra."

6. The client diagnosed with a myocardial infarction is receiving thrombolytic therapy. Which data would warrant immediate intervention by the nurse?
   1. The client's telemetry has reperfusion dysrhythmias.
   2. The client is oozing blood from the intravenous site.
   3. The client is alert and oriented to date, time, and place.
   4. The client has no signs of infiltration at the insertion site.

7. The nurse is completing A.M. care with a client diagnosed with angina when the client complains of chest pain. The client has a saline lock in the right forearm. Which intervention should the nurse at the bedside implement first?
   1. Assess the client's vital signs.
   2. Administer sublingual nitroglycerin (NTG).
   3. Administer intravenous morphine sulfate via saline lock.
   4. Administer oxygen via nasal cannula.

8. The client being discharged after sustaining an acute myocardial infarction is prescribed the ACE inhibitor lisinopril (Zestril). Which instruction should the nurse include when teaching about this medication?
   1. Instruct the client to monitor the blood pressure weekly.
   2. Encourage the client to take medication on an empty stomach.
   3. Discuss the need to rise slowly from lying to a standing position.
   4. Teach the client to take the medication at night only.

9. The client calls the clinic and says, "I am having chest pain. I think I am having another heart attack." Which intervention should the nurse implement first?
   1. Call 911 emergency medical services.
   2. Instruct the client to take an aspirin.
   3. Determine if the client is at home alone.
   4. Ask if the client has any sublingual nitroglycerin.

10. The nurse is administering 0.5 inch of nitropaste, a coronary vasodilator. How much paste should the nurse apply to the application paper?

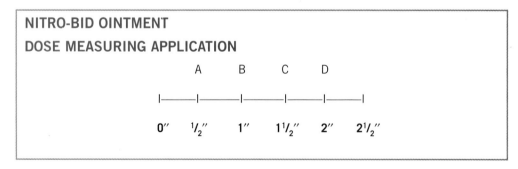

   1. A
   2. B
   3. C
   4. D

A Client with Coronary Artery Disease

11. The client diagnosed with coronary artery disease is prescribed atorvastatin (Lipitor), an HMG-CoA reductase inhibitor. Which statement by the client would warrant the nurse notifying the health-care provider?
    1. "I really haven't changed my diet, but I am taking my medication every day."
    2. "I am feeling pretty good except I am having muscle pain all over my body."
    3. "I am swimming at the local pool about three times a week for 30 minutes."
    4. "I am taking this medication first thing in the morning with a bowl of oatmeal."

12. The client diagnosed with coronary artery disease is instructed to take 81 mg of aspirin ("children's aspirin" or "adult low-dose aspirin") daily. Which statement best describes the scientific rationale for prescribing this medication?
    1. This medication will help thin the client's blood.
    2. Daily aspirin will decrease the incidence of angina.
    3. This medication will prevent platelet aggregation.
    4. Baby aspirin will not cause gastric distress.

13. The client with coronary artery disease is prescribed cholestyramine, a bile-acid sequestrant. Which intervention should the nurse implement when administering the medication?
    1. Administer the medication with fruit juice.
    2. Explain to decrease fiber when taking the medication.
    3. Monitor the cholesterol level before giving medication.
    4. Assess the client for upper-abdominal discomfort.

14. The elderly client diagnosed with coronary artery disease has been taking aspirin daily for more than a year. Which data would warrant notifying the health-care provider?
    1. The client has lost 5 pounds in the last month.
    2. The client has trouble hearing low tones.
    3. The client reports having a funny taste in the mouth.
    4. The client has hard, dark, tarry stools.

15. Which data would indicate to the nurse that simvastatin (Zocor), an HMG-CoA reductase inhibitor, is effective?
    1. The client's blood pressure is 132/80.
    2. The client's cholesterol level is 180 mg/dL.
    3. The client's LDL is 180 mg/dL.
    4. The client's HDL is 35 mg/dL.

16. The client with coronary artery disease is prescribed nicotinic acid (Niacin). The client complains of flushing of the face, neck, and ears. Which priority action should the nurse implement?
    1. Instruct the client to stop taking the medication immediately.
    2. Encourage the client to take the medication with meals only.
    3. Discuss that this is a normal side effect and will decrease with time.
    4. Tell the client to take 325 mg of aspirin 30 minutes before taking medication.

17. The client with a serum cholesterol level of 320 mg/dL is taking the antihyperlipidemic medication ezetimibe (Zetia). Which statement by the client indicates the client needs more teaching concerning this medication?
    1. "This medication helps decrease the absorption of cholesterol in my intestines."
    2. "I cannot take this medication with any other cholesterol-lowering medication."
    3. "I need to eat a low-fat, low-cholesterol diet even when taking the medication."
    4. "It will take a few months for my cholesterol level to get down to normal levels."

18. The client newly diagnosed with coronary artery disease is being prescribed a daily aspirin. The client tells the nurse, "I had a bad case of gastritis last year." Which action should the nurse implement first?
    1. Ask the client if he or she informed the HCP of the gastritis.
    2. Explain that regular aspirin could cause gastric upset.
    3. Instruct the client to take an enteric-coated aspirin.
    4. Determine if the client is taking any antiulcer medication.

19. The nurse is preparing to administer clopidogrel bisulfate (Plavix), an antiplatelet medication, to the client with coronary artery disease. The client asks the nurse, "Why am I getting this medication?" Which statement by the nurse would be most appropriate?
    1. "It will help decrease your chance of developing deep vein thrombosis."
    2. "Plavix will help decrease your LDL cholesterol levels in about 1 month."
    3. "This medication will help prevent your blood from clotting in the arteries."
    4. "The medication will help decrease your blood pressure if you take it daily."

20. The nurse is assessing the preprinted Medication Administration Record (MAR) for a client admitted with angina. Which medication order would the nurse discuss with the pharmacist?

Client Name: ABCD	Client Number: 1234567	Allergies: NKA	Diagnosis: Angina
Medication	0701–1500	1501–2300	2301–0700
Regular insulin subcutaneously ac and hs 0–60: 1 amp D_{50} 61–150: 0 units 151–300: 5 units 301–450: 10 units >450: Call HCP	0730 1130	1630 2100	
Metformin (Glucophage) 500 mg po b.i.d.	0800	1700	
Atorvastatin (Lipitor) 20 mg po every day	0900		
Digoxin (Lanoxin) 0.125 mg po every day	0900		
Nitroglycerin (Nitro-Dur) 0.4 mg/hr on in A.M.	0900		
Nitroglycerin (Nitro-Dur) 0.4 mg/hr off in P.M.		2100	

    1. The 1130 regular insulin order.
    2. The 0800 Glucophage order.
    3. The 0900 Lipitor order.
    4. The 2100 nitroglycerin order.

A Client with Congestive Heart Failure

21. The home health nurse is caring for a client diagnosed with congestive heart failure (CHF) who has been prescribed the cardiac glycoside digoxin (Lanoxin) and the loop diuretic furosemide (Lasix). Which statement by the client indicates the medications are effective?
    1. "I am able to walk next door now without being short of breath."
    2. "I keep my feet propped up as much as I can during the day."
    3. "I have gained 3 pounds since my last visit here."
    4. "I am staying on my diet, and I don't salt my foods anymore."

22. The female client diagnosed with congestive heart failure (CHF) tells the nurse that she has been taking hawthorn extract, an over-the-counter medication, since the HCP told her that she had heart problems. Which statement by the nurse would be appropriate?
    1. "You need to take garlic supplements with hawthorn for it to be effective."
    2. "You should stop taking this herb immediately because it can cause more problems."
    3. "This herb can cause bleeding if you take it with your other medications."
    4. "Some clients find this is helpful, but make sure your HCP is aware of the medication."

23. The client diagnosed with stage D congestive heart failure (CHF) has a brain natriuretic peptide (BNP) level greater than 1500. Which medication would the nurse anticipate the HCP prescribing?
    1. Captopril (Capoten), an angiotensin-converting enzyme inhibitor, orally.
    2. Digoxin (Lanoxin), a cardiac glycoside, IVP.
    3. Dobutamine (Dobutrex), a synthetic catecholamine, IV.
    4. Metoprolol (Lopressor), a beta blocker, orally.

24. The client diagnosed with congestive heart failure (CHF) is prescribed the angiotensin-converting enzyme (ACE) inhibitor enalapril (Vasotec). Which statement explains the scientific rationale for administering this medication?
    1. ACE inhibitors increase the levels of angiotensin II in the blood vessels.
    2. ACE inhibitors dilate arteries, which reduces the workload of the heart.
    3. ACE inhibitors decrease the effects of bradykinin in the body.
    4. ACE inhibitors block the action of antidiuretic hormone in the kidney.

25. The nurse is providing discharge instructions for a client prescribed the thiazide diuretic hydrochlorothiazide (Diuril). Which instruction should the nurse include?
    1. Drink at least 8 to 10 glasses of water a day.
    2. Weigh monthly and report the weight to the HCP.
    3. Eat bananas or oranges regularly.
    4. Try to sleep in an upright position.

26. The nurse in the HCP's office is completing an assessment on a client who has been prescribed the cardiac glycoside digoxin (Lanoxin) for congestive heart failure (CHF). Which data indicates the medication has been effective?
    1. The client's sputum is pink and frothy.
    2. The client has 2+ pitting edema of the sacrum.
    3. The client has clear breath sounds bilaterally.
    4. The client's heart rate is 78 beats per minute.

27. Which medication would the nurse question administering?
    1. Lisinopril (Zestril), an ACE inhibitor, to a client with a BP of 118/84.
    2. Carvedilol (Coreg), a beta blocker, to a client with an apical pulse of 62.
    3. Verapamil (Calan), a calcium channel blocker, to a client with angina.
    4. Furosemide (Lasix), a loop diuretic, to a client complaining of leg cramps.

28. The nurse is administering digoxin (Lanoxin), a cardiac glycoside, to a client diagnosed with congestive heart failure (CHF). Which interventions should the nurse implement? Select all that apply.
    1. Assess the client's carotid pulse for 1 full minute.
    2. Check the client's current potassium level.
    3. Ask the client if he or she is seeing a yellow haze around objects.
    4. Have the client squeeze the nurse's fingers.
    5. Teach the client to get up slowly from a sitting position.

29. Which medication should the nurse question administering to a client diagnosed with stage C congestive heart failure (CHF)?
    1. Ibuprofen (Motrin), a nonsteroidal anti-inflammatory drug (NSAID).
    2. Amlodipine (Norvasc), a calcium channel blocker.
    3. Spironolactone (Aldactone), a potassium-sparing diuretic.
    4. Atenolol (Tenormin), a beta blocker.

30. The HCP prescribed an angiotensin-converting enzyme (ACE) inhibitor for a client diagnosed with congestive heart failure (CHF). Which instruction should the nurse provide?
    1. Eat a banana or drink orange juice at least twice a day.
    2. Notify the HCP if you develop localized edematous areas that itch.
    3. A dry cough is expected early in the morning on arising.
    4. The symptoms of CHF should improve rapidly.

A Client with Dysrhythmias and Conduction Problems

31. The client is exhibiting the following telemetry reading. Which PRN medication should the nurse anticipate the health-care provider ordering?

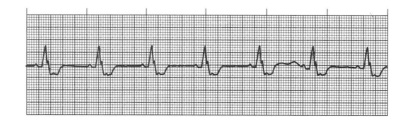

    1. The beta blocker atenolol (Tenormin).
    2. The calcium channel blocker verapamil (Calan).
    3. The coronary vasodilator nitroglycerin (NTG).
    4. The angiotensin-converting enzyme inhibitor captopril (Capoten).

32. Which assessment data should the nurse obtain prior to administering a calcium channel blocker?
    1. The serum calcium level.
    2. The client's radial pulse.
    3. The current telemetry reading.
    4. The client's blood pressure.

33. Which medication should the nurse prepare to administer to the client exhibiting the following telemetry strip?

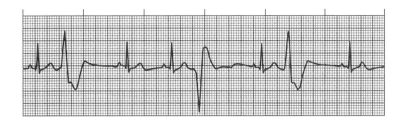

   1. The miscellaneous antidysrhythmic adenosine (Adenocard).
   2. The potassium channel blocker amiodarone (Cordarone).
   3. The cardiac glycoside digoxin (Lanoxin).
   4. The inotropic medication dopamine (Intropin).

34. The client complaining of weakness, dizziness, and lightheadedness is exhibiting the following telemetry strip. The nurse administered the antidysrhythmic medication atropine sulfate intravenously. Which data best indicates the medication was effective?

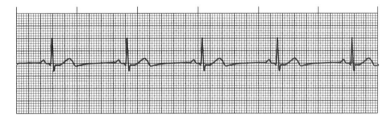

   1. The client's apical pulse rate is 68.
   2. The client's blood pressure is 110/70.
   3. The client's oral mucosa is moist.
   4. The client ambulates to the bathroom safely.

35. The nurse is preparing to administer the antidysrhythmic adenosine (Adenocard) for the client diagnosed with supraventricular tachycardia (SVT). Which assessment finding would indicate the effectiveness of the medication?
   1. The client's ECG tracing shows normal sinus rhythm.
   2. The client's apical pulse is within normal limits.
   3. The client's blood pressure is above 100/60.
   4. The client's serum adenosine level is 1.8 mg/dL.

36. The nurse is caring for clients on the telemetry unit. Which medication should the nurse administer first?
   1. The antidote Digibind for the client whose digoxin level is 1.9 mg/dL.
   2. The narcotic morphine IVP to the client who has pleuritic chest pain.
   3. The sodium channel blocker lidocaine to the client exhibiting bigeminy.
   4. The ACE inhibitor lisinopril (Zestril) to the client with a B/P of 170/90.

37. The client who is 1-day postoperative open-heart surgery is exhibiting the following strip and has a T 101.6, P 110, R 24, and B/P 128/92. Based on the data provided, which action should the nurse implement?

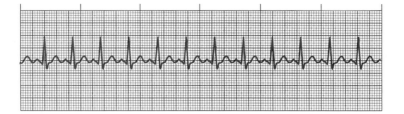

1. Continue to monitor the client and take no action.
2. Administer the antipyretic acetaminophen (Tylenol).
3. Administer the antidysrhythmic quinidine sulfate (Quindex).
4. Administer the sodium channel blocker disopyramide (Norpace).

38. The nurse is preparing to administer 2 g/500 mL of lidocaine, an antidysrhythmic, after administering a 100 mg intravenous bolus to a client with multifocal premature ventricular contractions (PVC). Which intervention should the nurse implement?
   1. Cover the intravenous bag and tubing with tin foil.
   2. Monitor the brain natriuretic peptide (BNP) daily.
   3. Hold the lidocaine drip if no PVCs are noted.
   4. Obtain an infusion pump to administer the medication.

39. The client who has been exhibiting the following telemetry reading for the last 6 months is being discharged. Which instruction will the nurse discuss with the client?

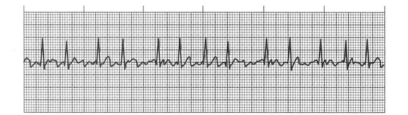

1. The importance of monitoring the client's urinary output.
2. The need to monitor the PTT level while taking aspirin.
3. Dietary restrictions while taking the anticoagulant warfarin (Coumadin).
4. The need to take the cardiac glycoside digoxin on an empty stomach.

40. The client is exhibiting the following telemetry strip. Which interventions should the nurse implement? Select all that apply.

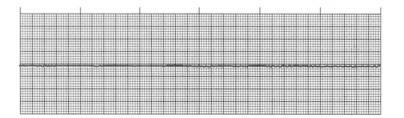

1. Administer the antidysrhythmic atropine.
2. Assess the client's apical heart rate.
3. Administer epinephrine, a sympathomimetic.
4. Initiate cardiopulmonary resuscitation.
5. Administer lidocaine, an antidysrhythmic.

A Client with Inflammatory Cardiac Disorders

41. The client is diagnosed with subacute bacterial endocarditis (SBE). Which health-care provider order should the nurse question?
1. Initiate the antibiotic penicillin intravenously.
2. Obtain a blood culture and sensitivity.
3. Administer a positive protein derivative (PPD) intradermal.
4. Place patient on bed rest with bathroom privileges.

42. The client is diagnosed with subacute bacterial endocarditis (SBE) and is prescribed intravenous antibiotic therapy. Which assessment data indicates the client is ready for home therapy?
1. The client's insurance will no longer pay for hospitalization.
2. The client is afebrile and has no signs of heart failure.
3. The client's white blood cell count is 20,000 mm.
4. The client is asymptomatic while taking oral antibiotics.

43. The nurse is preparing to administer the initial intravenous antibiotic to a client diagnosed with bacterial endocarditis. Which priority intervention should the nurse implement?
1. Determine if the client has any known allergies.
2. Assess the client's intravenous site.
3. Monitor the client's vital signs.
4. Take the medication bag out of the refrigerator.

44. The nurse is preparing to administer the nonsteroidal anti-inflammatory drug (NSAID) ibuprofen (Motrin) to a client diagnosed with pericarditis. Which intervention should the nurse include in the plan of care?
1. Monitor the blood glucose level.
2. Have the client sit upright for 30 minutes after taking the medication.
3. Instruct the client to drink a full glass of water.
4. Administer the medication with food.

45. The clinic nurse is assessing a client diagnosed with pericarditis. The client reports to the nurse, "I take an aspirin every morning to help prevent a heart attack." Which statement would be the nurse's best response based on the client's medical diagnosis?
1. "Aspirin is known to prevent heart attacks. It is excellent that you take it."
2. "Have you noticed that you are bruising more easily since you started taking it?"
3. "I would recommend taking the enteric-coated aspirin to prevent gastric upset."
4. "You should quit taking the aspirin immediately, and I will talk to your HCP."

46. The nurse is administering methylprednisolone sodium succinate (Solu-Medrol), a glucocorticoid, intravenous push to a client diagnosed with pericarditis. The client has a saline lock in the left forearm. After the nurse reconstitutes the powdered medication in the Act-O-Vial, which intervention should the nurse implement?
1. Dilute the medication and flush the saline lock with 10 mL of normal saline before and after administration.
2. Administer the medication undiluted and flush the saline lock with 3 mL of normal saline.
3. Flush the saline lock, administer the diluted medication, and flush the saline lock.
4. Initiate an intravenous line of D_5W and administer the medication through the intravenous tubing.

47. The client diagnosed with pericarditis is a taking a nonsteroidal anti-inflammatory drug (NSAID). Which statement by the client would warrant immediate intervention by the nurse?
1. "I just spit up a small amount of bright red blood."
2. "This medication really doesn't help my pain."
3. "My mother is really allergic to NSAIDs."
4. "My bowel movements have been clay-colored."

48. The client diagnosed with bacterial endocarditis is being discharged home receiving intravenous antibiotic therapy. Which interventions should the nurse implement? Select all that apply.
    1. Refer the client to home health-care services.
    2. Teach the client to report an elevated temperature.
    3. Explain how to use the intravenous pump.
    4. Contact the hospital pharmacy to provide an intravenous pump.
    5. Discuss the need for prophylaxis before dental procedures.

49. The client diagnosed with bacterial endocarditis develops a rash and complains of itching. Which medication would the nurse discuss with the health-care provider?
    1. Intravenous clindamycin (Cleocin), an antibiotic.
    2. Intravenous furosemide (Lasix), a loop diuretic.
    3. The oral glucocorticoid prednisone.
    4. The bacterial agent *Lactobacillus acidophilus*.

50. The client diagnosed with bacterial endocarditis is prescribed gentamycin intravenous piggyback (IVPB). The IVPB comes in 100 mL of fluid to be administered over 1 hour on an intravenous pump. At what rate should the nurse administer the medication?

    Answer _____

A Client with Arterial Occlusive Disease

51. The client with arterial occlusive disease is prescribed pentoxifylline (Trental), a hemorrheologic agent. Which information should the nurse discuss with the client?
    1. Explain that the medication should be taken on an empty stomach.
    2. Instruct the client to avoid smoking when taking this medication.
    3. Discuss that common side effects are flushing of the skin and sedation.
    4. Encourage the client to wear long sleeves and a hat when in the sunlight.

52. The client diagnosed with the peripheral vascular disease Raynaud's disease is prescribed isoxsuprine (Vasodilan), a peripheral vasodilator. Which statement indicates the client understands the discharge teaching?
    1. "I will probably have palpitations and episodes of low blood pressure."
    2. "I should take the medication when I go outside in the cold weather."
    3. "I need to take an enteric-coated aspirin every morning with food."
    4. "This medication will help increase blood flow to my extremities."

53. The client diagnosed with chronic venous insufficiency has a venous stasis ulcer that is being treated with autolytic medication for debridement and an occlusive dressing. The nurse notices a foul-smelling odor. Which action should the nurse take?
    1. Assess the client's vital signs, especially the temperature.
    2. Obtain a culture and sensitivity of the venous stasis ulcer.
    3. Document the finding and take no further action.
    4. Ask the health-care provider to discontinue the medication.

54. The wound care nurse is applying an enzyme debridement ointment to a client with a venous stasis ulcer on the left ankle. Which priority intervention should the nurse implement?
    1. Cover the wound with wrung out saline-soaked gauze.
    2. Place dry gauze and a loose bandage over the wound.
    3. Do not allow any ointment on the normal surrounding skin.
    4. Apply the ointment with a sterile tongue blade.

55. The client with a venous stasis ulcer has exudate. A calcium alginate dressing is applied to the draining ulcer. The client asks the nurse, "How often will the dressing be changed?" Which statement is the nurse's best response?
    1. "The dressing will have to be changed daily."
    2. "It will be changed when the exudate seeps through."
    3. "The doctor will determine when the dressing is changed."
    4. "It will not be changed until the wound is healed."

56. The client with arterial occlusive disease is taking clopidogrel (Plavix), an antiplatelet medication. Which statement by the client would warrant intervention by the nurse?
    1. "I am taking the herb ginkgo to help improve my memory."
    2. "I am a vegetarian and eat a lot of green, leafy vegetables."
    3. "I have not had any blood drawn in more than a year."
    4. "I always use a soft-bristled toothbrush to brush my teeth."

57. The client with arterial occlusive disease has been taking 325 mg of aspirin daily for 1 month. The client tells the nurse, "I have been having a lot of stomach pain." Which priority intervention should the nurse implement?
    1. Instruct the client to take a non–enteric-coated aspirin.
    2. Encourage the client to take the medication with food.
    3. Discuss the need to take only one 81-mg aspirin a day.
    4. Tell the client to notify the health-care provider.

58. The client with a venous stasis ulcer is being treated with the debriding agent dextranomer (Debrisan), highly porous special beads. The nurse notes the beads are a grayish-yellow color. Which action should the primary nurse implement?
    1. Flush the beads with normal saline and apply a new layer of beads.
    2. Take no action because this is the normal color of the beads.
    3. Apply a new layer of beads without removing the grayish-yellow beads.
    4. Prepare the client for surgical debridement of the wound.

59. The client with arterial occlusive disease is postoperative right femoral–popliteal bypass surgery. Which health-care provider's order should the nurse question?
    1. D_5W 1000 mL to infuse at 75 mL/hr.
    2. Ceftriaxone (Rocephin) 500 mg every 12 hours.
    3. Dipyridamole (Persantine) 50 mg three times a day.
    4. Meperidine (Demerol) 25 mg IVP every 4 hours.

60. The nurse is preparing to administer the initial intravenous antibiotic to a client with an arterial ulcer on the right ankle. The client has a saline lock in the right forearm. In which order should the nurse prepare to administer the medication? Select all that apply. Rank in order of performance.
    1. Inject 3 mL of normal saline into the saline lock.
    2. Check to see if a culture and sensitivity test has been done.
    3. Flush the intravenous tubing with the antibiotic.
    4. Determine if the client has any known allergies.
    5. Connect the antibiotic medication to the saline lock.

A Client with Arterial Hypertension

61. The client with essential hypertension is prescribed the beta blocker metoprolol (Lopressor). Which assessment data would make the nurse question administering this medication?
    1. The client's blood pressure is 112/90.
    2. The client's apical pulse is 56.
    3. The client has an occipital headache.
    4. The client is complaining of a yellow haze.

62. The client diagnosed with arterial hypertension is receiving furosemide (Lasix), a loop diuretic. Which data indicates the medication is effective?
    1. The client's 8-hour intake is 1800 mL and the output is 2300 mL.
    2. The client's blood pressure went from 144/88 to 154/96.
    3. The client's has had a weight loss of 1.3 kg in 7 days.
    4. The client reports occasional lightheadedness and dizziness.

63. The client diagnosed with high blood pressure is ordered the angiotensin-converting enzyme inhibitor captopril (Capoten). Which statement by the client indicates to the nurse that the discharge teaching has been effective?
    1. "I should get up slowly when I am getting out of my bed."
    2. "I should check and record my blood pressure once a week."
    3. "If I get leg cramps, I should increase my potassium supplements."
    4. "If I forget to take my medication, I will take two doses the next day."

64. The nurse is preparing to administer the following medications. Which medication would the nurse question administering?
    1. The vasodilator hydralazine (Apresoline) to the client with a blood pressure of 168/94.
    2. The alpha blocker prazosin (Minipress) to the client with a serum sodium level of 137 mEq/L.
    3. The calcium channel blocker diltiazem (Cardizem) to the client with a glucose level of 280 mg/dL.
    4. The loop diuretic furosemide (Lasix) to the client with a serum potassium level of 3.1 mEq/L.

65. The nurse is discussing the thiazide diuretic chlorothiazide (Diuril) with the client diagnosed with essential hypertension. Which discharge instruction should the nurse discuss with the client?
    1. Encourage the intake of sodium-rich foods.
    2. Instruct the client to drink adequate fluids.
    3. Teach the client to keep strict intake and output.
    4. Explain to take the medication at night only.

66. The client diagnosed with essential hypertension is taking the loop diuretic bumetanide (Bumex). Which statement by the client would warrant notifying the client's health-care provider?
    1. "I really wish my mouth would not be so dry."
    2. "I get a little dizzy when I get up too fast."
    3. "I usually have one or two glasses of wine a day."
    4. "I have been experiencing really bad leg cramps."

67. The male client diagnosed with essential hypertension tells the nurse, "I am not able to make love to my wife since I started my blood pressure medications." Which statement by the nurse would be most appropriate?
    1. "You are concerned that you cannot make love to your wife."
    2. "I will refer you to a psychologist so that you can talk about it."
    3. "You need to discuss this with your health-care provider."
    4. "Ask your wife to come in and we can discuss it together."

68. The health-care provider prescribed a beta blocker for the client diagnosed with arterial hypertension. Which is the scientific rationale for administering this medication?
    1. This medication decreases the sympathetic stimulation to the heart, thereby decreasing the client's heart rate and blood pressure.
    2. This medication prevents the calcium from entering the cell, which helps decrease the client's blood pressure.
    3. This medication prevents the release of aldosterone, which deceases absorption of sodium and water, which, in turn, decreases blood pressure.
    4. This medication will cause an increased excretion of water from the vascular system, which will decrease the blood pressure.

69. The nurse is preparing to administer a calcium channel blocker, a loop diuretic, and a beta blocker to a client diagnosed with arterial hypertension. Which action should the nurse implement?
   1. Hold the medication and notify the HCP on rounds.
   2. Check the client's blood pressure.
   3. Contact the pharmacist to discuss the medication.
   4. Double-check the health-care provider's orders.

70. The nurse is administering the combination medication Tenoretic (clorthalidone and atenolol), a thiazide diuretic and beta blocker, to a client diagnosed with chronic hypertension. Which interventions should the nurse implement? Select all that apply.
   1. Do not administer if the client's B/P is less than 90/60.
   2. Do not administer if the client's apical pulse is less than 60.
   3. Teach the client how to prevent orthostatic hypotension.
   4. Encourage the client to eat potassium-rich foods.
   5. Monitor the client's oral intake and urinary output.

A Client with Deep Vein Thrombosis

71. The nurse is preparing to administer warfarin (Coumadin), an anticoagulant. The client's current laboratory values are as follows:

PT38   PTT 39
Control 12.9   Control 36
INR 5.9

Which action should the nurse implement?
   1. Discontinue the intravenous bag immediately.
   2. Prepare to administer AquaMEPHYTON (vitamin K).
   3. Notify the health-care provider to increase the dose.
   4. Administer the medication as ordered.

72. The nurse is discharging the female client diagnosed with deep vein thrombosis (DVT) who is prescribed the anticoagulant warfarin (Coumadin). Which statement indicates the client needs more teaching concerning this medication?
   1. "I should wear a MedicAlert bracelet in case of an emergency."
   2. "If I get cut, I will apply pressure for at least 5 minutes."
   3. "I will increase the amount of green, leafy vegetables I eat."
   4. "I will have to see my HCP regularly while taking this medication."

73. The nurse is preparing to hang the next bag of heparin to a client diagnosed with deep vein thrombosis. The client's current laboratory values are as follows:

PT 12.7   PTT 62
Control 12.9   Control 36
INR 1

Which intervention should the nurse implement?
   1. Hang the intravenous bag at the same rate.
   2. Order a STAT PT/INR/PTT.
   3. Notify the health-care provider.
   4. Assess the client for abnormal bleeding.

74. The client diagnosed with a deep vein thrombosis (DVT) asks the nurse, "Why do I have to take my Coumadin in the evening?" Which statement would be the nurse's best response?
   1. "The medication works more effectively while you are sleeping."
   2. "The medicine should be given with the largest meal of the day."
   3. "The side effects of the Coumadin are less if you take it in the evening."
   4. "This allows for a more accurate INR level when we draw your morning labs."

75. The client has had a total right hip replacement. Which medication should the nurse anticipate the HCP prescribing?
    1. The oral anticoagulant warfarin (Coumadin).
    2. The intravenous anticoagulant heparin.
    3. The thrombolytic alteplase (Activase).
    4. The low molecular weight heparin enoxaparin (Lovenox).

76. The client has petechiae on the anterior lateral upper-abdominal wall. The Medication Administration Record (MAR) indicates the client is receiving a daily baby aspirin, an intravenous narcotic, and a low molecular weight heparin. Which action should the nurse implement?
    1. Request an order to discontinue the 81-mg aspirin.
    2. Assess the client's pain level on a 1–10 scale.
    3. Document the finding and take no action.
    4. Put cool compresses on the abdominal wall.

77. The client on strict bed rest is prescribed subcutaneous heparin. Which data indicates the medication is effective?
    1. The client's current PT is 22, the INR is 2.4, and the PTT is 70.
    2. The client's calves are normal size, are normal skin color, and are nontender.
    3. The client performs active range-of-motion exercises every 4 hours.
    4. The client's varicose veins have reduced in size and appearance.

78. The client is immobile. In which area should the nurse administer the subcutaneous heparin injection?

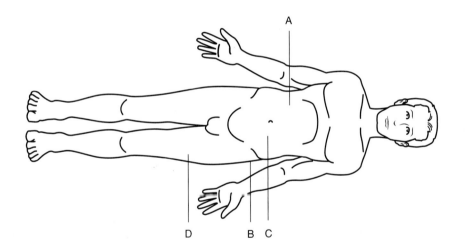

    1. A
    2. B
    3. C
    4. D

79. The client is receiving an intravenous infusion of heparin. The bag hanging has 20,000 units of heparin in 500 mL of D₅W at 22 mL per hour via an intravenous pump. How many units of heparin is the client receiving every hour?

    Answer _____

80. The client is receiving an intravenous infusion of heparin. The bag hanging has 10,000 units of heparin in 100 mL of D₅W. The HCP has ordered the medication to be delivered at 1000 units per hour. At what rate would the nurse set the intravenous pump?

    Answer _____

A Client with Anemia

81. The 28-year-old client diagnosed with sickle cell anemia has been admitted to the medical unit for a vasoocclusive crisis. Which intervention should the nurse implement first?
    1. Elevate the head of the client's bed.
    2. Administer the narcotic analgesic.
    3. Apply oxygen via nasal cannula.
    4. Initiate intravenous fluids.

82. The nurse is caring for a client diagnosed with sickle cell disease (SCD). Which medication would the nurse question?
    1. Morphine sulfate, a narcotic analgesic, IVP.
    2. Fentanyl (Duragesic), a narcotic agonist, patch.
    3. Epoetin (Procrit), a biologic response modifier, SQ.
    4. Piperacillin and tazobactam (Zosyn), an antibiotic combination, IVPB.

83. The client who has had a gastric bypass surgery asks the nurse, "Why do I need to take vitamin B_{12} injections?" Which statement is the nurse's best response?
    1. "You have pernicious anemia, and the injections will cure the problem."
    2. "Your body cannot absorb the vitamin from the food you eat."
    3. "Since the surgery you cannot eat enough food to get the amount you need."
    4. "You will need to take the injections daily until your body begins to make B_{12}."

84. The client diagnosed with iron-deficiency anemia is being discharged. Which discharge instruction should the nurse include regarding the oral iron preparation prescribed?
    1. Teach the client to perform a fecal occult blood test daily.
    2. Demonstrate how to crush the tablets and mix with pudding.
    3. Inform the client to take the medication at night.
    4. Tell the client that his or her stools will be greenish black.

85. The nurse is administering iron dextran (Imferon), an iron preparation, to a client diagnosed with iron-deficiency anemia. Which intervention should the nurse implement?
    1. Make sure the client is well-hydrated.
    2. Give the medication subcutaneously in the deltoid.
    3. Check for allergies to fish or other seafood.
    4. Administer the medication by the Z-tract method.

86. The client diagnosed with polycythemia vera is being discharged. Which discharge instruction should the nurse teach the client?
    1. Take the anticoagulant warfarin (Coumadin) as ordered.
    2. Do not abruptly stop taking prednisone, a steroid.
    3. Rise slowly from a seated position to prevent hypotension.
    4. Restrict fluids to 1000–1500 mL per day.

87. The health-care provider ordered a transfusion to be administered to a client diagnosed with aplastic anemia. Which intervention should the nurse implement? Rank in order of performance.
    1. Obtain informed consent to administer blood.
    2. Make sure the client understands the procedure.
    3. Check the blood out from the laboratory.
    4. Perform a pre-blood assessment.
    5. Start an IV with an 18-gauge catheter.

88. The client is diagnosed with folic acid deficiency anemia and Crohn's disease. Which medication would the nurse anticipate being prescribed?
    1. Oral folic acid.
    2. Cyanocobalamin, vitamin B_{12} IM.
    3. B complex vitamin therapy orally.
    4. Intramuscular folic acid.

89. The male client at the outpatient client was diagnosed with folic acid deficiency anemia and was given a sample of oral folic acid. At the follow-up visit the nurse assesses the client to determine effectiveness of the treatment. Which data indicates the treatment is effective?
    1. The client has gained 2 pounds and has pink buccal mucosa.
    2. The client does not have any paresthesias of the hands and feet.
    3. The client stopped drinking any alcoholic beverage.
    4. The client can tolerate eating green, leafy vegetables.

90. The nurse is caring for a client newly diagnosed with immunohemolytic anemia. Which medication should the nurse anticipate the HCP ordering?
    1. Filgrastim (Neupogen), a hematopoietic growth factor.
    2. Methylprednisolone (Solu-Medrol), a glucocorticoid.
    3. A transfusion of red blood cells.
    4. Leucovorin (folinic acid), a blood former.

A Client with Angina/Myocardial Infarction

1. 1. If the NTG is not kept in a dark-colored bottle, it will lose its potency. This statement shows the client's understanding of the medication teaching and that more teaching on that topic is not necessary.
   2. Sublingual NTG is placed under the client's tongue when chest pain first occurs. The patient understands the teaching.
   3. **The client should put one tablet under the tongue every 5 minutes and, if the chest pain is not relieved after taking three tablets, the client should seek medical attention. This statement indicates the client needs more teaching about the medication.**
   4. Nitroglycerin causes vasodilatation and will cause a headache. The client understands this.

2. 1. Nitroglycerin causes hypotension and the nurse should question administering a transdermal patch if the client's blood pressure is less than 90/60 but not if it is less than 110/70.
   2. The nurse should use gloves when applying nitroglycerin paste, not a transdermal patch. The patch will not cause any medication to be absorbed through the nurse's skin
   3. **The nurse should remove the old patch, wash the client's skin, note the date and time the new patch is applied, and apply it in a new area that is not hairy.**
   4. The transdermal patch must be rotated so that skin irritation will not occur.

3. 1. Morphine sulfate should not be administered intramuscularly to a client with a suspected MI because it will take longer for the medication to take effect and it can skew the cardiac enzyme results.
   2. **Morphine sulfate is the drug of choice for chest pain, and it is administered intravenously so that it acts as soon as possible, within 10–15 minutes. Intravenous push medications should be diluted to help decrease the pain when it is administered and to prevent irritation to the vein. An intravenous push also allows the nurse to inject the medication more accurately over the 5-minute administration time.**
   3. Morphine sulfate should not be questioned; it is the medication of choice and the nurse should know it is always administered intra-

venously for a client with a myocardial infarction.
   4. The nurse should not assess the pain any further; the pain medication should be administered immediately.

4. 1. **The client receiving a calcium channel blocker (CCB) should avoid grapefruit juice because it can cause the CCB to rise to toxic levels.**
   2. The apical heart rate should be greater than 60 beats per minute before a beta blocker is administered; because the apical pulse is 62, the nurse should administer this medication.
   3. The nitroglycerin patch should be held if the client's blood pressure is less than 90/60; because it is above that, the nurse should not question administering this medication.
   4. The client's platelet count is not monitored when administering medication.

MEDICATION MEMORY JOGGER: Grapefruit juice can inhibit the metabolism of certain medications. Specifically, grapefruit juice inhibits cytochrome P450-3A4 found in the liver and the intestinal wall. The nurse should investigate any medications the client is taking if the client drinks grapefruit juice.

5. 1. **Life-threatening hypotension can result with concurrent use of nitroglycerin and sildenafil (Viagra).**
   2. This is a therapeutic response, which is not appropriate because the nurse must make sure the client understands the importance of not taking the medications together.
   3. The client should not take Viagra within 24 hours of taking nitrates, but the client should be instructed not to take Viagra at all while taking Nitrobid, which is an oral medication taken daily.
   4. The nurse should provide the client with correct information about medication and should not rely on the HCP for medication teaching.

6. 1. Reperfusion dysrhythmias indicate the thrombolytic therapy is effective; it indicates that the cardiac tissue is being perfused.
   2. **Any bleeding from the intravenous site, gums, rectum, or vagina should be reported to the HCP. The HCP may not be able to take action to prevent the bleeding during therapy, but it warrants notifying the HCP.**
   3. Being alert and oriented would not warrant intervention by the nurse. However, the

nurse should monitor the patient's level of consciousness because cerebral hemorrhage is a major concern when a client is being given thrombolytic therapy.

4. The nurse should monitor the intravenous site for signs of infiltration, which could lead to tissue damage. If there are no signs of infiltration, intervention by the nurse is not warranted.

7. 1. The client is having chest pain with activity; therefore, the nurse should treat the client.
   2. Administering sublingual NTG would be appropriate, but unless the nurse has the NTG in the room, the nurse should not leave the client alone.
   3. Administering morphine sulfate would be appropriate, but the nurse at the bedside would not have MS at the bedside and it would take time to prepare.
   4. The nurse would have oxygen at the bedside, and applying it would be the first intervention the nurse could implement at the bedside.

MEDICATION MEMORY JOGGER: When answering test questions or when caring for clients at the bedside, the nurse should remember assessing the client may not be the correct action to take when the client is in distress. The nurse may need to intervene directly to help the client.

8. 1. The client is taking the ACE inhibitor to improve survival following an acute MI, and the blood pressure should be monitored daily, not weekly.
   2. The client can take the medication with food to help decrease gastric distress.
   3. **This medication causes orthostatic hypotension, and the client should be instructed to rise slowly from lying to sitting to standing position to prevent falls and injury.**
   4. There is no reason for the medication to be taken at night; it is usually taken in the morning.

9. 1. This should be done, but the nurse should not hang up the phone until taking other actions.
   2. The client should take an aspirin because aspirin has been shown to be effective in decreasing the mortality rate of death from myocardial infarction, but the client should not walk to get the aspirin.
   3. This should be the second intervention; the nurse needs to assess the situation to

determine if the client has anyone who can get the aspirin and let the EMS personnel in when they arrive at the home.

4. **Because the client has had one myocardial infarction, the client may have sublingual NTG in a pocket and can take it immediately. If the client does not have any on the body, then the nurse should determine if there is anyone in the home that can help the client.**

10. 1. A. **The line is in increments of 0.5 (1/2 inch) and the order is 0.5 inch, or 1/2 inch; therefore, the nurse should apply this much paste.**
    2. B. This would be 1 inch, which is twice the prescribed dose of medication.
    3. C. This would be 1 1/2 inches, which is not the correct dose.
    4. D. This would be 2 inches, which is not the correct dose.

A Client with Coronary Artery Disease

11. 1. The client should adhere to a low-fat, low-cholesterol diet, and the nurse is able to teach the client about diet; therefore, the HCP does not need to be notified.
    2. **Statins can cause muscle injury, which can lead to myositis, fatal rhabdomyolysis, or myopathy. Muscle pain or tenderness should be reported to the HCP immediately; usually the medication is discontinued.**
    3. Sedentary lifestyle is a risk factor for developing atherosclerosis; therefore, exercising should be praised and does not need to be reported to the HCP.
    4. The medication should not be taken in the morning, but the nurse can teach this and there is no need to notify the health-care provider.

MEDICATION MEMORY JOGGER: If the client verbalizes a complaint, if the nurse assesses data, or if laboratory data indicates an adverse effect secondary to a medication, the nurse must intervene. The nurse must implement an independent action during intervention or notify the health-care provider because medications can result in serious or even life-threatening complications.

12. 1. Aspirin does not thin the blood. It prevents platelet aggregation. The nurse

must understand the correct rationale for administering medications even if the client may say it "thins the blood."

2. Angina is a complication of atherosclerosis, and aspirin may help decrease angina, but that is not the scientific rationale as to why it is prescribed.

3. **When a baby aspirin is taken daily, it helps prevent platelet aggregation, which, in turn, helps the blood pass through the narrowed arteries more easily.**

4. Baby aspirin can cause gastric distress, but the question is asking for the scientific rationale for taking this medication.

13. 1. **This medication should be administered with water, fruit juice, soup, or pulpy fruit (applesauce, pineapple) to reduce the risk of esophageal irritation and impaction.**

2. The client should increase, not decrease, fiber consumption while taking this medication to help decrease constipation.

3. The cholesterol level is initially monitored monthly and then at longer intervals.

4. There is no reason for the nurse to assess the client for upper-abdominal discomfort because this is not a potential complication of this medication.

14. 1. A 5-pound weight loss in 1 month would not make the nurse suspect the client is experiencing any long-term complications from taking daily aspirin.

2. Elderly clients often have a loss of hearing, but it is not a complication of long-term aspirin use. Tinnitus is, however, a possible complication of aspirin use.

3. Elderly clients often lose taste buds, which may cause a funny taste in the mouth, but it is not a complication of taking daily aspirin.

4. **A complication of long-term aspirin use is gastric bleeding, which could result in dark, tarry stools. This data would warrant further intervention.**

15. 1. The client's blood pressure is within normal limits, but that does not indicate that the medication is effective.

2. **A cholesterol level less than 200 mg/dL is desirable and indicates the medication is effective.**

3. The client's optimal LDL is less than 100 mg/dL, and greater than 200 mg/dL is considered very high. A level of 180 mg/dL is high.

4. HDL promotes cholesterol removal, and the level should be greater than 60 mg/dL. The client's HDL is low, less than 40 mg/dL, which indicates the medication is not effective.

16. 1. This is an expected side effect of the medication, and there is no need to quit taking the medication.

2. Taking the medication with meals will not stop the flushing of the face, neck, and ears.

3. The flushing of the face, neck, and ears may or may not decrease with time, but the nurse should address the client's complaints first.

4. **Taking an aspirin prior to the medication will help reduce the flushing of the face, neck, and ears.**

17. 1. This is a true statement; therefore, the client does not need more teaching.

2. **This is not a true statement; therefore, the client needs more teaching. Zetia acts by decreasing cholesterol absorption in the intestine and is used together with statins to help lower cholesterol in clients whose cholesterol levels cannot be controlled by taking statins alone.**

3. This is a true statement; therefore, the client does not need more teaching.

4. This is a true statement; therefore, the client does not need more teaching.

18. 1. If the HCP is not aware of this significant history, then the HCP should be informed, but it is not the first nursing intervention.

2. Teaching is important, but it is not the first intervention.

3. Enteric-coated aspirin is appropriate for this client to take, but it is not the first intervention.

4. **Assessment is the first part of the nursing process, and determining if the client is taking any antiulcer medication is the first question the nurse should ask the client.**

19. 1. Anticoagulants, not antiplatelets, help prevent deep vein thrombosis.

2. Plavix decreases platelet aggregation, not LDL cholesterol levels.

3. **This medication works in the arteries to prevent platelet aggregation and is prescribed for a client diagnosed with arteriosclerosis.**

4. Plavix is not an antihypertensive medication; it an antiplatelet medication.

20. 1. There is no reason for the nurse to discuss the insulin order with the pharmacist.
    2. There is no reason for the nurse to discuss the Glucophage order with the pharmacist.
    3. **Lipitor should be administered in the evening (not at 0900) so that it will enhance the enzyme that works in the gastrointestinal system to help eliminate cholesterol. The nurse should notify the pharmacist and request a change in the time of administration.**
    4. A nitroglycerin patch is removed during nighttime hours; therefore, the nurse would not discuss the medication with the pharmacist.

A Client with Congestive Heart Failure

21. 1. **A symptom of CHF is shortness of breath. The fact that the client can ambulate without being short of breath is an improvement of symptoms, which shows that the medications are effective.**
    2. This statement indicates compliance with treatment guidelines, not effectiveness of a medication.
    3. Weight gain would indicate that the client is retaining fluid and the medications are not effective.
    4. This statement indicates compliance with treatment guidelines, not effectiveness of a medication.

MEDICATION MEMORY JOGGER: The nurse determines the effectiveness of a medication by assessing for the symptoms, or lack thereof, for which the medication was prescribed.

22. 1. Garlic does not need to be taken for hawthorn to be effective. Both herbs lower blood pressure, so one or the other should be taken.
    2. Many clients use herbs, vitamins, and minerals. The nurse should not be judgmental in responses to clients who confide in the nurse. Doses of ACE inhibitors, cardiac glycosides, and beta blockers may need to be modified if they are taken in combination with some herbs.
    3. The herb does not interfere with platelet aggregation or have any anticoagulant effect, so it will not cause bleeding.

4. Hawthorn dilates the peripheral blood vessels, increases coronary circulation, improves cardiac oxygenation, acts as an antioxidant, has a mild diuretic effect, and is used to treat CHF and HTN. Doses of ACE inhibitors, cardiac glycosides, and beta blockers may need to be modified if taken in combination with hawthorn.

23. 1. ACE inhibitors should be prescribed for clients with diabetes, hyperlipidemia, and hypertension when in stage A heart failure.
    2. Digoxin is prescribed in stage C heart failure.
    3. **Dobutamine is given for short-term IV therapy for clients in stage D CHF and is preferred to dopamine because it does not increase vascular resistance. Dobutamine increases myocardial contractility and cardiac output.**
    4. Beta blockers are prescribed in stage C heart failure. The client may not see an improvement of symptoms, but research has demonstrated that beta blockers can prolong life even in the absence of clinical improvement.

24. 1. ACE inhibitors decrease the level of angiotensin in the body by blocking the conversion from angiotensin I to angiotensin II.
    2. **By reducing the levels of angiotensin II, ACE inhibitors dilate blood vessels, reduce blood volume, and prevent or reverse angiotensin II pathologic changes in the heart and kidneys.**
    3. ACE inhibitors increase bradykinin levels.
    4. ACE inhibitors have no effect on the action of the antidiuretic hormone.

25. 1. The client should drink enough fluid to replace insensible losses (e.g., through perspiration and in feces) or the client will become dehydrated; however, the client should not drink 8–10 glasses of water per day. The medication is being given to reduce the amount of fluid in the body.
    2. The client should weigh himself or herself daily in the same amount of clothes and at approximately the same time for accuracy in weight measurement. The client should report a weight gain of 3 pounds within a week.
    3. Loop and thiazide diuretics cause the body to excrete potassium in the urine. The client should attempt to replace

the potassium by eating potassium-rich foods such as bananas and orange juice.
4. The client does not need to sleep in an upright position if the CHF is being controlled. If the client has to sleep in an upright position to breathe, the HCP should be notified.

26. 1. Pink, frothy sputum indicates that the client's lungs are filling with fluid. This indicates the client's condition is becoming worse.
2. Pitting edema of the sacrum would be seen in clients on bed rest. This is a symptom of CHF and would only indicate the client is getting better if the client had 3+ or 4+ edema initially.
3. Clear lung sounds bilaterally indicate the treatment is effective. The nurse assesses for the signs and symptoms of the disease for which the medication is being administered. If the symptoms are resolving, then the medication is effective.
4. The client's heart rate must be 60 or above to administer digoxin safely, but the heart rate does not indicate the client with CHF is getting better.

27. 1. The blood pressure is above 90/60; there is no reason for the nurse to question administering an ACE inhibitor in this situation.
2. The apical pulse is above 60, so the nurse would not question administering a beta blocker in this situation.
3. Calcium channel blockers are prescribed to treat angina, so there is no reason for the nurse to question the medication.
4. Leg cramps may indicate a low blood potassium level; the nurse should hold the medication until the potassium level can be checked. Loop diuretics cause the kidneys to excrete potassium. Hypokalemia can cause life-threatening dysrhythmias.

28. 1. The client's apical pulse, not the carotid pulse, should be assessed.
2. The client's potassium level, as well as the digoxin level, is monitored because high levels of potassium impair therapeutic response to digoxin and low levels can cause toxicity. The most common cause of dysrhythmias in clients receiving digoxin is hypokalemia from diuretics that are usually given simultaneously.

3. Yellow haze indicates the client may have high serum digoxin levels. The therapeutic range for digoxin is relatively small (0.5 to 1.2), and levels of 2.0 or greater are considered toxic.
4. This is part of a neurological assessment and not needed for digoxin.
5. This would be an intervention to prevent orthostatic hypotension. Digoxin does not affect blood pressure.

29. 1. NSAIDs promote sodium retention and peripheral vasoconstriction—actions that can make CHF worse. Additionally, they reduce the efficacy and intensify the toxicity of diuretics and ACE inhibitors. The nurse should question this medication.
2. As a category of medications, calcium channel blockers are contraindicated in a client diagnosed with CHF; however, the calcium channel blocker Norvasc is an exception: it alone among the calcium channel blockers has been shown not to reduce life expectancy. Norvasc may be given to the client safely.
3. Spironolactone is prescribed for clients in stage C congestive heart failure in addition to loop diuretics for its diuretic effect without causing potassium loss.
4. Beta blockers have been shown to improve life expectancy, although clinical symptoms may not improve. The nurse would not question administering this medication.

30. 1. ACE inhibitors have a side effect of hyperkalemia. The client should not be encouraged to eat potassium-rich foods.
2. A condition in which there are localized edematous areas (wheals), accompanied by intense itching of the skin and mucous membranes, is called angioedema. This is an adverse reaction to an ACE inhibitor and should be reported to the HCP.
3. An intractable dry cough is a reason for discontinuing the ACE inhibitor and should be reported to the HCP.
4. Symptomatic improvement may take weeks to months to develop for a client diagnosed with CHF.

A Client with Dysrhythmias and Conduction Problems

31. 1. Beta blockers are commonly prescribed for heart failure, hypertension, and

tremors; this medication is not ordered PRN because the medication must be tapered off.

2. Calcium channel blockers are usually ordered for hypertension or certain dysrhythmias but not for a bundle branch block.

3. The telemetry reading shows a bundle branch block (BBB) that occurs when the right or left ventricle depolarizes late in the cardiac cycle. BBB commonly occurs in clients diagnosed with coronary artery disease. Nitroglycerin (NTG) dilates coronary arteries to allow increased blood flow to the myocardium; therefore, the nurse would anticipate the HCP prescribing this medication.

4. ACE inhibitors are prescribed for a variety of conditions, including myocardial infarction and heart failure, and to prevent cardiac or renal damage in clients diagnosed with diabetes, but they are not usually prescribed for bundle branch block.

MEDICATION MEMORY JOGGER: Typically medications ending in "ol" or "al" are in the beta blocker classification. Typically medications ending in "il" are ACE inhibitors, but verapamil is the exception to the rule; it is a calcium channel blocker.

32. 1. The client's serum calcium level is not affected by this medication; calcium levels would be monitored for clients taking calcium supplements.

2. The nurse should assess the client's apical pulse before administering any medication that affects the heart rate; the client should be taught to check the radial pulse when taking the medication at home.

3. The client's telemetry reading would not affect the nurse administering this medication.

4. The nurse should not administer this medication if the client's blood pressure is less than 90/60 because it will further decrease the blood pressure, resulting in the brain not being perfused with oxygen.

33. 1. Adenosine (Adenocard) is use to treat supraventricular tachycardia, not premature ventricular contractions.

2. This potassium channel blocker slows repolarization of both the atria and

ventricles and is the drug of choice for prevention and treatment of ventricular dysrhythmia. The strip shows multifocal PVCs in which two or more areas of the ventricle are initiating beats. This is potentially life threatening.

3. Digoxin (Lanoxin) slows the heart rate and increases the contractility of the cardiac muscle and is used to treat atrial dysrhythmias or congestive heart failure, not premature ventricular contractions.

4. Dopamine (Intropin) is used to increase blood pressure or to maintain renal perfusion, but it is not used to treat dysrhythmias.

34. 1. Atropine decreases vagal stimulation, increases the heart rate, and is the medication of choice to treat symptomatic bradycardia—weakness, dizziness, and lightheadedness. An increased heart rate indicates the medication is effective.

2. Atropine has little or no effect on the client's blood pressure other than when the pulse increases the cardiac output should increase.

3. A side effect of this medication is a dry mouth, but a moist oral mucosa would not determine if the medication was effective.

4. The client ambulating safely does not determine if the medication is effective.

MEDICATION MEMORY JOGGER: The nurse determines the effectiveness of a medication by assessing for the symptoms, or lack thereof, for which the medication was prescribed.

35. 1. The client with SVT must be continuously monitored on telemetry when this medication is being administered. When the SVT converts to normal sinus rhythm, the nurse knows the medication has been effective.

2. The apical pulse can be monitored, but when administering medications for a dysrhythmia, a change in the electrical conductivity of the heart to normal sinus rhythm is the best way to determine the effectiveness of the medication. The normal apical pulse rate is 60 to 100 beats per minute.

3. The blood pressure would not indicate if this medication was effective.

4. The client's serum adenosine level would not indicate the medication was effective.

36. 1. The digoxin level is within therapeutic range; therefore, the antidote Digibind would not be administered to this client.
    2. Pleuritic pain is pain involving the thoracic pleura and should be addressed, but it is not a priority over a life-threatening dysrhythmia.
    3. **A client with bigeminy, a life-threatening ventricular dysrhythmia, must be assessed first and treated; an intravenous bolus of lidocaine, followed by an intravenous drip, is the treatment of choice.**
    4. This blood pressure is elevated, but it is not at a life-threatening level; therefore, this client would not be assessed or treated first.

37. 1. This client's elevated temperature and sinus tachycardia require intervention by the nurse.
    2. **Sinus tachycardia may be caused by elevated temperature, exercise, anxiety, hypoxemia, hypovolemia, or cardiac failure. Because the client's temperature is elevated, an antipyretic should be administered.**
    3. Quinidine is used to treat ventricular or atrial dysrhythmias, and the word "sinus" means the beat originates at the sinoatrial node; therefore, the nurse must treat the cause.
    4. Norpace is used to treat PVC, SVT, or ventricular tachycardia, and this telemetry strip is sinus tachycardia.

38. 1. Light does not affect the lidocaine; therefore, the nurse does not have to protect the bag and tubing.
    2. The BNP is monitored for a client diagnosed with congestive heart failure and is not monitored for a client receiving lidocaine.
    3. The lidocaine drip must be administered even if the client has no PVCs in order to prevent and stabilize ventricular irritability because the half-life of lidocaine is very short.
    4. **Lidocaine is a very potent medication and is administered in this concentration by an intravenous pump to maintain a constant rate of administration. The pump also ensures that too much medication is not administered at one time, which can result in death.**

39. 1. The client with atrial fibrillation would not necessarily be taking a diuretic, which would require the client to monitor fluid status.
    2. The PTT level is monitored for a client who is receiving heparin intravenously.
    3. **Atrial fibrillation causes pooling of the blood in the atria, which could lead to the development of a blood clot, and the client is prescribed Coumadin to decrease the probability of developing a thrombus/embolus. Green, leafy vegetables are high in vitamin K, which is the antidote for Coumadin overdose and should be limited in the client's diet.**
    4. Digoxin should be administered after meals or with meals to decrease gastric irritability.

40. 1. Atropine decreases vagal stimulation, increases the heart rate, and is the drug of choice for a client exhibiting asystole.
    2. **The nurse should determine if the telemetry reading is artifact or if the client is in asystole before administering any treatment.**
    3. Intravenous epinephrine vasoconstricts the peripheral circulation and shunts the blood to the central circulation (brain, heart, lungs) in clients who do not have a heartbeat.
    4. Asystole (no heartbeat) requires the nurse to start CPR.
    5. Lidocaine is the drug of choice for a client with a ventricular dysrhythmia, but it will not help convert asystole into normal sinus rhythm.

A Client with Inflammatory Cardiac Disorders

41. 1. Antibiotics are the mainstay of treatment for SBE, and in most cases the ideal antibiotic is one of the penicillins. The nurse would not question this order.
    2. A positive blood culture is a prime diagnostic indicator of SBE, and both aerobic and anaerobic specimens are obtained for culture. The nurse would not question this order.
    3. **The nurse would question why the HCP is ordering a PPD, which is a tuberculosis skin test. TB is not a risk factor for developing SBE.**
    4. Complete bed rest is not enforced unless the client with SBE has a fever or signs of

heart failure; therefore, bed rest with bathroom privileges would not be questioned by the nurse.

MEDICATION MEMORY JOGGER: The nurse must be knowledgeable about accepted standards of practice for disease processes and conditions. If the nurse administers a medication the health-care provider has prescribed and it harms the client, the nurse could be held accountable. Remember that the nurse is a client advocate.

42. 1. The client's ability to pay for the hospitalization is not an indicator of when the client should be discharged for home therapy.
2. **The client is ready for home therapy when the client is afebrile, has negative blood cultures, and has no signs of heart failure or embolization. Home therapy consists of approximately 5 more weeks of intravenous antibiotic therapy.**
3. The WBC level is elevated, which indicates the medication is not effective and the client is not ready for home therapy.
4. The client is receiving intravenous antibiotic therapy for up to 6 weeks and will not be taking oral antibiotic therapy after discharge.

43. 1. **This is priority because if the client is allergic to the antibiotic and the nurse administers it to the client, the client could go into anaphylactic shock and die.**
2. Even if the antibiotic infiltrates into the client's tissues, it is not a life-threatening emergency.
3. The client's vital signs should be monitored for elevated temperature and signs of heart failure, but this is not priority over checking for allergies because this is the first dose of antibiotics to be given.
4. The medication should be administered at room temperature, but this is not priority over determining if the client is allergic to any antibiotics.

44. 1. The blood glucose level is not affected by an NSAID.
2. There is no reason the client should have to sit up after taking an NSAID.
3. Drinking a full glass of water will not increase or decrease the efficacy of an NSAID.

4. NSAIDs interfere with the prostaglandin production in the stomach, which can result in erosion of the protective mucosal barrier causing an ulcer; this can be prevented by taking the NSAID with food.

45. 1. This is a true statement, but it is not appropriate for a client diagnosed with pericarditis.
2. Clients taking one aspirin a day should not notice an increase in bleeding.
3. This is a true statement, but it is not appropriate for clients diagnosed with pericarditis.
4. **The client with pericarditis should avoid taking aspirin and anticoagulants because they may increase the possibility of cardiac tamponade.**

46. 1. The saline lock does not need to be flushed with 10 mL of normal saline; it should be flushed with 2–3 mL, depending on hospital policy.
2. Intravenous push medication should be diluted to ensure correct rate of administration, to protect the vein, and to decrease the client's pain during administration.
3. **The medication should be diluted (see # 2 rationale), then the saline lock should be flushed before administration of the medication to ensure vein patency, and then it should be flushed after administration to ensure all medication was delivered.**
4. There is no reason the medication cannot be administered safely through the saline lock.

47. 1. NSAIDs interfere with the prostaglandin production in the stomach, which can result in erosion of the protective mucosal barrier, causing an ulcer. Bright-red bleeding requires immediate further assessment.
2. Pericarditis causes pain, which is expected, but hemorrhaging could be an adverse effect of NSAIDs and warrants immediate intervention.
3. A family member's allergy does not affect the client who has been taking the medication.
4. Clay-colored stools are not indicative of an adverse or side effect of NSAIDs and would not warrant immediate intervention.

MEDICATION MEMORY JOGGER: If the client verbalizes a complaint, if the nurse assesses data, or if laboratory data indi-

cates an adverse effect secondary to a medication, the nurse must intervene. The nurse must implement an independent action during the intervention or notify the health-care provider because medications can result in serious or even life-threatening complications.

48. 1. Intravenous antibiotics are prescribed for up to 6 weeks. The client is discharged home and will receive this therapy with the assistance of a home health-care nurse.
2. The nurse must teach the client self-monitoring for manifestations of endocarditis. The client should take his or her temperature daily and report an elevated temperature.
3. The nurse would not explain how to use the IV pump in the hospital because it probably will not be the same equipment provided by the home health-care agency; the home health-care nurse will be responsible for this intervention.
4. Hospital pharmacies do not provide intravenous pumps for home use.
5. Prophylactic antibiotics are administered prior to invasive procedures (such as teeth cleaning) so that there will not be an exacerbation of the endocarditis.

49. 1. Antibiotics are well-known for causing allergic reactions; a rash and itching should make the nurse suspect that the client is experiencing an allergic reaction.
2. The nurse should not question a loop diuretic as the first medication causing the clinical manifestations of an allergic reaction.
3. The nurse should not question a steroid, which is a hormone produced by the body, as causing an allergic reaction.
4. *Lactobacillus acidophilus* is used to replace good bacteria destroyed by the antibiotics and to prevent or treat diarrhea or secondary yeast infection.

50. 100 mL. The pump administers medication at a rate per hour; therefore, 100 mL would infuse over 1 hour.

A Client with Arterial Occlusive Disease

51. 1. The medication should be taken with food to prevent gastric upset.

2. The client should avoid smoking because nicotine increases vasoconstriction.
3. Flushing of the skin, faintness, sedation, and gastrointestinal disturbances are signs of an overdose of this medication, **not common side effects,** and should be reported to the health-care provider.
4. This medication does not cause photosensitivity, so there is no need for the client to wear long sleeves and a hat.

52. 1. Adverse effects of this medication are hypotension, tachycardia, and palpitations; the client should notify the health-care provider so that the medication can be discontinued. This statement indicates the client does not understand the teaching.
2. This medication should be taken on a regular basis at least three to four times a day, not only when going outside in cold weather. The client does not understand the teaching.
3. This medication is contraindicated in clients with bleeding disorders; therefore, the client should not take daily aspirin, an antiplatelet medication.
4. **This medication increases blood flow, which is restricted in peripheral vascular diseases, such as Raynaud's disease and atherosclerosis obliterans. This statement indicates the client understands the discharge teaching.**

53. 1. The foul odor does not indicate an infection; therefore, the client's vital signs do not need to be assessed.
2. A culture and sensitivity would only be taken if the nurse suspected an infection, and this foul odor does not indicate a wound infection.
3. **This is an expected reaction. The foul odor is produced by the breakdown of cellular debris and does not indicate that the wound is infected.**
4. There is no need to discontinue the medication; the foul odor indicates the medication is working effectively.

54. 1. The wound should be covered with a thoroughly wrung out saline-soaked gauze, but this is not the priority intervention.
2. After applying the ointment and then the saline-soaked gauze, a dry gauze should be applied to the wound, but this is not the priority intervention.
3. **The most important intervention is not to allow any of the enzymatic ointment to be placed on the normal surround-**

ing skin because it will cause necrosis of the normal skin.

4. The ointment should be applied with a sterile tongue blade to prevent any type of bacteria from entering the stasis ulcer, but this is not the priority intervention.

55. 1. The dressing is changed at least every 7 days or when the exudate seeps through the dressing.
2. **The dressing is changed when the exudate seeps through the dressing or at least every 7 days.**
3. The doctor does not determine when the dressing will be changed.
4. The dressing will be changed many times before the wound is healed.

56. 1. **Ginkgo, an herb, can increase bleeding when taken with an antiplatelet medication such as aspirin or Plavix. Therefore, this statement warrants intervention and the nurse should encourage the client to quit taking ginkgo. Ginkgo has been shown to have a beneficial effect of increasing blood flow to the brain, but in this case, the risk of bleeding warrants the nurse's intervention.**
2. Green, leafy vegetables would interfere with warfarin (Coumadin) anticoagulant therapy, not with antiplatelet medications; therefore, this would not warrant intervention by the nurse.
3. Antiplatelet medication does not require routine bloodwork to determine effectiveness; therefore, this would not warrant intervention by the nurse.
4. Soft-bristled toothbrushes should be used to help prevent abnormal bleeding.

MEDICATION MEMORY JOGGER: Some herbal preparations are effective, some are not, and a few can be harmful or even deadly. If a client is taking an herbal supplement and a conventional medicine, the nurse should investigate to determine if there is a possible interaction that could cause harm to the client. The nurse should always be the client's advocate.

57. 1. Aspirin causes gastric irritation and the best way to prevent this is to take enteric-coated aspirin, not a non–enteric-coated aspirin. Enteric-coated aspirin will be absorbed in the intestines and not in the stomach.
2. **The client should take the aspirin with food to help prevent gastric irritation,**

and the nurse should instruct the client to take an enteric-coated aspirin.
3. A baby aspirin or a regular aspirin can cause gastric irritation, so the nurse should instruct the client to take an enteric-coated aspirin.
4. The nurse can provide correct information about the client's complaint. The nurse is not prescribing it because the client is already taking the medication.

58. 1. **The grayish-yellow color indicates the beads are saturated, at which point their cleansing action stops. The beads should be flushed from the wound with normal saline and a fresh layer should be applied.**
2. This is not the normal color of the beads.
3. The grayish-yellow beads must be removed before a new layer is applied.
4. This is a debriding agent that is working effectively; therefore, no surgical debridement is necessary.

59. 1. This intravenous order would be an expected order for a client who has undergone surgery; therefore, the nurse would not question this order.
2. This is an antibiotic that would be expected for a client who has just had surgery; therefore, the nurse would not question this order.
3. **This is an antiplatelet medication that should have been discontinued 5–7 days prior to surgery because it may cause bleeding in the postoperative client; therefore, the nurse would question why the client is receiving this medication.**
4. This is a pain medication that would be ordered for a client who has undergone surgery; therefore, the nurse would not question this medication.

MEDICATION MEMORY JOGGER: The nurse must be knowledgeable about accepted standards of practice for disease processes and conditions. If the nurse administers a medication the health-care provider has prescribed and it harms the client, the nurse could be held accountable. Remember that the nurse is a client advocate.

60.   **2, 4, 3, 1, 5**
2. If a culture and sensitivity (C&S) has been ordered and the nurse administers the antibiotic, the C&S will be

skewed and an accurate result will not be available.

4. **The nurse should always check to see if a client has any known allergies before administering the initial medication, especially an antibiotic.**

3. **The nurse should prepare the intravenous antibiotic in the medication room—not at the bedside—and should always flush the tubing so that air will not be injected into the client's vein.**

1. The nurse must determine if the saline lock is patent; this is done by injecting normal saline into the lock.

5. After all the previously listed interventions are completed, then the nurse can infuse the medication.

A Client with Arterial Hypertension

61. 1. The nurse would question administering a beta blocker if the client's blood pressure was less than 90/60 because this medication would further lower the blood pressure.

2. **The nurse would question administering a beta blocker if the client's apical pulse was less than 60 because this medication decreases the heart rate.**

3. An occipital headache could be a sign of high blood pressure; therefore, the nurse would administer the medication.

4. A yellow haze is a common symptom of a client who is exhibiting digoxin (a cardiac glycoside) toxicity.

62. 1. **The client has had 500 mL (2300–1800 = 500) excess urinary output. This indicates the medication is effective— the diuretic is causing an increase in urinary output.**

2. This blood pressure has increased; therefore, the medication is not effective.

3. A weight loss of 1.3 kg (2.6 pounds) in 7 days would not indicate a loss of fluid; it could be a loss of fat. Remember 1000 mL equals about 1 kg (2.2 pounds).

4. These are signs of orthostatic hypotension and do not indicate the medication is effective.

MEDICATION MEMORY JOGGER: The nurse determines the effectiveness of a medication by assessing for the symptoms, or lack thereof, for which the medication was prescribed.

63. 1. **Antihypertensive medications in general cause orthostatic hypotension. Therefore, the client should be taught to get up slowly from lying to sitting and sitting to a standing position to help prevent dizziness and lightheadedness.**

2. The blood pressure must be checked more than once a week; it should be checked daily.

3. ACE inhibitors do not require potassium supplements.

4. The client should never make up doses of medication missed; that may cause hypotension.

64. 1. The blood pressure (168/94) is elevated; therefore, the nurse should administer this medication without questioning it.

2. The normal serum sodium level is 135–145 mEq/L. Therefore, the nurse should administer this medication without questioning.

3. The glucose level is not pertinent when administering this medication. Although the glucose level is elevated (70–110 mg/dL is normal), it would not cause the nurse to question administering this medication.

4. **The serum potassium level is low (normal is 3.5–5.0 mEq/L). Therefore, because a loop diuretic will cause further potassium loss, the nurse should question administering this medication and obtain a potassium supplement for the client.**

MEDICATION MEMORY JOGGER: The nurse must be knowledgeable about accepted standards of practice for medication administration, including which client assessment data and laboratory data should be monitored prior to administering the medication.

65. 1. The client should be discouraged from eating sodium-rich foods and encouraged to increase intake of potassium-rich food.

2. **The client should drink adequate amounts of fluids to replace insensible loss of fluids and to help prevent dehydration.**

3. To ask the client to keep strict intake and output is unrealistic; this would be done in the hospital, but not in the client's home.

4. The medication should be taken in the morning to prevent nocturia.

66. 1. The nurse should instruct the client to increase fluids or suck on hard candy, but

the HCP does not need to be notified because dry mouth is an expected side effect of this medication.

2. The nurse should discuss how to prevent orthostatic hypotension, but the HCP does not need to be notified because this is an expected side effect.

3. The client should not be drinking alcohol because it may potentiate orthostatic hypotension, but the nurse should discuss this with the client and not necessarily notify the HCP.

4. **Leg cramps could indicate hypokalemia, which is potentially life threatening secondary to cardiac dysrhythmias. This needs to be reported to the HCP so that the dosage can be reduced or potassium supplements can be ordered for the client.**

MEDICATION MEMORY JOGGER: If the client verbalizes a complaint, if the nurse assesses data, or if laboratory data indicates an adverse effect secondary to a medication, the nurse must intervene. The nurse must implement an independent action or notify the health-care provider because medications can result in serious or even life-threatening complications.

67. 1. This is a therapeutic response that helps the client to ventilate feelings, but the impotence may be a side effect of the medication and the HCP should be notified.
2. This may be a side effect of the medication and the HCP should be notified.
3. **This may be a side effect of the medication and is a reason for noncompliance in male clients. The HCP should be notified so that the HCP can discuss the situation and possibly prescribe a different medication.**
4. This may be a side effect of the medication and the HCP should be notified.

68. 1. **This is the correct scientific rationale for administering this medication.**
2. This is the scientific rationale for a calcium channel blocker.
3. This is the scientific rationale for an angiotensin-converting enzyme (ACE) inhibitor.
4. This is the scientific rationale for a diuretic.

69. 1. Many clients with hypertension are prescribed multiple medications to help decrease the blood pressure. There is no need to hold the medication or notify the HCP.
2. **These medications all work in different parts of the body to help decrease the client's blood pressure. The nurse should realize the HCP is having difficulty controlling the client's blood pressure and should monitor the client's blood pressure prior to administering.**
3. Multiple antihypertensive medications are prescribed to help control a client's blood pressure; therefore; there would be no need for the nurse to contact the pharmacist.
4. The nurse should not question administering multiple antihypertensive medications that work on different parts of the body; this is an accepted standard of care.

70. 1. If the client's blood pressure is less than 90/60, the medication should be held so that the client will not experience profound hypotension.
2. If the client's apical pulse is less than 60, the medication should be held so that the client's pulse will not plummet to less than 60, which is sinus bradycardia.
3. A side effect of antihypertensive medications is orthostatic hypotension, and the nurse should discuss how to prevent episodes.
4. Thiazide diuretics do not cause excess loss of potassium, but the client should be encouraged to eat potassium-rich foods to prevent hypokalemia, which may occur as a result of increased urination.
5. The nurse should monitor the client's intake and output to determine if the medication is effective.

A Client with Deep Vein Thrombosis

71. 1. Coumadin is administered orally. There is no reason to discontinue an IV.
2. **AquaMEPHYTON is the antidote for Coumadin toxicity. The therapeutic range for the INR is 2–3. With an INR of 5.9, this client is at great risk for hemorrhage and should be given the vitamin K.**
3. The dose should not be administered because it is above the therapeutic range.

The dose should be held until the therapeutic range is obtained.

4. Administering this medication is a medication error that could possibly result in the death of the client.

MEDICATION MEMORY JOGGER: When trying to remember which laboratory value correlates with which anticoagulant, follow this helpful hint: "PT boats go to war (warfarin) and if you cross the small "t's" in "Ptt" with one line it makes an "h" (heparin).

72. 1. The client is at risk for bleeding and should wear a medical alert bracelet to notify HCPs about the anticoagulant; therefore, the client understands the medication teaching.
2. If the client cuts himself or herself, the client should apply direct pressure for 5 minutes without peeking at the cut. If the cut is still bleeding after this time, the client should continue to apply pressure and seek medical attention. This statement indicates the client understands the medication teaching.
3. **Green, leafy vegetables are high in vitamin K, which is the antidote for Coumadin toxicity. AquaMEPHYTON is the chemical name for vitamin K. Green, leafy vegetables would interfere with the therapeutic effects of Coumadin. This statement indicates the client does not understand the medication teaching.**
4. The client's PT/INR is monitored at routine intervals to determine if the medication is within the therapeutic range: an INR of 2–3 should be maintained. The client should regularly see the HCP. This statement indicates the client understands the medication teaching.

73. 1. **The therapeutic range for heparin is 1.5 to 2.0 times the control, or 54 to 72. The client's PTT of 62 indicates the client is within therapeutic range and the next bag should be administered at the same rate.**
2. The client's PTT is within therapeutic range; therefore, there is no need to order any further laboratory studies.
3. The HCP need not be notified of the client's situation because the client's PTT is within therapeutic range.
4. The client's PTT is within therapeutic range. This level does not indicate a potential for abnormal bleeding.

74. 1. This is a false statement; this medication does not work better during the night.
2. This medication can be taken on an empty stomach or with food.
3. There are not any side effects of Coumadin that would be decreased by taking the medication in the evening.
4. **Routine laboratory tests are drawn in the morning. If Coumadin is administered in the morning, the International Normalized Ratio (INR) will be lower as a result of the medication's effects wearing off. If the Coumadin is taken in the evening, then the INR level will reflect more accurately the peak blood level.**

75. 1. The nurse would not anticipate the HCP prescribing a medication that would cause bleeding for a client who has had surgery.
2. The nurse would not anticipate the HCP prescribing a medication that would cause bleeding for a client who has had surgery. Intravenous heparin is only used to treat clients with actual clotting problems.
3. Thrombolytic medications would destroy thrombus formations and would not be prescribed for a surgical client.
4. **Lovenox is prescribed for clients who are immobile, such as this surgical client, to help prevent deep vein thrombosis; therefore, the nurse should anticipate this medication being prescribed.**

76. 1. A baby aspirin would not cause the client to have petechiae.
2. Petechiae have nothing to do with the client's pain level.
3. **The petechiae, tiny purple or red spots that appear on the skin as a result of minute hemorrhages within the dermal or submucosal areas, are secondary to subcutaneous injections of Lovenox, a low molecular weight heparin.**
4. Cool compresses cause vasoconstriction, but this would not help prevent or treat petechiae.

77. 1. Heparin has a very short half-life, and to achieve a therapeutic level it must be administered intravenously. Subcutaneous heparin is used prophylactically to prevent deep vein thrombosis (DVT). Laboratory tests are not monitored for this route.
2. **Subcutaneous heparin is used prophylactically to prevent deep vein thrombosis. Symptoms of a DVT include calf edema, redness, warmth, and pain on**

dorsiflexion. Lack of these symptoms indicates the client does not have a DVT and that, therefore, the medication is effective.

3. ROM exercise is an intervention and does not indicate the medication is effective.

4. In most people, the appearance of varicose veins will improve when the legs are elevated. Remember, however, that varicose veins are superficial veins and that subcutaneous heparin is not used to treat this condition.

MEDICATION MEMORY JOGGER: The nurse determines the effectiveness of a medication by assessing for the symptoms, or lack thereof, for which the medication was prescribed.

78. 1. This is the area called the "love handles," and low molecular weight heparin, Lovenox, is administered here to prevent abdominal wall trauma.

2. This is the area where intramuscular injections are primarily administered.

3. **Subcutaneous heparin is administered in the lower abdomen for better absorption and should be at least 2 inches away from the umbilicus.**

4. If subcutaneous heparin is administered in the thigh area, it could possibly result in large hematoma formation secondary to leg movement.

79. **880 units of heparin are being infused every hour.** When determining the units, the nurse must first determine how many units are in each mL.

$$\frac{20,000 \text{ units}}{500 \text{ mL}} = 40 \text{ units per mL}$$

40 units per mL × 22 mL per hour = 880 mL per hour

80. **10 mL per hour.** When setting the intravenous pump the nurse must first determine the number of units per mL.

$$\frac{10,000 \text{ units}}{100 \text{ mL}} = 100 \text{ units per mL}$$

Then divide the desired number of units per hour by the units per mL.

$$1000 \div 100 = 10$$

A Client with Anemia

81. 1. Elevating the head of the client's bed would assist with dyspnea but would not help the client's pain, which is priority, along with reversing the sickling process.

2. Pain medication is administered intravenously; therefore, the first intervention would be to initiate intravenous fluids and then administer pain medication.

3. Oxygen is usually administered, but the best method of promoting oxygenation is the reversal of sickling, which is accomplished by administering IV fluids.

4. **Intravenous fluids help reverse the sickling process, which is priority; this reversal will relieve the pain and increase the oxygenation to the cells.**

82. 1. The nurse would not question administering morphine to a client subject to painful infarcts of organs and infiltrations of the joints.

2. The nurse would not question administering a sustained-release medication for pain to a client subject to painful infarcts of organs and infiltrations of the joints.

3. **Procrit stimulates the bone marrow to produce red blood cells (erythropoiesis). The client with sickle cell disease produces red blood cells that "sickle," increasing the levels of hemoglobin S (HbS). The client does not need more RBCs; therefore, the nurse would question administering this medication.**

4. Clients diagnosed with sickle cell disease may go into a crisis situation for several reasons, including dehydration and infection. The nurse would not question an antibiotic.

MEDICATION MEMORY JOGGER: The nurse must be knowledgeable about accepted standards of practice for disease processes and conditions. If the nurse administers a medication the health-care provider has prescribed and it harms the client, the nurse could be held accountable. Remember that the nurse is a client advocate.

83. 1. Pernicious anemia is a disease caused by the body's lack of intrinsic factor needed to absorb vitamin B_{12} from the food ingested. There is no cure for the disease; there is only treatment with cyanocobalamin, vitamin B_{12}. This client has not been identified as having pernicious anemia.

2. **The rugae in the stomach produce intrinsic factor, which is necessary for the absorption of vitamin B_{12} from the food eaten. A gastric bypass surgery eliminates much of the surface area of**

the stomach and the rugae so the client cannot absorb vitamin B_{12}. The client will need to replace vitamin B_{12}, which is needed for the production of red blood cells.

3. The problem is not in the amount of food eaten; it is the lack of rugae in the stomach lining.

4. The injections are given on a weekly or monthly schedule depending on the severity of the deficit of the vitamin. The body does not make vitamin B_{12} on its own; the body absorbs the vitamin from the foods ingested.

84. 1. Health-care providers sometimes ask clients to obtain fecal occult blood test specimens, usually once a year. The client brings the card to the HCP's office for the test to be completed. This is not a daily test the client performs at home.

2. The tablets should not be crushed; they are enteric-coated. If the client cannot swallow tablets, liquid iron preparations are available.

3. The medication should not be taken with food if the client can tolerate it, but it does not need to be taken at night.

4. Iron causes the stool to turn a greenish-black and can mask the appearance of blood in the stool. The client should know that this will occur.

85. 1. The client's hydration status will not affect the medication.

2. The medication is black and will stain the skin, sometimes permanently. It is never given in the upper extremities or subcutaneously.

3. Knowledge of allergies to seafood is important when administering any preparation of iodine, not iron.

4. Iron is black and stains the skin. The medication is administered deep IM in the dorsogluteal muscle in adults and the lateral thigh in small children. It is given by the Z-tract method to trap the medication in the deep tissues and prevent leakage back into the shallow tissues.

86. 1. Polycythemia vera is a malignant overproduction of red blood cells. The blood becomes viscous and has a tendency to clot. Anticoagulants are ordered to prevent clot formation.

2. Steroids are not ordered for polycythemia vera.

3. Clients diagnosed with polycythemia vera develop hypertension as a result of the increased red blood cell volume. The viscosity of the blood causes increased resistance in the blood vessels.

4. The blood is "thick" (viscous) so fluids are increased, not limited.

87. **2, 1, 4, 5, 3**

2. **The nurse should determine that the client understands the procedure prior to having the client sign the permission form for receiving blood or blood products. The HCP is responsible for informing the client about the procedure, but the nurse should make sure the client understands before witnessing the signature.**

1. **The administration of blood or blood products requires that the client sign a consent form. If the client does not consent, the procedure is stopped at this point until or if the client decides to agree.**

4. **A preblood assessment should be performed to determine preexisting conditions or problems. The nurse uses this information to guide the safe administration of the blood.**

5. **An 18-gauge catheter is preferred to administer blood so that the cells are not broken (lysed) during the transfusion.**

3. **The blood is not retrieved from the laboratory until the nurse is ready to transfuse it. The nurse has 30 minutes from the time the blood is checked out from the laboratory until the initiation of the infusion.**

88. 1. Oral preparations of folic acid are administered to clients diagnosed with a folic acid deficiency who do not have a malabsorption problem, such as Crohn's disease.

2. A vitamin B_{12} deficiency is not the problem for this client.

3. B complex vitamins are not folic acid.

4. Crohn's disease is the second most common cause of folic acid deficiency anemia. Crohn's disease is a malabsorption syndrome of the small intestines. The client must receive the medication via the parenteral route.

89. 1. Symptoms of folic acid deficiency include pallor, pale mucous membranes, fatigue, and weight loss. A weight gain and pink buccal mucosa indicate an

improvement in the client's condition and that the medication is effective.

2. Paresthesias of the hands and feet are symptoms of vitamin B_{12} deficiency, not of folic acid deficiency. The lack of neurological symptoms is the differentiating factor used to diagnosis folic acid deficiency because the anemias share most other symptoms.

3. One of the main causes of folic acid deficiency anemia is chronic alcoholism, but abstaining from alcohol would not indicate the anemia is better.

4. The client should be encouraged to eat green, leafy vegetables, but tolerance of foods does not indicate effectiveness of the medication.

MEDICATION MEMORY JOGGER: The nurse determines the effectiveness of a medication by assessing for the symptoms, or lack thereof, for which the medication was prescribed.

90. 1. In immunohemolytic anemias, the client's own immune system attacks and destroys red blood cells. The client does not have leukopenia (low white blood cells) for which Neupogen is administered.

2. **The first-line therapy for immunohemolytic anemia is steroids, which are temporarily effective in most clients. Splenectomy followed by immune suppressive therapy usually follows. Plasma exchange therapy may be done if immune suppressive therapy is not successful.**

3. Red blood cells are seen by the body as nonself and are attacked. A transfusion is not indicated for this client.

4. Leucovorin is administered in megaloblastic anemia or as rescue factors for methotrexate toxicity, not for immunohemolytic anemias.

1. The client in congestive heart failure is prescribed milrinone lactate (Primacor), a phosphodiesterase inhibitor. Which priority intervention should the nurse implement?
   1. Assess the client's respiratory status.
   2. Monitor the client's telemetry strip.
   3. Check the client's apical pulse rate.
   4. Evaluate the brain natriuretic peptide (BNP).

2. The nurse is preparing to administer medications to the following clients. Which client would the nurse question administering the medication?
   1. The client receiving the angiotensin-receptor blocker losartan (Cozaar) who has a B/P of 168/94.
   2. The client receiving the calcium channel blocker diltiazem (Cardizem) who has 1+ nonpitting edema.
   3. The client receiving the alpha blocker terazosin (Hytrin) who is complaining of a headache.
   4. The client receiving the thiazide diuretic hydrochlorothiazide (HCTZ) who is complaining of leg cramps.

3. The client taking digoxin (Lanoxin), a cardiac glycoside, has a serum digoxin level of 4.2 ng/mL. Which medication should the nurse anticipate the HCP prescribing?
   1. The digitalis binder Fab antibody fragments (Digibind).
   2. The loop diuretic furosemide (Lasix).
   3. None.
   4. The cardiac glycoside digoxin (Lanoxin).

4. The nurse is preparing to administer the alpha-beta blocker labetalol (Normodyne) intravenous push (IVP) to a client diagnosed with hypertensive crisis. Which intervention should the nurse implement?
   1. Monitor the client's labetalol serum drug level.
   2. Keep the medication covered with tin foil.
   3. Administer the medication slow IVP over 5 minutes.
   4. Teach the client signs/symptoms of hypertension.

5. The nurse is preparing to administer spironolactone (Aldactone), a potassium-sparing diuretic. Which priority intervention should the nurse implement?
   1. Check the client's potassium level.
   2. Monitor the client's urinary output.
   3. Encourage consumption of potassium-rich foods.
   4. Give the medication with food.

6. The nurse is preparing to administer medication to the following clients. Which medication should the nurse question?
   1. The biguanide metformin (Glucophage) to a client with Type 1 diabetes who is receiving insulin.
   2. The loop diuretic bumetanide (Bumex) to a client diagnosed with essential hypertension.
   3. The biologic response modifier erythropoietin (Procrit) to a client diagnosed with end-stage renal failure.
   4. The central-acting alpha agonist clonidine (Catapres) to a client diagnosed with heart failure.

7. According to the American Heart Association, which medication should the client suspected of having a myocardial infarction take immediately when having chest pain?
   1. Morphine, a narcotic analgesic.
   2. Acetaminophen (Tylenol), a nonnarcotic analgesic.
   3. Acetylsalicylic acid (aspirin), an antiplatelet.
   4. Nitroglycerin paste, a coronary vasodilator.

8. The client diagnosed with congestive heart failure is taking digoxin (Lanoxin), a cardiac glycoside. Which data indicates the medication is effective?
   1. The client's blood pressure is 110/68.
   2. The client's apical pulse rate is regular.
   3. The client's potassium level is 4.2 mEq/L.
   4. The client's lungs are clear bilaterally.

9. Which client would the nurse most likely suspect will require polypharmacy to control essential hypertension?
   1. The 84-year-old white male client.
   2. The 22-year-old Hispanic female client.
   3. The 60-year-old Asian female client.
   4. The 46-year-old African American male client.

10. Which statement indicates to the nurse that the client with coronary artery disease (CAD) understands the medication teaching for taking aspirin, an antiplatelet, daily?
    1. "I will probably have occasional bleeding when taking this medication."
    2. "I will call 911 if I have chest pain unrelieved and I will chew an aspirin."
    3. "If I have any ringing in my ears, I will call my health-care provider."
    4. "I should take my daily aspirin on an empty stomach for better absorption."

11. The client on telemetry is showing multifocal premature ventricular contractions. Which antidysrhythmic medication should the nurse administer?
    1. Lidocaine.
    2. Atropine.
    3. Adenosine.
    4. Epinephrine.

12. The nurse is preparing to administer digoxin (Lanoxin), a cardiac glycoside, to a client diagnosed with congestive heart failure. Which area should the nurse assess prior to administering the medication?

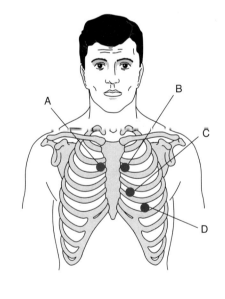

    1. A
    2. B
    3. C
    4. D

13. The mother of a child diagnosed with strep throat asks the nurse, "Why do you have to give my child that antibiotic shot?" Which statement by the nurse is the best response?
    1. "You sound concerned. Are you worried about your child getting a shot?"
    2. "This injection may keep your child from getting rheumatic fever."
    3. "Strep throat always results in children developing heart problems."
    4. "I am giving this medication because the throat culture showed a viral infection."

14. The home health-care nurse is visiting a client diagnosed with deep vein thrombosis who is taking warfarin (Coumadin), an oral anticoagulant. The nurse assesses a large hematoma on the abdomen and multiple small ecchymotic areas scattered over the body. Which action should the nurse implement?
    1. Send the client to the emergency department immediately.
    2. Encourage the client to apply ice to the abdominal area.
    3. Inform the client that this is expected when taking this medication.
    4. Instruct the client to wear a MedicAlert bracelet at all times.

15. The emergency department nurse received a client with multiple hematomas and has an International Normalized Ratio (INR) of 7.2. Which medication should the nurse prepare to administer?
    1. Protamine sulfate.
    2. Heparin.
    3. AquaMEPHYTON.
    4. Vitamin C.

16. The nurse is caring for the clients on the telemetry unit. Which medication should the nurse administer first?
    1. The antiplatelet medication clopidogrel (Plavix) to the client with arterial occlusive disease.
    2. The cardiac glycoside digoxin (Lanoxin) to the client diagnosed with congestive heart failure.
    3. The iron dextran infusion to the client diagnosed with iron-deficiency anemia who has pale skin.
    4. The antidysrhythmic amiodarone (Cordarone) to the client in ventricular bigeminy on the telemetry monitor.

17. The elderly client diagnosed with iron-deficiency anemia has been prescribed an oral iron preparation. Which information should the nurse teach the client?
    1. Instruct the client to take the medication with food
    2. Teach the client to take the iron with milk products.
    3. Explain that this medication may discolor the teeth.
    4. Discuss taking the medication 2 hours after a meal.

18. The nurse is discharging a client who has undergone surgery for a mechanical valve replacement. Which statement indicates the client needs more discharge teaching?
    1. "I will have to take an anticoagulant the rest of my life."
    2. "I don't have to take any medications after this surgery."
    3. "I must take antibiotics prior to all dental procedures."
    4. "I must go to my HCP for routine bloodwork."

19. The client is being prepared for a cardiac catheterization. Which statement by the client would warrant immediate intervention by the nurse?
    1. "I took my blood pressure medications yesterday."
    2. "I broke out in an awful rash after eating oysters."
    3. "I have not had my daily aspirin in more than a week."
    4. "I am highly allergic to poison ivy or oak."

20. The nurse is preparing to administer a nitroglycerin patch to a client diagnosed with coronary artery disease. Which interventions should the nurse implement? Rank in order of performance.
    1. Date and time the nitroglycerin patch.
    2. Remove the old patch.
    3. Clean the site of the old patch.
    4. Apply the nitroglycerin patch.
    5. Check the patch against the MAR.

1. 1. The client's respiratory status should be evaluated, but the cardiac status is priority for this medication.
   2. **Primacor inhibits the enzyme phosphodiesterase, thus promoting a positive inotropic response and vasodilatation. Severe cardiac dysrhythmias may result from this medication; therefore, the client's telemetry should be monitored.**
   3. The client's cardiac status, including pulse rate, heart sounds, and blood pressure, should be monitored, but the client's telemetry reading is priority.
   4. The BNP is a laboratory test that is useful as a marker in the diagnosis of congestive heart failure. Normal is less than 100 pg/mL. However, this test is not priority when giving a patient Primacor for already-diagnosed CHF.

2. 1. The nurse would want to give this antihypertensive medication to a client with an elevated blood pressure; the nurse would question the medication if the B/P were low, which it is not.
   2. The client with 1+ nonpitting edema would not be affected by a calcium channel blocker.
   3. Hytrin is not contraindicated in a client who has a headache; the apical pulse should be greater than 60.
   4. Leg cramps could indicate hypokalemia, which may lead to life-threatening cardiac dysrhythmias. Therefore, the nurse should question administering this medication until a serum potassium level is obtained.

   MEDICATION MEMORY JOGGER: The nurse must be knowledgeable about accepted standards of practice for medication administration, including which client assessment data and laboratory data should be monitored prior to administering the medication.

3. 1. When digoxin overdose is suspected, as it would be with a digoxin level of 4.2 ng/mL, Fab antibody fragments bind digoxin and prevent it from acting. The therapeutic range of digoxin is 0.5 to 1.2 ng/mL and toxic range is 2.0 ng/mL or higher.
   2. This digoxin level is extremely high and requires stopping the medication and prescribing the antidote. Lasix is not an antidote for digoxin.
   3. The nurse should anticipate the HCP prescribing a medication to lower the digoxin level.
   4. The level is above the toxic range, and the nurse should not administer any more digoxin—it could be fatal.

4. 1. Labetalol does not have a serum drug level.
   2. Only medications that are inactivated or weakened by exposure to light would have to be covered; this medication is not affected by light.
   3. **Medications that directly affect the cardiac muscle or vasculature are administered slowly over a minimum of 5 minutes for safety reasons. Many medications require dilution with normal saline to have sufficient volume for a smooth equal delivery to prevent cardiac dysrhythmias.**
   4. The nurse should teach the client about possible signs or symptoms of hypertension, but remember, clients with hypertension are often asymptomatic. Hypertension is the "silent killer."

5. 1. **When preparing to administer a potassium-sparing diuretic, the nurse should check the potassium level because both hyperkalemia and hypokalemia can result in cardiac dysrhythmias that are life threatening. Therefore, checking potassium level is a priority nursing intervention.**
   2. Monitoring the client's output is more appropriate for determining the effectiveness of the medication. It is not data that would prevent the nurse from administering the medication.
   3. The client should not eat potassium-rich foods because this medication retains potassium.
   4. This medication can be administered with or without food; therefore, this is not a priority intervention.

6. 1. Glucophage acts on the liver to prevent gluconeogenesis and is often prescribed along with insulin for Type 1 or Type 2 diabetes.
   2. A client with hypertension would be prescribed a diuretic; therefore, the nurse would not question administering this medication.
   3. Procrit is administered to stimulate the bone marrow to produce red blood cells

and is often prescribed for clients with chronic kidney disease.

4. The nurse would question administering Catapres to a client with decreased cardiac output (heart failure) because this medication acts within the brain stem to suppress sympathetic outflow to the heart and blood vessels. The result is vasodilatation and reduced cardiac output, both of which lower blood pressure.

7. 1. Morphine must be administered intravenous push to achieve rapid relief of chest pain; therefore, the client could not administer this medication to himself or herself.
2. A nonnarcotic analgesic will not help the client having a "heart attack."
3. **The AHA recommends that a client having chest pain chew two baby aspirins or one 325-mg tablet immediately to help prevent platelet aggregation and further extension of a coronary thrombosis.**
4. Nitroglycerin must be taken sublingually, not as a paste, during acute chest pain to achieve rapid effect of the medication.

8. 1. Digoxin does not affect the client's blood pressure; therefore, it cannot be used to determine the effectiveness of the medication.
2. The client's apical pulse must be assessed prior to administering the medication, but this data is not used to determine the effectiveness of the medication.
3. The client's potassium level must be assessed prior to administering the medication, but it is not used to determine the effectiveness of the medication.
4. **Signs and symptoms of CHF are crackles in the lungs, jugular vein distention, and pitting edema. Therefore, if the client has clear lung sounds, the nurse can assume the medication is effective.**

MEDICATION MEMORY JOGGER: The nurse determines the effectiveness of a medication by assessing for the symptoms, or lack thereof, for which the medication was prescribed.

9. 1. The elderly client is often prescribed multiple medications, but people who are white usually respond well to one antihypertensive medication.
2. A young Hispanic female would not be considered high risk for hypertension and would probably not require multiple antihypertensive medications.
3. The Asian diet is high in omega-3 fatty acid, which decreases atherosclerosis, a risk factor for hypertension; this population usually does not require multiple antihypertensive medications.
4. **Ethnically and racially, African Americans have poorer responses to ACE inhibitors, beta blockers, and other antihypertensive medications than do people of other backgrounds. There is no specific reason known for this, but it is empirically and scientifically documented. Polypharmacy is using multiple medications to medically treat a client, and African Americans often require this to treat hypertension.**

10. 1. If the client experiences any abnormal bleeding, the HCP should be notified.
2. **Aspirin is administered as an antiplatelet to prevent coronary artery occlusion. It is not administered for chest pain. If the client has chest pain that is not relieved with NTG, the client should call the Emergency Medical Services (EMS) and get medical treatment immediately. Taking an extra aspirin may prevent further cardiac damage.**
3. Tinnitus, ringing in the ears, is a symptom of aspirin toxicity, but the client taking one aspirin a day would not be at risk for this symptom.
4. Aspirin is very irritating to the gastric mucosa and should be taken with food to help prevent gastric irritation resulting in ulcers. Enteric-coated aspirin is used to help prevent this complication.

11. 1. **Lidocaine suppresses ventricular ectopy and is a first-line drug for the treatment of ventricular dysrhythmias.**
2. Atropine decreases vagal stimulation, which increases the heart rate and is the drug of choice for asystole, complete heart block, and symptomatic bradycardia.
3. Adenosine is the drug of choice for terminating paroxysmal supraventricular tachycardia by decreasing the automaticity of the sinoatrial node and slowing conduction through the AV node.
4. Epinephrine constricts the periphery and shunts the blood to the central trunk and is the first medication administered to a client in a code.

12. 1. This is the second intercostal space right sternal notch, which is one of the two areas used to auscultate the aortic valve, but it is not where the apical pulse is assessed.
    2. This is the second intercostal space left sternal notch, which is used to auscultate the pulmonic valve, but it is not where the apical pulse is assessed.
    3. This is the fourth and fifth intercostal space to the left of the sternum and is where the tricuspid valve is best heard.
    4. **The apical pulse located at the fifth intercostal midclavicular space must be assessed for 1 minute prior to administering digoxin. If the apical pulse is less than 60 beats per minute, the nurse should hold the medication.**

13. 1. This is a therapeutic response and does not answer the mother's question. This type of response is used to encourage the client to ventilate feelings.
    2. **Antibiotics will treat the strep throat, which will decrease the child's fever and pain. If untreated, strep throat can lead to the development of rheumatic fever, which can result in rheumatic endocarditis in future years.**
    3. This is a false statement.
    4. Strep throat is a bacterial infection, not a viral infection.

14. 1. **Abnormal bleeding is a sign of Coumadin overdose; the client needs to be assessed immediately and have a STAT International Normalized Ratio laboratory test.**
    2. Ice causes vasoconstriction, but this bleeding is abnormal and will not stop without medical treatment.
    3. Abnormal bleeding to this extent is not expected while receiving Coumadin therapy.
    4. This is an appropriate teaching intervention for clients receiving Coumadin, but this is not an appropriate action at this time.

15. 1. Protamine sulfate is the antidote for heparin toxicity.
    2. Heparin is a parenteral anticoagulant and would not be administered for Coumadin toxicity.
    3. **AquaMEPHYTON, vitamin K, is the antidote for Coumadin toxicity, which is supported by an INR of 7.2 and the bruising. The therapeutic range is 2–3.**
    4. The antidote is vitamin K, not vitamin C.

16. 1. This medication can be administered after the nurse treats the client with a life-threatening dysrhythmia.
    2. Digoxin is not a priority medication over treating a client with a life-threatening dysrhythmia.
    3. An iron dextran infusion must be administered and closely monitored. The nurse must treat the client with a life-threatening dysrhythmia before being able to devote time to the administration of the medication.
    4. **Ventricular bigeminy is a life-threatening dysrhythmia that must be treated immediately to prevent cardiac arrest.**

17. 1. The medication should be taken on an empty stomach because food interferes with the absorption of iron.
    2. Milk products would interfere with the absorption of the medication.
    3. Oral medication (pill) will not stain the teeth, but liquid iron preparations would stain the teeth. Just because the client is elderly does not mean the client cannot take pills.
    4. **The medication should be taken on an empty stomach or 2 hours after a meal because food interferes with the absorption of iron.**

18. 1. The client will be taking warfarin (Coumadin), an anticoagulant, the rest of his or her life. This statement indicates the client understands the teaching.
    2. **The client with a mechanical valve replacement will be taking anticoagulants and periodic antibiotics. The client needs more discharge teaching.**
    3. If antibiotics are not taken prior to dental procedures, the client may develop strep infections leading to vegetative growth on cardiac structures. The client understands this.
    4. The client must have regular INR labs drawn to determine if anticoagulant levels are within therapeutic range. Therapeutic INR for a client with a mechanical valve replacement is 2.0–3.5.

19. 1. The client should take his or her blood pressure medication prior to the cardiac catheterization; therefore, this statement does not warrant intervention.
    2. **This may indicate the client is allergic to iodine, a component of the cardiac catheterization dye, and warrants further assessment by the nurse.**

3. The client should stop any medication that interferes with clot formation, so this statement does not require intervention by the nurse.
4. An allergy to poison ivy or oak would not interfere with this procedure.

MEDICATION MEMORY JOGGER: The nurse must be knowledgeable about diagnostic tests and surgical procedures. If the client provides information that would indicate a potential harm to the client, then the nurse must intervene. Iodine is found in many types of seafood and is used in many diagnostic tests.

20.   5, 1, 2, 4, 3
5. The nurse should implement the five rights of medication administration, and the first is to make sure it is the right medication and the right client.
1. Before applying the nitroglycerin paste, the nurse should date and time the application paper prior to putting it on the client so that the nurse is not pressing on the client when writing on the patch.
2. The nurse should have the gloves on when removing the old application paper for the above reason.
4. Last, the nurse should administer the nitro patch application paper in a clean, dry, nonhairy place.
3. The nurse should make sure no medication remains on the client's skin.

Pulmonary System

There is no such thing as a safe drug. All drugs have the ability to cause injury.

—Richard A. Lehne

PRACTICE QUESTIONS

A Client with an Upper Respiratory Infection

1. The client diagnosed with arterial hypertension develops a cold. Which information regarding over-the-counter medications should the nurse teach?
   1. Try to find a medication that will not cause drowsiness.
   2. Over-the-counter medications are not as effective as a prescription.
   3. Over-the-counter medications are more expensive than prescriptions.
   4. Do not take over-the-counter medication unless approved by the HCP.

2. The client with the flu is prescribed the over-the-counter cough suppressant dextromethorphan. Which information should the nurse teach regarding this medication?
   1. Take the medication every 4–8 hours as needed for cough.
   2. The medication can cause addiction if taken too long.
   3. Do not drive or operate machinery while taking the drug.
   4. Do not take a beta blocker while taking this medication.

3. The HCP prescribed amoxicillin/clavulanate (Augmentin), an antibiotic, for a client diagnosed with chronic obstructive pulmonary disease (COPD) who has a cold. Which intervention should the nurse implement?
   1. Discuss the prescription with the HCP because antibiotics do not help viral infections.
   2. Teach the client to take all the antibiotics as ordered.
   3. Encourage the client to seek a second opinion before taking the medication.
   4. Ask the client if he or she is allergic to sulfa drugs or shellfish.

4. The female client asks the nurse why her teenage child would have many boxes of Sudafed, an over-the-counter cold and allergy medication, in her room. Which would be the nurse's first response?
   1. "Has your child always had allergy problems?"
   2. "Teenagers will try to take care of their own health problems."
   3. "Has the teenager's behavior at school or at home changed recently?"
   4. "Remove the medication and say nothing to the teenager about it."

5. The client with the flu has been taking acetylcysteine (Mucomyst), a mucolytic. Which adverse effect would the nurse assess for?
   1. Bronchospasm.
   2. Nausea.
   3. Fever.
   4. Drowsiness.

6. Which over-the-counter herb should the nurse recommend for a client with a cold who has mild hypertension?
   1. *Crataegus laevigata*, hawthorn.
   2. *Zingiber officinale*, ginger.
   3. *Allium sativum*, garlic.
   4. *Hydrastis canadensis*, goldenseal.

7. The client who has been using oxymetazoline (Afrin) nasal spray for several weeks complains to the nurse that the spray no longer seems to work to clear the nasal passages. Which information should the nurse teach?
   1. Increase the amount of sprays used until the desired effect has been reached.
   2. This type of medication can cause rebound congestion if used too long.
   3. Alternate the Afrin with a saline nasal spray every 2 hours.
   4. Place the Afrin nasal spray in a vaporizer at night for the best results.

8. Which is the scientific theory for prescribing zinc preparations for a client with a cold?
   1. Zinc binds with the viral particle and reduces the symptoms of a cold.
   2. Zinc decreases the immune system's response to a virus.
   3. Zinc activates viral receptors in the body's immune system.
   4. Zinc blocks the virus from binding to the epithelial cells of the nose.

9. The client diagnosed with the flu is prescribed the cough medication hydrocodone. Which information should the nurse teach the client regarding this medication?
   1. Teach the client to monitor the bowel movements for constipation.
   2. Driving or operating machinery is all right while taking this medication.
   3. This medication usually causes insomnia, so plan for rest periods.
   4. This medication is more effective when taken with a mucolytic.

10. The nurse on a medical unit is administering 0900 medications. Which medication should the nurse question administering?
    1. Acetylcysteine (Mucomyst), a mucolytic, to a client who is coughing forcefully.
    2. Cefazolin (Ancef), an antibiotic, IVPB to a client diagnosed with the flu.
    3. Diphenhydramine (Benadryl), an antihistamine, to a client who is congested.
    4. Dextromethorphan (Robitussin), an antitussive, to a client who has pneumonia.

A Client with Lower Respiratory Infection

11. The male client diagnosed with chronic obstructive pulmonary disease (COPD) tells the nurse that he has been expectorating "rusty-colored" sputum. Which medication would the nurse anticipate the HCP prescribing?
    1. Prednisone, a glucocorticoid.
    2. Habitrol, a transdermal nicotine system.
    3. Dextromethorphan (Robitussin), an antitussive.
    4. Ceftriaxone (Rocephin), a cephalosporin.

12. The female client is being admitted to a medical unit with a diagnosis of pneumonia. Which intervention would the nurse implement? Rank in order of implementation.
    1. Start an intravenous access line.
    2. Administer the IVPB antibiotic.
    3. Teach to notify the nurse of any vaginal itching.
    4. Obtain sputum and blood cultures.
    5. Place an identity band on the client.

13. The client diagnosed with emphysema is admitted to the surgical unit for a cholecystectomy (gallbladder removal). Which postoperative intervention should the nurse implement?
    1. Have the patient turn, cough, and breathe deeply every shift.
    2. Administer oxygen to the client at 4 L/min.
    3. Assess the surgical site for delayed healing.
    4. Medicate frequently with morphine 15 mg IVP.

14. The nurse is discharging a client diagnosed with chronic obstructive pulmonary disease (COPD). Which discharge instructions should the nurse provide regarding the client's prescription for prednisone, a glucocorticoid?
    1. Take all the prednisone as ordered until the prescription is empty.
    2. Take the prednisone on an empty stomach with a full glass of water.
    3. Stop taking the prednisone if a noticeable weight gain occurs.
    4. The medication should never be abruptly discontinued.

15. The nurse is preparing to administer medications on a pulmonary unit. Which medication should the nurse administer first?
    1. Prednisone, a glucocorticoid, for a client diagnosed with chronic bronchitis.
    2. Oxygen via nasal cannula at 2 L/min for a client diagnosed with pneumonia.
    3. Lactic acidophilus (Lactinex) to a client receiving IVPB antibiotics.
    4. Cephalexin (Keflex), an antibiotic, to a client being discharged.

16. The client diagnosed with chronic obstructive pulmonary disease (COPD) is prescribed morphine sulfate (MS Contin). Which statement is the scientific rationale for prescribing this medication?
    1. MS Contin will depress the respiratory drive.
    2. Morphine dilates the bronchi and improves breathing.
    3. MS Contin is not addicting, so it can be given routinely.
    4. Morphine causes bronchoconstriction and decreased sputum.

17. The client diagnosed with adult respiratory distress syndrome (ARDS) has been found to have a disease-causing organism resistant to the antibiotics being given. Which intervention should the nurse implement?
    1. Monitor for therapeutic blood levels of the aminoglycoside antibiotic prescribed.
    2. Prepare to administer the glucocorticoid medication ordered intramuscularly.
    3. Obtain an order for repeat cultures to confirm the identity of the resistant organism.
    4. Place the client on airborne isolation precautions.

18. The client diagnosed with chronic obstructive pulmonary disease is prescribed methylprednisolone (Solu-Medrol), a glucocorticoid, IVP. Which laboratory test should the nurse monitor?
    1. The white blood cell (WBC) count.
    2. The hemoglobin and hematocrit.
    3. The blood glucose level.
    4. The BUN and creatinine.

19. Which data would indicate that the antibiotic therapy has not been successful for a client diagnosed with a bacterial pneumonia?
    1. The client's hematocrit is 45%.
    2. The client is expectorating thick, green sputum.
    3. The client's lung sounds are clear to auscultation.
    4. The client has no complaints of pleuritic chest pain.

20. The nurse is preparing to administer an IVPB antibiotic to a client diagnosed with pneumonia; 10 mL of the medication is mixed in 100 mL of saline. At what rate would the nurse set the pump to infuse the medication in 30 minutes?

    Answer _____

A Client with Reactive Airway Disease

21. Which information should the nurse discuss with the client diagnosed with reactive airway disease who is prescribed theophylline (Slo-Phyllin), a xanthine bronchodilator?
    1. Instruct the client to take the medication on an empty stomach.
    2. Explain that an increased heart rate and irritability are expected side effects.
    3. Discuss the need to avoid large amounts of caffeine-containing drinks.
    4. Tell the client to double the next dose if a dose is missed.

22. The client with chronic reactive airway disease is taking the leukotriene receptor inhibitor montelukast (Singulair). Which statement by the client would warrant intervention by the nurse?
    1. "I have been having a lot of headaches lately."
    2. "I have started taking an aspirin every day."
    3. "I keep this medication up on a very high shelf."
    4. "I must protect this medication from extreme temperatures."

23. The client with reactive airway disease is taking the oral sympathomimetic bronchodilator metaproterenol (Alupent) three times a day. Which intervention should the nurse implement?
    1. Instruct the client to take the last dose a few hours before bedtime.
    2. Teach the client to decrease the fluid intake when taking this medication.
    3. Have the client demonstrate the correct way to use the inhaler.
    4. Encourage the client to take the medication with an antacid.

24. The client is prescribed albuterol (Ventolin), a sympathomimetic bronchodilator, metered-dose inhaler. Which behavior indicates the teaching concerning the inhaler is effective?
    1. The client holds his or her breath for 5 seconds and then exhales forcefully.
    2. The client states the canister is full when it is lying on top of the water.
    3. The client exhales and then squeezes the canister as the next inspiration occurs.
    4. The client connects the oxygen tubing to the inhaler before administering the dose.

25. The client admitted for an acute exacerbation of reactive airway disease is receiving intravenous aminophylline. The client's serum theophylline level is 28 μg/mL. Which action should the nurse implement first?
    1. Continue to monitor the aminophylline drip.
    2. Assess the client for nausea and restlessness.
    3. Discontinue the aminophylline drip.
    4. Notify the health-care provider immediately.

26. Which assessment data best indicates the client with reactive airway disease has "good" control with the medication regimen?
    1. The client's peak expiratory flow rate (PEFR) is greater than 80% of his or her personal best.
    2. The client's lung sounds are clear bilaterally, both anterior and posterior.
    3. The client has only had three acute exacerbations of asthma in the last month.
    4. The client's monthly serum theophylline level is 18 μg/mL.

27. The client with an acute exacerbation of reactive airway disease is prescribed a nebulizer treatment. Which statement best describes how a nebulizer works?
    1. Nebulizers are small, handheld pressurized devices that deliver a measured dose of an antiasthma drug with activation.
    2. A nebulizer is an inhaler that delivers an antiasthma drug in the form of a dry, micronized power directly to the lungs.
    3. A nebulizer is a small machine used to convert an antiasthma drug solution into a mist that is delivered though a mouthpiece.
    4. Nebulizers are small devices that are used to crush glucocorticoids so that the client can place them under the tongue for better absorption.

28. Which information should the nurse teach the client who is prescribed a glucocorticoid inhaler?
    1. Advise the client to gargle after each administration.
    2. Instruct the client to use the inhaler on a PRN basis.
    3. Encourage the client not to use a spacer when using the inhaler.
    4. Teach the client to check his or her forced expiratory volume daily.

29. The 28-year-old female client with chronic reactive airway disease is taking the leukotriene receptor inhibitor montelukast sodium (Singulair). Which statement by the client indicates the client teaching is effective?
    1. "I will not drink coffee, tea, or any type of cola drinks."
    2. "I will take this medication at the beginning of an asthma attack."
    3. "It is all right to take this medication if I am trying to get pregnant."
    4. "I should not decrease the dose or suddenly stop taking this medication."

30. Which medical treatment is recommended for the client who is diagnosed with mild intermittent asthma?
    1. This classification of asthma requires a combination of long-term control medication plus a quick-relief medication.
    2. Mild intermittent asthma needs a routine glucocorticoid inhaler and a sustained-relief theophylline.
    3. This classification requires daily inhalation of an oral glucocorticoid and daily nebulizer treatments.
    4. Mild intermittent asthma is treated on a PRN basis and no long-term control medication is needed.

A Child with Reactive Airway Disease

31. The 8-year-old male child diagnosed with reactive airway disease is prescribed a cromolyn (Intal) inhaler. The child shares with the nurse that he wants to play baseball but can't because of his asthma. Which intervention should the nurse discuss with the child and parents?
    1. Instruct the child to take the medication as soon as shortness of breath starts.
    2. Teach the child to take a puff of the cromolyn inhaler 15 minutes before playing ball.
    3. Encourage the child to play another sport that does not require running outside.
    4. Inform the parents to notify the pediatrician if the child complains of a yellow haze.

32. The 6-year-old child is experiencing an acute exacerbation of reactive airway disease. The child passed out, and the parents brought the child to the emergency department. Which intervention should the nurse implement first?
    1. Administer subcutaneous epinephrine via a tuberculin syringe.
    2. Administer a beta$_2$-adrenergic agonist, albuterol (Ventolin), via nebulizer.
    3. Administer intravenous methylprednisolone, a glucocorticoid.
    4. Administer oxygen to maintain oxygen saturation above 95%.

33. The clinic nurse is teaching the parent of a child with reactive airway disease about nebulizer treatments. Which statement indicates the teaching has been effective?
    1. "I will use half the medication in the nebulizer at each treatment."
    2. "The nebulizer treatment will take about 30 minutes or longer."
    3. "I will use a disinfectant solution weekly when cleaning the nebulizer."
    4. "I will rinse the nebulizer in clean water after each breathing treatment."

34. The child with an acute asthma attack is prescribed a 7-day course of the systemic corticosteroid prednisolone. The mother asks the nurse, "Doesn't this medication cause serious side effects?" Which statement is the nurse's best response?
    1. "Yes, this medication does have serious side effects, but your child needs the medication."
    2. "The doctor would not have ordered a medication that has serious side effects."
    3. "A short-term course of steroids will not cause serious side effects."
    4. "There may be serious side effects if your child takes the medication for a long time."

35. The child diagnosed with reactive airway disease is prescribed a cromolyn inhaler. The mother asks the nurse to explain how this medication helps control her child's asthma. Which statement is the best explanation to give to the mother?
    1. This medication diminishes the mediator action of leukotrienes.
    2. This medication blocks the release of mast cell mediators.
    3. This medication causes relaxation of the bronchial smooth muscle.
    4. This medication decreases bronchial airway inflammation.

36. Which statement indicates to the nurse that the 13-year-old child understands the zone system for monitoring the treatment of asthma?
    1. "When I am in the green zone, it means good control and I do not need any medication."
    2. "If I am in the black zone, it means I should go to the emergency department."
    3. "If I am in the red zone, it means I should take my cromolyn and steroid inhaler."
    4. "The yellow zone means I tell my mom so she can give me a nebulizer treatment."

37. The pediatric nurse is caring for a 7-year-old child with chronic reactive airway disease who is being discharged. The nurse must evaluate the breathing capacity of the child to determine the effectiveness of the medication regimen. Which interventions should the nurse implement when using the peak flow meter? Select all that apply.
    1. Instruct the child to lie down in the bed in the supine position.
    2. Tell the child to seal the lips tightly around the mouthpiece.
    3. Note the number on the scale after the client gives a sharp, short breath.
    4. Blow into the peak flow meter one time and obtain the results.
    5. Move the pointer on the peak flow meter to zero.

38. The 10-year-old child is being prescribed a cromolyn inhaler. Which statement indicates the child needs more teaching concerning the cromolyn inhaler?
    1. "If I cannot take a deep breath, I will not use my cromolyn inhaler."
    2. "I should not exhale into my inhaler after I have finished taking a puff."
    3. "I should wait at least 1 hour to rinse my mouth after taking my inhaler."
    4. "I should not stop taking my inhaler because I might have an asthma attack."

39. The nurse is teaching the mother of a 9-year-old child with severe reactive airway disease. The child is prescribed theophylline (Bronkodyl) 100 mg po every 12 hours. Which instructions should the nurse include when discussing the medication with the mother?
    1. Instruct the mother to perform and record a daily theophylline level
    2. Inform the mother to notify the HCP if the child vomits or becomes irritable.
    3. Tell the mother to give the medication at 8:00 A.M. and 8:00 P.M.
    4. Recommend that the medication be refrigerated at all times.

40. The health-care provider has ordered theophylline 5 mg/kg/q 6 hrs for a child who weighs 35 lbs. How much medication would the nurse administer in each dose?

    Answer _____

A Client with Pulmonary Embolus

41. The client diagnosed with rule-out deep vein thrombosis (DVT) is experiencing dyspnea and chest pain on inspiration. On assessment, the nurse finds a respiratory rate of 40. Which medication should the nurse anticipate the health-care provider ordering?
    1. Warfarin (Coumadin), an oral anticoagulant.
    2. Enoxaparin (Lovenox), a low molecular weight heparin.
    3. Heparin, an intravenous anticoagulant.
    4. Ticlopidine (Ticlid), an antiplatelet medication.

42. The nurse is preparing to administer warfarin (Coumadin), an anticoagulant. The client's current laboratory values are as follows:

    PT 22   PT 39
    Control 12.9   Control 36
    INR 2.6

    Which action should the nurse implement?
    1. Question administering the medication.
    2. Prepare to administer AquaMEPHYTON (vitamin K).
    3. Notify the health-care provider to increase the dose.
    4. Administer the medication as ordered.

43. The HCP has ordered streptokinase (Streptase), a thrombolytic, intravenously for the client diagnosed with a pulmonary embolus. The client has intravenous heparin infusing at 1600 units per hour via a 20-gauge angiocath. Which intervention should the nurse implement?
    1. Administer the streptokinase via a Y-tubing.
    2. Start a second intravenous site to infuse the streptokinase.
    3. Discontinue the heparin and infuse streptokinase via the 20-gauge angiocath.
    4. Piggyback the streptokinase through the heparin line at the port closest to the client.

44. The client diagnosed with a massive pulmonary embolus is ordered the thrombolytic streptokinase. The nurse notes on the Medication Administration Record that the client is allergic to the "-mycin" medications, including streptomycin. Which action should the nurse implement?
    1. Call the HCP to report the allergy.
    2. Administer the medication as ordered.
    3. Call the pharmacist to substitute medication.
    4. Check the bleeding-time laboratory values.

45. The nurse is discharging the female client diagnosed with a pulmonary embolus (PE) who is prescribed the anticoagulant warfarin (Coumadin). Which statement indicates the client understands the medication teaching?
    1. "I should use a straight razor when I shave my legs."
    2. "I will use a hard-bristled toothbrush to clean my teeth."
    3. "An occasional nosebleed is common with this drug."
    4. "It will be important for me to have regular bloodwork done."

46. The client diagnosed with a pulmonary embolus (PE) is receiving intravenous heparin, and the HCP prescribes 5 mg warfarin (Coumadin) orally once a day. Which statement best explains the scientific rationale for prescribing these two anticoagulants?
    1. Coumadin interferes with production of prothrombin.
    2. It takes 3–5 days to achieve a therapeutic level of Coumadin.
    3. Heparin is more effective when administered with warfarin.
    4. Coumadin potentiates the therapeutic action of heparin.

47. The nurse is administering alteplase (Activase), a thrombolytic, to a client diagnosed with massive pulmonary emboli (PE). Which data indicates the medication is effective?
    1. The client's PTT level is within therapeutic range.
    2. The client is able to ambulate to the bathroom.
    3. The client denies chest pain on inspiration.
    4. The client's chest x-ray is normal.

48. The nurse is preparing to hang the next bag of heparin. The client's current laboratory values are as follows:

PT 13.4   PTT 92
Control 12.9   Control 36
INR 1

Which intervention should the nurse implement first?
1. Discontinue the heparin infusion.
2. Prepare to administer protamine sulfate.
3. Notify the health-care provider.
4. Assess the client for bleeding.

49. The client is receiving an intravenous infusion of heparin. The bag hanging has 25,000 units of heparin in 500 mL of D_5W at 14 mL per hour via an intravenous pump. How many units of heparin is the client receiving every hour?

Answer _____

50. The client is receiving an intravenous infusion of heparin. The bag hanging has 40,000 units of heparin in 500 mL of D_5W. The HCP has ordered the medication to be delivered at 1200 units per hour. At what rate would the nurse set the intravenous pump?

Answer _____

A Client with an Upper Respiratory Infection

1. 1. The client should be informed about the dangers of self-medicating with over-the-counter (OTC) medications. Many OTC medications work by causing vasoconstriction, which will increase the client's hypertension.
   2. Efficacy of medications depends on the medication and strength. Most OTC medications were at one time prescription medications. There are many variables, and this statement is too general to be true.
   3. The expense of the medications is not the relevant point for this client. The problem is to inform the client about the actions of many OTC medications and the effect on the client's hypertension.
   4. **Many OTC medications work by causing vasoconstriction, which will increase the client's hypertension; the client should only take medications (approved by the HCP) that will not affect the client's hypertension.**

2. 1. **Dextromethorphan is relatively safe in the recommended dose range of 10–30 mg every 4–8 hours. At these levels it does not produce respiratory depression and side effects are not common.**
   2. This medication does not have the potential to cause addiction.
   3. This medication does not produce drowsiness, so driving or operating machinery while taking dextromethorphan is acceptable.
   4. The medication does not slow the heart rate, and there is no reason for a client not to take a prescribed beta blocker medication while taking dextromethorphan.

3. 1. Antibiotics do not treat viral infections, but HCPs will frequently prescribe prophylactic antibiotics for clients with comorbid conditions (such as COPD) to prevent a secondary bacterial infection.
   2. **Clients prescribed antibiotics should always be taught to take all the medication as ordered to prevent resistant strains of bacteria from developing.**
   3. There is no reason for a second opinion; this is standard medical practice.
   4. This is a penicillin preparation, not a sulfa medication or iodine.

4. 1. These may be allergy medications when used legally, but they are also the ingredients in illegal methamphetamine production. Quantities of any medication in a teenager's room should be investigated.
   2. Teenagers do try to develop independence, but it is always the parent or guardian's responsibility to monitor the child's health.
   3. **This situation could indicate the teenager is involved with the drug culture, taking or manufacturing drugs. The nurse should assess for signs of drug involvement.**
   4. The parent is responsible for determining the teenager's activities; the situation should be discussed with the teenager.

5. 1. **Mucomyst can cause bronchospasm, which will impair the client's breathing, not improve it. An adverse reaction is a reason to immediately discontinue the medication.**
   2. Nausea is a side effect of many medications and can usually be managed by taking the medication with food. A side effect is not an adverse effect.
   3. Fever would result from the cold, flu, or infection, not from the medication.
   4. Drowsiness is caused by some cold and flu preparations, usually the antihistamines. Mucomyst causes the client to expectorate secretions, which will keep the client awake.

6. 1. Hawthorn is used for mild hypertension, congestive heart failure, and angina, but it does nothing for a cold or the flu.
   2. Ginger is used to stimulate digestion and to help ease nausea and motion sickness. It does nothing for hypertension or the flu or colds.
   3. **Garlic is used for colds and the flu and can also be given for hypertension. It causes mild vasodilation and will not make hypertension worse.**
   4. Goldenseal is used for respiratory, digestive, and urinary infections, but it increases the effectiveness of some antihypertensive medications, beta blockers, and antidysrhythmics. It should be used with caution in clients who have cardiovascular disease, diabetes mellitus, or glaucoma.

MEDICATION MEMORY JOGGER: Some herbal preparations are effective, some are not, and a few can be harmful or even deadly. If a client is taking an herbal supplement and a conventional medicine, the nurse should investigate to determine if the combination will cause harm to the client. The nurse should always be the client's advocate.

7. 1. Increasing the number of sprays will only increase the problem. This medication is for short-term use only (that is, a few days). Longer use can cause a rebound congestion that can be difficult to resolve.
    2. **Afrin is recommended for short-term relief of nasal congestion for clients older than the age of 6 years. Longer use can cause a rebound congestion that can be difficult to resolve.**
    3. Afrin should be used every 10–12 hours only; using it more often increases the chance of developing a dependence on the medication and rebound congestion.
    4. Afrin nasal spray is to be used intranasally; it is not an additive for a vaporizer.

8. 1. Zinc does not bind the viral particle. Symptoms are diminished by blocking the ability of the virus to bind with the nasal lining.
    2. Zinc is a micronutrient found in the body that helps to increase the body's immune system.
    3. Activating viral receptors would increase the symptoms of a cold.
    4. **Theoretically, zinc blocks viral binding to nasal epithelium. Observation has shown that increased amounts of zinc can prevent the binding and prevent the development of symptoms of the rhinovirus.**

9. 1. **Hydrocodone is an opioid and can slow the peristalsis of the bowel, resulting in constipation. The client should be aware of this and increase the fluid intake and use bulk laxatives and stool softeners, if needed.**
    2. Opioids can cause drowsiness, so driving or operating machinery should be discouraged.
    3. Opioids usually cause the client to be drowsy, not have insomnia.
    4. Hydrocodone is a cough suppressant and a mucolytic is an expectorant. These are opposite-acting medications.

10. 1. **An adverse effect of Mucomyst is bronchospasm. This client should be assessed for bronchospasm before administering a dose of Mucomyst.**
    2. Antibiotics are frequently administered to clients with viral infections to prevent secondary bacterial infections. This client is considered at risk or the client would not be in a hospital receiving care. There is no reason to question this medication.

3. Antihistamines are prescribed for congestion; there is no reason to question this medication.
4. A symptom of pneumonia is a cough. There is no reason to question this medication.

A Client with Lower Respiratory Infection

11. 1. Clients diagnosed with COPD are commonly prescribed a steroid (glucocorticoid) medication to decrease inflammation in the lungs. This client should already be taking this or a similar medication. The client's "rusty-colored" sputum indicates an infection and an antibiotic should be ordered.
    2. The client should quit smoking if still smoking, but the client's "rusty-colored" sputum indicates an infection and an antibiotic should be ordered.
    3. The client may require an antitussive but more likely would require a mucolytic to help to expectorate the thick tenacious sputum associated with COPD.
    4. **The client's "rusty-colored" sputum indicates an infection and an antibiotic should be ordered. Rocephin is a broad-spectrum antibiotic.**

12. 5, 4, 1, 2, 3
    5. The laboratory technician that will draw the blood cultures will need the band to identify the client before drawing the specimen, and the nurse will need the band before administering the medication. Checking for the right client is one of the five rights of medication administration.
    4. Cultures are obtained prior to the initiation of antibiotics to prevent skewing of the results.
    1. An intravenous line must be initiated before the nurse can administer IV medications.
    2. Intravenous antibiotics should be administered within 1–2 hours of the order being written. This should always be considered a "now" medication.
    3. Superinfections are a potential complication of antibiotic therapy. Vaginal yeast infections occur when the good bacteria are killed off by the antibiotic. Diarrhea from destruction of intestinal flora is also a possibility.

13. 1. Clients undergoing surgery are encouraged to turn, cough, and deep breathe (TC&DB) a minimum of every 2 hours. Clients with emphysema should TC&DB more often than every 2 hours.
    2. The client should be administered oxygen at 1–3 L/min. Clients with chronic lung disease have developed carbon dioxide narcosis; high levels of carbon dioxide have destroyed the client's first stimulus for breathing. Oxygen hunger is the body's backup system for sustaining life. Administering oxygen at levels above 2 L/min at rest and 3 L/min during activity may cause the client to stop breathing.
    3. **Clients diagnosed with chronic lung disease are frequently prescribed long-term steroid therapy. Steroids delay wound healing. The nurse should assess the wound to determine that the surgical incision is healing as desired.**
    4. Morphine can cause respiratory compromise, especially when given frequently and in large doses. This client is already at risk for respiratory complications from the emphysema.

14. 1. This is instruction for an antibiotic. Prednisone is not abruptly discontinued because cortisol (a glucocorticoid) is necessary to sustain life and the adrenal glands will stop producing cortisol while the client is taking it exogenously.
    2. Prednisone can produce gastric distress; it is given with food to minimize the gastric discomfort.
    3. Weight gain is a side effect of steroid therapy, and the client should not stop taking the medication if this occurs. This medication must be tapered off if the client is to stop the medication—if the client is able to discontinue the medication at all.
    4. **Prednisone is not abruptly discontinued because cortisol (a glucocorticoid) is necessary to sustain life and the adrenal glands stop producing cortisol while the client is taking it exogenously. The medication must be tapered off to prevent a life-threatening complication.**

15. 1. This is an oral preparation and one that can be given daily; this is not the first medication to be administered.
    2. **Oxygen is considered a medication and should be a priority whenever it is ordered. A client diagnosed with pneu-**monia will have some amount of respiratory compromise, and the ordered 2 L/min indicates a client with a chronic lung disease. This is the priority medication.
    3. Lactinex is administered to replace the good bacteria in the body destroyed by the antibiotic, but it does not need to be administered first.
    4. Keflex is an oral antibiotic, but this client is being discharged, indicating the client's condition has improved. This client could wait until the oxygen is initiated.

MEDICATION MEMORY JOGGER: Oxygen is a medication, and the nurse should remember basic principles that apply to oxygen administration. The test taker could choose the correct answer based on Maslow's Hierarchy of Needs and breathing/oxygen is the priority.

16. 1. The nurse does not administer medications to decrease the respiratory drive for any client—especially not one diagnosed with pulmonary disease.
    2. **Morphine is a mild bronchodilator, and the continuous-release formulation provides a sustained effect for the client.**
    3. All forms of morphine can be addicting.
    4. Bronchoconstriction would increase the client's difficulty in breathing and trap sputum below the constricted bronchus.

17. 1. **Currently the medications used to treat resistant bacteria are the aminoglycoside antibiotics. Vancomycin is the drug of choice, but gentamycin may also be used. These medications can be toxic to the auditory nerve and to the kidneys. The therapeutic range is 10–20 mg/dL. The nurse should monitor the blood levels.**
    2. If ordered, the steroid would be given intravenously, not intramuscularly.
    3. The culture does not need to be repeated; this would add unnecessary expense to the client.
    4. The client should be placed on contact and possibly droplet precautions. Airborne isolation is required for tuberculosis.

18. 1. White blood cells are monitored to detect the presence of an infection, not for steroids.
    2. The hemoglobin and hematocrit are monitored to detect blood loss, not for steroid therapy.

3. Steroid therapy interferes with glucose metabolism and increases insulin resistance. The blood glucose levels should be monitored to determine if an intervention is needed.
4. The BUN and creatinine levels are monitored to determine renal status. The adrenal glands produce cortisol.

MEDICATION MEMORY JOGGER: The nurse must be knowledgeable about accepted standards of practice for medication administration including which client assessment data and laboratory data should be monitored prior to administering the medication.

19. 1. This hematocrit is normal, but this does not indicate that the client is responding to the antibiotics.
2. Thick, green sputum is a symptom of pneumonia, which indicates the antibiotic therapy is not effective. If the sputum were changing from a thick, green sputum to a thinner, lighter-colored sputum, it would indicate an improvement in the condition.
3. The symptoms of pneumonia include crackles and wheezing in the lung fields. Clear lung sounds indicate an improvement in the pneumonia and that the medication is effective.
4. Pleuritic chest is a symptom of pneumonia, and no chest pain indicates the medication is effective.

MEDICATION MEMORY JOGGER: The nurse determines the effectiveness of a medication by assessing for the symptoms, or lack thereof, for which the medication was prescribed.

20. 220 mL/hour. The nurse should set the pump at 220 mL/ hour.
Pumps are set at an hourly rate.
60 minutes divided by 30 equals 2.
100 + 10 = 110
110 multiplied by 2 = 220.

A Client with Reactive Airway Disease

21. 1. The client should take the medication with a glass of water or with meals to avoid an upset stomach.
2. The client should notify the health-care provider of a rapid or irregular heartbeat, vomiting, dizziness, or irritability because these are not expected side effects.

3. The client should avoid drinking large amounts of caffeine-containing drinks such as tea, coffee, cocoa, and cola drinks.
4. If a dose is missed within an hour, the client should take the dose immediately, but if it is more than 1 hour, the client should skip the dose and stay on the original dosing schedule. The client should not double the dose.

22. 1. These drugs are generally safe and well-tolerated, with a headache being the most common side effect; therefore, this statement would not warrant intervention by the nurse.
2. This medication interacts with aspirin, warfarin, erythromycin, and theophylline; therefore, this statement warrants further intervention by the nurse.
3. All medications should be kept out of the reach of children, and keeping the medication on a high shelf would not warrant intervention by the nurse.
4. This medication does not need to be kept from extreme temperatures; it is the anti-asthmatic zafirlukast (Accolate) that must be protected from extremes of temperature, light, and humidity.

MEDICATION MEMORY JOGGER: If the client verbalizes a complaint, if the nurse assesses data, or if laboratory data indicates an adverse effect secondary to a medication, the nurse must intervene. The nurse must implement an independent action during intervention or notify the health-care provider because medications can result in serious or even life-threatening complications.

23. 1. The client should take the last dose a few hours before bedtime so that the medication does not produce insomnia.
2. The client should increase fluid intake, especially water, because it will make the mucus thinner and help the medication work more effectively.
3. This medication is taken orally; therefore, there is no reason for the client to demonstrate the correct way to use an inhaler.
4. Antacids decrease the absorption of medication; therefore, the medication should not be taken with or within 2 hours of taking an antacid.

24. 1. The client should hold his or her breath as long as possible before exhaling to allow the medication to settle before

administering another dose; 5 seconds is not long enough.

2. The client can check how much medication is in a metered-dose canister by placing the canister in a glass of water; if the canister stays under water, the canister is full, and if it floats on top of the water, it is empty.

3. **This is the correct way to use an inhaler because it will carry the medication down into the lung.**

4. Oxygen is not used when using an inhaler; oxygen is used to deliver the medication when using an aerosol.

25. 1. The therapeutic level for theophylline is 10–20 μg/mL; therefore, the nurse should take action.

2. As the serum theophylline level rises above 20 μg/mL, the client will experience nausea, vomiting, diarrhea, insomnia, and restlessness. This theophylline level may result in serious effects, such as convulsion and ventricular fibrillation. Therefore, the client should not be assessed first.

3. **The client has the potential for having convulsions and ventricular fibrillation because the theophylline level is too high; therefore, the nurse should discontinue the aminophylline drip first.**

4. After discontinuing the aminophylline drip and then assessing the client for potential life-threatening complications, the nurse should notify the health-care provider.

MEDICATION MEMORY JOGGER: The nurse must be knowledgeable about accepted standards of practice for medication administration, including which client assessment data and laboratory data should be monitored prior to administering the medication.

26. 1. **The PEFR is defined as the maximal rate of airflow during expiration in a relatively inexpensive, handheld device. If the peak flow is less than 80% of personal best, more frequent monitoring should be done. The PEFR should be measured every morning.**

2. A normal respiratory assessment does not indicate that the medication regimen is effective and has "good" control.

3. Three asthma attacks in the last month would not indicate the client has "good" control of the reactive airway disease.

4. A serum theophylline level between 10 and 20 μg/mL indicates the medication is within the therapeutic range, but it is not the best indicator of the client's control of the signs or symptoms.

27. 1. This is the description of how a metered-dose inhaler works.

2. This is the description of how a dry-powder inhaler works.

3. **This is the description of how a nebulizer works. Nebulizers take several minutes to deliver the same amount of drug contained in one puff from an inhaler. They are usually used at home but can be used in the hospital.**

4. This is not the description of how a nebulizer works. Glucocorticoids are not used sublingually to treat acute or chronic asthma.

28. 1. **Gargling after each administration will help decrease the development of oropharyngeal yeast infections.**

2. Glucocorticoids are intended for preventive therapy, not for aborting an ongoing asthma attack, and they should not be taken on a PRN basis.

3. A spacer, a device that attaches directly to the metered-dose inhaler, should be used because a spacer increases the delivery of the drug to the lungs and decreases deposition of the drug on the oropharyngeal mucosa.

4. Forced expiratory volume (FEV) is the single most useful test of lung function, but the instrument required is a spirometer, which is expensive, cumbersome, and not suited for home use.

29. 1. This medication does not stimulate the central nervous system; therefore, the client does not need to avoid caffeine-containing products. This statement indicates that the teaching is not effective.

2. These medications are not used to treat an acute exacerbation of reactive airway disease. They are adjunctive drugs given as part of the asthma regimen. This statement indicates the teaching is not effective.

3. The safety of these drugs has not been established in pregnancy and breastfeeding. This statement indicates that the teaching has not been effective.

4. **The client should not suddenly stop taking the medication or decrease the dose. This statement indicates the**

teaching has been effective. Singulair is used with other types of asthma medications and should be continued if the client has an acute asthma attack.

30. 1. This type of medical treatment would be used for a client with mild persistent asthma.
    2. This medical treatment would be prescribed for a client with moderate persistent asthma.
    3. The most severe class, severe persistent asthma, is managed with daily inhalation of a glucocorticoid (high dose), plus salmeterol, a long-acting inhaled agent.
    4. **Mild intermittent asthma is treated on a PRN basis; long-term control medication is not needed. The occasional acute attack is managed by inhaling a short-acting beta$_2$ agonist. If the client needs the beta$_2$ agonist more than twice a week, moving to Step 2 (mild persistent asthma) may be indicated.**

A Child with Reactive Airway Disease

31. 1. Cromolyn is a safe and effective drug for prophylaxis of asthma, but it is not useful for aborting an ongoing attack.
    2. **Cromolyn can prevent bronchospasm in children subject to exercise-induced asthma. It should be administered 15 minutes prior to anticipated exertion.**
    3. The child with a chronic illness should be encouraged to live as normal a life as possible; therefore, encouraging the child to not play ball is not appropriate.
    4. Cromolyn is devoid of significant adverse effects and drug interactions. A yellow haze is not an expected side effect or adverse effect of cromolyn.

32. 1. Because the child is unconscious the nurse should prepare to administer epinephrine, a beta$_2$-adrenergic agonist, but this is not the first action.
    2. The client is unconscious; therefore, a nebulizer could not be administered to the child. It would be administered as soon as the child is conscious.
    3. If there is no response to the nebulizer, then the child should receive an intravenous glucocorticoid.
    4. **The first intervention should be administering oxygen to the child and**

then administering medication. Oxygen is considered a medication.

33. 1. All the medication in the nebulizer should be used during the treatment; medication should not be stored in the nebulizer for later use.
    2. The length of treatment is usually 10 to 15 minutes. If it takes longer, the parent should check the nebulizer equipment or compressor for defects or problems.
    3. The nebulizer should be cleaned daily (not weekly) using a disinfecting solution or a solution containing one part white vinegar and four parts water.
    4. **The nebulizer should be cleaned with water after each treatment and allowed to air dry after loosely covering it with a clean paper towel. Storing the equipment wet promotes the growth of mold and bacteria.**

34. 1. Prolonged glucocorticoid therapy can cause serious adverse effects such as adrenal suppression, osteoporosis, hyperglycemia, and peptic ulcer disease. Short-term use does not cause these adverse effects.
    2. Doctors often order medications that have serious side effects, but it must be done to treat the client. This statement is false and is not appropriate.
    3. **This is a true statement and the nurse's best response.**
    4. This is not the best response to the mother's question about her son's use of the medication. Prolonged glucocorticoid therapy can cause serious adverse effects, but short-term use does not cause these adverse effects.

35. 1. This is the explanation for administering leukotriene blockers.
    2. **This is the correct explanation for administering a cromolyn inhaler; it prevents the asthma attack by blocking the release of mast cell mediators.**
    3. This is the explanation for administering theophylline, a bronchial dilator.
    4. This is the explanation for administering glucocorticoids, such as prednisone.

36. 1. **The zone system is used to help children monitor their treatment. The child uses a peak flow meter, which monitors breathing capacity and shows which zone—green, yellow, or red—the child's peak flow is in. Treatment, if**

4. Theophylline does not need to be refrigerated.

40. **79.5 mg.** 35 divided by 2.2 equals 15.9 kg; 15.9 times 5 equals 79.5 mg per dose.

A Client with Pulmonary Embolus

41. 1. An oral anticoagulant would not be prescribed in an acute situation.
2. Lovenox is prescribed prophylactically to prevent deep vein thrombosis. The client is currently experiencing a complication of DVT; therefore, the nurse should not anticipate an order for this medication.
3. **Heparin is the medication of choice for treating a pulmonary embolus, which the nurse should suspect with these signs and symptoms. Intravenous heparin will prevent further clotting.**
4. Ticlid is a medication used to treat arterial, not venous, conditions.

MEDICATION MEMORY JOGGER:
Remember that antiplatelets work in the arteries and anticoagulants work in the veins.

42. 1. The INR is within therapeutic range; therefore, the nurse should not question administering this medication.
2. Vitamin K is the antidote for Coumadin toxicity, but the client is not in a toxic state.
3. There is no reason to notify the HCP to request an increase in the dose because the client is in the therapeutic range.
4. **When the nurse is administering Coumadin, the International Normalized Ratio (INR) must be monitored to determine therapeutic level, which is 2–3. Because the INR is 2.6, the nurse should administer this medication.**

MEDICATION MEMORY JOGGER: When trying to remember which laboratory value correlates with which anticoagulant, here's a helpful hint: "PT boats go to war (warfarin), and if you cross the small 't's' in 'Ptt' with one line it makes an 'h' (heparin)."

43. 1. Blood or blood products are the only fluids infused through Y-tubing.
2. **Heparin and streptokinase cannot be administered in the same intravenous line because they are incompatible.**

needed, is then based on which zone the peak flow meter shows. Green zone means all clear; no asthma symptoms are present.
2. There is no such zone as the black zone.
3. The red zone indicates a medical alert—a bronchodilator should be taken and the child should seek medical attention for acute severe asthma. The cromolyn and steroid inhaler are not used for an acute asthma attack.
4. The yellow zone indicates caution because an acute episode may be present. The control is insufficient. The child should inhale a short-acting beta$_2$ agonist. If this fails to return the child to the green zone, a short course of oral glucocorticoids may be needed.

37. 1. The child should be standing up at the bedside, not lying down.
2. **This is the correct way to obtain the peak flow meter results.**
3. **This is the correct way to take a reading from the peak flow meter.**
4. The peak flow meter should be repeated three times, waiting at least 10 seconds between each attempt. The highest reading of the three attempts is recorded.
5. **The pointer should be at zero every time the child attempts to blow into the peak flow meter.**

38. 1. The cromolyn inhaler should be taken routinely and is not used for an acute asthma attack; therefore, the child understands the teaching.
2. Moisture (from exhaled air) will interfere with proper use of the inhaler; therefore, the child understands the teaching.
3. **The child should rinse the mouth with water immediately after using the inhaler to help prevent throat irritation, dry mouth, and hoarseness.**
4. Discontinuing the medication quickly can cause the child to have an acute attack of asthma. The child understands this.

39. 1. Serum theophylline levels are obtained routinely but not on a daily basis.
2. **Theophylline toxicity can occur, and it requires medical intervention. Signs and symptoms include vomiting, dizziness, irritability, rapid or irregular heartbeat, and seizure activity.**
3. The evening dose should be administered earlier, around 5:00 P.M. with a meal, to help prevent insomnia.

The nurse must start a second line to administer the streptokinase simultaneously with the heparin. The nurse does not need an order to do this.

3. The client needs both of these medications; therefore, the nurse cannot discontinue the heparin. Streptokinase is a thrombolytic, which will dissolve the clot in the pulmonary artery, but heparin, an anticoagulant, is prescribed to prevent reformation of the clot.

4. Heparin and streptokinase cannot be administered in the same intravenous line because they are incompatible. The nurse must start a second line to administer the streptokinase simultaneously with the heparin. The nurse does not need an order to do this.

44. 1. **Streptokinase is a foreign protein extracted from the cultures of streptococci bacteria, and streptomycin is derived from *Streptomyces*. As a result, this could possibly cause the client to have an allergic reaction. The nurse should discuss this allergy with the HCP.**

2. The nurse should not administer this medication until determining if the client is at risk for an allergic reaction.

3. The pharmacist is not licensed to change an HCP order.

4. Bleeding times could be assessed after it is determined that the streptokinase will not cause the client to have an allergic reaction.

45. 1. The client is at risk for bleeding and should be encouraged to use an electric razor.

2. The client is at risk for bleeding, and a soft-bristled toothbrush should be used.

3. Any abnormal bleeding, such as a nosebleed, is not expected and should be reported to the HCP. Unexplained bleeding is a sign of toxicity.

4. **The client's International Normalized Ratio (INR) is monitored at routine intervals to determine if the medication is within the therapeutic range, INR 2–3.**

46. 1. This is the scientific rationale for why Coumadin is prescribed to prevent thrombus formation, but it is not the rationale for why the medications are administered together.

2. **Heparin has a short half-life and is prescribed as soon as a PE is suspected. The client must go home having taken an oral anticoagulant such as Coumadin, which has a long half-life and needs at least 3–5 days to reach a therapeutic level. Discontinuing the heparin prior to achieving a therapeutic level of Coumadin places the client at risk for another PE.**

3. Heparin and warfarin work in different steps in the bleeding cascade.

4. This is a false statement; heparin and warfarin work in different steps in the bleeding cascade.

47. 1. The PTT test is used to monitor the anticoagulant heparin, not the thrombolytic Activase.

2. A client with a massive PE would be on bed rest; therefore, ambulating would not indicate the medication is effective.

3. **To determine if the medication is effective, the nurse must assess for an improvement in the signs or symptoms for the condition for which the medication was ordered. Chest pain is one of the most common symptoms of PE; denial of chest pain would indicate the medication is effective.**

4. In the client diagnosed with a PE the chest x-ray is usually normal; therefore, it would not be used to determine if the thrombolytic is effective.

48. 1. **This would be the first intervention because the client is above the therapeutic range. The therapeutic range for heparin is 1.5 to 2.0 times the control, or 54 to 72. The client's PTT of 92 places the client at risk for bleeding. Therefore, the nurse must prevent further infusion of medication.**

2. This is the antidote for heparin, but the nurse would not administer this first. Discontinuing the infusion of heparin for a few hours may be sufficient to correct the overdose.

3. The HCP should be notified of the client's situation, but it is not the first intervention.

4. Assessment is the first step in the nursing process, but if the client is in "distress" or experiencing a complication, the nurse should first treat the client.

MEDICATION MEMORY JOGGER: When trying to remember which laboratory value correlates with which anticoagulant, here's a helpful hint: "PT boats go to war (warfarin), and if you cross the small 't's' in 'Ptt' with one line it makes an 'h' (heparin)."

49. **700 units of heparin are being infused every hour.** When determining the units, the nurse must first determine how many units are in each milliliter.

$$\frac{25{,}000 \text{ Units}}{500 \text{ mL}} = 50 \text{ units per mL}$$

50 units per mL $\times$ 14 mL per hour = 700 mL per hour

50. **15 mL per hour.** When setting the intravenous pump, the nurse must first determine the number of units per milliliter.

$$\frac{40{,}000 \text{ units}}{500 \text{ mL}} = 80 \text{ units per mL}$$

$$\frac{1200 \text{ units per hour}}{80 \text{ units per mL}} = 15 \text{ mL}$$

1. The 34-year-old female client who is para 2, gravida 1 is prescribed the narcotic antitussive hydrocodone (Hycodan). Which information should the nurse discuss with client?
   1. Explain that this medication can be taken when pregnant.
   2. Teach that this medication will not cause any type of addiction.
   3. Instruct the client to take 1 teaspoon after every cough.
   4. Discuss keeping the medication away from children.

2. The client with asthma asks the nurse, "Why should I use the corticosteroid inhaler instead of prednisone?" Which statement by the nurse would be most appropriate?
   1. "The lungs are incapable of utilizing prednisone to decrease inflammation."
   2. "The inhaler costs less than the prednisone, which is why it should be used."
   3. "The inhaler will not cause the systemic problems that prednisone does."
   4. "Prednisone is not on your insurance formulary and the inhaler is."

3. The pediatric clinic nurse is assessing the routine medications for a child with cystic fibrosis. Which medication would the nurse question?
   1. The oral aminoglycoside antibiotic tobramycin.
   2. The daily pancreatic enzyme Pancrease.
   3. The nonnarcotic antitussive Tessalon Perles.
   4. The mucolytic agent Pulmozyme.

4. The client diagnosed with tuberculosis is administered rifampin (Rifadin), an antitubercular medication. Which information should the nurse discuss with the client?
   1. Instruct the client to consume fewer dark-green, leafy vegetables.
   2. Explain that the client's urine and other body fluids will turn orange.
   3. Encourage the client to stop smoking cigarettes while taking this medication.
   4. Tell the client to increase fluid intake to 3000 mL a day.

5. The client is having an acute exacerbation of asthma. The health-care provider has prescribed epinephrine (adrenaline) subcutaneously. Which intervention should the nurse implement when administering this medication?
   1. Administer the medication using a tuberculin syringe.
   2. Dilute the medication to a 5-mL bolus prior to administering.
   3. Perform a complete respiratory assessment.
   4. Monitor the client's serum epinephrine level.

6. The nurse is preparing to administer the following medications. Which client would the nurse question administering the medication?
   1. The client receiving prednisone, a glucocorticoid, who has a glucose level of 140 mg/dL.
   2. The client receiving ceftriaxone (Rocephin), an antibiotic, who has a white blood cell count of 15,000.
   3. The client receiving heparin, an anticoagulant, who has a PTT of 78 seconds with a control of 39.
   4. The client receiving theophylline (Theo-Dur) who has a theophylline level of 25 mg/dL.

7. The nurse is discussing health-promotion activities with a client diagnosed with chronic obstructive pulmonary disease (COPD). What information should the nurse discuss with the client?
   1. Instruct the client to get the influenza vaccine semi-annually.
   2. Teach the client to continue taking low-dose antibiotics at all times.
   3. Encourage the client to get the pneumococcal vaccine every 5 years.
   4. Discuss the need to receive three doses of the hepatitis B vaccine.

8. The nurse and the unlicensed assistive personnel (UAP) are caring for a client diagnosed with chronic pulmonary disease (COPD). Which action by the UAP warrants immediate intervention by the nurse?
   1. The UAP encourages the client to wear the nasal cannula at all times.
   2. The UAP calculates the client's fluid intake after the lunch meal.
   3. The UAP increases the oxygen to 5 L/min while ambulating the client.
   4. The UAP obtains the client's pulse oximeter reading.

9. The client with active tuberculosis is prescribed antitubercular medications. Which intervention will the public health nurse implement?
   1. Request the client come to the public health clinic weekly for sputum cultures.
   2. Place the client and family in quarantine while the client takes the medication.
   3. Inform the neighbors and coworkers that the client has been diagnosed with TB.
   4. Arrange for a health-care professional to observe the client taking the medication daily.

10. Which statement by the nurse best describes the scientific rationale for how a nonnarcotic antitussive medication works in the body?
    1. It suppresses the cough reflex by directly acting on the medulla of the brain.
    2. It reduces the cough reflex by anesthetizing stretch receptors in the respiratory passages.
    3. Nonnarcotic antitussives slow down the destruction of sensitized mast cells.
    4. It acts to block receptors for cysteinyl leukotrienes that prevent bronchoconstriction.

11. The client with an acute exacerbation of asthma is being treated with asthma medications. Which assessment data indicates the medication is effective?
    1. The client has bilateral wheezing.
    2. The client's lung sounds are clear.
    3. The client's pulse oximeter reading is 90%.
    4. The client has no peripheral clubbing.

12. The child with cystic fibrosis is taking high-dose intravenous antibiotic therapy, cephalosporin (Ancef), and is getting progressively worse. Which medication would the intensive care nurse anticipate being added to the medication regimen?
    1. An intravenous corticosteroid.
    2. An intravenous aminoglycoside antibiotic.
    3. An oral proton-pump inhibitor.
    4. An oral mucolytic agent.

13. The client with tuberculosis is prescribed isoniazid (INH). Which diet selection indicates the client needs more teaching?
    1. Tuna fish sandwich on white bread, potato chips, and iced tea.
    2. Pot roast, mashed potatoes with brown gravy, and a light beer.
    3. Fried chicken, potato salad, corn on the cob, and white milk.
    4. Caesar salad with chicken noodle soup and water.

14. The client's arterial blood gas results are pH 7.48, PaO_2 98, PCO_2 30, and HCO_3 24. Which action would be most appropriate for this client?
    1. Administer oxygen 10 L/min via nasal cannula.
    2. Administer an antianxiety medication.
    3. Administer 1 amp of sodium bicarbonate IVP.
    4. Administer 30 mL of an antacid.

15. The 3-year-old child is admitted to the emergency department with an acute episode of laryngotracheobronchitis (LTB). The health-care provider has prescribed racemic epinephrine nebulized with oxygen. Which intervention should the nurse implement?
    1. Administer the epinephrine with a tuberculin syringe.
    2. Ensure that antibiotics are given simultaneously.
    3. Notify the pediatric floor of the child's admission.
    4. Obtain a culture and sensitivity of the throat.

16. Which intervention is priority when administering intravenous (IV) fluids to a 2 year old diagnosed with acute epiglottitis?
    1. Label the intravenous fluid with the client's name.
    2. Obtain the daily weight and post at the head of the bed.
    3. Assess the child's intravenous site for redness and warmth.
    4. Administer the IV fluids with a volume-control chamber.

17. The 8-year-old male child diagnosed with asthma is prescribed theophylline (Theo-Dur). The child tells the nurse that if he is good at the doctor's visit, his mom is going to get a hamburger, French fries, and a cola for him. Which action should the nurse implement?
    1. Encourage the child to be good so he can go get his meal.
    2. Tell the mother not to use food as a reward for visiting the doctor.
    3. Suggest drinking a Sprite or 7-Up with his lunch instead of cola.
    4. Explain that the child should not eat foods high in salt such as fries.

18. The health-care provider has ordered theophylline 3 mg/kg/q 6 hrs for a child who weighs 20 lbs. How much medication would the nurse administer to the child in a 24-hour time period?
    Answer _____

19. The nurse is preparing to administer the first dose of antibiotics to the client diagnosed with pneumonia. Which intervention should the nurse implement first?
    1. Check the white blood cell count.
    2. Determine if a C&S was obtained.
    3. Check the client's identification band.
    4. Teach the client about suprainfection.

20. The nurse is reading this intradermal positive protein derivative (PPD) skin test 72 hours after it was administered.

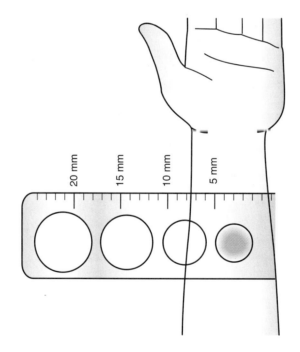

What would the nurse document based on this result?
    1. Significant but not at risk.
    2. Not significant.
    3. Undetermined reaction.
    4. Significant and at risk.

1. 1. This medication is a pregnancy risk category C, which is questionable when administered to a client who is pregnant. Pregnancy risk category A is the least dangerous to the fetus; categories B, C, and D are progressively more dangerous than category A, and category X is known to cause harm to the fetus.
   2. This cough syrup (antitussive) is similar to codeine and is a narcotic and has addictive properties.
   3. This medication should be taken every 4–6 hours to help prevent coughing but should not be taken after every cough; the client could experience excessive drowsiness, constipation, and nausea.
   4. **This medication is a narcotic and, because the client is 34 years old and has at least one child, the nurse should discuss proper storage of the medication to prevent accidental poisoning of any children.**

2. 1. Prednisone, frequently prescribed, is a systemic anti-inflammatory medication that has many side effects. The inhaler does not have systemic effects, which is why the inhaler is preferred.
   2. The cost of the medication does not have a bearing on why one route of medication should be used instead of another.
   3. **The steroid inhaler does not cause the systemic problem of suppression of the adrenal gland and exposure of cells of the body to excess cortisol. The inhaler delivers the anti-inflammatory medication directly to the lungs, where effects are desired.**
   4. Insurance should not be the reason for deciding which route of medication a client should be prescribed.

3. 1. The child with cystic fibrosis (CF) may be receiving routine daily doses of antibiotics; therefore, the nurse would not question the medication.
   2. Pancreatic enzymes are administered with every meal and snack to a child with CF to aid in digestion, so the nurse would expect this medication to be ordered.
   3. **An antitussive medication would suppress the cough reflex, which would result in stasis of thick tenacious secretions remaining in the lung and predispose the child to lung infections and possibly respiratory failure. The nurse would question this medication.**
   4. Mucolytic agents are administered to break down the thick sputum and to assist the child to expectorate the secretions. The nurse would expect this medication for a child with CF.

4. 1. The consumption of dark-green, leafy vegetables will not affect this medication.
   2. **The client should be informed that this medication turns the urine and body secretions orange and can discolor contact lenses. This is not harmful to the client.**
   3. The client should be encouraged to stop smoking for general health reasons, but smoking will not affect this medication.
   4. Increasing fluid intake has no bearing on taking this medication.

5. 1. **The medication is prescribed in very low doses of 0.2 to 1.0 mg for an adult. The dosage of a sympathomimetic must be carefully monitored to prevent tachycardia, decreased or increased blood pressure, nausea, headache, and other central nervous system symptoms. A tuberculin syringe should be used to help ensure accuracy of dosage administered.**
   2. The medication is being administered subcutaneously; therefore, the nurse will not dilute the medication.
   3. The client is in distress with an acute exacerbation of asthma. Therefore, the nurse should not assess but should treat the client because delaying the medication may result in a respiratory arrest.
   4. There is no such laboratory test as a serum epinephrine level.

6. 1. This blood glucose is elevated, but this is an expected side effect of prednisone; therefore, the nurse would not question administering this medication.
   2. A client receiving an antibiotic would be expected to have an elevated white blood cell count; therefore, the nurse would not question administering this medication.
   3. A PTT of 78 seconds is 1.5 to 2 times the control; therefore, the nurse would not question administering this medication.
   4. **The therapeutic serum theophylline level is 10–20 mg/dL, and the client has a higher level. Therefore, the nurse should question administering this medication and hold the dose.**

MEDICATION MEMORY JOGGER: The nurse must be knowledgeable about accepted standards of practice for disease processes and conditions. If the nurse administers a medication the health-care provider has prescribed and it harms the client, the nurse could be held accountable. Remember that the nurse is a client advocate.

7. 1. The influenza vaccine should be taken yearly, not semi-annually (every 6 months).
   2. The client may develop resistance to antibiotics if they are taken all the time; antibiotics will be prescribed during times of infection.
   3. The pneumococcal vaccine titers persist in most adults for 5 years; the vaccine protects against pneumonia and clients with COPD should receive it to prevent lung infections.
   4. The hepatitis B vaccine is not specifically recommended to promote health in clients with COPD.

8. 1. The client should wear the nasal cannula at all times; therefore, the nurse would not need to intervene.
   2. The UAP can calculate the fluid intake, but the nurse must evaluate it to determine if it is adequate for the client's disease process.
   3. **Long-term oxygen therapy has been shown to improve the client's quality of life and survival. The oxygen must be kept between 1 and 3 L/min to prevent respiratory failure, which occurs when the oxygen level is increased and the client's hypoxic drive is no longer active. Carbon dioxide narcosis occurs in clients with COPD and eliminates that stimulus for breathing.**
   4. The UAP can obtain a pulse oximeter reading, but the nurse must evaluate the result to determine if it is normal for the disease process.

9. 1. The client will not have to go to the clinic weekly. Sputum cultures are done to diagnose TB and to determine when the client's illness is no longer communicable. Three negative sputum cultures taken for 3 consecutive days 10–14 days after starting medication indicate the client's illness is no longer communicable.
   2. This medication will be administered for 9–12 months, and the client is quarantined for 10–14 days until negative sputum cultures are obtained. Family members are not quarantined unless they have active TB.
   3. The public health nurse will notify the people who have been in contact with the client during the infectious stage, but the nurse will not divulge the client's name, which would be a violation of HIPAA. The nurse will explain that the individual may have come into contact with a person recently diagnosed with TB and the person should receive a PPD skin test.
   4. **Tuberculosis is a communicable disease that is a detriment to the community; therefore, the client is mandated to take the antitubercular medication and will be observed daily for the duration of the regimen, which may be 9–12 months. The risk of drug resistance is extremely high if the regimen is not strictly and continuously followed. This will result in multi–drug–resistant TB in the community.**

10. 1. Narcotic antitussives suppress the cough reflex by acting directly on the cough center in the medulla of the brain.
    2. **Nonnarcotic antitussives reduce the cough reflex at its source by anesthetizing stretch receptors in the respiratory passages, lungs, and pleura and by decreasing their activity.**
    3. Slowing down the destruction of sensitized mast cells is the scientific rationale for administering Cromolyn, a mast cell inhibitor given to prevent asthma attacks.
    4. Blocking receptors for cysteinyl leukotrienes is the scientific rationale for administering leukotrienes to reduce the symptoms of asthma.

11. 1. Wheezing, a musical respiratory sound made when air is forced out through the small, mucus-lined passages during respiration, does not indicate the medication is effective.
    2. **Clear lung sounds would indicate that the asthma medications are effective.**
    3. The client's pulse oximeter should be greater than 93% to indicate the client is being adequately oxygenated.
    4. Clubbing does not occur with clients diagnosed with asthma. It occurs in clients with chronic hypoxia such as occurs with chronic obstructive pulmonary disease (COPD) or cystic fibrosis (CF).

12. 1. Steroids are sometimes prescribed when pulmonary symptoms are unresponsive to antibiotics because corticosteroids decrease inflammation in the lungs.
    2. The child should have cultures and sensitivities to determine resistance and sensitivity to an antibiotic. Changing an antibiotic depends on C&S results. Based on the information provided, there is no need to change antibiotics.
    3. A proton-pump inhibitor decreases gastric secretions, but it is not indicated to improve pulmonary symptoms.
    4. The client will be receiving inhaled mucolytic therapy in the intensive care unit. There is no reason to add an oral agent.

13. 1. Tuna, foods with yeast extracts, aged cheese, red wine, and soy sauce contain tyramine and histamine, which interact with INH and result in a headache, flushing, hypotension, lightheadedness, palpitations, and diaphoreses.
    2. Red wine, not beer, can cause a reaction with INH.
    3. Fried foods and whole milk may not be a healthy diet, but they are not contraindicated with INH.
    4. Soup is high in sodium content, but it is not contraindicated in clients taking INH.

14. 1. This client is in respiratory alkalosis, which is caused by hyperventilating. Oxygen would not be helpful in treating this client.
    2. This client is in respiratory alkalosis, which is caused by hyperventilating and could be the result of anxiety, elevated temperature, or pain. The nurse should assess the cause and administer the appropriate medication.
    3. Sodium bicarbonate is the drug of choice for metabolic acidosis and this is respiratory alkalosis. This medication is an alkaline substance and would increase the client's alkalosis.
    4. An antacid would not help treat respiratory alkalosis because it is also an alkaline substance.

15. 1. The child is 3 years old and the medication is being administered with a nebulizer, not via the parenteral route.
    2. Antibiotics are not indicated unless a bacterial infection has been confirmed.
    3. **The child taking this medication must be hospitalized to monitor for changes**

in respiratory status and should not be treated with epinephrine on an outpatient basis because the effects of epinephrine are temporary and respiratory distress may return.
    4. A throat culture is not required prior to administering epinephrine; this would be appropriate when administering an antibiotic for the first time.

16. 1. This is an acceptable practice, but it is not priority when administering fluids to a child.
    2. The weight is important when administering medication to a child, but it is not priority when administering IV fluids.
    3. Redness and warmth at the intravenous site indicate phlebitis, which requires the IV to be discontinued, but this is not the priority intervention.
    4. A volume-control chamber (Buretrol) is a special IV tubing device that allows for 1 hour of fluid to potentially infuse at any one time. It is a safety device to prevent fluid overload in a child. This is the priority intervention because fluid-volume overload in a 2 year old could be fatal.

17. 1. The nurse should teach the child about food preferences because the child has a chronic disease; caffeine-containing drinks should be discouraged.
    2. The nurse should not be judgmental about the mother's parenting skills.
    3. The child should avoid drinking large amounts of caffeine-containing drinks such as tea, cocoa, and cola drinks; Sprite and 7-Up do not contain caffeine.
    4. This is an untrue statement; children rarely have problems with sodium intake.

18.   **108 mg/24 hours.** First, determine the child's weight in kilograms: 20 lb divided by 2.2 kg is equal to 9.09 kg. Then, determine how many milligrams should be given with each dose: 9.09 kg times 3 mg is equal to 27.27 mg. Because it is below 0.5, the nurse should round down to 27. Because the dose is to be given every 6 hours, the child will be receiving 4 doses in a 24-hour time period: 27 mg times 4 is equal to 108 mg/per 24 hours.

19. 1. The client's WBC count will not affect whether the nurse administers the medication; therefore, it is not priority.

2. This must be implemented first because if the culture and sensitivity (C&S) is obtained after the antibiotic is administered, the results will be skewed and useless. This is usually checked at the nurse's station before entering the client's room to give the medication.

3. This should be checked before administering the medication, but if the C&S is not checked, then the nurse should not administer the medication.

4. The nurse should teach about the antibiotic destroying the good flora resulting in a suprainfection, but it is not the first intervention.

20. 1. A wheal 5 mm or greater may be significant in individuals who are considered at risk.

2. A wheal measuring 5 mm or less is considered not significant, and this client's reaction is less than 5 mm induration.

3. This would indicate the reaction is not readable and could result from poor administration technique of the intradermal injection.

4. A wheal of 10 mm or greater is significant in individuals with normal immunity.

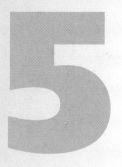

Gastrointestinal System

"There is no future in any job. The future lies in the man who holds the job."

—George Crane

PRACTICE QUESTIONS

A Client with Gastroesophageal Reflux

1. The client complaining of "acid" when lying down at night asks the nurse if there is any medication that might help. Which statement is the nurse's best response?
   1. "There are no medications to treat this problem, but losing weight will sometimes help the symptoms."
   2. "There are several over-the-counter and prescription medications available to treat this. You should discuss this with the HCP."
   3. "Have you had any x-rays or other tests to determine if you have cancer or some other serious illness?"
   4. "Acid reflux at night can lead to serious complications. You need to have tests done to determine the cause."

2. The nurse on a medical unit has received the morning report. Which medication should the nurse administer first?
   1. The proton-pump inhibitor pantoprazole (Protonix) to a client on call to surgery.
   2. The antacid calcium carbonate (TUMS) to a client complaining of indigestion.
   3. The antimicrobial bismuth (Pepto Bismol) to a client diagnosed with an ulcer.
   4. The H_2 blocker famotidine (Pepcid) to a client diagnosed with GERD.

3. Which statement is the scientific rationale for administering a proton-pump inhibitor (PPI) to a client diagnosed with gastrointestinal reflux disease (GERD)?
   1. PPI medications neutralize the gastric secretions.
   2. PPI medications block H_2 receptors on the parietal cells.
   3. PPI medications inhibit the enzyme that generates gastric acid.
   4. PPI medications form a protective barrier against acid and pepsin.

4. Which statement is an advantage to administering a histamine$_2$ blocker rather than an antacid to a client diagnosed with gastroesophageal reflux disease (GERD)?
   1. Antacids are more potent than H_2 blockers in relieving the symptoms of GERD.
   2. Histamine$_2$ blockers have more side effects than antacids.
   3. Histamine$_2$ blockers are less expensive than antacids.
   4. Histamine$_2$ blockers require less frequent dosing than antacids.

5. Which side effects would the nurse explain to the male client who is prescribed cimetidine (Tagamet), a histamine$_2$ blocker?
   1. The medication can cause indigestion and heartburn.
   2. The medication can cause impotence and gynecomastia.
   3. The medication can cause insomnia and hypervigilance.
   4. The medication can cause Zollinger-Ellison syndrome.

6. The home health nurse is caring for a male client diagnosed with a hiatal hernia and reflux. Which data indicates the medication therapy has been effective?
   1. The client takes the antacid 1 hour before and 3 hours after a meal.
   2. The client complains of indigestion after eating a large meal.
   3. The client states that he did not wake up with heartburn during the night.
   4. The client has lost 3 pounds in the last 2 weeks.

7. The nurse is preparing to administer the proton-pump inhibitor esomeprazole (Nexium). Which intervention should the nurse implement?
   1. Order an infusion pump for the client.
   2. Elevate the client's foot of the bed.
   3. Check for allergies to cephalosporin.
   4. Ask the client his or her date of birth.

8. The nurse is discharging a client diagnosed with gastroesophageal reflux disease (GERD). Which information should the nurse include in the teaching?
   1. There are no complications of GERD as long as the client takes the medications.
   2. Notify the health-care provider if the medication does not resolve the symptoms.
   3. Immediately after a meal, lie down for at least 45 minutes.
   4. If any discomfort is noted, take an NSAID for the pain.

9. The nurse is discharging a client 2 days postoperative hiatal hernia repair. Which discharge instructions should the nurse include? Select all that apply.
   1. Take all the prescribed antibiotic.
   2. Eat six small meals per day.
   3. Use the legs to bend down, not the back.
   4. Take esomeprazole (Nexium) twice a day.
   5. Use the pain medication when the pain is an 8–10.

10. The adult client recently has been diagnosed with asthma. Which medication would be recommended to treat this problem?
    1. Omeprazole (Prilosec), a proton-pump inhibitor, daily.
    2. Amoxicillin (Amoxil), an antibiotic, twice daily.
    3. Loratadine (Claritin), an antihistamine, twice daily.
    4. Prednisone, a glucocorticoid, daily.

A Client with Inflammatory Bowel Disease

11. The client diagnosed with ulcerative colitis is prescribed mesalamine (Asacol), an aspirin product. Which information should the nurse discuss with the client?
    1. Explain to the client that undissolved tablets may be expelled in stool.
    2. Discuss the importance of taking the medication on an empty stomach only.
    3. Tell the client to avoid drinking any type of carbonated beverages.
    4. Instruct the client not to crush, break, or chew the tablets or capsules.

12. The client with inflammatory bowel disease is prescribed sulfasalazine (Azulfidine), a sulfonamide antibiotic. Which intervention should the nurse implement when administering this medication?
    1. Ensure the client drinks at least 2000 mL of water daily.
    2. Administer the medication once a day with breakfast.
    3. Explain that the medication may cause slight bruising.
    4. Assess the client's stool for steatorrhea and mucus.

13. The client diagnosed with severe ulcerative colitis is prescribed azathioprine (Imuran), an immunosuppressant. Which assessment data concerning the medication would warrant immediate intervention by the nurse?
    1. Complaints of a sore throat, fever, and chills.
    2. Reports of 10–20 loose stools a day.
    3. Complaints of abdominal pain and tenderness.
    4. Reports of dry mouth and oral mucosa.

14. The client with a severe acute exacerbation of Crohn's disease is prescribed total parenteral nutrition (TPN). Which interventions should the nurse implement when administering TPN? Select all that apply.
    1. Monitor the client's glucose level every 6 hours.
    2. Administer the TPN on an intravenous pump.
    3. Assess the peripheral intravenous site every 4 hours.
    4. Check the TPN according to the five rights prior to administering.
    5. Encourage the client to eat all of the food offered at meals.

15. The client diagnosed with inflammatory bowel disease taking mesalamine (Asacol), an aspirin product, has complaints of nausea, vomiting, and diarrhea. Which action should the clinic nurse take?
    1. Instruct the client to quit taking the medication immediately.
    2. Tell the client to take Prevacid, a proton-pump inhibitor, with the medication.
    3. Advise the client to keep taking the medication, but notify the HCP.
    4. Explain that these symptoms are expected and will resolve with time.

16. Which statement indicates to the nurse that the client with Crohn's disease understands the medication teaching concerning sulfasalazine (Azulfidine), a sulfonamide antibiotic?
    1. "I will take an antacid 30 minutes before taking my medication."
    2. "I may get a slight red rash when taking this medication."
    3. "I need to keep a strict record of my urinary output."
    4. "I should avoid direct sunlight and use sunblock when outside."

17. The client with inflammatory bowel disease has been on hyperalimentation, total parenteral nutrition (TPN), for 2 weeks. The health-care provider has written orders to discontinue TPN. Which action should the nurse implement?
    1. Notify the health-care provider and question the order.
    2. Discontinue the TPN and flush the subclavian port.
    3. Do not implement the order and talk to the HCP on rounds.
    4. Discuss the order with the pharmacist before discontinuing.

18. Which laboratory data should the nurse monitor for the client with inflammatory bowel disease who is prescribed sulfasalazine (Azulfidine), a sulfonamide antibiotic?
    1. The client's liver function tests.
    2. The client's serum potassium level.
    3. The client's serum creatinine level.
    4. The client's International Normalized Ratio (INR).

19. The client diagnosed with inflammatory bowel disease is prescribed mesalamine (Asacol), an aspirin product, suppositories. Which statement indicates the client understands the medication teaching?
    1. "I should retain the suppository for at least 15 minutes."
    2. "The suppository may stain my underwear or clothing."
    3. "I should store my medication in the refrigerator."
    4. "I should have a full rectum when applying the suppository."

20. The client with inflammatory bowel disease is prescribed the glucocorticoid prednisone. Which priority intervention should the nurse implement?
    1. Monitor the client's blood glucose level.
    2. Discuss the long-term side effects of prednisone.
    3. Administer the medication with food.
    4. Explain that the prednisone will be tapered when it is to be discontinued.

A Client with Peptic Ulcer Disease

21. The nurse is administering 0800 medications. Which medication would the nurse question?
    1. Misoprostol (Cytotec), a prostaglandin analog, to a 29-year-old female with an NSAID-produced ulcer.
    2. Omeprazole (Prilosec), a proton-pump inhibitor, to a 68-year-old male with a duodenal ulcer.
    3. Furosemide (Lasix), a loop diuretic, to a 56-year-old male with a potassium level of 4.2 mEq/L.
    4. Acetaminophen (Tylenol), a nonnarcotic analgesic, to an 84-year-old female with a frontal headache.

22. The client diagnosed with severe congestive heart failure is complaining of indigestion. Which antacid medication should the nurse administer?
    1. Sodium bicarbonate.
    2. Amphogel.
    3. Riopan.
    4. Mylanta DS.

23. The female client diagnosed with low back pain has been self-medicating with ibuprofen (Motrin), a nonsteroidal anti-inflammatory drug (NSAID), around the clock. The client calls the clinic and tells the nurse that she has been getting dizzy and lightheaded. Which action would be the nurse's best response?
    1. Tell the client to get up from a sitting or lying position slowly.
    2. Have the client come to the clinic for lab work immediately.
    3. Suggest the client take the ibuprofen with food or an antacid.
    4. Discuss changing to a different nonsteroidal anti-inflammatory medication.

24. The client is diagnosed with a *Helicobacter pylori* infection and peptic ulcer disease (PUD). Which discharge instructions should the nurse teach?
    1. Discuss placing the head of the bed on blocks to prevent reflux.
    2. Teach to never use nonsteroidal anti-inflammatory drugs again.
    3. Encourage the client to limit smoking to half a pack per day.
    4. Take the combination of medications for 14 days as directed.

25. The intensive care nurse is preparing to administer the H_2 receptor blocker ranitidine (Zantac) IVPB to a client with severe burns. Which statement is the scientific rationale for administering this medication?
    1. Zantac will prevent an *H. pylori* infection.
    2. The client has a history of ulcer disease.
    3. It is for prophylaxis to prevent Curling's ulcer.
    4. There is no rationale; the nurse should question the order.

26. The male client diagnosed with peptic ulcer disease (PUD) has been taking magnesium hydroxide (Milk of Magnesia) for indigestion. The client complains that he has been having diarrhea. Which action would be the nurse's best response?
    1. Suggest that the client use magnesium hydroxide with aluminum hydroxide (Mylanta).
    2. Encourage the client to discuss the problem with the health-care provider.
    3. Tell the client to take loperamide (Imodium), over the counter.
    4. Discuss why the client is concerned about experiencing diarrhea.

27. The client diagnosed with peptic ulcer disease is admitted to the medical unit with a hemoglobin level of 6.2 g/dL and a hematocrit level of 18%. Which intervention should the nurse prepare to implement first?
    1. Obtain an order for an oral proton-pump inhibitor.
    2. Instruct the client to save all stools for observation.
    3. Initiate an IV with 0.9% NS with an 18-gauge catheter.
    4. Place a bedside commode in the client's room.

28. The nurse is preparing to administer pantoprazole (Protonix), a proton-pump inhibitor, IVPB, in 50 mL of fluid over 20 minutes to a client diagnosed with peptic ulcer disease. The IVPB set delivers 20 drops per mL. At what rate would the nurse set the infusion set?
    Answer _____

29. The nurse is administering 0900 medications to a client diagnosed with peptic ulcer disease (PUD). Which medication would the nurse question?
    1. Metronidazole (Flagyl), an anti-infective.
    2. Bismuth subsalicylate (Pepto Bismol), an antibiotic.
    3. Lansoprazole (Prevacid), a proton-pump inhibitor.
    4. Sucralfate (Carafate), a mucosal barrier agent.

30. The client has been on a therapeutic regimen for an *H. pylori* infection. Which data suggest the medication is not effective?
    1. The client states that the midepigastric pain has been relieved.
    2. The client's hemoglobin is 15 g/dL and the hematocrit is 44%.
    3. The client has gained 3 pounds in 1 week.
    4. The client's pulse is 124 and blood pressure is 92/48.

An Elderly Client with Diverticulosis/Diverticulitis

31. The elderly client with diverticulosis is instructed to take the bulk laxative psyllium mucilloid (Metamucil). Which question would be most important for the nurse to ask the client?
    1. "When was your last bowel movement?"
    2. "Do you have any difficulty swallowing?"
    3. "How much fiber do you eat daily?"
    4. "Do you ever notice any abdominal tenderness?"

32. The 72-year-old client is admitted to the medical unit diagnosed with an acute exacerbation of diverticulosis. The health-care provider has prescribed the intravenous antibiotic ceftriaxone (Rocephin). Which intervention should the nurse implement first?
    1. Monitor the client's white blood cell count.
    2. Assess the client's most recent vital signs.
    3. Determine if the client has any known allergies.
    4. Send a stool specimen to the laboratory.

33. The nurse is transcribing the admitting health-care provider's orders for an elderly client diagnosed with diverticulitis. Which order would the nurse question?
    1. Administer one bisacodyl (Dulcolax), by mouth, daily.
    2. Insert a nasogastric tube to intermittent low suction.
    3. Administer morphine 2 mg intravenous push for pain every 4 hours.
    4. Infuse D5 0.45 NS at 100 mL an hour.

34. Which information should the nurse discuss with the 75-year-old client diagnosed with diverticulosis who is prescribed methylcellulose (Citrucel), a bulk laxative?
    1. Notify the health-care provider if abdominal cramping occurs.
    2. Explain that results should be evident within 24 hours.
    3. Encourage the client to increase the intake of fluids, especially water.
    4. Instruct the client to decrease fiber intake while taking this medication.

35. The 80-year-old client with diverticulosis is prescribed the stool surfactant docusate sodium (Colace). Which assessment data indicate the medication is effective?
    1. The client has a bowel movement within 8 hours.
    2. The client has soft, brown stools.
    3. The client has a soft, nontender abdomen.
    4. The client has bowel sounds in all four quadrants.

36. The 62-year-old client suspected of having diverticulosis is scheduled for a colonoscopy and is prescribed sodium biphosphate (Fleets Phospho-Soda) the night before the procedure. Which priority intervention should the nurse implement prior to the procedure?
    1. Assess the client's skin turgor and oral mucosa.
    2. Initiate intravenous therapy for the client.
    3. Determine if the client has iodine allergies.
    4. Monitor the client's bowel movements.

37. The client is prescribed a bulk-forming agent. Which statement best describes the scientific rationale for administering this medication?
    1. The medication acts by lubricating the stool and the colon mucosa.
    2. Bulk-forming agents irritate the bowel to increase peristalsis.
    3. The medication causes more water and fat to be absorbed into the stool.
    4. Bulk-forming agents absorb water, which adds size to the fecal mass.

38. The elderly female client with diverticulosis is taking docusate calcium (Surfak), a stool softener, daily. The client tells the clinic nurse that her daughter has her taking the herb cascara every day. Which action should the nurse take?
    1. Instruct the client to quit taking the herb immediately.
    2. Explain that the herb will help the diverticulosis.
    3. Tell the client to have her daughter call the nurse.
    4. Advise the client to inform her health-care provider.

39. The client diagnosed with diverticulitis is requesting pain medication. Which intervention should the medical nurse implement first?
    1. Administer the client's pain medication as requested.
    2. Check the client's serum sodium and potassium level.
    3. Determine when the last pain medication was administered.
    4. Assess the client's bowel sounds and abdomen for tenderness.

40. The male client who has essential hypertension tells the clinic nurse he is taking the over-the-counter stool softener docusate sodium (Colace). Which priority action should the clinic nurse implement?
    1. Determine how often the client has a bowel movement.
    2. Discuss the importance of not taking this stool softener.
    3. Ask the client what was his last blood pressure reading.
    4. Obtain a stool specimen for an occult blood test.

A Client with Liver Failure

41. The client in end-stage liver failure has an elevated ammonia level. The health-care provider prescribes lactulose (Cephulac), a laxative. Which intervention should the nurse implement to determine the effectiveness of the medication?
    1. Monitor the client's intake and output.
    2. Assess the client's neurological status.
    3. Measure the client's abdominal girth.
    4. Document the number of bowel movements.

42. The client in end-stage liver failure is prescribed neomycin sulfate. Which statement best describes the scientific rationale for administering this medication?
    1. Neomycin sulfate helps lower the hepatic venous pressure.
    2. It helps increase the excretion of fluid through the kidneys.
    3. Neomycin is administered to help prevent a systemic infection.
    4. It reduces the number of ammonia-forming bacteria in the bowel.

43. The client in end-stage liver failure is prescribed vitamin K. The client asks the nurse, "Why do I have to take vitamin K?" Which statement is the nurse's best response?
1. "It will help your blood to clot so you won't have spontaneous bleeding."
2. "It may help prevent eye and skin changes along with night blindness."
3. "Vitamin K helps prevent skin and mucus membrane lesions."
4. "It prevents a complication called Wernicke-Korsakoff psychosis."

44. The client in end-stage liver failure is experiencing esophageal bleeding. The health-care provider has prescribed vasopressin (Pitressin). Which statement is the scientific rationale for administering this medication?
1. It lowers portal pressure by venodilation and decreased cardiac output.
2. Vasopressin produces constriction of the splanchnic arterial bed.
3. This medication causes vasoconstriction of the coronary arteries.
4. Vasopressin causes the liver to decrease in size and vascularity.

45. The nurse is preparing to administer medications to the following clients. To which client would the nurse question administering the medication?
1. Lactulose (Cephulac), a laxative, to a client who has an ammonia level of 50 μg/dL.
2. Furosemide (Lasix), a loop diuretic, to a client who has a potassium level of 3.7 mEq/L.
3. Spironolactone (Aldactone), a potassium-sparing diuretic, to a client with a potassium level of 5.9 mEq/L.
4. Vasopressin (Pitressin) to a client with a serum sodium level of 137 mEq/L.

46. The client in end-stage liver failure is being admitted to the medical floor. Which health-care provider's order would the nurse question?
1. Prepare the client for a paracentesis.
2. Administer vitamin C 100 mg po daily.
3. Administer morphine 2 mg IVP for pain.
4. Give D_5W 0.9 NS at 25 mL/hour.

47. The client with esophageal varices undergoes endoscopic sclerotherapy. Which post-procedure intervention will the nurse implement?
1. Administer the proton-pump inhibitor omeprazole (Prilosec).
2. Do not allow the client to eat or drink anything for 24 hours.
3. Administer promethazine (Phenergan), an antiemetic.
4. Administer the antacid aluminum hydroxide (Maalox).

48. The client in end-stage liver failure is complaining of pruritus. Which information should the nurse discuss with the client?
1. Encourage the client to sit in a hot spa before going to bed.
2. Instruct the client to not use emollients or lotions on the skin.
3. Explain the need to take the prescribed antihistamine as directed.
4. Apply hydrocortisone 1.0% cream to the affected areas.

49. The client in end-stage liver failure is taking the laxative lactulose (Cephulac). Which statement indicates the client needs more teaching concerning this medication?
1. "I will notify my doctor if I have any watery diarrhea."
2. "If I get nauseated, I will quit taking the lactulose."
3. "I will take my lactulose with fruit juice."
4. "I should have two or three soft stools a day."

50. The client in end-stage liver failure with ascites is prescribed spironolactone (Aldactone). Which interventions should the nurse implement? Select all that apply.
1. Check the serum potassium level.
2. Weigh the client daily at the same time.
3. Assess the client's bowel sounds.
4. Monitor the client's intake and output.
5. Monitor the client's abdominal girth.

A Client with Hepatitis

51. The public health nurse is administering the hepatitis A vaccine to a client. Which statement indicates the client understands the medication teaching about the vaccine?
    1. "I will not need to have another dose of the vaccine."
    2. "I will notify the clinic if there is pain at the injection site."
    3. "This vaccine will provide long-term protection against hepatitis A."
    4. "This medication will be injected in my buttocks."

52. The employee health nurse is preparing to administer the first dose of hepatitis B vaccine to an employee. Which question would be most important for the nurse to ask the employee before administering this medication?
    1. "Do you have any known allergies to medications?"
    2. "Are you allergic to yeast or any type of yeast products?"
    3. "Have you ever had an allergic reaction to egg yolks?"
    4. "Are you allergic to any type of milk or milk products?"

53. The client exposed to hepatitis A calls the clinic and wants to know if anything can be done to prevent getting hepatitis A. Which information should the nurse tell the client?
    1. Explain that there is a hepatitis A vaccine available that the client can receive.
    2. Inform the client that there is nothing available to help prevent hepatitis A.
    3. Instruct the client to get an immune globulin injection within 2 weeks.
    4. Tell the client to go to the nearest emergency department as soon as possible.

54. The client diagnosed with chronic hepatitis C who is taking interferon alfacon (Infergen), an antiviral medication, reports having fever, muscle pain, and headaches to the nurse. Which action should the nurse take?
    1. Instruct the client to taper off the medications immediately.
    2. Encourage the client to take acetaminophen (Tylenol).
    3. Explain that the client will just have to live with these side effects.
    4. Recommend that the client see the health-care provider.

55. The client tells the nurse, "I would like to get the vaccine for hepatitis C." Which response would be most appropriate by the nurse?
    1. "There is no vaccination against hepatitis C."
    2. "The vaccination must be administered in two doses."
    3. "Have you received the hepatitis B vaccination?"
    4. "Why are you interested in receiving this vaccine?"

56. The male client diagnosed with chronic hepatitis C tells the nurse that he is taking the herb St. John's wort for depression. Which action should the nurse implement?
    1. Tell the client to quit taking the herb immediately.
    2. Document the information and take no action.
    3. Encourage the client to take a prescribed antidepressant.
    4. Determine if the herb has hepatotoxic properties.

57. The public health nurse notified a young woman that one of her sexual contacts was positive for hepatitis B. The woman denied ever having hepatitis B or having received the hepatitis B vaccinations. Which information is most important for the nurse to discuss with the woman?
    1. Instruct the woman not to have unprotected sexual intercourse.
    2. Advise the woman not to drink any type of alcoholic beverage.
    3. Tell the woman to get hepatitis B immune globulin (HBIG).
    4. Encourage the client to get the hepatitis B vaccination.

58. The male client with chronic hepatitis C is being prescribed ribavirin (Virazole), an antiviral medication. Which information should the nurse discuss with the client?
    1. Discuss the importance of using two reliable forms of birth control.
    2. Explain the need to eat a diet high in vitamin K during treatment.
    3. Instruct the client to avoid direct sunlight for long periods.
    4. Teach the client that the medication might cause temporary impotence.

59. The clinic nurse is preparing to administer the hepatitis B vaccine to the client. Which information should the nurse discuss with the client?
    1. Instruct the client to come back to the clinic in 2 months for the last injection.
    2. Teach the client not to wash the injection site for at least 24 hours.
    3. Encourage the client to rotate the arms when receiving the hepatitis B vaccine.
    4. Explain that the client must have two more doses of the vaccine at 1 and 6 months.

60. The client who is homeless comes to the free clinic. During the interview the client admits to using illegal intravenous drugs. Which intervention would the nurse recommend to the client?
    1. Recommend the combined hepatitis A and B vaccine (Twinrix).
    2. Recommend the client receive the hepatitis B vaccination.
    3. Recommend the client go to the county rehabilitation center.
    4. Recommend that the client receive the HIV vaccination.

A Child with Gastroenteritis

61. The pediatric clinic nurse is assessing the 4-year-old child with gastroenteritis. The mother tells the nurse that she has been using bilberry herbs to help the child. Which statement would assess the effectiveness of the herb?
    1. "Did your child vomit after you administered the bilberry?"
    2. "Does this herb help your child's allergy to milk and milk products?"
    3. "What was the child's temperature when you administered the herb?"
    4. "How many diarrhea stools has your child had since taking the bilberry?"

62. The child diagnosed with infectious gastroenteritis is prescribed Bactrim, a sulfa antibiotic, 10 mg/kg/day in divided doses twice a day. The child weighs 60 pounds. The medication comes 100 mg/5 mL. How many milliliters will the nurse administer with the morning dose?
    Answer _____

63. The child with chronic kidney infections develops *Clostridium difficile*. Which medication would the nurse administer first to decrease the amount of diarrhea?
    1. Penicillin (Ampicillin), an antibiotic.
    2. Cholestyramine (Questran), an antilipemic.
    3. Trimethoprim sulfa (Bactrim), a sulfa drug.
    4. Diphenoxylate (Lomotil), an antidiarrheal.

64. The 3-year-old child weighing 37.5 pounds is diagnosed with mild to moderate diarrhea and placed on oral replacement therapy (ORT). Which information should the nurse teach the parent?
    1. "Try to get your child to drink about 1000 mL of Pedialyte over 4 hours."
    2. "The child should drink 100 mL of homemade rice water every 2 hours."
    3. "Get the child to drink apple juice or a lemon-lime soda every 3–4 hours."
    4. "Do not let the child eat any solid foods for a few days. Just give the liquids."

65. The HCP wrote an order for "0.33% dextrose solution IV" for a 6-year-old child diagnosed with gastroenteritis. Which interventions should the nurse implement? Select all that apply.
    1. Monitor the serum sodium and potassium levels.
    2. Check the fontanels for the hydration status.
    3. Discuss the order with the health-care provider.
    4. Use a chamber infusion device on the IV pump.
    5. Assess the intravenous site every hour.

66. The child diagnosed with gastroenteritis is scheduled for an endoscopic examination of the stomach and duodenum. Which intervention is priority for the nurse assisting with the procedure?
    1. Watch the screen for abnormal data.
    2. Hand the physician the instruments.
    3. Monitor the child's respiratory status.
    4. Clean the instruments between clients.

67. The 8-year-old child diagnosed with gastroenteritis is admitted to the pediatric unit. The nurse administered prochlorperazine (Compazine), an antiemetic, rectally. Which side effects should the nurse assess for?
    1. Nausea, vomiting, and diarrhea.
    2. Tremors, involuntary twitching, and restlessness.
    3. Diplopia, ptosis, and urinary retention.
    4. Myalgias, hallucinations, and weakness.

68. The 10-year-old client is diagnosed with an *Escherichia coli* infection after being at a day camp. Which discharge instructions should the nurse teach the parent?
    1. Give the child an antiemetic suppository before each meal.
    2. Have anyone in contact with the child wear a mask.
    3. Be sure the child takes all the antibiotic medication.
    4. Administer an antidiarrheal after each loose stool.

69. Which is the scientific rationale for administering acidophilus capsules to a child diagnosed with a Shigella infection?
    1. The acidophilus capsule will treat the Shigella infection.
    2. The acidophilus will help the child develop an immunity to Shigella.
    3. The acidophilus will prevent a complication of the antibiotics.
    4. The acidophilus is the antibiotic of choice for Shigella.

70. The toddler diagnosed with rotavirus is admitted to the hospital. Which intervention should the nurse implement?
    1. Schedule the antibiotic for around-the-clock dosing.
    2. Teach the parent to discard the diapers in a biohazard can.
    3. Initiate intravenous fluids with a controlled chamber device.
    4. Administer the rotavirus vaccine in the toddler's thigh.

A Client Who Is Obese

71. The client who is obese is prescribed medication therapy to aid in weight reduction. Which information should the nurse teach the client?
    1. While taking the medications, the client does not need to limit caloric intake.
    2. The medications cannot be taken with antihypertensive medications.
    3. The medications will not result in the loss of large amounts of weight.
    4. The client will be taking the medications for 2–3 weeks at a time.

72. The client with a body mass index (BMI) of 35 is prescribed sibutramine (Meridia), an antiobesity medication. Which statement is the scientific rationale for prescribing this medication?
    1. Sibutramine works by increasing the production of thyroid hormone.
    2. Sibutramine works by treating the depression associated with obesity.
    3. Sibutramine works by causing diarrhea and weight loss through the bowel.
    4. Sibutramine works by suppressing the client's appetite.

73. The client is prescribed orlistat (Xenical), a lipase inhibitor. Which statement by the client indicates the client requires more teaching?
    1. "It does not matter what I eat because I will still lose weight."
    2. "I will limit the amount of fat in my diet to 30%."
    3. "I may need to take Metamucil daily with the orlistat."
    4. "I will take a daily multivitamin supplement."

74. The client diagnosed with Type 2 diabetes mellitus and a body mass index (BMI) of 29 is prescribed the hormone leptin. Which intervention should the nurse implement?
1. Administer the medication subcutaneously in the deltoid.
2. Determine if the client is taking OTC oral leptin supplements.
3. Have an EpiPen ready for possible allergic reaction.
4. Teach that flulike symptoms are a side effect of leptin.

75. The female client tells the clinic nurse that she has been taking Dexedrine, an over-the-counter medication, for weight loss. Which statement would be the nurse's best response?
1. "This is a dangerous medication and you should not take it."
2. "What other things have you tried to lose weight?"
3. "Your HCP can prescribe a better weight loss program."
4. "Tell me how you feel about being overweight."

76. Which medication would be the most appropriate medication for the client who is obese who is trying to quit smoking?
1. Orlistat (Xenical), a lipase inhibitor.
2. Sibutramine (Meridia), an appetite suppressant.
3. Bupropion (Zyban), an antidepressant.
4. Olestra (Olean), a fat substitute.

77. The nurse is discussing weight loss therapy with a client who is obese who has been prescribed sibutramine (Meridia). Which information should the nurse provide? Select all that apply.
1. Do not take Meridia on an empty stomach.
2. Exercise for 20 minutes 3–4 times a week.
3. An appropriate goal is a 1–2–pound loss weekly.
4. Meridia can cause orthostatic hypotension.
5. Do not take OTC cold remedies while taking Meridia.

78. The client who is obese is participating in an investigational study using metformin (Glucophage), a biguanide antidiabetic medication, for weight loss. Which data should the nurse monitor?
1. The hemoglobin A_1C every 2 months.
2. Daily fasting glucose levels.
3. The urine ketones every 2 weeks.
4. The client's weight every month.

79. The client taking orlistat (Xenical), a lipase inhibitor, reports copious frothy diarrhea stools. What would the nurse suspect is the cause of the diarrhea?
1. The client has consumed an excessive amount of fats.
2. The client is also taking a lipid-lowering medication.
3. This is a desired effect of the medication.
4. The client has developed a chronic bowel syndrome.

80. The nurse is administering morning medications. Which medication would the nurse question administering?
1. Bupropion (Zyban), an antidepressant, to a client who has chronic obstructive pulmonary disease (COPD).
2. Meperidine (Demerol), a narcotic analgesic, to a client who has had gastric bypass surgery for obesity.
3. Loperamide (Imodium), an antidiarrheal, to a client who has irritable bowel syndrome (IBS).
4. Sibutramine (Meridia), an appetite suppressant, to a client receiving fluoxetine (Prozac) for depression.

A Client Experiencing Constipation or Diarrhea

81. The elderly client is discussing complaints of constipation with the clinic nurse. The client tells the nurse, "I take a laxative every day so that I will have a bowel movement every day." Which statement should the nurse respond to first?
    1. "Do you have heart problems or diabetes?"
    2. "Have you ever had a rash or itching when you took a laxative?"
    3. "You should not use laxatives every day."
    4. "Most people don't have to have bowel movements daily."

82. The client is complaining of not having a bowel movement in 4 days and is having abdominal discomfort. Which intervention should the nurse recommend to the client?
    1. Instruct the client to take methylcellulose (Citrucel), a bulk-forming laxative.
    2. Encourage the client to make an appointment with the health-care provider.
    3. Explain to the client the need to take docusate sodium (Colace), a stool softener.
    4. Tell the client to take the lubricant laxative castor oil 2 hours after the next meal.

83. The client taking antibiotics calls the clinic and tells the nurse that the client has diarrhea. Which action should the nurse implement?
    1. Recommend the client take lactobacillus (Bacid), an antidiarrheal agent.
    2. Explain that this is a side effect of antibiotics and nothing can be done.
    3. Ask the client if he or she has had any type of bad-tasting or -smelling food.
    4. Instruct the client to quit taking the antibiotic for 24 hours, and then start taking again.

84. The female client calls the clinic complaining of diarrhea and reports that she just came back from vacation in Mexico. Which action should the nurse implement first?
    1. Instruct the client to take loperamide (Imodium), an antidiarrheal medication.
    2. Ask how long the client has had the diarrhea and when did she get back from Mexico.
    3. Explain that an antibiotic should be prescribed and that the client needs to see the HCP.
    4. Tell the client this is probably traveler's diarrhea and it will run its course.

85. The elderly client calls the clinic and is complaining of loose, watery stools. Which interventions should the nurse implement? Select all that apply.
    1. Instruct the client to take the antidiarrheal exactly as recommended.
    2. Recommend the client drink clear liquids only, such as tea or broth.
    3. Determine how long the client has been having the loose, watery stool.
    4. Tell the client to go to the emergency department as soon as possible.
    5. Ask the client what other medications he or she has taken in the last 24 hours.

86. The female nurse is working at a senior citizen center. She is giving a lecture on health-promotion activities for the elderly. Which information should the nurse discuss with the group to help prevent constipation?
    1. The antispasmodic dicyclomine (Bentyl), taken every morning with the breakfast meals, will help prevent constipation.
    2. Eating five to six small meals a day including low-residue foods will help prevent the development of constipation.
    3. Taking a daily stool softener along with daily exercise, increased fluids, and a high-fiber diet will help prevent constipation from developing.
    4. Elderly clients must have at least one bowel movement a day to prevent the development of constipation.

87. The client with diarrhea is taking diphenoxylate (Lomotil). Which intervention should the nurse discuss with the client?
    1. Instruct the client to take one pill after each loose stool until the diarrhea stops.
    2. Discuss the need to decrease fluid intake to help decrease loose, watery stool.
    3. Explain that the medication should be taken once a day for 1 week.
    4. Tell the client not to take more than eight tablets in a 24-hour period.

88. The client calls the clinic and reports large amounts of watery stool for the last 3 days. Which action should the clinic nurse implement?
    1. Instruct the client to take diphenoxylate (Lomotil) after each loose stool.
    2. Recommend the client eat some cheese or constipating-type food.
    3. Request that the client write down all foods ingested in the last 3 days.
    4. Make an appointment for the client to come to the clinic today.

89. The nurse is discussing the problem of constipation with an elderly client. Which information should the nurse discuss with the client concerning laxative abuse?
    1. Explain that stimulant laxatives, the chewing gum and chocolate types, are the kind most often abused.
    2. Discuss that laxative abuse can occur if the client takes bulk-forming laxatives on a daily basis.
    3. Tell the client that taking a Fleets enema daily will help prevent the client from becoming dependent on laxatives.
    4. Recommend to the client that eating a high-fiber diet and increasing fluid consumption will ensure the client will not get constipated.

90. The client is prescribed the stimulant laxative senna (Senokot) for constipation. The client calls the clinic and reports yellow-green–colored feces. Which action should the clinic nurse implement?
    1. Have the client come to the clinic immediately.
    2. Explain that this is a common side effect of Senokot.
    3. Instruct the client to get a stool specimen to bring to the clinic.
    4. Determine if the client has eaten any type of yellow or green food.

A Client Undergoing Abdominal Surgery with General Anesthesia

91. The day surgery nurse is admitting a client for repair of an inguinal hernia. Which information provided by the client would be important to report to the surgical team?
    1. The client has never had surgery before.
    2. The client is allergic to shellfish.
    3. The client has not eaten since midnight.
    4. The client had a sinus infection last month.

92. The client is being prepped for an open cholecystectomy. Which preoperative instructions would be important for the nurse to teach?
    1. There will be an upper-left abdominal incision.
    2. The client will be turned to the left side every hour.
    3. The client will be placed on total parenteral nutrition.
    4. Discuss pain medications and the 1–10 pain scale.

93. The client is scheduled for an exploratory laparotomy in the morning. Which order has priority?
    1. Prepare the preoperative injection for when the OR notifies the floor.
    2. Document the client's hemoglobin and hematocrit on the checklist.
    3. Be sure the client has taken the preoperative pHisoHex shower.
    4. Ambulate the client in the hallway at least two times.

94. The client who has had an abdominal surgery has returned from the post-anesthesia care unit (PACU) with a patient-controlled analgesia (PCA) pump. Which intervention should the nurse implement?
    1. Check the PCA setting with another nurse.
    2. Administer a bolus by pushing the button.
    3. Teach the family to push the button for the client.
    4. Change the cartridge with a new PCA medication.

95. The client had a general anesthetic for an abdominal surgery. When taking off the postoperative orders the charge nurse notes that there is no antiemetic medication ordered. Which action should the charge nurse take?
    1. Continue transcribing the orders and do nothing.
    2. Ask the anesthesiologist if the client was nauseated during surgery.
    3. Contact the surgeon and request an order for an antiemetic.
    4. Tell the client's nurse to notify the charge nurse if there is nausea.

96. The client in the post-anesthesia care unit (PACU) has an order for meperidine (Demerol), an opioid, 75 mg IVP every 2–3 hours PRN for pain. The nurse working in the PACU administers Demerol 50 mg IM and 25 mg IVP. How should the nurse chart the medication?
    1. Demerol administered IM and IVP, incident report completed.
    2. Demerol 50 mg IM in R gluteus maximus and 25 mg slow IVP.
    3. Demerol 75 mg administered by slow intravenous route.
    4. Demerol 25 mg IM in L ventrogluteal and 50 mg slow IVP.

97. The client who has had abdominal surgery has an IV at 150 mL/hour for 12 hours and two IVPBs of 50 mL each. How much fluid would the nurse document on the intake and output (I & O) record?
    Answer _____

98. The client is on call for surgery. Which order would the nurse implement when the operating room nurse notifies the floor that the orderly is on the way to pick up the client?
    1. Have the client sign the operative permit.
    2. Teach the client to turn, cough, and deep breathe.
    3. Notify the family to wait in the OR waiting room.
    4. Administer the preoperative antibiotic IVPB.

99. The client postgastrectomy has a patient-controlled analgesia (PCA) pump. Which data would require immediate intervention by the nurse?
    1. The client complains that the pain is still a "3."
    2. The client has serous drainage on the dressing.
    3. The client's has a T 99.2, P 78, R 10, and BP 110/82.
    4. The client splints the incision before trying to cough.

100. The client who had an elective cholecystectomy is receiving a prophylactic antibiotic. Which information indicates the medication is not working?
    1. The client's white blood cell (WBC) count is 18,000.
    2. The client refuses to turn, cough, and deep breathe.
    3. The client's sodium level is 139 mEq/L.
    4. The client's nasogastric tube has green drainage.

A Client with Gastroesophageal Reflux

1. 1. There are several classifications of medications used to treat acid reflux problems. Sometimes losing weight will help relieve symptoms, but the client did not ask about lifestyle modifications.
   2. **Proton-pump inhibitors, histamine$_2$ blockers, and antacids all treat the symptoms of acid reflux. The nurse should encourage the client to discuss which medication is best with the HCP.**
   3. The symptoms do not indicate cancer. The nurse should not scare the client.
   4. Acid reflux can lead to complications, including adult-onset asthma, that should be treated, but most HCPs will empirically treat the symptoms of acid reflux before ordering tests to determine the cause or possible complications.

2. 1. **A medication for a client on call to surgery is a priority; the client's surgery could be delayed if the medication has not been administered when the call to surgery comes.**
   2. This would be the second medication to administer; this client has a complaint of discomfort.
   3. This medication is a routine medication and could be administered at any time.
   4. This medication is a routine medication and could be administered at any time.

3. 1. Antacids, not proton-pump inhibitors, neutralize gastric secretions.
   2. Histamine$_2$ blockers block receptors on the parietal cells.
   3. **Proton-pump inhibitors inhibit the enzyme that generates gastric acid.**
   4. Mucosal barrier agents form a protective barrier against acid and pepsin.

4. 1. H$_2$ blockers actually block the production of gastric acid; they have a longer effect than an antacid.
   2. An increase in side effects would not be an advantage.
   3. Antacids are usually less expensive than H$_2$ blockers.
   4. **H$_2$ blockers require less frequent administration than do antacids, which require frequent administration, seven or more times a day, for therapeutic effects. The fewer times a client is expected to take a medication, the more likely the client is to comply with a medication regimen.**

5. 1. Tagamet is used to treat indigestion and heartburn (pyrosis).
   2. **Over time, Tagamet can cause males to become impotent, have decreased libido, and have breast development (gynecomastia).**
   3. Tagamet can cause lethargy and somnolence, not insomnia and hypervigilance.
   4. Tagamet is used to treat Zollinger-Ellison syndrome, a syndrome characterized by hypersecretion of gastric acid and the formation of peptic ulcers.

6. 1. This indicates client compliance with the dosing regimen for antacids, not that the medication is effective.
   2. The return of symptoms indicates the medication is not effective.
   3. **This indicates an improvement in symptoms and that the medication is effective.**
   4. Losing weight would not indicate that a medication for hiatal hernia is effective.

MEDICATION MEMORY JOGGER: The nurse determines the effectiveness of a medication by assessing for the symptoms, or lack thereof, for which the medication was prescribed.

7. 1. Nexium is an oral medication; an intravenous pump is not needed.
   2. The head of the bed, not the foot of the bed, would be elevated for the client to be able to swallow.
   3. Nexium is not a cephalosporin. The cephalosporins are a class of antibiotics.
   4. **The Joint Commission requires that two patient identifiers be used to determine the "right patient." Most health-care facilities use the client's name and date of birth as these identifiers.**

8. 1. There may be several complications of GERD. Adult-onset asthma and Barrett's esophagus leading to cancer of the esophagus are two complications of GERD. The chance of developing these problems is less if the GERD is adequately treated, but there are no guarantees.
   2. **The client should always be informed of what symptoms to report to the HCP.**
   3. The client should be instructed to sit upright for at least 60 minutes following a meal to prevent reflux from occurring.

4. NSAIDs can increase gastric distress. Ulcers caused by NSAID use may be asymptomatic, or the symptoms may be attributed to the GERD. The client should use the prescribed H$_2$ receptor blocker, proton-pump inhibitor, or an antacid to relieve the discomfort associated with GERD.

9. 1. Prophylactic antibiotics are frequently prescribed both presurgery and post-surgery. The client should be instructed to take all the medication as directed.
   2. Hiatal hernia repair may not last and the client should continue the recommended lifestyle modifications, such as eating small meals.
   3. Part of the lifestyle modifications for hiatal hernia is to limit pressure on the abdominal cavity, especially after a meal. Using the leg muscles to bend down, rather than bending over, should be taught to the client.
   4. Nexium is administered daily, not twice a day.
   5. For best relief, pain medication should be taken at the onset of the pain. The client should not wait until the pain is an 8–10 before taking the pain medication.

10. 1. Up to 90% of adult-onset asthma is the result of gastroesophageal reflux disease (GERD). Treating the gastric reflux will treat the asthma.
    2. The client is diagnosed with asthma, not an infection. There is no reason to administer an antibiotic.
    3. Antihistamines such as Claritin are used to treat allergic reactions to pollens, dust, or other irritating substances. They are not effective against asthma.
    4. Glucocorticoids are prescribed daily for clients with chronic lung diseases, such as emphysema or chronic bronchitis. A client with asthma would not be prescribed a daily steroid.

A Client with Inflammatory Bowel Disease

11. 1. The client should notify the health-care provider if undissolved tablets or capsules are found in the stool because this is not expected.
    2. This medication can be taken with or without food; food does not affect the effectiveness of the medication.

3. There are no restrictions on foods, beverages, or activities when taking this medication unless the health-care provider directs otherwise.
4. **The tablets must be swallowed whole because they are specially formulated to release the medication after it has passed through the stomach.**

12. 1. Increasing fluid intake dilutes the drug, which helps to prevent crystalluria (crystals in the urine) from occurring.
    2. The medication is administered every 6–8 hours, not once a day.
    3. Instruct the client to report any bruising or bleeding because it could be a sign of a drug-induced blood disorder (agranulocytosis).
    4. This medication will not cause fat, frothy stools; therefore, the nurse does not need to assess the stool.

13. 1. Azathioprine can cause a decrease in the number of blood cells in the bone marrow (agranulocytosis). Signs or symptoms that would warrant intervention by the nurse include sore throat, fever, chills, unusual bleeding or bruising, pale skin, headache, confusion, tachycardia, insomnia, and shortness of breath.
    2. Ten to 20 loose watery stools a day are characteristic of an acute exacerbation of ulcerative colitis and would not warrant intervention by the nurse secondary to the medication.
    3. Abdominal pain and tenderness are characteristic of an acute exacerbation of ulcerative colitis and would not warrant intervention by the nurse secondary to the medication.
    4. Dehydration may occur with ulcerative colitis, but it does not warrant intervention by the nurse secondary to the medication.

MEDICATION MEMORY JOGGER: If the client verbalizes a complaint or if the nurse's assessment data or laboratory data indicates an adverse effect secondary to a medication, the nurse must intervene. The nurse must implement an independent intervention or notify the health-care provider because medications can result in serious or even life-threatening complications.

14. 1. TPN is 50% dextrose; therefore, the client's blood glucose level should be

checked every 6 hours; sliding-scale regular insulin coverage is usually ordered.

2. TPN should always be administered using an intravenous pump and not via gravity; fluid volume resulting from an overload of TPN could cause a life-threatening hyperglycemic crisis.

3. TPN must be administered via a subclavian line because a peripheral line will collapse as a result of the hyperosmolarity of the TPN and phlebitis may occur.

4. TPN is considered a medication and should be administered as any other medication.

5. The client with severe acute exacerbation of Crohn's is NPO to rest the bowel. When on TPN, the client is usually NPO because the TPN provides all necessary nutrients; therefore, the nurse would not encourage the client to eat food.

15. 1. The client should not quit taking the medication abruptly because that would result in an acute exacerbation of the inflammatory bowel disease.

2. A PPI will not help treat these symptoms.

3. **These are side effects of the medication, and the HCP should be notified, but the client should not stop taking the medication.**

4. These symptoms will not resolve with time and should be reported to the HCP.

16. 1. The client should not take an antacid with this medication because it will decrease the absorption rate of the medication.

2. Any type of rash should be considered a possible allergic reaction and should be reported to the health-care provider immediately.

3. The client should drink several quarts of water a day to prevent the formation of crystals in the urine, but a strict record of urinary output is not required or needed.

4. **The client should avoid direct sunlight, use sunblock, and wear protective clothing to decrease the risk of photosensitivity reactions to the medication.**

17. 1. **TPN must be tapered off because of its high glucose content; if TPN is not tapered, the client may experience hypoglycemia. Therefore, the nurse should call the HCP to request an order to taper the TPN.**

2. TPN must be tapered; therefore, the nurse should not discontinue the TPN abruptly.

3. If the nurse is not going to implement the order as written, the nurse should notify the HCP immediately and not wait for the HCP to make rounds. TPN is a medication and the client should not be taking it any longer than necessary.

4. The pharmacist cannot change a health-care provider's order; therefore, there is no reason for the nurse to talk to the pharmacist.

18. 1. There is no indication that sulfasalazine is hepatotoxic; therefore, liver function tests do not need to be monitored when administering this medication.

2. The serum potassium level is not affected by sulfasalazine; therefore, the nurse does not need to monitor this laboratory data.

3. **Sulfasalazine is insoluble in acid urine and can cause crystalluria and hematuria, resulting in kidney damage. Therefore, the nurse should monitor the serum creatinine level, which is normally 0.5 to 1.5 mg/dL.**

4. Sulfasalazine may cause abnormal bleeding and bruising, but the INR is monitored for clients taking the oral anticoagulant warfarin (Coumadin).

MEDICATION MEMORY JOGGER: The nurse must be knowledgeable about accepted standards of practice for medication administration, including which client assessment data and laboratory data should be monitored prior to and during the use of the medication.

19. 1. The suppository should be retained for 1–3 hours if possible to get the maximum benefit of the medication.

2. **The client should use caution when using the suppository because it may stain clothing, flooring, painted surfaces, vinyl, enamel, marble, granite, and other surfaces. This statement indicates the client understands the teaching.**

3. The medication should be stored at room temperature away from moisture and heat.

4. The client should empty the bowel just before inserting the rectal suppository.

20. 1. Prednisone may increase the glucose level, but no matter what the glucose level, the nurse must administer the

medication; therefore, this is not the priority intervention.

2. Long-term side effects occur, but teaching about them is not priority when administering the medication.

3. **Steroids are notorious for causing gastric irritation that may result in peptic ulcers; therefore, administering the prednisone with food is priority.**

4. Tapering the medication is important, but it is not priority when administering the medication.

A Client with Peptic Ulcer Disease

21. 1. **A 29-year-old female is of childbearing age. The nurse should determine that the client is not pregnant before administering this medication. Misoprostol can be used in a combination with mifepristone to produce an abortion.**

2. Prilosec is prescribed to treat duodenal and gastric ulcers; the nurse would not question this medication.

3. The potassium level is within normal range (3.5–5.5 mEq/L); the nurse would not question this medication.

4. Tylenol is frequently administered for headaches; the nurse would not question this medication.

MEDICATION MEMORY JOGGER: Whenever an age is mentioned in the stem of the question or in the answer options, one or more of the ages will be important. The only option that gives the test taker a clue regarding the correct answer is the 29 year old, and the test taker should also note that it is a female client. Twenty-nine-year-old females are of childbearing age, so the nurse has two potential clients to consider.

22. 1. Clients with congestive heart failure are limited in the amount of sodium they should consume. Sodium bicarbonate has sodium as an ingredient.

2. Amphogel is not a low-sodium preparation. This client requires a low-sodium antacid.

3. **Riopan is the antacid of choice for clients who need to limit their sodium intake.**

4. Mylanta is not a low-sodium preparation. This client requires a low-sodium antacid.

MEDICATION MEMORY JOGGER: The nurse must always be aware of comorbid conditions when administering medications. The two key words or phrases in this question are "severe congestive heart failure" and "indigestion."

23. 1. This is information to teach when the client is taking antihypertensive medications, not NSAIDs.

2. **A life-threatening complication of NSAID use is the development of gastric ulcers that can hemorrhage; dizziness and lightheadedness could indicate a bleeding problem. The client has been taking the medications "around the clock," indicating use during the night when it would be unusual for the client to consume food along with the medication.**

3. NSAID medications should be taken with food or something to coat the stomach lining, but this client is symptomatic and should be seen by an HCP.

4. There is no reason to suggest a change in NSAID; the nurse should be concerned that the client has developed an NSAID-produced ulcer.

24. 1. The client has peptic ulcer disease (PUD), not gastroesophageal reflux disease (GERD), for which elevating the head of the bed would be recommended.

2. The client's ulcer is caused by a bacterial infection, not NSAID use. The client should limit use of NSAIDs until the ulcer has healed to prevent complicating the healing process, but the client should be able to use NSAID medications once the *H. pylori* infection has been treated.

3. Smoking decreases prostaglandin production and results in decreased protection of the mucosal lining. Smoking should be stopped, not decreased.

4. ***H. pylori* is a bacterial infection that is treated with a combination of medications. At least two antibiotics and an antisecretory medication will be ordered. As with all antibiotic prescriptions, the client should be taught to take all the medications as ordered. Resistant strains of *H. pylori* are being documented in clients who have not been compliant with the treatment program.**

25. 1. *H. pylori* is a bacterial infection. Zantac is not an antibiotic and would not prevent an infection.

2. In this situation, Zantac or a proton-pump inhibitor would be administered to all clients, not just those with a history of ulcer disease.

3. Because of the fluid shifts that occur as a result of severe burn injuries, the blood supply to the gastrointestinal tract is diminished while the stress placed on the body increases the gastric acid secretion, leading to gastric ulcers, a condition called Curling's ulcer. Zantac would be administered to decrease the production of gastric acid.

4. The nurse should request an H_2 receptor blocker or a proton-pump inhibitor if one is not ordered; the nurse would not question the order.

26. 1. **Milk of Magnesia is the most potent antacid, but it is usually used as a laxative because of the actions of magnesium hydroxide on the bowel. A combination antacid—magnesium hydroxide (produces diarrhea) and aluminum hydroxide (produces constipation)—is preferred to balance the side effects.**

2. The nurse can answer the client's question. It is only necessary to discuss this with the health-care provider if antacids are not resolving the client's complaints of indigestion.

3. The Milk of Magnesia is causing the problem, and changing antacids should resolve the situation.

4. Most clients are concerned about diarrhea, and the nurse should be concerned about fluid and electrolyte imbalances resulting from diarrhea.

27. 1. The client would need an intravenous proton-pump inhibitor at first and then later could be changed to an oral PPI. The client may also need a nasogastric tube or to be NPO. This client has a very low hemoglobin and hematocrit level, indicating active bleeding and the need for a fast route for the delivery of fluids and medications.

2. The nurse should observe the stool for color (black) and consistency (tarry) indicating blood, but this is not the first action.

3. This client has very low blood counts; is at risk for shock; and should be assessed for hypotension, tachycardia, and cold clammy skin. The client will

need fluid and blood cell replacement. The nurse should start the IV as soon as possible.

4. The client should have a bedside commode for safety, but it is not the first intervention. Prevention of or treating shock is the first intervention.

MEDICATION MEMORY JOGGER: The stem told the test taker the client's hemoglobin and hematocrit levels, which were levels indicating a "crisis" situation. The first step in many crises is to make sure that an IV access is available to administer fluids and medications.

28. **50 gtts per minute.** The nurse must first determine the rate per hour; 20 minutes into 60 minutes equals 3 (20-minute time segments).
50 mL of fluid multiplied by 3 equals 150 mL per hour.
150 divided by 60 equals 2.5 mL/min to infuse.
2.5 multiplied by 20 equals 50 gtts per minute.

29. 1. Flagyl is administered in combination with Pepto Bismol, Prevacid, and one other antibiotic to treat PUD; the nurse would not question this medication.

2. Pepto Bismol is administered in combination with Flagyl, Prevacid, and one other antibiotic to treat PUD; the nurse would not question this medication.

3. Prevacid is administered with a combination of antibiotics to treat PUD; the nurse would not question this medication.

4. Sucralfate (Carafate) is a mucosal barrier agent and must be administered on an empty stomach for the medication to coat the stomach lining. The nurse should question the time the medication is scheduled for and arrange for the medication to be administered at 0730.

30. 1. A lack of epigastric pain would indicate the medication is effective. The question asks for which data indicates the medication is not effective.

2. A hemoglobin of 15 g/dL and hematocrit of 44% are within normal limits and would indicate that the client is not bleeding as a result of the ulcer.

3. Clients who experience a gastric ulcer lose weight because of the pain associated with eating. A weight gain would indicate less

pain and the client being able to consume nutrients.

4. The client has a rapid pulse and low blood pressure, which indicate shock. This could be caused by hemorrhage from the ulcer. This client's treatment has not been effective.

MEDICATION MEMORY JOGGER: The nurse determines the effectiveness of a medication by assessing for the symptoms, or lack thereof, for which the medication was prescribed.

An Elderly Client with Diverticulosis/Diverticulitis

31. 1. This is a question that the nurse could ask the client, but it is not specific or important to ask for a client taking Metamucil; therefore, it is not the most important question to ask the client.
    2. **Bulk laxatives can swell and cause obstruction of the esophagus; therefore, the most important question to ask the client is if he or she has difficulty swallowing. If the client has difficulty swallowing, the nurse should question the client taking Metamucil.**
    3. Fiber helps decrease constipation, but fiber does not affect the effectiveness of Metamucil; therefore, it is not the most important question the nurse should ask the client.
    4. Metamucil may cause abdominal cramping, but abdominal tenderness is not pertinent information regarding taking a bulk laxative daily; therefore, it is not the most important question for the nurse to ask the client.

32. 1. The white blood cell count is monitored to determine the effectiveness of the medication and would not be checked prior to administering the first dose of the antibiotic medication.
    2. The nurse should monitor the client's vital signs, especially the temperature, but it would not affect the nurse administering the first dose of antibiotics.
    3. **Antibiotics are notorious for causing allergic reactions, and the nurse should make sure the client is not allergic to any antibiotics prior to administering this medication. Therefore, this is the first intervention.**
    4. Stool specimens are sent to the laboratory to detect ova or parasites. Diverticulitis is not the result of ova or parasites; therefore, there is no need for the client to have a stool specimen sent to the laboratory.

33. 1. **The client should be NPO and not have any fecal matter going through an inflamed descending and sigmoid bowel; therefore, the nurse would question administering a stimulant laxative, which would cause the client to have a bowel movement.**
    2. Because the client is NPO, a nasogastric tube is inserted to remove gastric acid and decompress the bowel.
    3. The client would have pain medication; therefore, this order would not be questioned.
    4. Because the client is NPO the nurse would not question an order for intravenous fluids.

MEDICATION MEMORY JOGGER: The nurse must be knowledgeable about accepted standards of practice for disease processes and conditions. If the nurse administers a medication the health-care provider has prescribed and it harms the client, the nurse could be held accountable. Remember that the nurse is a client advocate.

34. 1. Abdominal cramping is expected when this medication is first started; therefore, the client would not need to notify the HCP.
    2. It takes 2–3 days after the initial dose for the medication to work.
    3. **Esophageal or intestinal obstruction may result if the client does not take in adequate amounts of fluid with the medication.**
    4. When taking this medication, the client should increase dietary fiber, such as whole grains, fibrous fruits, and vegetables.

35. 1. A stool surfactant or softener does not stimulate a bowel movement.
    2. **Colace is a stool softener; if the client has soft brown stools, the medication is effective.**
    3. The abdomen should be soft and nontender, but this does not indicate that the medication is effective.
    4. The client should have bowel sounds in all four quadrants of the abdomen, but this does not indicate the medication is effective.

MEDICATION MEMORY JOGGER: To determine if the medication is effective the nurse should think about why the medication is being administered. Consider what disease process or condition the medication is being prescribed to treat.

36. 1. In addition to being given an osmotic laxative, such as Fleets Phospho-Soda, the client will be NPO. This can lead to dehydration. Skin turgor and the condition of the oral mucosa should be monitored to assess for dehydration.
    2. The client will need an intravenous line, but it is not priority over assessing the client.
    3. Iodine is not used in a colonoscopy, so the nurse need not ask this question.
    4. The client should not be having any bowel movements at this time; the bowel should be cleaned out prior to the colonoscopy.

37. 1. Lubricating the stool and colon mucosa is the rationale for administering mineral oil.
    2. Irritating the bowel to increase peristalsis is the rationale for administering stimulants.
    3. Stool softeners or surfactants cause more water and fat to be absorbed into the stool.
    4. **Bulk-forming agents absorb water and swell, thus increasing the size of the fecal mass. The larger the fecal mass, the more the defecation reflex is stimulated and the passage of stool is promoted.**

38. 1. **When docusate and certain herbs, such as senna, cascara, rhubarb, or aloe, are taken simultaneously, it will increase their absorption and the risk of liver toxicity. The nurse should tell the client to stop taking the herb.**
    2. The herb will not help the diverticulitis and could cause complications.
    3. The nurse cannot talk to the client's daughter because of HIPAA regulations.
    4. The nurse can discuss herbs and prescribed medications with the client; there is no specific reason for the client to notify the HCP.

MEDICATION MEMORY JOGGER: Some herbal preparations are effective, some are not, and a few can be harmful or even deadly. If a client is taking an herbal supplement and a conventional medicine, the nurse should investigate to determine if the herb will interact with the conventional medicine or in any way possibly cause harm to the client. The nurse should always be the client's advocate.

39. 1. The nurse should not administer pain medication without first assessing the client for any complications.
    2. Electrolyte levels do not need to be monitored prior to administering pain medication for clients with diverticulitis.
    3. The nurse should determine when the next pain medication could be administered, but the first intervention is always assessing the client.
    4. **The nurse must assess the client to determine if the pain is pain expected with diverticulitis or if it is a result of a complication of diverticulitis, such as bowel obstruction or bowel perforation. Remember that the first intervention is assessment.**

MEDICATION MEMORY JOGGER: Remember that pain may be expected as a result of the disease process or the condition, but it may also indicate a complication. Assessment is the first intervention when addressing the client's complaints of pain.

40. 1. Stool softeners do not increase the number of bowel movements; they make the stool softer and easier to pass. Therefore, determining how often the client has a bowel movement is not priority.
    2. **A client with essential hypertension would be on a low-sodium diet; docusate sodium (Colace) should not be given to clients on sodium restriction.**
    3. The client's current blood pressure should be assessed; the client's last blood pressure would not be priority.
    4. There is nothing to indicate that the client is at risk for gastrointestinal bleeding; therefore, this is not a priority intervention.

A Client with Liver Failure

41. 1. Lactulose will not affect the client's urinary output.
    2. **An elevated ammonia level affects the client's neurological status. Lactulose is prescribed to remove ammonia through the intestinal tract. Assessing the client's neurological status will determine the effectiveness of the medication.**

3. Lactulose is not administered to treat the client's ascites; therefore, measuring the abdominal girth will not help determine the effectiveness of lactulose.

4. Lactulose is a laxative and will cause the client to have bowel movements, but the bowel movements will not determine the effectiveness of this medication.

MEDICATION MEMORY JOGGER: The nurse determines the effectiveness of a medication by assessing for the symptoms, or lack thereof, for which the medication was prescribed.

42. 1. Neomycin does not help reduce hepatic venous pressure.
   2. Diuretics, not the antibiotic neomycin, help increase the excretion of fluid through the kidneys.
   3. Neomycin is an antibiotic, but it is not administered to help prevent a systemic infection.
   4. **Neomycin sulfate is administered to help reduce the ammonia level by reducing the number of ammonia-forming bacteria in the bowel.**

43. 1. **End-stage liver failure causes inadequate absorption of vitamins. Vitamin K deficiency results in hypoprothrombinemia, which results in spontaneous bleeding and ecchymosis.**
   2. Night blindness and eye and skin changes result from a deficiency of vitamin A, not of vitamin K.
   3. Skin and mucous membrane lesions are caused by deficiency of riboflavin and pyridoxine, not of vitamin K.
   4. This psychosis, along with beriberi and polyneuritis, results from a deficiency of thiamine, not of vitamin K.

44. 1. Venodilation is the scientific rationale for administering nitrates such as isosorbide (Isordil), not vasopressin.
   2. **Vasopressin is prescribed for a client with end-stage liver failure because it produces constriction of the splanchnic arterial bed, resulting in a decrease in portal pressure, which will help decrease esophageal bleeding. Vasopressin is administered intravenously or by intraarterial infusion.**
   3. Vasoconstriction of the coronary arteries is a side effect of vasopressin. It is treated by administering nitroglycerin in combination with the vasopressin.

4. Vasopressin does not affect the size or vascularity of the liver.

45. 1. The normal plasma ammonia level is 15–45 µg/dL (varies with method), and this client's level is above normal so the nurse would not question administering this medication, which is prescribed to remove ammonia from the intestinal tract.
   2. This client's potassium level is within normal limits (3.5–5.5 mEq/L); therefore, the nurse should not question the administration of the diuretic.
   3. **This client's potassium level is above normal level (3.5–5.5 mEq/L); therefore, the nurse should question administering this potassium-sparing diuretic.**
   4. This client's sodium level is within normal limits (135–145 mEq/L); therefore, the nurse would not question administering the medication. Clients taking vasopressin may, however, develop hyponatremia, or below-normal sodium levels.

MEDICATION MEMORY JOGGER: The nurse must be knowledgeable about accepted standards of practice for disease processes and conditions. If the nurse administers a medication the health-care provider has prescribed and it harms the client, the nurse could be held accountable. Remember that the nurse is a client advocate.

46. 1. Paracentesis is the removal of fluid (ascites) from the peritoneal cavity through a small incision or puncture through the abdominal wall under aseptic conditions. This would be an expected procedure for a client in end-stage liver failure.
   2. Liver failure causes a decrease in the absorption of vitamins; therefore, an order for vitamin C to help prevent hemorrhagic lesions of scurvy would be an expected order.
   3. **The client in end-stage liver failure would have hepatic encephalopathy, which affects the client's neurological status. Therefore, sedatives, tranquilizers, and analgesic medications are not administered to the client. The nurse would question this order.**
   4. Glucose is administered intravenously to clients with end-stage liver disease to minimize protein breakdown. Because the client is third spacing, the IV rate will be low.

47. 1. Proton-pump inhibitors are not routine medications prescribed after endoscopic sclerotherapy.
    2. The client does not have to be NPO for 24 hours after endoscopic sclerotherapy.
    3. Endoscopic sclerotherapy does not cause nausea or vomiting; therefore, there is no need to administer an antiemetic.
    4. **Antacids may be administered after the procedure to counteract the effect of gastric reflux.**

48. 1. The client should use warm water, rather than hot water, when bathing. Hot water increases pruritus.
    2. Emollient or lubricants should be used to keep the skin moist to prevent dry skin.
    3. **Antihistamines are prescribed to help the itching (pruritus) but should be used as directed because decreased liver function increases the risk for altered drug responses.**
    4. Hydrocortisone cream will not help this type of itching because the itching is not secondary to a rash or skin irritation. Severe jaundice with bile salt deposits on the skin causes the pruritus.

49. 1. Diarrhea indicates an overdose of the medication and the client should call the HCP for a decrease in the dosage; therefore, this comment indicates the client understands the teaching.
    2. **Although the drug may cause nausea, the client should keep taking it because it decreases the ammonia level. The nurse should instruct the client to take the medication with crackers or a soft drink, which may decrease the nausea. This statement indicates the client does not understand the medication teaching and needs more teaching.**
    3. To mask the sweet taste, lactulose can be diluted with fruit juice. This statement indicates the client understands the medication teaching.
    4. Having two to three soft stools a day indicates the medication is working to help decrease the ammonia level.

50. 1. **Aldactone addresses one of the causes of ascites, which is increased aldosterone levels that cause water retention. Aldactone is a potassium-sparing diuretic; therefore, the client should be monitored for hyperkalemia.**
    2. **Diuretics cause excretion of fluid, and a daily weight check is an excellent**

assessment of the effectiveness of the medication. Also, 1000 mL is approximately 1 pound.
    3. Diuretics do not affect the client's gastrointestinal system, so there is no need to monitor the client's bowel sounds.
    4. **Diuretics cause excretion of fluid, and intake and output levels evaluate the effectiveness of the diuretic therapy.**
    5. **Diuretic therapy is prescribed to help decrease ascites, which results from third spacing; assessing the abdominal girth will help determine if the medication is effective.**

A Client with Hepatitis

51. 1. Usually adults achieve immunity after one dose of the vaccine, but two doses are recommended for full protection.
    2. The nurse should inform the client that pain is expected at the injection site, and there is no reason to notify the clinic.
    3. **Hepatitis A vaccine provides long-term protection against hepatitis A infection, which is transmitted by the fecal–oral route via contaminated shellfish or other food or water and by direct contact with an infected person.**
    4. This vaccine is administered intramuscularly into the deltoid muscle.

52. 1. This is a question that a nurse should ask any client before giving a medication, but it is not the most important question when administering the hepatitis B vaccine.
    2. **A yeast-recombinant hepatitis B vaccine (Recombivax HB) is used to provide active immunity; therefore, the nurse should specifically ask the employee if he or she is allergic to yeast.**
    3. The hepatitis B vaccine is not made with egg yolks; therefore, this would not be an important question.
    4. The hepatitis B vaccine is not made with any type of milk; therefore, this would not be an important question.

MEDICATION MEMORY JOGGER: The nurse must be knowledgeable about accepted standards of practice for medication administration, including which client assessment data and laboratory data should be monitored prior to administering the medication.

53. 1. Once the client has been exposed to the hepatitis A virus, the hepatitis A vaccine will not help prevent the client from getting hepatitis A.
    2. This is providing incorrect information to the client because there is something available to prevent the client from getting hepatitis A.
    3. **This is correct information. An immune globulin injection within 2 weeks of exposure will help prevent the client from getting hepatitis A.**
    4. There is no reason for the client to go to the emergency department. The client can come to the clinic and receive the injection.

54. 1. Flulike symptoms, including fever, fatigue, myalgia, headache, and chills, are the most common side effects of Infergen and do not require discontinuing the medication.
    2. **Some of the flulike symptoms (fever, headache, myalgia) can be reduced with acetaminophen.**
    3. These flulike symptoms tend to diminish with continued therapy; therefore, the client will not have to live with these side effects.
    4. The nurse must be knowledgeable about the expected side effects of medications and is responsible for teaching the client. These side effects are common and the client does not need to see the health-care provider.

MEDICATION MEMORY JOGGER: If the client verbalizes a complaint, if the nurse assesses data, or if laboratory data indicates an adverse effect secondary to a medication, the nurse must intervene. The nurse must implement an independent intervention or notify the health-care provider because medications can result in serious or even life-threatening complications.

55. 1. **At this time, there is no vaccination for the prevention of hepatitis C; therefore, this is the nurse's best response.**
    2. There are vaccines to prevent hepatitis A and B, but there is no vaccination for hepatitis C.
    3. This question does not have any relevance to the client's request.
    4. This question may be construed as challenging by the client, and the nurse should give the client factual information.

56. 1. The nurse should first determine if the medication will affect liver function before telling the client to quit taking the medication. The herb may need to be tapered.
    2. The nurse should investigate to determine if the medication will damage the client's liver before taking any action.
    3. If the herb is treating the client's depression and is not hepatotoxic, then there is no reason for the client to take a prescribed antidepressant. Prescribed antidepressants may be hepatotoxic and usually cost more than herbs.
    4. **The nurse should advise the client to avoid substances (medications, herbs, illicit drugs, and toxins) that may affect liver function; therefore, the nurse should determine if St. John's wort is hepatotoxic.**

57. 1. This is information the woman should be told, but it is not priority at this time; getting the woman medical treatment for the virus is priority.
    2. This information should be discussed with the woman, but the most important intervention is to provide medical treatment.
    3. **Hepatitis B immune globulin (HBIG) provides passive immunity against hepatitis B and is indicated for people exposed to the hepatitis B virus who have never had hepatitis B and have never received the hepatitis B vaccination.**
    4. Prompt immunization with hepatitis B vaccine (within a few hours or days after exposure to hepatitis B) increases the likelihood of protection. Because the incubation period for hepatitis B is on the average 70–80 days, it would be too late for the woman to receive the immunization because her partner has just been diagnosed with hepatitis B. The client would have to have been vaccinated within 2–3 days after exposure from her partner.

58. 1. **During ribavirin treatment, pregnancy must be ruled out. During treatment, pregnancy must be avoided both by females and by female partners of men taking ribavirin. To avoid pregnancy, couples should use two reliable forms of birth control during treatment and for 6 months after treatment.**
    2. There is no vitamin requirement for clients taking ribavirin.
    3. Sunlight does not cause complications when taking this medication.

4. This medication does not cause impotence in men.

59. 1. This vaccine must be administered in three doses, not two doses. Therefore, requesting the client to come back in 2 months and telling the client it is the last dose is incorrect information.
2. There is no reason why the client cannot wash the injection site.
3. There is no reason to rotate arms because there is 1 month and 6 months between the injections.
4. **The hepatitis B vaccine must be administered intramuscularly in three doses, with the second and third doses at 1 and 6 months after the first dose. The third dose is very important in producing prolonged immunity.**

60. 1. **The U.S. Food and Drug Administration (FDA, 2001) has approved a combined hepatitis A and B vaccine (Twinrix) for vaccination of persons 18 years of age and older with indications for both hepatitis A and B vaccination. The Twinrix vaccination consists of three doses, given on the same schedule as that used for single-antigen hepatitis B vaccine—that is, initial dose, after 1 month, and at 6 months.**
2. Because the client is homeless and uses illegal IV drugs, the nurse should recommend both the hepatitis A and B combined vaccination.
3. The client needs to quit using the illegal drugs, but recommending the rehabilitation center may not lead to the client agreeing to go and receiving the hepatitis vaccination to prevent a chronic potentially life-threatening disease.
4. At this time, there is no HIV vaccination available.

A Child with Gastroenteritis

61. 1. Bilberry is used to treat diarrhea in children and is not an emetic.
2. Bilberry does not treat lactose intolerance.
3. Bilberry is not an antipyretic and would not treat a fever.
4. **Bilberry is used to treat diarrhea. This question would assess the effectiveness of the herb.**

MEDICATION MEMORY JOGGER: Some herbal preparations are effective, some are not, and a few can be harmful or even

deadly. **If a client is taking an herbal supplement and a conventional medicine, the nurse should investigate to determine if the herb will cause harm to the client. The nurse should always be the client's advocate.**

62. **6.8 mL per dose.** The first step is to determine the body weight in kilograms.
60 pounds divided by 2.2 conversion factor is 27.272, or 27.27 kg.
Multiply 27.27 times 10 equals 272.2 or 272 mg of medication each 24 hours.
Divide 272 by 2 to determine the amount of medication to be administered each dosing time; this equals 136 mg per dose.

To set up the algebraic formula:
$136 : x = 100 : 5$
Then cross multiply:
$100x = 680$

To solve for x, divide each side of the equation by 100:
$$\frac{100x}{100} = \frac{680}{100}$$
$x = 6.8$ mL per dose

63. 1. The most likely cause of the child's developing the diarrhea is the administration of antibiotic medications. The antibiotics kill the "good" bacteria in the bowel that are needed for digestion. Penicillin would increase the diarrhea.
2. **Cholestyramine is used to enhance mucosal recovery and decrease the length of the diarrhea.**
3. The most likely cause of the child's developing the diarrhea is the administration of antibiotic medications. The antibiotics kill the "good" bacteria in the bowel needed for digestion. Trimethoprim would increase the diarrhea.
4. Diphenoxylate is an opioid that contains atropine; use of this medication should be limited in children. This would not be the first medication administered.

64. 1. **The American Academy of Pediatrics recommends 50 mL/kg body weight over 4 hours for mild diarrhea and 100 mL/kg for moderate diarrhea. The child is 37.5 pounds, or 17.04 kg ($35 \div 2.2 = 17.04$) or 17 kg; 17 times 50 equals 850 mL and 17 times 100 mL equals 1700 mL. Pedialyte or Rehydralyte is recommended because they contain electrolytes that should be replaced. The recommended schedule for ORT is given in the following table.**

Oral Replacement Therapy in Children with Vomiting or Diarrhea*

	Not Dehydrated	Mild Dehydration	Moderate Dehydration	Severe Dehydration
Oral replacement therapy (ORT)	Not necessary unless not taking other fluids well	50 mL/kg of ORT + replace ongoing losses over a 4-hour period	100 mg/kg of ORT + replace ongoing losses over a 4-hour period	IV therapy bolus of 20 mL/kg of normal saline or lactated Ringer's
Ongoing losses	10 mL/kg of ORT for each stool or emesis. Volume is estimated and replaced.	10 mL/kg of ORT for each stool or emesis. Volume is estimated and replaced.	10 mL/kg of ORT for each stool or emesis. Volume is estimated and replaced.	—
Feeding	Continue age-appropriate diet	Resume age-appropriate diet as soon as dehydration is corrected	Resume age-appropriate diet as soon as dehydration is corrected	Begin ORT when child is stable and alert; keep IV line until child is drinking well; resume diet as soon as dehydration is corrected
Reevaluate hydration, and estimate ongoing fluid losses	As necessary	Every 2 hours	Every hour	Continuous evaluation; must evaluate after each bolus of IV solution

*Modified from the American Academy of Pediatrics Provisional Committee on Quality Improvement; Subcommittee on Acute Gastroenteritis.

2. This would only be 200 mL over 2 hours and not enough to treat the diarrhea. Homemade rice water does not contain replacement electrolytes.
3. Because juices and soft drinks have high carbohydrate content and because the osmotic effect in the intestine can increase the diarrhea, they are not recommended.
4. The child should resume an age-appropriate diet as soon as the fluids have been replaced. Current research indicates that resuming solid food actually reduces the duration of the diarrhea.

65. 1. The client is receiving IV fluids and the nurse should monitor the child's electrolytes.
2. A 6-year-old child's fontanels have closed; the child is assessed for dehydration by checking skin turgor on the abdomen.
3. The order is incomplete. No rate has been given. The nurse should clarify the order with the HCP.
4. All pediatric intravenous infusions require safety measures to make sure the child is not fluid overloaded. Using a pump is a method of ensuring that the rate of infusion is maintained and that too much fluid is not infused at one time. Most hospitals also require simultaneous use of a chambered infusion device (Buretrol).
5. The nurse should assess pediatric IV sites at least every hour.

66. 1. The HCP is responsible for identifying abnormal data noted during the procedure.
2. The instrument being used is a fiberoptic scope, and it will be in the HCP's hands during the procedure. The instrument that might be handed is the biopsy instrument, but this is not a priority over the respiratory function of the client.
3. The child will have received conscious sedation; the nurse should monitor the child's respiratory status to make sure that respiratory depression leading to respiratory failure does not occur.
4. The nurse or a technician will clean the instruments after a procedure, but this is not priority over monitoring the client.

67. 1. Compazine is an antiemetic and should relieve nausea and vomiting; it is not known to cause diarrhea.
2. Tremors, involuntary twitching, and restlessness are signs of an extrapyramidal reaction. Children, the elderly, and clients who are dehydrated are especially susceptible. If these symp-

toms occur, the medication is held and the HCP is notified.

3. Compazine does not cause diplopia (double vision), ptosis (drooping eyelids), or urinary retention. It can cause blurred vision.

4. Compazine does not cause myalgias (muscle aches), hallucinations, or weakness.

68. 1. Antiemetic suppositories are not administered on this schedule for clients with gastroenteritis. They are administered on a PRN basis. Suppositories are manufactured in a set mg/suppository (25 mg); this could be an excessive amount of medication depending on the weight of the child.

2. The bacteria are transmitted by an oral route. The child should be in contact precautions in the hospital and the family should be cautious with handwashing and sharing glasses or eating utensils at home, but wearing a mask is not necessary.

3. **E. coli is a bacterium and is treated with antibiotics. The nurse should teach the parents to make sure that the child takes all the antibiotics as prescribed.**

4. Current research indicates that taking antidiarrheal medications when an infectious bacterium is present only delays healing because the bacteria cannot be eliminated from the body through the stool.

69. 1. Acidophilus is not an antibiotic and will not treat a bacterial infection.

2. Acidophilus will not increase the child's ability to develop immunity to Shigella.

3. **Acidophilus is a bacterium that replaces the normal intestinal flora and helps to prevent secondary diarrhea caused by destroying this flora.**

4. Acidophilus is not an antibiotic.

70. 1. The rotavirus is a virus and antibiotics do not treat a virus.

2. The parents should not discard the diapers until the nurse has weighed the diapers to determine the toddler's hydration status.

3. **The purpose of admitting a child with rotavirus is to ensure that dehydration is prevented or treated. The nurse should start the IV and use a controlled IV chamber device.**

4. At this time there is no vaccine for rotavirus. If there were a vaccine it would not help once the child has the infection. Vaccines are administered prior to the infection to prevent an infection from occurring.

A Client Who Is Obese

71. 1. Medications alone will not guarantee weight loss. The client should exercise regularly and limit calories to lose an appreciable amount of weight.

2. Some of the medications have drug interactions with selective serotonin reuptake inhibitors, MAO inhibitors, triptans, and some opioids, but not with antihypertensive medications.

3. **Weight loss attributable to drug therapy is usually between 4.4 and 22 pounds over a 6-month time period.**

4. The medications are prescribed for up to a year at a time.

72. 1. Sibutramine does not act on the thyroid gland.

2. Sibutramine is not an antidepressant. Caution is used when prescribing sibutramine to a client taking an SSRI or MAO inhibitor antidepressant because a potentially life-threatening serotonin syndrome can occur.

3. Sibutramine can cause constipation, not diarrhea.

4. **Sibutramine works by suppressing the client's appetite and possibly by increasing the client's metabolism by blocking serotonin and norepinephrine uptake.**

73. 1. **Xenical acts by inhibiting the absorption of fats and cholesterol in the GI tract. The client should eat a reduced-calorie diet with no more than 30% of the calories coming from fats. Increasing the fat intake can result in foul-smelling, frothy, diarrhea stools. The client needs more teaching.**

2. The client should eat a reduced-calorie diet with no more than 30% of the calories coming from fats. Increasing the fat intake can result in foul-smelling, frothy, diarrhea stools. This statement does not require intervention.

3. Metamucil will add bulk to the stool and limit the diarrhea that can occur with Xenical. This statement does not require intervention.

4. Xenical can interfere with the absorption of needed vitamins and minerals. This statement does not require intervention.

74. 1. **Leptin is administered subcutaneously daily and can suppress the appetite to achieve a moderate weight loss. Weight loss resulting from leptin is almost all fat.**

2. Leptin is given by the parenteral route, not orally.
3. The risk of an allergic reaction is rare. EpiPens are used by clients who are allergic to bee stings or wasp venom.
4. The most common side effect of leptin is a localized itching or swelling at the injection site.

75. 1. This is an over-the-counter preparation that can be used safely, if used as directed by the manufacturer. All medications can be abused if taken incorrectly, but the client did not say that she was abusing the drug.
 2. **The nurse should portray a nonjudgmental attitude when discussing treatments and medications or herbs the client has used to treat any health problem. The nurse should assess what else the client has tried for weight loss.**
 3. This is a judgmental statement, and the nurse does not know what the HCP will prescribe.
 4. The question does not require a therapeutic response from the nurse. The question requires a factual response.

76. 1. Xenical will decrease the absorption of fats and cholesterol in the GI tract, but it will not help the client to quit smoking.
 2. Meridia can suppress the appetite, but it will not address the smoking.
 3. **Zyban is an antidepressant that is used to assist clients to quit smoking. It has also been shown to suppress the appetite by suppressing the uptake of norepinephrine and serotonin.**
 4. Olean is a nonabsorbable fat substitute; it does not help with nicotine withdrawal or suppress the appetite.

77. 1. Meridia can be taken at any time, with food or on an empty stomach.
 2. **All weight loss programs include some type of exercise. Exercise for at least 20 minutes 3–4 times a week is recommended**
 3. **An appropriate weight loss goal is 1–2 pounds per week. Many Americans want a quick-fix solution to obesity, but a slow weight loss program that includes reduced calories, exercise, and behavior modification is the only proven method of sustained weight loss other than surgery.**
 4. Meridia can cause a mild elevation in the blood pressure, not orthostatic hypotension.

5. **Meridia can cause a mild elevation in the blood pressure; the client should avoid medications that contain ephedrine or pseudoephedrine, which are found in many OTC cold remedies and which can raise the blood pressure.**

78. 1. Glucophage is being investigated for weight loss in clients who do not have diabetes. There is no need to monitor the hemoglobin A$_1$C. Glucophage acts on the liver to prevent gluconeogenesis; it does not increase insulin levels.
 2. Glucophage is being investigated for weight loss in clients who do not have diabetes. There is no need to monitor daily fasting blood glucose levels. Glucophage acts on the liver to prevent gluconeogenesis; it does not increase insulin levels.
 3. Urine ketones are monitored when a client diagnosed with diabetes has a high glucose level and sometimes by clients on the Atkins diet to monitor if they are having success. Normal diets do not monitor urine ketones.
 4. **The medication is being administered for weight loss; the client's weight should be monitored.**

79. 1. **If a client consumes more than 30% of daily calories in fats while taking Xenical, the fats will not be absorbed by the gastrointestinal tract and the result is foul-smelling, frothy, diarrhea stools.**
 2. The "statins," or lipid-lowering medications, would not cause this response.
 3. This is an uncomfortable and sometimes embarrassing possibility with this medication; it is not desired.
 4. The foul-smelling, frothy, diarrhea stool indicates that the stool contains undigested fats. This is not a symptom of a chronic bowel syndrome.

80. 1. Zyban is listed as an antidepressant, but it has proven efficacy for nicotine withdrawal. The main risk factor for developing COPD is smoking; therefore, the nurse would not question administering this medication.
 2. Clients who have had surgery have significant pain; the nurse would not question administering a narcotic medication.
 3. Clients diagnosed with IBS experience frequent diarrhea. The nurse would not question this medication.

4. Combining Meridia with any other serotonergic medication, such as Prozac, can cause serotonin syndrome, a potentially life-threatening reaction characterized by incoordination, hyper-reflexia, myoclonus, fever, tremors, sweating, and mental changes. The nurse should hold the medication and discuss this with the HCP.

A Client Experiencing Constipation or Diarrhea

81. 1. Some laxatives are high in sodium or glucose and the contents of the laxative should be checked, but this should not be the nurse's first response.
    2. Rash or itching is indicative of an allergic reaction that can occur with laxatives, but because the client has been taking the laxatives daily this should not be the nurse's first response.
    3. **Laxatives are indicated for short-term use only and overuse of laxatives robs the bowel of its ability to perform well on its own. Laxative dependency is a very serious and common problem of the elderly; therefore, this should be the nurse's first response. The nurse should teach the client safety.**
    4. This is a true statement, but the nurse should first teach the client about safety, specifically the importance of not taking laxatives daily.

82. 1. Bulk laxatives add fiber to the diet and should be taken daily, but it may take from 12 hours to 3 days for the laxative to work. Therefore, this should not be recommended to the client.
    2. The nurse cannot prescribe medications, but laxatives are over-the-counter medications and the nurse can recommend one to the client. Constipation is not a condition that requires an appointment with an HCP unless a laxative does not work or if the stool is abnormal.
    3. A stool softener takes from 24 to 48 hours to work and this client needs something that will work immediately.
    4. **A stimulant laxative usually acts within 6–10 hours. However, castor oil acts within 1–3 hours. Therefore, this should be recommended because the client has not had a bowel movement in 4 days and is symptomatic.**

83. 1. Bacid is a nonprescription product specifically used to treat diarrhea caused by antibiotics. It reestablishes normal intestinal flora and may be used prophylactically in clients with a history of antibiotic-induced diarrhea.
    2. Diarrhea is a side effect of some antibiotics because antibiotics kill the good flora in the bowel, but the nurse must do something about the diarrhea.
    3. The nurse should realize that antibiotics can cause diarrhea and should not assess for possible gastroenteritis.
    4. The client should not quit taking the antibiotic because there may be a relapse of the infection for which the antibiotic was prescribed and the full dosage of antibiotic prescribed should always be taken.

84. 1. This is known as traveler's diarrhea caused by *Escherichia coli* bacteria. If the client takes an antidiarrheal agent, it will slow peristalsis, delay export of the causative organism, and prolong the infection. Therefore, this should not be the nurse's first intervention.
    2. **Tourists are often plagued by infectious diarrhea, known as traveler's diarrhea, Montezuma's revenge, or Aztec two-step, which is caused by the bacteria *Escherichia coli*. As a rule, treatment is not necessary and the diarrhea is self-limiting. If diarrhea is severe, it is treated with an antibiotic. Therefore, the nurse should assess the severity of the diarrhea first.**
    3. This is probably traveler's diarrhea, and as a rule treatment is not necessary because it is self-limiting. If diarrhea is severe, it is treated with an antibiotic. Therefore, the nurse should assess the severity of the diarrhea first.
    4. This is a possibility, but the nurse should assess the severity, length of time of diarrhea, and whether the client is dehydrated before making this statement.

MEDICATION MEMORY JOGGER: When answering test questions or when caring for clients at the bedside, the nurse should remember that assessing the client is usually the first intervention, but when the client is in distress, the nurse may need to intervene directly to help the client.

85. 1. Some antidiarrheal medications contain habit-forming drugs and should be used as directed only.

2. Clear liquids allow the bowel to rest. A client with diarrhea should be consuming clear liquids only for 24 hours, then move on to eating a bland diet, and after that progress to eating more solid food if the diarrhea does not reoccur.

3. If the client has had diarrhea more than 48 hours, the nurse should recommend the client come to the office because an elderly client is at risk for dehydration.

4. The client does not need to go to the emergency department but may need to be seen in the clinic if the diarrhea has occurred for longer than 24 hours or the client shows signs of dehydration.

5. **The nurse should determine what other medications the client is taking because diarrhea is a side effect of digoxin toxicity and may be a side effect of many other medications. The nurse should always ask what other medications the client is taking.**

86. 1. An antispasmodic medication controls spasms of the gastrointestinal tract and may help with irritable bowel syndrome, but it does not help prevent constipation.

2. Low-residue foods have low fiber and will cause the client to become constipated.

3. **Getting daily exercise, increasing fluid intake, eating a high-fiber diet, and using a stool softener that lubricates the stool lead to regular bowel movements, which, in turn, prevent constipation.**

4. A daily bowel movement is not required to prevent constipation, some clients have bowel movements every other day, which is fine as long as the bowel movements are regular. Regular bowel movements prevent the development of constipation.

87. 1. Because Lomotil has atropine and is a Schedule V controlled substance, the client should not take more than eight in a 24-hour period.

2. The client should drink clear liquids and increase fluid intake to help prevent dehydration.

3. Lomotil should not be taken for more than 2–3 days. If the diarrhea persists more than 48 hours, the client should notify the health-care provider.

4. **An adult should take two tablets and then one tablet after each loose stool up to a maximum of eight tablets in 24 hours. Atropine in the medication**

helps prevent narcotic abuse, but atropine is an anticholinergic medication, which dries up secretions.

88. 1. Lomotil is an antidiarrheal medication, but because the client has had diarrhea the last 3 days, the nurse should have the client come to the clinic.

2. The client with diarrhea should be restricted to clear liquids such as tea, gelatin, or broth.

3. Determining what the client has eaten may help determine the cause of the diarrhea, but 3 days is too long to have diarrhea. The client may become dehydrated.

4. **Diarrhea that persists for more than 48 hours should not be self-treated. The client should be seen by the HCP for further evaluation and diagnosis.**

89. 1. **This information is true and should be shared with the client. Chronic exposure to laxatives can diminish defecatory reflexes, leading to further reliance on laxatives. It may also cause serious pathologic changes, including electrolyte imbalance, dehydration, and colitis.**

2. Bulk-forming laxatives increase fiber, which will help decrease constipation, but they do not cause laxative abuse.

3. A daily Fleets enema should be discouraged because it causes laxative dependency and can irritate the rectum and anal area.

4. The nurse should recommend a high-fiber diet and an increase in fluid intake, but that does not ensure that an elderly client will not get constipated. The client may need laxatives occasionally, and the nurse should always provide correct information to the client.

90. 1. Senna may cause the stool to turn this color; therefore, there is no need for the client to come to the clinic.

2. **Senna (Senokot, Ex-Lax, and Agoral) may cause a yellow or yellow–green cast to feces; it may cause a red–pink discoloration of alkaline urine or yellow–brown color in acid urine. The nurse should teach the client about this when the medication is prescribed.**

3. Because this change in the color of the stool is common with senna, there is no need for the client to bring a stool specimen to the clinic.

4. Some foods can cause a discoloration of feces, but yellow–green feces are a side effect of the medication.

MEDICATION MEMORY JOGGER: If the client verbalizes a complaint, if the nurse assesses data, or if laboratory data indicates an adverse effect secondary to a medication, the nurse must intervene. The nurse must implement an independent intervention or notify the health-care provider because medications can result in serious or even life-threatening complications.

A Client Undergoing Abdominal Surgery with General Anesthesia

91. 1. This does not need to be reported to the surgical team.
    2. Allergy to shellfish usually indicates an allergy to iodine, the active ingredient in povidone (Betadine) surgical scrub. The nurse should place an allergy alert on the front of the client's chart, put an allergy bracelet on the client, and document the finding on the preoperative checklist.
    3. This is standard procedure and does not need to be reported to the surgical team.
    4. An infection last month should be cleared by now; this does not need to be reported to the surgical team.

    MEDICATION MEMORY JOGGER: The nurse must be knowledgeable about diagnostic tests and surgical procedures. If the client provides information that would cause harm to the client, then the nurse must intervene.

92. 1. The incision is a right upper-abdominal incision for a gallbladder.
    2. Clients should be turned every 2 hours, not every hour, and will be turned from side to side and to the back.
    3. The client will be NPO for a day or two and will have intravenous fluids, but unless complications occur there is no reason for total parenteral nutrition (TPN).
    4. The nurse should discuss pain control procedures with all clients having surgery.

93. 1. This is an intervention that will be done the morning of surgery, not the evening before.
    2. This is important, but it can be done at any time prior to surgery. The night nurse or the nurse completing the checklist form in the morning could do this.

3. Preoperative scrubs are ordered to cleanse the skin of bacteria. This should be done the evening before and also may be done the morning of surgery.
4. This is an important intervention for postoperative care, but it is not necessary the evening before surgery.

94. 1. For safety the nurse should doublecheck PCA settings with another nurse. This ensures that the correct dosage is being administered when the client pushes the PCA button.
    2. The initial bolus should have been administered by the PACU nurse; the PCA button should be controlled by the client and no one else.
    3. The family should be instructed to not push the button.
    4. The client is returning from PACU. The cartridge holds 30 mL of medication and should not have been completely used in the PACU.

95. 1. The client who has had general anesthesia frequently experiences nausea while the effects of the anesthetic agents are wearing off. The charge nurse should anticipate the client's needs and prepare for them.
    2. The client would have been "asleep" while under general anesthesia and could not complain of nausea to the anesthesiologist.
    3. The surgeon may have overlooked the need for an antiemetic while writing the orders; the nurse should contact the surgeon and ask for the order.
    4. The charge nurse should not have to request a primary nurse to keep the charge nurse informed of the client's condition.

96. 1. The nurse should never write "incident report" in a client's chart; this sends a red flag to an attorney that an error has been made. When an error is made, the facts should be charted honestly and succinctly.
    2. Many PACU nurses are given standing orders to use their judgment about the route of administration of postoperative pain medications. The theory of administering the medications by both routes is that the client will receive immediate relief from the IV route and the IM route will provide relief when the IV medication has worn off. The nurse should always chart accurately what was done and how.

3. This would be dishonest and could cost the nurse his or her license.

4. The number of milligrams of medication has been reversed in this option.

97. **1900 mL of IV fluid.**
    150 mL multiplied by 12 equals 1800 mL, plus 100 mL of IVPB fluid, equals 1900 mL of IV fluid.

98. 1. The client should have signed the consent form before the call that the orderly is coming to get the client for surgery is placed. Waiting until this point does not give the client time to ask questions and get clarification of concerns.

    2. This should have been done the night before or at least earlier on the day of surgery.

    3. The family can walk with the client to the operating room entrance and then be escorted or guided to the waiting room.

    4. **This is the appropriate time to administer any preoperative medication.**

99. 1. The client's pain level is in the mild range. The nurse can discuss nonpharmacological methods to decrease the pain further, such as distraction or guided imagery, but this level of pain is not a reason for immediate intervention.

    2. Serous drainage is expected after a surgery and does not warrant immediate intervention.

3. **The client's respiration rate is low, indicating a potential overdose of narcotic medication depressing the respiratory drive. This situation requires immediate intervention.**

4. The client should splint the incision prior to coughing. The nurse should praise the client.

100. 1. **The WBC count is elevated, indicating an infection. The surgeon would not have performed an elective surgery if the client had an infection at the time. This indicates the antibiotic is not working.**

    2. This might indicate that the pain medication is not relieving the client's pain, but it does not provide information about the antibiotic.

    3. The sodium level is within normal limits; it does not provide information about the antibiotic.

    4. This is normal color of drainage of a nasogastric tube, but it does not provide information about the antibiotic.

MEDICATION MEMORY JOGGER: The nurse determines the effectiveness of a medication by assessing for the symptoms, or lack thereof, for which the medication was prescribed.

1. The client diagnosed with gastroenteritis was admitted to the medical floor yesterday and has just had another loose, watery stool. Based on the following Medication Administration Record (MAR), which action should the nurse implement?

Client Name:	Account Number: 0 1234 56		Allergies: NKDA	
Date of Birth: 01 01	Weight: 165 lbs		Height: 70 inches	
Date	**Medication**	**2301–0700**	**0701–1500**	**1501–2300**
	Acetaminophen (Tylenol) 325 mg tab ii every 4 hours PRN temp or mild pain			
	Promethazine (Phenergan) 6.25 mg IVP PRN nausea			
	Diphenoxylate (Lomotil) 2.5 mg I tab after each loose stool PRN	0045 NN 0200 NN 0545 NN	0700 DN 0815 DN 1030 DN	1540 DN 1610 DN
	0.9% saline IV continuous infusion @ 125 mL/hour	0200 NN	1000 DN	
Sig: Night Nurse RN/NN		Sig: Day Nurse RN/DN		

   1. Administer a diphenoxylate (Lomotil) tablet.
   2. Increase the intravenous fluid rate.
   3. Notify the health-care provider.
   4. Send a stool specimen to the lab.

2. The client diagnosed with inflammatory bowel disease (IBD) has been prescribed the oral glucocorticosteroid prednisone daily. The client has pyrosis. Which statement would be the clinic nurse's best response?
   1. "What type of diet are you currently following?"
   2. "When do you take your prednisone?"
   3. "Have you had a change in your weight?"
   4. "Have you discussed this with your health-care provider?"

3. The African American mother brought her 3-year-old son to the clinic because the child has had diarrhea since last night. The mother tells the nurse, "My mother was giving my son cornstarch in a glass of warm water to help stop the diarrhea, but it didn't stop the diarrhea completely." Which statement is the clinic nurse's best response?
   1. "Cornstarch will not hurt your son and we need to let the diarrhea run its course."
   2. "You must tell your mother not to give your son anything the doctor has not ordered."
   3. "Why does the grandmother think that cornstarch will help your son's diarrhea?"
   4. "I hope that the cornstarch has not made your son's diarrhea get worse."

4. The client with gastroenteritis is being discharged from the emergency department with a prescription for promethazine (Phenergan), an antiemetic. Which information should the nurse discuss with the client?
   1. Explain that a sore throat and mouth sores are expected side effects.
   2. Tell the client to call the doctor if the urine turns light-amber colored.
   3. Encourage the client to drink carbonated beverages.
   4. Instruct the client not to drink alcohol with the medication.

5. The client with hepatitis is being treated with interferon alfa (Roferon), a biologic response modifier. Which information should the clinic nurse discuss with the client?
   1. Explain that if flulike symptoms occur, the client must stop taking the medication.
   2. Discuss that the client may experience some abnormal bruising and bleeding.
   3. Tell the client that the skin will become yellow while taking this medication.
   4. Recommend taking acetaminophen (Tylenol), two tablets, before the injection.

6. To which client would the nurse question administering the antidiarrheal medication diphenoxylate (Lomotil)?
   1. The 68-year-old client diagnosed with glaucoma.
   2. The 78-year-old client with traveler's diarrhea.
   3. The 44-year-old client with coronary artery disease.
   4. The 28-year-old client receiving aminoglycoside antibiotics.

7. The female client is diagnosed with irritable bowel syndrome (IBS). The health-care provider prescribes tegaserod (Zelnorm), a gastrointestinal agent. Which assessment data indicates the medication is effective?
   1. The client reports daily bowel movements.
   2. The client complains of "passing gas."
   3. The client reports a decrease in loose stools.
   4. The client is able to eat high-fiber foods.

8. The elderly client diagnosed with irritable bowel syndrome (IBS) is prescribed propantheline (Pro-Banthine), an antispasmodic. Which signs or symptoms indicate an adverse reaction to the medication?
   1. Flatus, abdominal pain, and cramping.
   2. Agitation, confusion, and drowsiness.
   3. Diarrhea alternating with constipation.
   4. Mucus in the stool and low-grade fever.

9. The charge nurse notices that the primary nurse is preparing to administer the antacid Maalox to the client receiving his routine morning medications. Which action should the charge nurse take first?
   1. Take no action because this is acceptable standard of practice.
   2. Discuss changing the administration time with the pharmacist.
   3. Inform the primary nurse to not administer the Maalox.
   4. Instruct the primary nurse to shake the Maalox container.

10. The nurse is administering the 0900 medications on the following Medication Administration Record (MAR). Which action should the nurse take?

Client Name:	Account Number: 0 1234 56		Allergies: NKDA	
Date of Birth: 01 01	Weight: 165 lbs		Height: 70 inches	
Date	Medication	2301–0700	0701–1500	1501–2300
	Omeprazole (Prilosec) po 40 mg every day		0900	
	Furosemide (Lasix) 90 20 mg every A.M.		0900	
	Acetylsalicylic acid (aspirin) E.C. po 325 mg daily		0900	
	Warfarin (Coumadin) po daily			1700
	Azithromycin (Zithromax) po 250 mg every 24 hours			1800
Sig: Night Nurse RN/NN			Sig: Day Nurse RN/DN	

1. Monitor the client's serum sodium level.
2. Check the client's International Normalized Ratio (INR).
3. Ensure that the client ate at least 75% of the breakfast meal.
4. Encourage the client to sit upright at least 30 minutes after taking Prilosec.

11. The client is scheduled for a bowel resection in the morning. The nurse administered one bottle of GoLYTELY. Which task should the nurse delegate to the unlicensed assistive personnel?
1. Remove the client's water pitcher from the room.
2. Take the client's vital signs every 2 hours.
3. Place a bedside commode in the client's room.
4. Administer moisture barrier cream to the anal area.

12. The client diagnosed with end-stage liver failure is taking lactulose (Chronulac), a laxative. Which assessment data indicate the medication is effective?
1. The client reports a decrease in pruritus.
2. The client's abdominal girth has decreased.
3. The client is experiencing diarrhea.
4. The client's ammonia level is decreased.

13. The client is 2 days post–gastric bypass surgery and is complaining of nausea. The nurse is preparing to administer promethazine (Phenergan) 12.5 mg intravenous push. The client has a peripheral IV line infusing normal saline at 100 mL/hour. Which intervention should the nurse implement?
1. Flush the peripheral IV and administer Phenergan undiluted.
2. Start a saline lock in the other arm to administer the medication.
3. Dilute the Phenergan with normal saline and administer slowly.
4. Administer the medication and elevate the client's arm.

14. The nurse is administering medications to the following clients. Which medication would the nurse question administering?
    1. Maalox, an antacid, to a client diagnosed with chronic kidney disease.
    2. Prevacid, a proton-pump inhibitor, to a client diagnosed with ulcer disease.
    3. Surfak, a stool softener, to a client diagnosed with diverticulosis.
    4. Metamucil, a bulk laxative, to a client diagnosed with diarrhea.

15. The home health care nurse is discussing bowel elimination patterns with an elderly client. The client tells the nurse that he must take something to make his bowels move every day. Which information should the nurse discuss with the client?
    1. Tell the client to take a cathartic laxative daily.
    2. Encourage the client to take a bulk laxative daily.
    3. Demonstrate how to give a Fleets enema.
    4. Instruct the client not to take a stool softener.

16. The client with cancer is not eating and has lost 15 lbs in the last month. The health-care provider has prescribed the cannabinoid dronabinol (Marinol). Which statement indicates the client needs more teaching concerning this medication?
    1. "This medication will help stimulate my appetite."
    2. "It is not uncommon to get drowsy when taking this medication."
    3. "This is marijuana and I do not want to get addicted to it."
    4. "I should chew sugarless gum when taking this medication."

17. The client diagnosed with lactose intolerance is prescribed lactase (Lactaid), a digestive enzyme. Which intervention should the nurse implement when administering this medication?
    1. Administer the medication on an empty stomach.
    2. Administer the medication with a full glass of water.
    3. Administer the medication with the client's food.
    4. Administer the medication with vitamin D.

18. The client with an ileostomy is prescribed bismuth subcarbonate tablets orally four times a day. Which statement best describes the scientific rationale for administering this medication?
    1. This medication will help thicken the ileostomy output.
    2. This medication will help decrease the odor in the ileostomy pouch.
    3. This medication helps to change the pH of the ileostomy output.
    4. This medication coats the lining of the small intestine.

19. The client is diagnosed with end-stage liver disease and is prescribed hydroxyzine (Atarax), an antipruritic. Which assessment data indicates the medication is effective?
    1. The client reports a decrease in nausea.
    2. The client reports an increase in appetite.
    3. The client reports being more alert.
    4. The client reports a decrease in itching.

20. The female client tells the clinic nurse that she gets carsick every time the family goes on a vacation and the health-care provider prescribed the anticholinergic scopolamine (Transderm Scop). Which statement indicates the client understands the medication teaching?
    1. "I will put the Transderm Scop patch on my abdomen."
    2. "I will put the patch on for 12 hours and take it off at night."
    3. "If my carsickness does not go away, I will wear two patches."
    4. "I should leave the patch on for 3 days before changing it."

1. 1. Diphenoxylate is combined with atropine to form Lomotil. Diphenoxylate is an opioid whose only indication is to treat diarrhea, but atropine is added to discourage narcotic abuse. The client cannot have more than eight doses of Lomotil daily.
   2. The nurse should not increase the client's intravenous rate without an HCP's order.
   3. **The nurse should notify the health-care provider because the maximum dose of Lomotil is eight doses in 24 hours.**
   4. Sending a stool specimen will not treat the diarrhea.

2. 1. The client's diet does not have any bearing on the client's heartburn.
   2. **Pyrosis, or heartburn, could be secondary to the client's taking the prednisone on an empty stomach. Prednisone is very irritating to the stomach and must be taken with food to prevent severe heartburn and possible peptic ulcer.**
   3. A weight change is not significant to the client's complaint of heartburn.
   4. The nurse should assess the client's complaint before referring the client to the HCP. If the nurse can give factual information, the nurse should teach the client.

3. 1. **Cornstarch works by absorbing excess water in the intestines, thus stopping diarrhea. Therefore, this is the nurse's best response. In children, antidiarrheal medication is not prescribed because of possible adverse reactions. Pedialyte is prescribed to prevent dehydration, and the diarrhea usually subsides on its own.**
   2. This statement is judgmental, and many home remedies have produced valid results.
   3. A client often interprets a "why" question as judgmental, so this is not the best response.
   4. This statement has no factual basis, and even if the nurse were not aware of the effectiveness of cornstarch, the nurse should investigate before making the mother worry about her son's condition.

   MEDICATION MEMORY JOGGER: Some herbal preparations or alternative therapies are effective, some are not, and a few can be harmful or even deadly. If a client is taking a home remedy, the nurse should investigate. The nurse should always be the client's advocate.

4. 1. A sore throat and mouth sores could indicate that the client is experiencing agranulocytosis, which is a possible adverse effect of Phenergan and should be reported to the HCP. The HCP would have a complete blood cell count (CBC) drawn to evaluate for this adverse effect.
   2. Light-amber–colored urine indicates the client is no longer dehydrated and would not warrant notifying the HCP.
   3. Nonpharmacologic measures of alleviating nausea and vomiting, such as flattened carbonated beverages, weak tea, crackers, and dry toast, should be discussed with the client. Drinking carbonated beverages should be discouraged.
   4. **The client should not consume alcohol when taking antiemetics because it can intensify the sedative effect.**

   MEDICATION MEMORY JOGGER: Drinking alcohol is always discouraged when taking any prescribed or over-the-counter medication because of adverse interactions. The nurse should encourage the client not to drink alcoholic beverages.

5. 1. Flulike symptoms are expected and should be treated with Tylenol.
   2. Abnormal bleeding and bruising are not expected and should be reported to the HCP.
   3. The client may be jaundiced from the hepatitis but not from taking the medication.
   4. **Interferon is naturally produced by the body in response to a viral infection. The administration of synthetic interferon produces the same flulike symptoms and should be treated with Tylenol, which will help decrease the severity of the symptoms from the injection. After multiple interferon injections, the client will no longer have the flulike symptoms.**

   MEDICATION MEMORY JOGGER: Usually if a client is prescribed a new medication and has flulike symptoms within 24 hours of taking the first dose, the client should contact the HCP. These are signs of agranulocytosis, which indicates the medication has caused a sudden drop in the white blood cell count, which, in turn, leaves the body defenseless against bacterial invasion. Biologic response modifiers are the exception to the rule.

6. 1. **The client with glaucoma should not receive Lomotil because of the drug's anticholinergic effect, which will increase the intraocular pressure.**

2. Lomotil is prescribed for adult clients diagnosed with traveler's diarrhea. In children, diarrhea should be allowed to run its course.

3. Lomotil is not contraindicated in clients with coronary artery disease.

4. Antibiotics sometimes cause a suprainfection that kills the normal flora in the bowel, resulting in diarrhea. This client may receive an antidiarrheal medication.

MEDICATION MEMORY JOGGER: Glaucoma is a condition that the nurse should recognize. Its presence precludes the use of many medications.

7. **1. Zelnorm is prescribed for women with IBS who present with constipation as their primary complaint; it binds to 5HT receptors in the gastrointestinal tract to stimulate peristalsis. A daily bowel movement indicates the medication is effective.**

2. Flatus, or "passing gas," is a symptom of IBS and indicates the medication is not effective.

3. Zelnorm is not prescribed for diarrhea, so this response is not applicable.

4. The ability to eat high-fiber foods does not indicate the effectiveness of the medication.

8. 1. These are the signs or symptoms of IBS.

2. **Agitation, confusion, and drowsiness are signs or symptoms of an adverse reaction in the client who is elderly or debilitated that requires discontinuation of the medication.**

3. Diarrhea alternating with constipation is a sign of IBS, not an adverse reaction to the medication.

4. Mucus in the stool is a sign of IBS, but low-grade fever is not. However, neither of these indicates an adverse reaction to the medication.

9. 1. Taking antacids with other medications is not an acceptable standard of practice.

2. The charge nurse should discuss changing the times of Maalox administration to 1–2 hours before or after taking other drugs because Maalox could affect the absorption of the other drugs. However, this is not the first intervention.

3. **The client should not receive any oral medications 1–2 hours before or after taking an antacid because the antacid may interfere with absorption of the other medications.**

4. Maalox is a suspension and should be shaken, but this is not the first action the nurse should take.

10. 1. The nurse should monitor the client's serum potassium level, not sodium level, prior to administering the 0900 of Lasix.

2. **Prilosec interacts with warfarin and may increase the likelihood of bleeding; therefore, the nurse should check the client's INR.**

3. Prilosec can be taken on an empty stomach.

4. The client should sit up after eating a meal but not after taking Prilosec.

11. 1. The client would not be NPO at this time because the client will have to drink a gallon of GoLYTELY. There is no reason for the UAP to remove the water pitcher.

2. There is no reason for the client's vital signs to be taken every 2 hours preoperatively. Vital signs are tasks that can be delegated to a UAP.

3. **GoLYTELY is a colonic stimulant that is prescribed to cleanse the bowel prior to bowel surgery; therefore, the client should have a bedside commode readily available and the nurse can delegate the UAP to perform this task.**

4. The UAP is allowed to apply moisture barrier to excoriated perianal areas, but nothing in the stem indicates the client has this need.

12. 1. Lactulose is not administered to help with the client's complaints of itching.

2. Lactulose will not help decrease the client's ascites.

3. Diarrhea is a sign of medication toxicity and would warrant decreasing the medication dose.

4. **Lactulose is administered to decrease the client's serum ammonia level; the normal adult level is 19–60 mcg/dL.**

13. 1. Phenergan is caustic to peripheral veins and should be diluted prior to being administered.

2. Phenergan is compatible with normal saline; therefore, the nurse need not start a saline lock in the other arm, causing the patient discomfort.

3. **Phenergan is caustic to peripheral veins, is very painful when administered peripherally, and may result in a chemical phlebitis. The nurse must dilute the medication and push slowly to prevent pain and sclerosing of the vein.**

4. The only time the arm should be elevated after administering IVP medication is during a code.

14. 1. **Maalox should not be administered to a client with chronic kidney disease because it contains magnesium, and diseased kidneys are unable to excrete magnesium, resulting in the client developing hypermagnesemia. If the client needs an antacid, he or she should receive aluminum hydroxide (Amphogel) because it helps remove phosphates.**
    2. A proton-pump inhibitor decreases gastric secretion and would be prescribed for a client with PUD.
    3. A stool softener would be prescribed for a client with diverticulosis to help prevent constipation.
    4. A bulk laxative adds substance to the feces and will help decrease watery stools.

15. 1. A cathartic laxative is a stimulant laxative, and daily use can lead to laxative dependence. Elderly clients should be encouraged to use other methods to ensure a daily bowel movement.
    2. **A bulk laxative is recommended for daily use because it increases fiber and requires the colon to function normally. Stimulant laxatives may cause "laxative dependency," which is not healthy for the client.**
    3. The client should not be encouraged to take Fleets enemas unless recommended by an HCP because they may cause dependence. The nurse should encourage the use of medications that require the bowel to function normally.
    4. If the client needs to have a bowel movement daily, then a stool softener should be encouraged because it does not stimulate the bowel; it just softens the stool.

16. 1. This medication is prescribed to help stimulate the client's appetite; therefore, the client does not need more teaching.
    2. A side effect of this medication is drowsiness; therefore, the client does not need more teaching.
    3. **Cannabinoid, the active ingredient in marijuana, is frequently abused as an illegal drug, but it is not addicting.**
    4. A side effect of this medication is a dry mouth, so chewing sugarless gum indicates the client understands the medication teaching.

17. 1. Enzymes break down food; therefore, they must be administered with food.
    2. This medication does not need to be administered with water to be effective.
    3. **Lactaid is a gastrointestinal enzyme essential for the absorption of lactose from the intestines. It must be taken with food.**
    4. Vitamin D deficiency results from a lack of milk and milk products in the diet. Lactaid is administered so the client can tolerate milk products, but it does not need to be administered with vitamin D.

18. 1. A stool thickener, such as Lomotil, can be prescribed to thicken the watery ileostomy output, which will decrease the odor.
    2. **Decreasing odor is the scientific rationale for administering bismuth subcarbonate to a client with an ileostomy.**
    3. This medication does not affect the pH of the ileostomy output.
    4. This medication does not coat the lining of the small intestine.

19. 1. This medication is being used as an antipruritic; therefore, a decrease in nausea does not indicate the effectiveness of the medication.
    2. This medication does not stimulate the appetite; therefore, assessment of the appetite does not determine the effectiveness of the medication.
    3. Atarax will cause drowsiness and is not administered to increase the client's cognitive ability.
    4. **The client in end-stage liver disease often has jaundice, which causes pruritus (itching). A decrease in itching indicates the medication is effective.**

MEDICATION MEMORY JOGGER: The test taker must note the drug classification to determine the effectiveness of the medication. Many medications are administered for different reasons, which changes their drug classification.

20. 1. The Transderm Scop patch should be applied behind the ears, not on the abdomen.
    2. The patch can be left on for up to 3 days before changing, but it should not be alternated on and off.
    3. The client should not wear two patches at one time because of the anticholinergic effect of the medication.
    4. **The patch is effective up to 3 days; therefore, this indicates the client understands the medication teaching.**

Endocrine System

"Standards of care are the skills and learning commonly possessed by members of a profession."

—Michael Adams, Dianne Josephson, and Leland Holland

A Client with Type 1 Diabetes

1. The nurse administered 25 units of Humulin N to a client with Type 1 diabetes at 1600. Which intervention should the nurse implement?
   1. Assess the client for hypoglycemia around 1800.
   2. Ensure the client eats the nighttime snack.
   3. Check the client's serum blood glucose level.
   4. Serve the client the supper tray.

2. The nurse is teaching the client with Type 1 diabetes how to use an insulin pen injector. Which information should the nurse discuss with the client?
   1. Instruct the client to dial in the number of insulin units needed to inject.
   2. Demonstrate the proper way to draw up the insulin in an insulin syringe.
   3. Discuss that the insulin pen injector must be used in the abdominal area only.
   4. Explain that the traditional insulin syringe is less painful than the injector pen.

3. The nurse is teaching a client with newly diagnosed Type 1 diabetes about insulin therapy. Which statement indicates the client needs more teaching concerning insulin therapy?
   1. "If I have a headache or start getting nervous, I will drink some orange juice."
   2. "If I pass out at home, a family member should give me a glucagon injection."
   3. "Because I am taking my insulin daily I do not have to adhere to a diabetic diet."
   4. "I will check my blood glucose with my glucometer at least once a day."

4. The nurse administered 12 units of regular insulin to the patient with Type 1 diabetes at 0700. Which meal would prevent the client from experiencing hypoglycemia?
   1. Breakfast.
   2. Lunch.
   3. Supper.
   4. HS snack.

5. The client diagnosed with Type 1 diabetes is complaining of a dry mouth, extreme thirst, and increased urination. Which action should the nurse implement?
   1. Administer one amp of intravenous 50% glucose.
   2. Prepare to administer intravenous regular insulin.
   3. Inject Humulin N subcutaneously in the abdomen.
   4. Hang an intravenous infusion of D5W at a keep open rate.

6. The client newly diagnosed with Type 1 diabetes asks the nurse, "Why should I get an external portable insulin pump?" Which statement is the nurse's best response?
   1. "It will cause you to have fewer hypoglycemic reactions and it will control blood glucose levels better."
   2. "Insulin pumps provide an automatic memory of the date and time of the last 24 boluses."
   3. "The pump injects intermediate-acting insulin automatically into the vein to maintain a normal blood glucose level."
   4. "The portable pump is the easiest way to administer insulin to someone with Type 1 diabetes and is highly recommended."

7. The nurse in the medical department is preparing to administer Humalog, a rapid-acting insulin, to a client diagnosed with Type 1 diabetes. Which intervention should the nurse implement?
   1. Ensure the client is wearing a MedicAlert bracelet.
   2. Administer the dose according to the regular insulin sliding scale.
   3. Assess the client for hyperosmolar, hyperglycemic, nonketotic coma.
   4. Make sure the client eats the food on the meal tray that is at the bedside.

8. Which assessment data best indicate the client with Type 1 diabetes is adhering to the medical treatment regimen?
   1. The client's fasting blood glucose is 100 mg/dL.
   2. The client's urine specimen has no ketones.
   3. The client's glycosylated hemoglobin is 5.8%.
   4. The client's glucometer reading is 120 mg/dL.

9. The nurse is discussing storage of insulin vials with the client. Which statement indicates the client understands the teaching concerning the storage of insulin?
   1. "I will keep my unopened vials of insulin in the refrigerator."
   2. "I can keep my insulin in the trunk of my car so I will have it at all times."
   3. "It is all right to put my unopened insulin vials in the freezer."
   4. "If I prefill my insulin syringes, I must use them within 1–2 days."

10. Which statement best describes the pharmacodynamics of insulin?
    1. Insulin causes the pancreas to secrete glucose into the bloodstream.
    2. Insulin is metabolized by the liver and muscle and excreted in the urine.
    3. Insulin is needed to maintain colloidal osmotic pressure in the bloodstream.
    4. Insulin lowers blood glucose by promoting use of glucose in the body cells.

A Client with Type 2 Diabetes

11. The client diagnosed with Type 2 diabetes is prescribed the sulfonylurea glipizide (Glucotrol). Which statement by the client would warrant intervention by the nurse?
    1. "I have to eat my diabetic diet even if I am taking this medication."
    2. "I will need to check my blood glucose level at least once a day."
    3. "I usually have one glass of wine with my evening meal."
    4. "I do not like to walk every day, but I will if it will help my diabetes."

12. Which statement best describes the scientific rationale for prescribing the biguanide metformin (Glucophage)?
    1. This medication decreases insulin resistance, improving blood glucose control.
    2. This medication allows the carbohydrates to pass slowly through the large intestine.
    3. This medication will decrease the hepatic production of glucose from stored glycogen.
    4. This medication stimulates the beta cells to release more insulin into the bloodstream.

13. The nurse is discussing the oral hypoglycemic medication Micronase with the client diagnosed with Type 2 diabetes. Which information should the nurse discuss with the client?
    1. Instruct the client to take the oral hypoglycemic medication with food.
    2. Explain that hypoglycemia will not occur with oral medications.
    3. Tell the client to notify the HCP if a headache, nervousness, or sweating occurs.
    4. Recommend the client check the ketones in the urine every morning.

14. The client diagnosed with Type 2 diabetes is receiving the combination oral antidiabetic medication glyburide/metformin (Glucovance). Which data indicate the medication is effective?
    1. The client's skin turgor is elastic.
    2. The client's urine ketones are negative.
    3. The serum blood glucose level is 118 mg/dL.
    4. The client's glucometer level is 170 mg/dL.

15. The client with Type 2 diabetes is admitted into the medical department with a wound on the left leg that will not heal. The HCP prescribes sliding-scale insulin. The client tells the nurse, "I don't want to have to take shots. I take pills at home." Which statement would be the nurse's best response?
    1. "If you can't keep your glucose under control with pills, you must take insulin."
    2. "You should discuss the insulin order with your HCP because you don't want to take it."
    3. "You are worried about having to take insulin. I will sit down and we can talk."
    4. "During illness you may need to take insulin to keep your blood glucose level down."

16. The nurse is caring for the client diagnosed with Type 2 diabetes. The client is complaining of a headache, jitteriness, and nervousness. Which action should the nurse implement first?
    1. Check the client's serum blood glucose level.
    2. Give the client a glass of orange juice.
    3. Determine when the last antidiabetic medication was administered.
    4. Assess the client's blood pressure and apical pulse.

17. The overweight client diagnosed with Type 2 diabetes reports to the clinic nurse that he has lost 35 pounds in the last 4 months. Which action should the nurse implement first?
    1. Determine if the client has had an increase in hypoglycemic reactions.
    2. Instruct the client to make an appointment with the health-care provider.
    3. Ask the client if he has been trying to lose weight or has it happened naturally.
    4. Check the client's last weight in the chart with the weight obtained in the clinic.

18. The female client diagnosed with Type 2 diabetes tells the clinic nurse that she started taking ginseng to help increase her memory. Which action should the clinic nurse take?
    1. Take no action because ginseng does not affect Type 2 diabetes.
    2. Determine what type of memory deficits the client is experiencing.
    3. Explain that herbs are dangerous and she should not be taking them.
    4. Determine if the client is currently taking any type of antidiabetic medication.

19. The school nurse is teaching a class about Type 2 diabetes to elementary school teachers. Which information is most important for the nurse to discuss with the teachers?
    1. The importance of not allowing students to eat candy in the classroom.
    2. The increase in the number of students developing Type 2 diabetes.
    3. The signs and symptoms of hypoglycemia and the immediate treatment.
    4. The need to have the students run or walk for 20 minutes during the recess period.

20. The client newly diagnosed with Type 2 diabetes who has been prescribed an oral hypoglycemic medication calls the clinic and tells the nurse that the sclera has a yellow color. Which action should the clinic nurse implement?
    1. Ask the client if he or she has been exposed to someone with hepatitis.
    2. Determine if the client has a history of alcohol use or is currently drinking alcohol.
    3. Check to see if the client is taking the cardiac glycoside digoxin.
    4. Make an appointment for the client to come to the health-care provider's office.

A Client with Pancreatitis

21. The nurse is administering medications. Which medication would the nurse question administering?
    1. Morphine sulfate, an opioid, to a client diagnosed with pancreatitis.
    2. Diphenhydramine (Benadryl), an H_1 blocker, to a client with an allergic reaction.
    3. Methylprednisolone (Solu-Medrol), a glucocorticoid, to a client with Type 2 diabetes.
    4. Vasopressin (DDAVP), a hormone, to a client diagnosed with diabetes insipidus.

22. The nurse has received the morning report. Which medication should be administered first?
    1. Levothyroxine (Synthroid), a hormone, to a client diagnosed with hypothyroidism.
    2. Pantoprazole (Protonix), a proton-pump inhibitor, to a client diagnosed with GERD.
    3. Acetaminophen (Tylenol) to a client with a migraine headache of "7" on the pain scale.
    4. Pancreatin (Donnazyme), an enzyme, to a client diagnosed with chronic pancreatitis.

23. The client diagnosed with chronic pancreatitis has a nasogastric tube. The charge nurse observes the primary nurse instill an antacid down the tube and then clamp the tube. Which action should the charge nurse take?
    1. Tell the nurse to reconnect the tube to suction.
    2. Notify the unit manager of the nurse's actions.
    3. Do nothing because this is the correct procedure.
    4. Instruct the nurse to administer the medication orally.

24. The HCP prescribed chlordiazepoxide (Librium), a sedative hypnotic, for a 55-year-old male client diagnosed with chronic pancreatitis. Which statement is the scientific rationale for prescribing this medication?
    1. Librium acts as an adjunct to pain medication.
    2. Librium limits complications related to alcohol withdrawal.
    3. Librium prevents the nausea related to pancreatitis.
    4. Librium is used as a sleep aid for clients who are NPO.

25. The client diagnosed with acute pancreatitis is complaining of severe abdominal pain. Which interventions should the nurse implement? Select all that apply.
    1. Ask the client to rate the pain on a 1–10 pain scale.
    2. Determine when the client received the last dose of medication.
    3. Administer hydrocodone (Vicodin), a narcotic pain medication.
    4. Assist the client to a semi-Fowler's position.
    5. Apply oxygen at 4 L/minute via nasal cannula.

26. The client diagnosed with acute pancreatitis is placed on total parenteral nutrition (TPN). Which intervention should the nurse implement?
    1. Monitor blood glucose levels daily.
    2. Assess the peripheral intravenous site.
    3. Check the client's complete blood count.
    4. Change the tubing with every new bag of TPN.

27. The nurse is administering pancreatic secretin, a stimulatory hormone, to a client to rule out chronic pancreatitis. Which procedure should the nurse follow?
    1. Have the client lie on the right side during the administration of the medication.
    2. Make sure the client has signed a permit for an investigational procedure.
    3. Aspirate gastric and duodenal contents before and after the medication.
    4. Place the client in the Trendelenburg position before beginning the medication.

28. Which intervention should be implemented when discharging a client diagnosed with chronic pancreatitis who has been receiving high doses of meperidine (Demerol), an opioid, for the past 4 weeks?
    1. Tell the client to monitor his or her stools and to avoid constipation.
    2. Taper the medication slowly over several days prior to discharge.
    3. Refer the client to a drug withdrawal clinic to stop taking the Demerol.
    4. Discuss signs and symptoms of drug dependence to report to the HCP.

29. The male client diagnosed with pancreatitis is prescribed octreotide (Sandostatin), a hormone. Which data indicates the medication has been effective?
    1. The client reports that the diarrhea has subsided.
    2. The client states that he has grown 1 inch.
    3. The client has no muscle cramping or pain.
    4. The client has no complaints of heartburn.

30. The client diagnosed with pancreatitis is complaining of polydipsia and polyuria. Which medication should the nurse prepare to administer?
    1. Humalog, a fast-acting insulin intravenously, and then monitor glucose levels.
    2. Pancrelipase (Cotazym) sprinkled on the client's food with meals.
    3. Humulin R subcutaneously after assessing the blood glucose level.
    4. Ranitidine (Zantac), a histamine$_2$ receptor blocker, orally.

A Client with Adrenal Disorders

31. The client diagnosed with Addison's disease is being discharged. Which statement indicates the client needs more discharge teaching?
    1. "I will be sure to keep my dose of steroid constant and not vary."
    2. "I may have to take two forms of steroids to remain healthy."
    3. "I will get weak and dizzy if I don't take my medication."
    4. "I need to notify any new HCP of the medications I take."

32. The client diagnosed with Cushing's disease is prescribed alendronate (Fosamax), a bisphosphonate regulator, to prevent osteoporosis. Which information should the clinic nurse teach?
    1. Take the medication with food to prevent esophageal irritation.
    2. Take the medication just before going to bed.
    3. Take the medication with an antacid to alleviate gastric disturbances.
    4. Take the medication at least 30 minutes before breakfast.

33. The client is scheduled for a bilateral adrenalectomy for Cushing's disease. Which information regarding the prescribed glucocorticoid prednisone (Deltasone) should the nurse teach? Select all that apply.
    1. When discontinuing this medication, it must be tapered.
    2. Take the medication regularly; do not skip doses.
    3. Stop taking the medication if you develop a round face.
    4. Notify the HCP if you start feeling thirsty all the time.
    5. Wear a MedicAlert bracelet in case of an emergency.

34. The emergency department nurse is caring for a client in an Addisonian crisis. Which intervention should the nurse implement first?
    1. Draw serum electrolyte levels.
    2. Administer methylprednisolone (Solu-Medrol) IV.
    3. Start an 18-gauge catheter with normal saline.
    4. Ask the client what medications he or she is taking.

35. The client diagnosed with Cushing's disease is prescribed pantoprazole (Protonix), a proton-pump inhibitor. Which statement is the scientific rationale for prescribing this medication?
    1. Protonix increases the client's ability to digest food.
    2. Protonix decreases the excess amounts of gastric acid.
    3. Protonix absorbs gastric acid and eliminates it in the bowel.
    4. Protonix coats the stomach and prevents ulcer formation.

36. The client has developed Cushing's syndrome as a result of long-term steroid therapy. Which assessment findings would indicate this condition?
    1. The client is short of breath on exertion and has pale mucous membranes.
    2. The client has a round face and multiple ecchymotic areas on the arms.
    3. The client has pink, frothy sputum and jugular vein distention.
    4. The client has petechiae on the trunk and sclerosed veins.

37. The client has developed Cushing's syndrome as a result of an ectopic production of ACTH by a bronchogenic tumor. Which medication would the nurse anticipate the health-care provider prescribing?
    1. Ketoconazole (Nizoral), an anti-infective.
    2. Methylprednisolone (Solu-Medrol), a corticosteroid.
    3. Propylthiouracil (PTU), a hormone substitute.
    4. Vasopressin (DDAVP), an antidiuretic hormone.

38. The male client diagnosed with iatrogenic Cushing's disease calls the clinic nurse and informs the nurse that he has a temperature of 100.1°F. Which action should the nurse take?
    1. Tell the client to take acetaminophen and drink liquids.
    2. Instruct the client to come to the clinic for an antibiotic.
    3. Have the client go to the nearest emergency department.
    4. Encourage the client to discuss his feelings about the disease.

39. The client diagnosed with Addison's disease asks the nurse, "Why do I have to take fludrocortisone (Florinef), a mineral corticosteroid?" Which statement is the nurse's best response?
    1. "It will keep you from getting high blood sugars."
    2. "Florinef helps the body retain sodium."
    3. "Florinef prevents muscle cramping."
    4. "It stimulates the pituitary gland to secrete ACTH."

40. The client being admitted with primary adrenal insufficiency provides the nurse with a list of home medications. Which medication would the nurse question?
    1. Prednisone (Orasone).
    2. Ginseng.
    3. Mitotane (Lysodren).
    4. Testosterone.

A Client with Pituitary Disorders

41. The client diagnosed with diabetes insipidus is prescribed desmopressin (DDAVP). Which comorbid condition would warrant a change in medication?
    1. Renal calculi.
    2. Diabetes mellitus Type 2.
    3. Sinusitis.
    4. Hyperthyroidism.

42. The middle-aged client with a pituitary tumor has enlarged viscera and bone deformities. Which medication would the nurse administer?
    1. Octreotide (Sandostatin), a synthetic hormone analog.
    2. Somatrem (Protropin), a human growth hormone.
    3. Ketorolac (Toradol), a nonsteroidal anti-inflammatory drug.
    4. CortiTropin (ACTH), a pituitary hormone.

43. The client diagnosed with diabetes insipidus is admitted in acute distress. Which interventions would the nurse implement? Select all that apply.
    1. Start an IV with lactated Ringer's.
    2. Insert an indwelling catheter.
    3. Monitor the urine specific gravity.
    4. Administer furosemide (Lasix) IVP.
    5. Assess the intake and output every shift.

44. The client diagnosed with mild diabetes insipidus is prescribed chlorpropamide (Diabinese), a sulfonylurea. Which discharge instruction should the nurse teach the client?
    1. Discontinue the medication if feeling dizzy.
    2. Chew sugarless gum to alleviate dry mouth.
    3. Take the medication before meals.
    4. Discuss signs and symptoms of an insulin reaction.

45. The 30-year-old female client is prescribed chorionic gonadotrophin (Chorigon), a hormone substitute. Which intervention should the nurse implement?
    1. Have the lab draw an FSH level every week.
    2. Schedule for regular pelvic sonograms.
    3. Discuss not becoming pregnant while taking this drug.
    4. Teach to take the medication with food.

46. The HCP ordered furosemide (Lasix) for a client diagnosed with syndrome of inappropriate antidiuretic hormone (SIADH). Which laboratory test would be monitored to determine the effectiveness of the medication?
    1. Serum sodium levels.
    2. Serum potassium levels.
    3. Creatinine levels.
    4. Serum ACTH levels.

47. Which medication would the nurse administer to the client diagnosed with nephrogenic diabetes insipidus?
    1. Clofibrate (Atromid-S), an antilipemic.
    2. Ibuprofen (Motrin), a prostaglandin inhibitor.
    3. Furosemide (Lasix), a loop diuretic.
    4. Desmopressin (DDAVP), a pituitary hormone.

48. The female client diagnosed with Hodgkin's disease is prescribed vincristine (Oncovin), a vinca alkaloid. Since the last treatment the client complains that she cannot wear her rings or most of her shoes because of weight gain. Which action should the nurse take first?
    1. Administer a diuretic before the Oncovin to prevent fluid overload.
    2. Monitor the client for signs of infection.
    3. Discuss a low-sodium diet with the client.
    4. Weigh the client and report the findings to the oncologist.

49. The client diagnosed with neurogenic diabetes insipidus is prescribed vasopressin tannate in oil. Which instructions should the nurse teach?
    1. Sleep with the head of the bed elevated.
    2. Use a tuberculin syringe to administer medication.
    3. Administer the medication in the evening.
    4. Alternate nares when taking the medication.

50. The nurse is administering morning medications. Which medication would the nurse question?
    1. Black cohosh, an herb, to a client with dysmenorrhea and cramping.
    2. Desmopressin (DDAVP), to a client with diabetes insipidus and angina.
    3. Hydrochlorothiazide (Diuril), to a client with SIADH from a head injury.
    4. Calcitonin (Cibacalcin) a hormone, to a client with hypercalcemia from lung cancer.

A Client with Thyroid Disorders

51. The client diagnosed with hypothyroidism is prescribed levothyroxine (Synthroid). Which assessment data would support that the client is not taking enough medication?
    1. The client has a 2-kg weight loss.
    2. The client complains of being too hot.
    3. The client's radial pulse rate is 110 bpm.
    4. The client complains of being constipated.

52. Which complication should the nurse assess for in the elderly client newly diagnosed with hypothyroidism who has been prescribed levothyroxine (Synthroid)?
    1. Cardiac dysrhythmias.
    2. Respiratory depression.
    3. Paralytic ileus.
    4. Thyroid storm.

53. The client with hyperthyroidism is administered radioactive iodine (I-131). Which intervention should the nurse implement?
    1. Explain that the medication will destroy the thyroid gland completely.
    2. Instruct the client to avoid close contact with children for 1 week.
    3. Discuss the need to take the medication at night for 7 days.
    4. Administer the radioactive iodine in 8 ounces of cold orange juice.

54. The client with hyperthyroidism is prescribed the thioamide propylthiouracil (PTU). Which laboratory data should the nurse monitor?
    1. The client's arterial blood gases.
    2. The client's serum potassium level.
    3. The client's red blood cell count (RBC).
    4. The client's white blood cell count (WBC).

55. The nurse is preparing to administer liothyronine (Cytomel), a thyroid hormone, to a client diagnosed with hypothyroidism. Which data would cause the nurse to question administering the medication?
    1. The client is complaining of being nervous.
    2. The client's oral temperature is 98.9°F.
    3. The client's blood pressure is 110/70.
    4. The client is complaining of being tired.

56. The nurse is discussing the thyroid hormone levothyroxine (Synthroid) with the client diagnosed with hypothyroidism. Which intervention should the nurse discuss with the client?
    1. Encourage the client to decrease the fiber in the diet.
    2. Discuss the need to monitor the T3, T4 levels daily.
    3. Tell the client to take the medication with food only.
    4. Instruct the client to report any significant weight changes.

57. The client diagnosed with hyperthyroidism who received radioactive iodine, I-131, tells the nurse, "I don't think the medication is working. I don't feel any different." Which statement would be the nurse's best response?
    1. "You should notify your health-care provider immediately."
    2. "You may need to have two or three more doses of the medication."
    3. "It may take up to several months to get the full benefits of the treatment."
    4. "You don't feel any different. Would you like to sit down and talk about it?"

58. The nurse is discussing the thyroid hormone levothyroxine (Synthroid) with a client diagnosed with hypothyroidism. Which intervention should be included in the client teaching?
    1. Discuss the importance of not using iodized salt.
    2. Explain the importance of not taking medication with grapefruit juice.
    3. Instruct the client to take the medication in the morning.
    4. Teach the client to monitor daily glucose levels.

59. The client diagnosed with hyperthyroidism is prescribed the antithyroid medication propylthiouracil (PTU). Which statement by the client warrants immediate intervention by the nurse?
    1. "I seem to be drowsy and sleepy all the time."
    2. "I have a sore throat and have had a fever."
    3. "I have gained 2 pounds since I started taking PTU."
    4. "Since taking PTU I am not as hot as I used to be."

60. The client diagnosed with hyperthyroidism is prescribed an antithyroid medication. Which interventions should the nurse implement? Select all that apply.
    1. Monitor the client's thyroid function tests.
    2. Monitor the client's weight weekly.
    3. Monitor the client for gastrointestinal distress.
    4. Monitor the client's vital signs.
    5. Monitor the client for activity intolerance.

A Client with Type 1 Diabetes

1. 1. Humulin N is an intermediate-acting insulin that peaks 6–8 hours after administration; therefore, the client would experience signs of hypoglycemia around 2200–2400.
   2. **The nurse needs to ensure the client eats the nighttime (HS) snack to help prevent nighttime hypoglycemia.**
   3. A serum blood glucose level would have to be done with a venipuncture and the blood sample must be taken to the laboratory. If the client needed the blood glucose checked, it should be done with a glucometer at the bedside.
   4. The supper tray would not help prevent a hypoglycemic reaction because the Humulin N is an intermediate-acting insulin that peaks in 6–8 hours.

2. 1. **The insulin pen injector resembles a fountain pen. It contains a disposable needle and insulin-filled cartridge. When the client operates the insulin pen, the correct dose is obtained by turning the dial to the number of insulin units needed.**
   2. The insulin pen injector does not require drawing up insulin in a syringe.
   3. The insulin pen injector can be used in any subcutaneous site that traditional insulin can be injected.
   4. Most clients state that there is less injection pain associated with the insulin pen than with the traditional insulin syringe.

3. 1. Headache, nervousness, sweating, tremors, and rapid pulse are signs of a hypoglycemic reaction and should be treated with a simple-acting carbohydrate, such as orange juice, sugar-containing drinks, and hard candy. This statement indicates the client understands the teaching.
   2. If a client cannot drink or eat a simple carbohydrate for hypoglycemia, then the client should receive a glucagon injection to treat the hypoglycemic reaction. This indicates the client understands the teaching.
   3. **Even with insulin therapy the client should adhere to the American Diabetic Association diet, which recommends "carbohydrate counting." This statement indicates the client needs more teaching.**
   4. Monitoring and documenting the blood glucose level is encouraged to determine the effectiveness of the treatment regimen. This

indicates the client understands the client teaching.

4. 1. **Regular insulin peaks in 2–4 hours; therefore, the breakfast meal would prevent the client from developing hypoglycemia.**
   2. Lunch would cover a 0700 dose of Humulin N, an intermediate-acting insulin.
   3. Supper would cover a 1600 dose of Humulin R, a short-acting insulin.
   4. The HS (nighttime) snack would cover a 1600 dose of Humulin N, an intermediate-acting insulin.

5. 1. One amp of 50% glucose would be used to treat a severe hypoglycemic reaction, and this client does not have signs or symptoms that indicate hypoglycemia. In fact, the client has signs and symptoms of hyperglycemia.
   2. **The client's signs and symptoms indicate the client is experiencing diabetic ketoacidosis (DKA), which is treated with intravenous regular insulin.**
   3. Humulin N is an intermediate-acting insulin, which is not used to treat hyperglycemia.
   4. An IV of D5W would cause the client to have further signs and symptoms of diabetic ketoacidosis (DKA); therefore, the nurse should not administer the IV.

6. 1. **A portable insulin pump is a battery-operated device that uses rapid-acting insulin—Lispro, Humalog, or NovoLog. It delivers both basal insulin infusion (continuous release of a small amount of insulin) and bolus doses with meals. This provides fewer hypoglycemic reactions and better blood glucose levels.**
   2. The pumps do provide a memory of boluses, but that is not the nurse's best response to explain why a client should get an external portable insulin pump.
   3. External portable insulin pumps are only used to deliver rapid-acting insulin subcutaneously. Intermediate- and long-acting insulins are not used with an external portable insulin pump because of unpredictable control of blood glucose.
   4. The insulin pump is not recommended as the initial way to administer insulin because the success of the insulin pump depends on the client's knowledge and compliance. Initially most clients start injecting insulin with a syringe and then graduate to the pumps.

7. 1. Because the client is in the hospital the client must have a hospital identification band; a MedicAlert bracelet would be needed when the client is not in the hospital.
2. Humalog is not regular insulin; it is fast-acting insulin. It is not administered according to the regular insulin sliding scale. The peak time for Humalog is 30 minutes to 1 hour; regular insulin peaks in 2–4 hours.
3. A client with Type 1 diabetes will experience diabetic ketoacidosis; a client with Type 2 diabetes will experience hyperosmolar, hyperglycemic, nonketotic coma.
4. **Humalog peaks in 30 minutes to 1 hour; therefore, the client needs to eat when or shortly after the medication is administered to prevent hypoglycemia.**

MEDICATION MEMORY JOGGER: Remember that the different types of insulin peak at different times, and the nurse must be knowledgeable about the peak times to ensure that the client does not experience hypoglycemia. Only the insulin product Lantus has no peak time.

8. 1. The fasting blood glucose level is obtained after the client is NPO for 8 hours; this blood result does not indicate adherence to the treatment regimen.
2. If the client has no ketones in the urine, it indicates that the body is not breaking down fat for energy, but it does not indicate adherence to the treatment regimen.
3. A glycosylated hemoglobin (A1C) gives the average of the blood glucose level over the last 3 months and indicates adherence to the medical treatment regimen. A glycosylated hemoglobin level of 5.8% is close to normal and indicates that the client is adhering to the treatment regimen. The following table shows blood glucose levels and corresponding glycosylated hemoglobin results:

Blood Glucose Level	Glycosylated Hemo-globin Result
70–110	4.0–5.5% Normal
135	6%
170	7%
205	8%
240	9%
275	10%
310	11%
345	12%

4. A glucometer reading of 120 mg/dL indicates a normal blood glucose level, but it is a one-time reading and does not indicate adherence to the medical treatment regimen.

9. 1. **This statement indicates the client understands the medication teaching. Keeping the insulin in the refrigerator will maintain the insulin's strength and potency. Once the insulin vial is opened it may be kept at room temperature for 1 month.**
2. Insulin vials should not be placed in direct sunlight or in a high-temperature area, such as the trunk of a car, because it will lose its strength.
3. Insulin should not be kept in the freezer because freezing will cause the insulin to break down and lose its effectiveness.
4. Prefilled syringes should be stored in the refrigerator and should be used within 1–2 weeks, not 1–2 days.

10. 1. The pancreas does not secrete glucose. It secretes insulin, which is the key that opens the door to allow glucose to enter the body cells. Glucose enters the body through the gastrointestinal system.
2. This statement explains the pharmacokinetics of insulin and how the body metabolizes and excretes urine. Pharmacokinetics is the process of drug movement to achieve drug interaction.
3. Insulin does not maintain colloidal osmotic pressure. Albumin, a product of protein, maintains colloidal osmotic pressure.
4. **This is the statement that explains the pharmacodynamics, which is the drug's mechanism of action or way that insulin is utilized by the body. Over time, elevated glucose levels in the bloodstream can cause long-term complications, including nephropathy, retinopathy, and neuropathy. Insulin lowers blood glucose by promoting the use of glucose in body cells.**

A Client with Type 2 Diabetes

11. 1. The client with Type 2 diabetes must adhere to the prescribed diet to help keep the blood glucose level within the normal range. Delaying or missing a meal can cause hypoglycemia. This statement would not warrant intervention by the nurse.
2. The client should check blood glucose levels to determine if the medication is effective; therefore, this statement would not warrant intervention by the nurse.

3. Sulfonylureas and biguanides may cause an Antabuse-like reaction when taken with alcohol, causing the client to become nauseated and vomit. Advise the client to abstain from alcohol and to avoid liquid over-the-counter (OTC) medications that may contain alcohol. Alcohol also increases the half-life of the medication and can cause a hypo-glycemic reaction.

4. The client with Type 2 diabetes does not need to walk daily to keep the glucose level within normal limits; walking three times a week will help control stress and help decrease weight if the client is over-weight.

12. 1. A thiazolidinedione, pioglitazone (Actos) or rosiglitazone (Avandia), not a biguanide like metformin, is prescribed to decrease insulin resistance.

2. An alpha-glucosidase inhibitor, acarbose (Precose) or miglitol (Glyset), is adminis-tered to allow carbohydrates to pass slowly through the intestine. Glucophage does not do this.

3. The scientific rationale for administer-ing metformin (Glucophage) is that it diminishes the increase in serum glucose following a meal and blunts the degree of postprandial hyperglycemia by preventing gluconeogenesis.

4. A meglitinide, repaglinide (Prandin), sulfonylurea, or nateglinide (Starlix) is prescribed to stimulate the beta cells to release more insulin into the bloodstream.

13. 1. The oral hypoglycemic medication should be administered with food to decrease gastric upset.

2. The client receiving oral hypoglycemic medications can experience hypoglycemic reactions, as can clients receiving insulin.

3. These are signs or symptoms of hypo-glycemia, and the client should be able to treat this without notifying the health-care provider.

4. Ketones are a byproduct of the breakdown of fats, which usually does not occur in clients with Type 2 diabetes because the client has enough insulin to prevent break-down of fats but not enough to keep the blood glucose level within an acceptable level.

14. 1. An elastic skin turgor is expected and normal, but it does not indicate that the antidiabetic medication is effective.

2. Urine ketones should be negative because there should not be a breakdown of fat in clients with Type 2 diabetes, but this does not indicate the effectiveness of the medication.

3. The serum blood glucose level should be within normal limits, which is 70–110 mg/dL. A level of 118 mg/dL is close to normal; therefore, the medica-tion can be considered effective.

4. A self-monitoring blood glucose level of 170 mg/dL is above a normal glucose level; this indicates the medication is not effective.

MEDICATION MEMORY JOGGER: The nurse determines the effectiveness of a medication by assessing for the symp-toms, or lack thereof, for which the medication was prescribed.

15. 1. During illness, the client with Type 2 diabetes may need insulin to help keep glucose levels under control, but this is a threatening type of statement and is not the nurse's best response.

2. Insulin may need to be prescribed in times of stress, surgery, or serious infection; therefore, the nurse should explain this to the client and not refer the client to the HCP.

3. This is a therapeutic response and the client needs to have factual information. Therapeutic responses are used to encour-age the client to ventilate feelings.

4. Blood glucose levels elevate during times of stress, surgery, or serious infection. The client with Type 2 diabetes may need to be given insulin temporarily to help keep the blood glucose level with normal limits.

16. 1. The client's serum blood glucose level is checked by drawing a venipuncture blood sample and sending it to the laboratory. This would take too long. The nurse must take care of the client; therefore, drawing a blood sample and awaiting results is not the first intervention.

2. The client is experiencing signs of a hypoglycemic reaction and the nurse must treat the client by administering some type of simple-acting glucose. This is the first intervention.

3. Determining when the last oral hypo-glycemic medication was administered is an intervention that could be imple-mented, but it is not the first intervention. The nurse needs to take care of the client.

4. The nurse could assess the client's vital signs, but this is not the first intervention; the nurse should take care of the client's signs and symptoms.

MEDICATION MEMORY JOGGER: When answering test questions or when caring for clients at the bedside, the nurse should remember that assessing the client might not be the first action to take when the client is in distress. The nurse may need to intervene directly to help the client.

17. 1. Changes in weight will affect the amount of medication needed to control blood glucose. The nurse should determine if the client's medication dose is too high by determining if the client has had an increase in hypoglycemic reactions. This is the nurse's first intervention.
    2. A significant weight loss may require a decrease or discontinuation of oral hypoglycemic medication, but the nurse should first determine if the client has had symptoms of hypoglycemia before referring him or her to the HCP.
    3. Determining if the client was deliberately losing weight or was losing without trying is significant because a 35-pound weight loss in 4 months would warrant intervention, depending on what caused the weight loss. However, this should not be the nurse's first intervention.
    4. The nurse should confirm the client's weight loss with the clinic scale and the last weight in the client's chart, but it is not the clinic nurse's first intervention.

MEDICATION MEMORY JOGGER: Remember that the first step in the nursing process is assessment. Words such as check, monitor, determine, ask, take, auscultate, and palpate indicate that the nurse is assessing the client. Assessment should be done before implementing an independent nursing action or notifying the health-care provider, except in certain serious or life-threatening situations.

18. 1. The nurse should investigate any herb the client is taking because most herbs do affect a disease process or the medication being taken for the disease process.
    2. The nurse should determine if ginseng affects the client's Type 2 diabetes or medications that the client is taking for the disease process.

3. This is a negative, judgmental statement. Many herbs are beneficial to the client. The nurse should always assess the client and determine if the herb is detrimental to the client's disease process or affects the client's routine medication regimen prior to making this type of statement.
4. The nurse should determine if the client is taking any medication because many oral hypoglycemics interact with herbs. Ginseng and garlic may increase the hypoglycemic effects of oral hypoglycemics.

MEDICATION MEMORY JOGGER: Some herbal preparations are effective, some are not, and a few can be harmful or even deadly. If a client is taking an herbal supplement and a conventional medicine, the nurse should investigate to determine if the herbal preparation would cause harm to the client. The nurse should always be the client's advocate.

19. 1. The students with Type 2 diabetes should not eat candy, but it is not the most important intervention for the school nurse to teach.
    2. This is pertinent information, but it is not the most important information.
    3. **The most important information for the teachers to know is how to treat potentially life-threatening complications secondary to the medications used to treat Type 2 diabetes. The school nurse should discuss issues that keep the students safe.**
    4. Exercise is important in helping to control Type 2 diabetes, but empowering the teachers to be confident when handling complications secondary to medication is priority for the safety of the students.

20. 1. Jaundiced sclera may indicate the client has hepatitis, but because the client has been prescribed oral hypoglycemic medications, their possible role in the development of the jaundice should be assessed.
    2. The nurse should not jump to the conclusion that the client is an alcoholic just because the sclera is jaundiced.
    3. Digoxin toxicity results in the client having a yellow haze, not the client's sclera being yellow.
    4. **Oral hypoglycemics are metabolized in the liver and may cause elevations in liver enzymes; the client should be instructed to report the first signs of**

yellow skin, sclera, pale stools, or dark urine to the HCP.

A Client with Pancreatitis

21. 1. Morphine can cause spasm of the pancreatic ducts and the sphincter of Oddi. Therefore, the nurse would question administering this medication.
    2. Diphenhydramine is a histamine$_1$ blocker that blocks the release of histamine$_1$ that occurs during allergic reactions. The nurse would not question this medication.
    3. Clients with diabetes mellitus may at times have a need for a steroid medication. The medication may elevate the client's glucose levels, and these levels should be monitored. The nurse would not question this medication.
    4. Vasopressin is the hormone that is lacking in clients diagnosed with diabetes insipidus (DI) and is the treatment for DI. The nurse would not question administering this medication.

    MEDICATION MEMORY JOGGER: The nurse must be knowledgeable about accepted standards of practice for disease processes and conditions. If the nurse administers a medication the health-care provider has prescribed and it harms the client, the nurse could be held accountable. Remember that the nurse is a client advocate.

22. 1. Synthroid is a daily medication and can be administered at any time.
    2. Protonix is a daily medication and can be administered at any time.
    3. Tylenol is for mild to moderate pain; this client would require a more potent analgesic. The nurse should assess the client's medications and discuss other medications with the HCP. This would not be the first medication to administer.
    4. Pancreatic enzymes are administered with every meal and snack. The nurse should administer this medication so the medication and the breakfast foods arrive in the small intestine simultaneously.

23. 1. The nurse is following a correct procedure for administering medications through a nasogastric tube that is connected to suction. The tube should remain clamped for 1 hour before it is reconnected to suction.

2. The nurse followed correct procedure; there is no reason to notify the manager.
3. The nurse is following a correct procedure for administering medications through a nasogastric tube that is connected to suction. The tube should remain clamped for 1 hour before it is reconnected to suction to allow the medication to be absorbed.
4. The medication is ordered to be administered through the tube, not orally.

24. 1. The Librium may act as an adjunct to pain relief, but this is not the reason for prescribing the medication to this client.
    2. Librium is useful in preventing delirium tremens in clients withdrawing from alcohol. The majority of clients diagnosed with chronic pancreatitis (75%) are middle-aged males who also have chronic alcoholism.
    3. Librium may have some antiemetic properties, but this is not the reason for prescribing the medication to this client.
    4. Librium can cause drowsiness, but it is not the drug of choice as a sleep aid for a client who is NPO.

25. 1. Clients should be asked to rate their pain on a scale so the nurse can objectively evaluate the effectiveness of the interventions.
    2. The nurse abides by the five rights of medication administration, including the right time. Pain medication is prescribed at specific time intervals. The nurse must make sure the time interval has passed and it is time for more medication.
    3. A client diagnosed with severe acute pancreatitis will be NPO, and Vicodin is an oral narcotic medication. The nurse would administer an IV medication.
    4. The client should be placed in a semi-Fowler's position to relieve pressure on the abdomen, thereby decreasing the client's pain.
    5. There is no indication that the client requires oxygenation at this time.

26. 1. Blood glucose levels should be monitored every 4–6 hours, not daily.
    2. TPN requires a central line for administration, not a peripheral line. The high concentration of dextrose in TPN causes phlebitis in peripheral veins.

3. The client's electrolytes and magnesium levels are monitored, not the complete blood count.
4. **The TPN solution contains all the required nutrients to sustain life. It also makes an ideal medium for bacterial growth. Infection control safety measures include using new tubing with every bag of TPN.**

27. 1. The client will be in a Fowler's or semi-Fowler's position to use gravity to pool secretions near the gastric/duodenal tube.
2. This is not an investigational procedure. The general treatment permission form the client signed when entering the hospital is sufficient.
3. **The gastric and duodenal contents are aspirated and sent to the laboratory for analysis before and after the administration of secretin, which stimulates the pancreas to secrete enzymes.**
4. The client is not placed in a head-down position for this procedure.

28. 1. The nurse should have been monitoring the client for constipation while in the hospital. The client should not be discharged on Demerol.
2. **To prevent withdrawal after weeks of administration of Demerol, the client should be tapered off the medication over several days.**
3. The client should be tapered off the medication prior to leaving the hospital, not sent to a drug withdrawal center.
4. Withdrawal from the medication should be accomplished prior to discharging the client, so the symptoms of withdrawal should occur while the client is still in the hospital.

29. 1. **Octreotide stimulates fluid and electrolyte absorption from the gastrointestinal tract and prolongs intestinal transit time, thereby decreasing diarrhea.**
2. Octreotide is prescribed for clients with acromegaly to prevent growth, not stimulate it.
3. Octreotide is helpful in preventing or treating diarrhea and associated abdominal pain, but not muscle cramping or pain.
4. Octreotide does not treat acid reflux.

MEDICATION MEMORY JOGGER: The nurse determines the effectiveness of a medication by assessing for the symp-toms, or lack thereof, for which the medication was prescribed.

30. 1. Humalog is not administered intravenously, and glucose levels should be monitored prior to insulin administration.
2. The client's symptoms should indicate hyperglycemia to the nurse, not pancreatic enzyme deficiency.
3. **Humulin R insulin is administered by sliding scale to decrease blood glucose levels. Clients with pancreatitis should be monitored for the development of diabetes mellitus. Polydipsia and polyuria are classic signs of diabetes mellitus.**
4. Zantac would not treat the client's symptoms.

A Client with Adrenal Disorders

31. 1. **The dose of corticosteroids may have to be increased during the stress of an infection or surgery. It is imperative that under these circumstances the client receives enough medication to replicate the body's own responses to stress (see the table).**
2. The client usually will need to take mineral and glucocorticoid replacement therapy. This statement does not need more teaching.
3. The client will experience symptoms of adrenal insufficiency if not taking the medications. This statement does not need more teaching.
4. Clients should be taught to inform all health-care providers of all medications, prescribed and over the counter, that they are taking. This statement does not need more teaching.

32. 1. The medication should be taken at least 30 minutes before food or fluid is consumed for the day. The client should drink a full glass of water with the medication and remain in an upright position for at least 30 minutes after taking Fosamax to prevent esophageal erosion and ulceration.
2. The medication is taken the first thing in the morning when the stomach is empty. Taking Fosamax and then lying down would cause esophageal reflux, resulting in erosion and ulceration of the esophagus.
3. An antacid will interfere with the absorption of Fosamax.

Guidelines for Giving Supplemental Doses of Glucocorticoids at Times of Stress Related to Medical Conditions and Surgical Procedures

Medical Condition or Surgical Procedure	Supplemental Glucocorticoid Dosage
MINOR Inguinal hernia repair Colonoscopy Mild febrile illness Mild/moderate nausea and vomiting Gastroenteritis	25 mg of hydrocortisone (or 5 mg of methylprednisolone) IV on day of procedure
MODERATE Open cholecystectomy Hemicolectomy Significant febrile illness Pneumonia Severe gastroenteritis	50–75 mg of hydrocortisone (or 10–15 mg of methylprednisolone) IV on day of procedure Taper quickly over 1–2 days to usual replacement dose
SEVERE Major cardiothoracic surgery Whipple procedure Liver resection Pancreatitis	100–150 mg of hydrocortisone (or 20–30 mg of methylprednisolone) IV on day of procedure Rapid taper over 1–2 days to usual replacement dose
CRITICAL Sepsis-induced hypotension or shock	50–100 mg of hydrocortisone IV every 6–8 hours (or 0.18 mg/kg/hour as continuous infusion) plus 50 mg of fludrocortisone until shock resolves, which may take several days to a week or more. Then, taper gradually, monitoring vital signs and serum sodium levels.

From Lehne, Richard (2004). *Pharmacology for Nursing Care*, adapted from *JAMA 2002;* 287:236–240.

4. The medication should be taken at least 30 minutes before food or fluid is consumed for the day. The client should drink a full glass of water with the medication and remain in an upright position for at least 30 minutes after taking Fosamax to prevent esophageal erosion and ulceration.

33. 1. The medication cannot be discontinued; a bilateral adrenalectomy means that all the hormones normally produced by the adrenal glands must be replaced. The client now has adrenal insufficiency (Addison's disease).

2. The glucocorticosteroids and mineralocorticosteroids, as well as the androgens produced by the adrenal glands, must be replaced regularly; doses should not be skipped.

3. The client cannot stop taking the medication. Doing so could result in a life-threatening situation. The development of a round face is a side effect of glucocorticoids that may indicate that the dose is too high. The client should notify the HCP to review the dosage.

4. Excess glucocorticoids may induce diabetes mellitus; the HCP should be notified if the client experiences symptoms of diabetes such as feeling thirsty all the time.

5. All clients with a chronic medical condition should wear a MedicAlert bracelet or necklace.

34. 1. The nurse will monitor the client's electrolytes, especially sodium and potassium and glucose levels, but this is not the first action.

2. The nurse should be prepared to replace the corticosteroids, but this is not the first action.

3. The nurse must treat an Addisonian crisis as all other shock situations. An IV and fluid replacement are imperative to prevent or treat shock. This is the first action.

4. This is important, but it will not prevent or treat shock.

MEDICATION MEMORY JOGGER: The stem of the previous question told the test taker that the situation is a "crisis." The first step in many crises is to make sure that an IV access is available to administer fluids and medications.

35. 1. Protonix does not increase the ability to digest food.
    2. **Protonix decreases the production of stomach acid by inhibiting the proton-pump step in gastric acid production.**
    3. Protonix does not absorb gastric acid; it prevents its production.
    4. Sucralfate (Carafate) is a mucosal barrier agent that coats the stomach lining. Protonix does not coat the stomach.

36. 1. Shortness of breath and pale mucous membranes do not indicate long-term steroid use or Cushing's syndrome.
    2. **A round face (moon face) indicates a redistribution of fat from steroid therapy. Multiple ecchymotic areas on the arms indicate a redistribution of subcutaneous fats away from the arm (thin extremities). Both are side effects of long-term steroid therapy.**
    3. Pink, frothy sputum and jugular vein distention are symptoms of congestive heart failure, not long-term steroid therapy.
    4. Petechiae indicate a low platelet count, and sclerosed veins indicate the use of IV access for medication administration. These are not signs of steroid therapy.

37. 1. **Ketoconazole is an anti-infective that also suppresses the production of adrenal hormones. This side effect makes it useful in treating the overproduction of adrenal hormones that results from secretion of ACTH by tumors that cannot be removed surgically.**
    2. Methylprednisolone is a steroid, and ACTH stimulates the production of adrenal hormones. This would increase the client's symptoms.
    3. Propylthiouracil is used to suppress the production of thyroid hormones, not adrenal hormones.
    4. Vasopressin is a pituitary hormone that prevents diuresis; it is not an adrenal hormone.

38. 1. The client diagnosed with Cushing's disease is at risk for infections because of the immune suppression that occurs as a result of excess cortisol production. This client should be seen by the HCP.
    2. Clients diagnosed with Cushing's disease are at risk for developing infections related to the excess production of cortisol by the adrenal glands. The client must be seen by an HCP and antibiotics must be initiated.
    3. The client is not in an emergent situation; the client can go to an HCP office or clinic to be seen.
    4. The client has a physiological problem, not a psychosocial problem. The client does not need therapeutic conversation.

39. 1. Florinef is not an oral hypoglycemic medication. It is a steroid and may increase the blood glucose, not decrease it.
    2. **Mineral corticosteroids help the body to maintain the correct serum sodium levels. Florinef is the preferred medication for Addison's disease, primary hypoaldosteronism, and congenital adrenal hyperplasia when sodium wasting occurs.**
    3. Florinef does not prevent muscle cramps. If the Florinef dose is too high, then potassium wasting will occur, resulting in muscle cramping.
    4. Florinef does not stimulate the pituitary gland. The pituitary gland produces hormones that stimulate the adrenal gland. The adrenal gland does not produce hormones that stimulate the pituitary gland.

40. 1. Replacement corticosteroids are necessary for clients with adrenal insufficiency. The nurse would not question administering prednisone.
    2. Ginseng is an herb that enhances the adrenal function. The nurse would not question this medication.
    3. **Mitotane is a medication that suppresses adrenal functioning. The nurse would question this medication in a patient with adrenal insufficiency.**
    4. In both males and females, the adrenal glands produce androgens, including testosterone. Replacing this hormone would not be unusual in a client with adrenal insufficiency.

MEDICATION MEMORY JOGGER: The nurse must be knowledgeable about accepted standards of practice for disease processes and conditions. If the nurse administers a medication the health-care provider has prescribed and it harms the client, the nurse could be held account-

able. Remember that the nurse is a client advocate.

MEDICATION MEMORY JOGGER: Some herbal preparations are effective, some are not, and a few can be harmful or even deadly. If a client is taking an herbal supplement and a conventional medicine, the nurse should investigate to determine if the herbal preparation will cause harm to the client. The nurse should always be the client's advocate.

A Client with Pituitary Disorders

41. 1. DDAVP acts on the kidney to concentrate urine, but kidney stones would not warrant a change in the medication.
    2. Diabetes mellitus Type 2 would not be a reason to change the medication.
    3. **DDAVP is administered intranasally, and a sinus infection could interfere with absorption of the medication. Vasopressin comes in an intramuscular form, and the client may need to take this form of vasopressin until the sinus infection has resolved.**
    4. Hyperthyroidism would not warrant a change in medication or route.

42. 1. **Octreotide suppresses the pituitary gland's secretion of human growth hormone, which, in adults, causes enlarged viscera, bone deformities, and other signs and symptoms of acromegaly. The nurse would expect to administer this medication. (Acromegaly in children results in gigantism.)**
    2. Somatrem is a growth hormone and would increase the client's symptoms.
    3. NSAIDs are administered to clients diagnosed with nephrogenic diabetes insipidus to inhibit prostaglandin production.
    4. The client has symptoms of acromegaly, an overproduction of human growth hormone. ACTH would not suppress this production.

43. 1. The client diagnosed with diabetes insipidus is excreting large amounts of dilute urine because the body is unable to conserve water and concentrate the urine. The client requires fluid-volume replacement. The nurse would insert an IV. The client would have a high

sodium level (because of the lack of fluid in the vascular system); lactated Ringer's solution would be preferred to normal saline.
    2. The client should be on hourly output measurements. An indwelling catheter is needed to measure the client's output. The client requires rest, and voiding many liters of urine every day would leave the client exhausted from lack of sleep.
    3. The urine specific gravity indicates the client's ability to concentrate urine and should be monitored.
    4. Lasix would increase the client's urinary output; this is opposite to the effect that is needed.
    5. In this situation, intake and output measurements are monitored every hour, not every shift.

44. 1. Diabinese can cause weakness, jitteriness, nervousness, and other signs of a hypoglycemic reaction. The client should be aware of this and be prepared to treat the reaction with a source of simple carbohydrate. This is not a reason to discontinue the medication.
    2. Diabinese is not a cholinergic medication with a side effect of a dry mouth.
    3. Clients with Type 2 diabetes mellitus usually take the medication prior to meals. The effects of Diabinese can last 2–3 days. This client can take the medication after a meal.
    4. **Diabinese potentiates the action of vasopressin in clients with residual hypothalamic function. The sulfonylureas are used mostly to treat Type 2 diabetes mellitus because they stimulate the pancreas to secrete insulin. The client should be aware that an insulin reaction (hypoglycemic reaction) can occur.**

45. 1. This medication is given to cause maturation of the ovarian follicle and trigger ovulation. An FSH level would have been done prior to prescribing Chorigon.
    2. **This medication is given to cause maturation of the ovarian follicle and trigger ovulation. The client is monitored for overstimulation of the ovaries by pelvic sonograms.**
    3. The medication is a category X medication, which indicates that it is known to cause harm to fetuses, but it is given to stimulate ovulation to achieve a preg-

nancy. It also is given to maintain the corpus luteum after LH decreases during a normal pregnancy.
4. The medication is given parenterally, not orally.

46. 1. **In SIADH, the body retains too much water. Elevated fluid levels in the body result in dilutional hyponatremia. Hyponatremia can cause seizures and other central nervous system dysfunction. The sodium level is monitored to determine the effectiveness of the intervention.**
2. The serum potassium level is important to monitor, but it will not measure the effectiveness of Lasix in treating this condition.
3. The problem in SIADH is in the pituitary gland; it is not a kidney problem.
4. The pituitary gland produces ACTH, but ACTH production is not the problem in SIADH. SIADH is an overproduction of vasopressin, the antidiuretic hormone.

MEDICATION MEMORY JOGGER: The nurse must be knowledgeable about accepted standards of practice for medication administration, including which client assessment data and laboratory data should be monitored prior to administering the medication.

47. 1. Clofibrate is an antilipemic that has an antidiuretic effect on clients with neurogenic diabetes insipidus, but it would not have an effect on a client whose diabetes insipidus is caused by the kidney's inability to respond to the medication.
2. **NSAIDs inhibit prostaglandin production and are used to treat nephrogenic diabetes insipidus.**
3. Lasix is a diuretic and would increase the urinary output in a client whose problem is too much urinary output.
4. Desmopressin is a form of vasopressin, the antidiuretic hormone, but production of the hormone is not in question in nephrogenic diabetes insipidus; the pituitary gland is producing the hormone. The problem is that the kidneys are unable to respond to it.

48. 1. The problem is that the client is in fluid-volume overload probably as a result of the medication vincristine. A diuretic may be administered, but as a treatment, not as a prophylactic measure.
2. Weight gain is not a sign of an infection. These symptoms indicate SIADH.

3. The client's diet is not responsible for the fluid weight gain.
4. **Vincristine, the phenothiazines, antidepressants, thiazide diuretics, and smoking are known to stimulate the pituitary gland, resulting in an overproduction of vasopressin. The client's symptoms indicate SIADH. The nurse should assess the weight gain, hold the medication, and notify the HCP.**

49. 1. Sleeping with the head of the bed elevated will not affect this medication.
2. The medication is administered intramuscularly. A tuberculin syringe is used for subcutaneous or intradermal injections.
3. **The medication should be administered in the evening for maximum effect during the sleeping hours, so the client will not be up to void frequently.**
4. DDAVP, not vasopressin tannate in oil, is administered intranasally.

MEDICATION MEMORY JOGGER: The test taker could eliminate option 4 by reading "in oil." Oil preparations are not usually administered in the nose.

50. 1. Black cohosh is an over-the-counter herb that is sometimes used to treat dysmenorrhea, premenstrual syndrome (PMS), and menopausal symptoms. The nurse would not question this medication.
2. **Desmopressin causes vasoconstriction and is contraindicated in clients with angina because of the coronary vasoconstriction.**
3. Diuril would be administered to a client with SIADH. SIADH may be caused by a head injury, pituitary tumors, tumors that secrete hormones, some medications, and smoking. The nurse would not question this medication.
4. Calcitonin is administered to decrease calcium levels. The nurse would not question this medication.

MEDICATION MEMORY JOGGER: The nurse must be knowledgeable about accepted standards of practice for disease processes and conditions. If the nurse administers a medication the health-care provider has prescribed and it harms the client, the nurse could be held accountable. Remember that the nurse is a client advocate.

A Client with Thyroid Disorders

51. 1. The client would have signs or symptoms of hypothyroidism if the client is not taking enough medication. Weight loss is a sign of hyperthyroidism, which indicates the client is taking too much Synthroid.
2. The client would have signs or symptoms of hypothyroidism if the client is not taking enough medication. Intolerance to heat is a sign of hyperthyroidism and indicates the client is taking too much medication.
3. Tachycardia, a heart rate greater than 100, is a sign of hyperthyroidism and indicates the client is taking too much medication.
4. **Decreased metabolism and constipation indicate that the client is not taking enough of the thyroid hormone.**

52. 1. **Synthroid increases the basal metabolic rate, which can precipitate cardiac dysrhythmias in clients with undiagnosed heart disease, especially in elderly clients. Synthroid can also cause cardiovascular collapse. Therefore the client's cardiovascular function should be assessed by the nurse.**
2. Respiratory depression is not a complication of thyroid hormone therapy.
3. The client with hypothyroidism may experience a paralytic ileus due to decreased metabolism. This would not be an expected complication in a client taking Synthroid.
4. A thyroid storm may occur when the thyroid gland is manipulated during a thyroidectomy, not when the client starts taking Synthroid.

53. 1. The goal of radioactive iodine treatment is to destroy just enough of the thyroid gland so that the levels of thyroid function return to normal; it does not destroy the entire gland.
2. **The client should not be in close contact with children or pregnant women for 1 week following administration of the medication because the client will be emitting small amounts of radiation.**
3. Most clients require a single dose of radioactive iodine, but some may need additional treatments.
4. The radioactive iodine is a clear, odorless, tasteless liquid that does not need to be administered with cold orange juice.

54. 1. The client's arterial blood gases are not affected by PTU.
2. The client's potassium level is not affected by PTU.
3. The client's red blood cell count is not affected by PTU.
4. **The client receiving PTU is at risk for agranulocytosis; therefore, the client's white blood cell count should be checked periodically. Because agranulocytosis puts the client at greater risk for infection, efforts to control invasion of microbes should be strictly observed.**

55. 1. **Nervousness, jitteriness, and irritability are signs or symptoms of hyperthyroidism; therefore, the nurse should question administering thyroid hormone.**
2. A normal temperature would indicate the client is in a euthyroid state; therefore, the nurse would not question administering this medication.
3. A normal blood pressure would indicate the client is in a euthyroid state; therefore, the nurse would not question administering this medication.
4. The nurse would not question administering the medication because fatigue is a sign of hypothyroidism, which is why the client has been prescribed thyroid hormone.

MEDICATION MEMORY JOGGER: If the client verbalizes a complaint, if the nurse assesses data, or if laboratory data indicates an adverse effect secondary to a medication, the nurse must intervene. The nurse must implement an independent intervention or notify the health-care provider because medications can result in serious or even life-threatening complications.

56. 1. The nurse should discuss ways to help cope with the symptoms of hypothyroidism. The client should increase fiber intake to help prevent constipation.
2. The T3, T4, and TSH levels are monitored to help determine the effectiveness of the medication, but this is not done daily by the client. Serum blood levels are monitored monthly initially and then every 6 months.
3. The medication should be taken on an empty stomach because thyroid hormones have their optimum effect when taken on an empty stomach.

4. The client's weight should be monitored weekly. Weight loss is expected as a result of the increased metabolic rate, and weight changes help to determine the effectiveness of the drug therapy.

57. 1. There is no reason for the client to notify the HCP because it takes several months to attain the euthyroid state.
2. Most clients only need one dose of radioactive iodine, but it takes several months to attain the euthyroid state.
3. **The goal of radioactive therapy for hyperthyroidism is to destroy just enough of the thyroid gland so that levels of thyroid function return to normal. Full benefits may take several months.**
4. This is a therapeutic response, which is not appropriate because the client needs factual information.

58. 1. This would be appropriate if the client is taking antithyroid medication, not thyroid hormones. Iodine increases the production of thyroid hormones, which is not desirable in clients taking antithyroid medications.
2. Grapefruit juice is contraindicated when taking some medications, but not thyroid hormone therapy.
3. **The medication should be taken in the morning to decrease the incidence of drug-related insomnia.**
4. Thyroid medications do not affect the client's blood glucose level; therefore, there is no need for the client to monitor the glucose level.

MEDICATION MEMORY JOGGER: Grapefruit juice can inhibit the metabolism of certain medications. Specifically, grapefruit juice inhibits cytochrome P450-3A4 found in the liver and the intestinal wall. The nurse should investigate any medications the client is taking if the client drinks grapefruit juice.

59. 1. Antithyroid medications may cause drowsiness; therefore, this statement would not warrant immediate intervention by the nurse.
2. **The antithyroid medication may affect the body's ability to defend itself against bacteria and viruses; therefore, the nurse should intervene if the client has any type of sore throat, fever, chills, malaise, or weakness.**
3. As a result of slower metabolism from the PTU, weight gain is expected; therefore, this statement would not warrant intervention by the nurse.
4. This indicates the medication is effective; the signs of hyperthyroidism—which include feeling hot much of the time—are decreasing. This would not warrant immediate intervention by the nurse.

60. 1. **Thyroid function tests are used to determine the effectiveness of drug therapy.**
2. **Weight gain is expected as a result of a slower metabolism.**
3. **Antithyroid medication may cause nausea or vomiting.**
4. **Changes in metabolic rate will be manifested as changes in blood pressure, pulse, and body temperature.**
5. **Hyperthyroidism results in protein catabolism, overactivity, and increased metabolism, which lead to exhaustion; therefore, the nurse should monitor for activity intolerance.**

1. The client diagnosed with Addison's disease tells the clinic nurse that he is taking licorice every day to help the disease process. Which action should the nurse implement?
   1. Tell the client licorice is a candy and will not help Addison's disease.
   2. Praise the client because licorice increases aldosterone production.
   3. Ask the client why he thinks licorice will help the disease process.
   4. Determine if the licorice has caused any mouth ulcers or sores.

2. The client is diagnosed with primary hyperaldosteronism and prescribed the aldosterone agonist spironolactone (Aldactone). Which data would support that the medication is effective?
   1. The client's potassium level is 4.2 mEq/L.
   2. The client's urinary output is 30 mL/hr.
   3. The client's blood pressure is 140/96.
   4. The client's serum sodium is 137 mEq/L.

3. The client diagnosed with diabetes insipidus (DI) is receiving desmopressin (DDAVP), a pituitary hormone, intranasally. Which assessment data would warrant the client notifying the health-care provider?
   1. The client does not feel thirsty all the time.
   2. The client is able to sleep throughout the night.
   3. The client has gained 2 kg in the last 24 hours.
   4. The client has to urinate at least five times daily.

4. The 2-year-old child has just been diagnosed with cystic fibrosis (CF). Which intervention should the nurse discuss with the child's mother?
   1. Do not administer over-the-counter mucolytic agents.
   2. Administer cough suppressants at night only.
   3. Check the child's blood glucose level four times a day.
   4. Sprinkle pancreatic enzymes on the child's food.

5. The 36-year-old female client who had an abdominal hysterectomy is prescribed the estrogen hormone replacement Premarin. The client calls the nurse in the Women's Health Clinic and reports she is producing breast milk. Which intervention should the nurse tell the client?
   1. Explain that this is an expected side effect and it will stop.
   2. Determine if the client is having abdominal cramping.
   3. Ask if this mainly occurs during sexual intercourse.
   4. Discontinue taking the estrogen until seen by the HCP.

6. The 10-year-old male client is receiving the growth hormone somatropin (Humatrope). Which signs or symptoms would warrant intervention by the nurse?
   1. A 3-cm increase in height.
   2. A moon face and buffalo hump.
   3. Polyuria, polydipsia, and polyphagia.
   4. T 99.4°F, P 108, R 22, and B/P 121/70.

7. The female client has secondary adrenal insufficiency and is prescribed adrenocorticotrophic hormone ACTH (Acthar). Which information should the nurse discuss with client?
   1. Explain ACTH will increase metabolism.
   2. Instruct the client to limit dietary salt.
   3. Inform the client that an increase in growth may occur.
   4. Tell the client that normal menses is expected.

8. The client is diagnosed with hypothyroidism and is taking the thyroid hormone levothyroxine (Synthroid). Which data indicates the medication is effective?
   1. The client's apical pulse is 84 and the blood pressure is 134/78.
   2. The client's temperature is 96.7°F and respiratory rate is 14.
   3. The client reports having a soft, formed stool every 4 days.
   4. The client tells the nurse that the client only needs 3 hours of sleep.

9. The nurse is administering the following medications. Which medication would the nurse question administering?
   1. The sulfonylurea glyburide (Micronase) to a client with Type 1 diabetes.
   2. The loop diuretic furosemide (Lasix) to a client with SIADH.
   3. The narcotic analgesic meperidine (Demerol) to a client with pancreatitis.
   4. The sliding-scale regular insulin to a client with Type 2 diabetes.

10. The client with Type 1 diabetes is scheduled for a CT scan of the abdomen with contrast. The client is taking metformin (Glucophage), a biguanide, and 70/30 insulin 24 units at 0700 and 1600. Which instruction should the nurse give the client?
    1. Administer the 70/30 insulin the morning of the test.
    2. Take half the dose of the morning insulin on the day of the test.
    3. Do not take the Glucophage after the procedure until the HCP approves.
    4. Take the medications as prescribed because they will not affect the test.

11. The client with chronic pancreatitis is prescribed the pancreatic enzyme Pancrease. Which data indicate that the dosage should be increased?
    1. No bowel movement for 3 days.
    2. Fatty, frothy, foul-smelling stools.
    3. A decrease in urinary output.
    4. An increase in midepigastric pain.

12. The client with Addison's disease is prescribed prednisone. Which laboratory data would the nurse expect this medication to alter?
    1. Glucose.
    2. Sodium.
    3. Calcium.
    4. Creatinine.

13. The client is prescribed prednisone, a glucocorticoid, for poison ivy. Which information should the nurse discuss with the client? Select all that apply.
    1. Take the medication with food.
    2. The medication must be tapered.
    3. Avoid going in the sunlight.
    4. Monitor the blood glucose level.
    5. Do not eat green, leafy vegetables.

14. The client diagnosed with hyperthyroidism undergoes a bilateral thyroidectomy. Which statement indicates the client understands the discharge instructions?
    1. "I must take my PTU medication at night only."
    2. "I should not take my medication if I am nauseated."
    3. "I will take my thyroid hormone pill every day."
    4. "I need to check my thyroid level daily."

15. The unlicensed assistive personnel (UAP) notifies the primary nurse that the client is complaining of being jittery and nervous and is diaphoretic. The client is diagnosed with diabetes mellitus. Which interventions should the primary nurse implement? Rank in order of performance.
    1. Have the UAP check the client's glucose level.
    2. Tell the UAP to get the client some orange juice.
    3. Check the client's medication administration record.
    4. Immediately go to the room and assess the client.
    5. Assist the UAP in changing the client's bed linens.

16. The client with Type 1 diabetes is diagnosed with diabetic ketoacidosis. The HCP prescribes intravenous regular insulin by continuous infusion. Which intervention should the intensive care nurse implement when administering this medication?
    1. Flush the tubing with 50 mL of the insulin drip before administering to the client.
    2. Monitor the client's serum glucose level every hour and document it on the MAR.
    3. Draw the client's arterial blood gas results daily and document them in the client's chart.
    4. Administer the client's regular insulin drip via gravity at the prescribed rate.

17. The nurse is administering medications to a client diagnosed with Type 1 diabetes. The client's 1100 glucometer reading is 310. Which action should the nurse implement?

Client's Name:	Account Number: 123456			Allergies: NKDA
Height: 69 inches	Weight: 165 pounds			
Date	Medication	2301–0700	0701–1500	1501–2300
	Regular insulin by bedside glucose subcu ac & hs			
	<60 notify HCP 150 0 units 151–200 2 units		0730 DN BG 142 0 units	
	201–250 4 units 251–300 6 units			
	301–350 8 units 351–400 10 units >400 notify HCP			
Signature/Initials		Day Nurse RN, DN		

1. Have the laboratory verify the glucose results.
2. Notify the health-care provider of the results.
3. Administer 8 units of regular insulin subcutaneously.
4. Recheck the client's glucometer reading at 1130.

18. The client with Type 2 diabetes is prescribed exenatide (BYETTA), a subcutaneous antidiabetic medication. Which information should the nurse discuss with the client?
1. Keep the BYETTA pen at room temperature after opening the pen.
2. Instruct the client to notify the health-care provider if nauseated.
3. Tell the client to take the medication 1 hour before the morning and evening meals.
4. Explain that this medication is a type of regular-acting insulin.

19. Which statement by the client with Type 2 diabetes indicates the client understands the medication teaching concerning exenatide (BYETTA), a subcutaneous antidiabetic medication?
1. "I will throw away my pen in 30 days, even if there is medicine in the pen."
2. "I always keep the needle on my pen, even when it is in the refrigerator."
3. "This medication cost so much I use my pen past the expiration date."
4. "I should not take any other diabetic medication when I take BYETTA."

20. The client with diabetes is prescribed Exubera, insulin human (rDNA origin) inhalation powder. Which statement indicates the client needs more medication teaching?
1. "With this medication I will be taking 10 times my regular insulin dose."
2. "My medication will be in a large canister that I must carry with me."
3. "I am glad that I don't have to worry about an insulin reaction with Exubera."
4. "If I get a cold or pneumonia, I will call my health-care provider."

1. 1. This is a false statement, and the nurse should investigate any type of alternative treatment before making this statement.
   2. **Licorice is a flavoring for candy, but it is also used as an herbal medication in tablet, tea, or tincture form. Licorice increases the aldosterone effect, which helps treat Addison's disease.**
   3. This is an aggressive-type judgmental question, and the client does not owe the nurse an explanation.
   4. Licorice is used to treat mouth ulcers; it does not cause them.

   MEDICATION MEMORY JOGGER: Some herbal preparations are effective, some are not, and a few can be harmful or even deadly. If a client is taking an herbal supplement and a conventional medicine, the nurse should investigate to determine if the herbal preparation will cause harm to the client. The nurse should always be the client's advocate.

2. 1. **Hyperaldosteronism causes hypokalemia, metabolic alkalosis, and hypertension. Spironolactone, a potassium-sparing diuretic, normalizes potassium levels in clients with hyperaldosteronism within 2 weeks; therefore, a normal potassium level, which is 4.2 mEq/L, indicates the medication is effective.**
   2. The urinary output is not used to determine the effectiveness of this medication in a client with hyperaldosteronism.
   3. The client does have hypertension, but this blood pressure is above normal limits and does not indicate the medication is effective.
   4. The serum sodium level is not used to determine the effectiveness of this medication in a client with hyperaldosteronism.

   MEDICATION MEMORY JOGGER: The nurse determines the effectiveness of a medication by assessing for the symptoms, or lack thereof, for which the medication was prescribed.

3. 1. The major symptom with DI is polyuria resulting in polydipsia (extreme thirst); therefore, the client not being thirsty indicates the medication is effective.
   2. The client being able to sleep through the night indicates that he or she is not getting up to urinate because of polyuria and thus that the medication is effective.

3. A weight gain of 4.4 pounds indicates the client is experiencing water intoxication, which would indicate the client is receiving too much medication and the HCP should be notified.
   4. The client urinating five times a day indicates the medication is effective; therefore, the client would not have to notify the HCP.

   MEDICATION MEMORY JOGGER: If the client verbalizes a complaint, if the nurse assesses data, or if laboratory data indicates an adverse effect secondary to a medication, the nurse must intervene. The nurse must implement an independent intervention or notify the health-care provider because medications can result in serious or even life-threatening complications.

4. 1. Mucolytic medications are administered to help liquefy thick tenacious secretions characteristic of CF.
   2. The child would not receive cough suppressants (antitussives) because the thick tenacious secretions need to be expectorated, not suppressed.
   3. Eventually the beta cells will become clogged as a result of the thick tenacious secretions in the pancreas, but this would not be a problem in the initial stage after diagnosis.
   4. **The thick tenacious secretions clog the pancreatic ducts, resulting in a decrease of the pancreatic enzymes amylase and lipase in the small intestines. The mother must administer these enzymes with every meal or snack to ensure digestion of carbohydrates and fats.**

5. 1. This is not an expected side effect and is caused by the estrogen stimulating the hypothalamus to produce prolactin. The estrogen dosage must be adjusted or discontinued.
   2. Abdominal cramping is a symptom associated with menses and the client does not have a uterus; therefore, this is not an appropriate question.
   3. The breast discharge is unrelated to sexual intercourse.
   4. **The medication should be stopped until the HCP can be seen because this warrants a dosage adjustment or discontinuation permanently. The estrogen stimulates the hypothalamus to produce prolactin, which causes the breast milk.**

6. 1. The child has grown a little more than 1 inch (2.54 cm equals 1 inch). Because the child has been prescribed the growth hormone to increase growth, this would indicate that the medication is effective and no intervention on the part of the nurse is needed.
   2. These are side effects of steroid therapy, not growth hormones.
   3. **Growth hormone is diabetogenic; therefore, any signs of diabetes mellitus, such as polyuria, polydipsia, and polyphagia, should be reported to the HCP immediately. These are the 3 Ps of diabetes mellitus.**
   4. The nurse must know the normal parameters for children (T 97.5°F to 98.6°F), so a temperature of 99.4°F would not warrant notification of the HCP. Normal pulse rate is 70–110, respiratory rate is 16–22, systolic B/P is 83–121, and diastolic B/P is 43–79. These vital signs do not warrant notifying the HCP.

7. 1. Thyroid hormones, not ACTH, would increase the client's metabolism.
   2. **ACTH is administered as an adrenal stimulant when the pituitary gland is unable to perform this function. This medication will cause the absorption of sodium and cause edema; therefore, the client should decrease salt intake.**
   3. This medication may decrease the client's growth.
   4. This medication causes abnormal menses.

8. 1. **If the thyroid medication is effective, the client's metabolism should be within normal limits, and this pulse and blood pressure support this.**
   2. These vital signs are subnormal, indicating hypothyroidism.
   3. A stool every 4 days indicates constipation and constipation is a sign of hypothyroidism. This indicates the medication is not effective.
   4. Six to 8 hours of sleep would be normal. Three hours would indicate hyperactivity, which is a sign of hyperthyroidism; perhaps a dosage adjustment in the medication is needed.

9. 1. **The sulfonylureas stimulate beta-cell production of insulin. Clients diagnosed with Type 1 diabetes have no functioning beta cells; therefore, they cannot be stimulated. The nurse should question administering this medication.**

2. The client with SIADH would be receiving a loop diuretic to decrease excess fluid volume.
3. Demerol is the drug of choice to treat pain from pancreatitis. Morphine stimulates the sphincter of Oddi.
4. A client with Type 2 diabetes is often prescribed insulin during times of stress or illness.

MEDICATION MEMORY JOGGER: The nurse must be knowledgeable about accepted standards of practice for disease processes and conditions. If the nurse administers a medication the health-care provider has prescribed and it harms the client, the nurse could be held accountable. Remember that the nurse is a client advocate.

10. 1. Because the client is NPO for the test, the insulin should be held.
    2. Because the client is NPO for the test, the insulin should be held. In addition, the nurse cannot prescribe medication or change the dosage.
    3. **Glucophage has a potential side effect of producing lactic acid. When it is administered simultaneously or within a close time span of the contrast dye used for the CT scan, lactic acidosis could result. It is recommended to hold the medication prior to and up to 48 hours after the scan. The HCP should obtain a BUN and creatinine to determine kidney function prior to restarting Glucophage.**
    4. Insulin should be held when the client is NPO, and Glucophage will be held because of the contrast dye.

MEDICATION MEMORY JOGGER: Any time the client is having a diagnostic test the nurse should question administering any medication.

11. 1. Constipation does not determine the effectiveness of the Pancrease.
    2. **Steatorrhea (fatty, frothy, foul-smelling stools) or diarrhea indicates a lack of pancreatic enzymes in the small intestines. This would indicate the dosage is too small and needs to be increased.**
    3. Urine output does not determine effectiveness of Pancrease.
    4. An increase in midepigastric pain is a symptom of peptic ulcer disease or gastrointestinal reflux disease and does not indicate the effectiveness of the pancreatic enzyme. The client with chronic pancre-

atitis may have abdominal pain, but the pancreatic enzymes are administered for digestion of food, not to alleviate pain.

12. 1. **Prednisone is a glucocorticoid medication, which affects the glucose metabolism; therefore, the nurse should expect the glucose level to be altered.**
    2. Sodium is not affected by prednisone.
    3. Calcium is not affected by prednisone.
    4. Creatinine is not affected by prednisone.

13. 1. **Prednisone is very irritating to the stomach and must be taken with food to avoid gastritis or peptic ulcer disease.**
    2. **To avoid adrenal insufficiency or Addisonian crisis, the client must taper the medication.**
    3. Prednisone does not cause photosensitivity.
    4. Because the prednisone is used short term for treating poison ivy, the blood glucose level would not need to be monitored.
    5. Green, leafy vegetables are high in vitamin K and would be contraindicated in anticoagulant treatment with Coumadin but not with prednisone treatment.

14. 1. PTU is an antithyroid medication and the client has had the thyroid gland removed.
    2. The client must take the thyroid hormone daily or the client will experience signs of hypothyroidism.
    3. **Because the client's thyroid has been removed the client now has hypothyroidism and must take a thyroid replacement daily for the rest of his or her life.**
    4. There is no daily test for thyroid level; it is checked by a venipuncture test every few months.

15.   **4, 1, 2, 3, 5**
    4. **These are symptoms of a hypoglycemic reaction and the nurse should assess the client immediately; therefore, this is the first intervention.**
    1. **Because the nurse is assessing the client in the room, the UAP can take the glucometer reading. The nurse cannot delegate care of an unstable client but can delegate a task because the nurse is in the room with the client.**
    2. **The treatment of choice for a conscious client experiencing a hypoglycemic reaction is to administer food or a source of glucose. Orange juice is a source of glucose, and the UAP can get it.**

3. **The nurse should check the MAR to determine when the last dose of insulin or oral hypoglycemic medication was administered.**
5. **When the client has been stabilized, then the linens should be changed to make the client comfortable.**

16. 1. **The regular insulin adheres to the lining of the plastic intravenous tubing; therefore, the nurse should flush the tubing with at least 50 mL of the insulin solution so that insulin will adhere to the tubing before the prescribed dosage is administered to the client. If this is not done, the client will not receive the correct dose of insulin during the first few hours of administration.**
    2. To monitor serum glucose, the nurse would need to perform an hourly venipuncture. This is painful, is more expensive, and takes a longer time to provide glucose results. Therefore, a capillary (fingerstick) bedside glucometer will be used to monitor the client's blood glucose level every hour.
    3. The nurse does not draw arterial blood gases; this is done by the respiratory therapist or the HCP.
    4. A regular insulin drip must be administered by an infusion-controlled device (IV pump). It may not be given via gravity because it is a very dangerous medication and could kill the client if not administered correctly.

17. 1. According to the sliding scale, blood glucose results should be verified when less than 60 or greater than 400.
    2. The HCP does not need to be notified unless the blood glucose is greater than 400.
    3. **The client's reading is 310; therefore, the nurse should administer 8 units of regular insulin as per the HCP's order.**
    4. There is no reason for the nurse to recheck the results.

18. 1. All BYETTA pens, used and unused, must be kept refrigerated or kept cold at 36°F.
    2. **The most common side effects with BYETTA include nausea, vomiting, diarrhea, dizziness, headache, and jitteriness. Nausea is most common when first starting BYETTA, but it decreases over time in most clients.**

3. **BYETTA is injected twice a day, at any time within 1 hour of the client's morning and evening meal. The client should not take BYETTA after the meal.**

4. BYETTA is not insulin or a substitute for insulin. Clients whose diabetes requires insulin must not use BYETTA.

19. 1. **The BYETTA pen should only be used for 30 days. The client should throw away the used BYETTA pen after 30 days, even if some medicine remains in the pen.**

2. The needle should be removed from the pen when storing the medication in the refrigerator because some medicine may leak from the BYETTA pen or air bubbles may form in the cartridge.

3. The BYETTA pen should not be used after the expiration date printed on the label.

4. BYETTA is used with metformin (Glucophage) or other types of antidiabetic medicine called sulfonylureas.

20. 1. The client must take 10 times the amount of injectable insulin because only 10% of the medication is absorbed by the body. This statement indicates the client understands the medication teaching.

2. The medication comes in a very large canister with an inhalation mouthpiece; the client understands the medication teaching.

3. **This is insulin, and the client is still subject to hypoglycemia. This statement indicates the client needs more medication teaching.**

4. Because the medication is absorbed in the lungs the client should call the HCP if the lungs are unable to absorb the medication. This indicates the client understands the discharge teaching.

Genitourinary System

"Drug therapy in pregnancy presents a vexing dilemma. When drugs are used during pregnancy, risks apply to the fetus as well as the mother."

—Richard L. Lehne

PRACTICE QUESTIONS

A Client with Chronic Renal Failure

1. The client diagnosed with chronic renal failure is prescribed erythropoietin (Epogen), a biologic response modifier. Which statement best describes the scientific rationale for administering this medication?
   1. This medication stimulates red blood cell production.
   2. This medication stimulates white blood cell production.
   3. This medication is used to treat thrombocytopenia.
   4. This medication increases the production of urine.

2. Which intervention should the nurse implement when administering the biologic response modifier erythropoietin (Epogen) subcutaneously?
   1. Shake the dose well prior to preparing the injection.
   2. Apply a warm washcloth after administering the medication.
   3. Discard any unused portion of the vial after pulling up the correct dose.
   4. Keep the medication vials in the freezer until preparing to administer.

3. Which statement best describes the scientific rationale for administering aluminum hydroxide (Amphojel), an antacid, to a client in chronic renal failure (CRF)?
   1. This medication neutralizes gastric acid production.
   2. It binds to phosphorus to help decrease hyperphosphatemia.
   3. The medication is administered to decrease the calcium level.
   4. It will help decrease episodes of constipation in the client with CRF.

4. Which statement best describes the scientific rationale for administering calcitriol (Rocaltrol), a vitamin D analog, to a client in end-stage renal failure?
   1. This medication increases the availability of vitamin D in the intestines.
   2. This medication stimulates excretion of calcium from the parathyroid gland.
   3. The medication helps the body excrete calcium through the feces.
   4. This medication increases serum calcium levels by promoting calcium absorption.

5. The client in end-stage renal disease (ERSD) is taking calcitriol, a vitamin D analog. Which assessment data would warrant intervention by the nurse?
   1. The client complains of nausea.
   2. The client has had two episodes of diarrhea.
   3. The client has an increase in the serum creatinine level.
   4. The client has blood in the urine.

6. The client in end-stage renal disease is taking aluminum hydroxide (Amphojel), a liquid antacid. Which information should the nurse discuss with the client?
   1. Drink at least 500 mL of water after taking the medication.
   2. Do not drink any water for 1 hour after taking the medication.
   3. Drink 2–4 ounces of water after taking the medication.
   4. Eat 30 minutes prior to taking the aluminum hydroxide.

7. The client in end-stage renal disease is receiving oral Kayexalate, a cation exchange resin. Which assessment data indicates the medication is effective?
   1. The client's serum potassium level is 5.8 mEq/L.
   2. The client's serum sodium level is 135 mEq/L.
   3. The client's serum potassium level is 4.2 mEq/L.
   4. The client's serum sodium level is 147 mEq/L.

8. The nurse is administering the thiazide diuretic hydrochlorothiazide (HydroDIURIL) to a client diagnosed with end-stage renal disease (ESRD). Which assessment data would cause the nurse to question the administration of this medication?
   1. The urine output was 90 mL for the last 8 hours.
   2. The skin turgor is elastic and oral mucosa is moist.
   3. The client's has 3+ sacral and peripheral edema.
   4. The client's blood pressure is 90/60 in the left arm.

9. The client diagnosed with chronic kidney disease on hemodialysis is prescribed lanthanum (Fosrenol), an electrolyte- and water-balancing agent. Which laboratory data indicates the medication is effective?
   1. A decreased serum potassium level.
   2. A normal serum sodium level.
   3. A decreased serum blood urea nitrogen (BUN) level.
   4. A normal serum phosphorus level.

10. The client diagnosed with chronic kidney disease on hemodialysis is prescribed lanthanum (Fosrenol), an electrolyte- and water-balancing agent. Which intervention should the nurse discuss with the client?
    1. Chew the tablets completely before swallowing.
    2. Monitor the dialysis graft for bleeding.
    3. Take an over-the-counter proton-pump inhibitor.
    4. Check the radial pulse prior to taking the medication.

A Client with a Urinary Tract Infection

11. The nurse in the long-term care facility is caring for a client with an indwelling catheter. Which preparation should the nurse order for the client?
    1. Cranberry juice with breakfast daily.
    2. Nitrofurantoin (Macrodantin), a sulfa drug.
    3. Vitamin C, a vitamin supplement.
    4. Goldenseal, an herbal preparation.

12. The male client is admitted to the medical floor at 1200 with a diagnosis of pyelonephritis. Which intervention should the nurse implement first?
    1. Initiate an intravenous access with a 20-gauge catheter.
    2. Administer the IV antibiotic within 2 hours of admission.
    3. Obtain a urine specimen for culture and sensitivity.
    4. Notify the dietary department to order the client a regular diet.

13. The client diagnosed with glomerulonephritis is receiving trimethoprim sulfa (Bactrim DS). Which indicates the medication is effective?
    1. A urine specific gravity of 1.010.
    2. WBC of 35/hpf on the urinalysis.
    3. Urine pH of 6.9.
    4. Negative urine leukocyte esterase.

14. The nurse is administering medications to clients on a urology floor. Which medication would the nurse question?
    1. Ceftriaxone (Rocephin), a third-generation cephalosporin, to a client who is pregnant.
    2. Cephalexin (Keflex), a cephalosporin, to a client who is allergic to penicillin.
    3. Trimethoprim sulfa (Bactrim), a sulfa antibiotic, to a client post–prostate surgery.
    4. Nitrofurantoin (Macrodantin), a sulfa antibiotic, to a client with urinary stasis.

15. The nurse observes the unlicensed assistive personnel (UAP) performing delegated tasks. Which action by the UAP requires immediate intervention?
    1. The UAP measures the output of a client who had a transurethral resection of the prostate.
    2. The UAP tells the client whose urine is green that something must be wrong for the urine to be such an odd color.
    3. The UAP encourages the client to drink a glass of water after the nurse administered the oral antibiotic.
    4. The UAP assists the client diagnosed with a urinary tract infection to the bedside commode every 2 hours.

16. The male client is diagnosed with methicillin-resistant *Staphylococcus aureus* (MRSA) of the urine and is receiving vancomycin (IVPB). Which intervention should the nurse implement when administering this medication?
    1. Hold the medication if the trough level is 5 mg/dL.
    2. Ask the client if he is allergic to penicillin.
    3. Administer the medication via an infusion pump.
    4. Check the client's CPK-MB isoenzyme level.

17. The female client taking nitrofurantoin (Macrodantin) for a urinary tract infection calls the clinic and tells the nurse that her urine has turned dark. Which statement is the nurse's best response?
    1. "This is a side effect of the medication and is not harmful."
    2. "This means that you have cystitis and should come in to see the HCP."
    3. "If you take the medication with food, it causes this reaction."
    4. "There must be some other problem going on that is causing this."

18. The client diagnosed with a bladder infection is prescribed phenazopyridine (Pyridium). Which is the scientific rationale for prescribing this medication?
    1. Pyridium is used to treat gram-negative urinary tract infections.
    2. Pyridium stimulates a hypotonic bladder to increase urine output.
    3. Pyridium alleviates pain and burning during urination.
    4. Pyridium decreases urinary frequency to control an overactive bladder.

19. The client diagnosed with a urinary tract infection is prescribed aztreonam (Azactam) IVPB every 8 hours. Which data indicates the medication is not effective?
    1. The client is able to void 300–400 mL of urine each time.
    2. The client complains of urinary frequency and burning.
    3. The client's temperature is 99.0°F.
    4. The client's urine is a clear amber color.

20. The nurse is preparing the client for the placement of an indwelling urinary catheter. Which statement has priority for the nurse to ask the client?
    1. "Do you have a preference of which leg the tube is taped to?"
    2. "When did you last attempt to void?"
    3. "Do you have a feeling of needing to void?"
    4. "Are you allergic to iodine or Betadine?"

A Client with Benign Prostatic Hypertrophy and Spinal Anesthesia

21. The client diagnosed with mild benign prostatic hypertrophy (BPH) is prescribed the 5-alpha-reductase inhibitor finasteride (Proscar) to relieve symptoms of urinary frequency. Which intervention should the clinic nurse implement?
    1. Tell the client to drink at least 8–10 glasses of water a day.
    2. Schedule an appointment with the HCP for a 1-week follow-up examination.
    3. Have the laboratory draw a prostate-specific antigen level.
    4. Give the client a urinal to measure his daily output of urine.

22. The male client diagnosed with complaints of urinary frequency and nocturia tells the nurse he is taking the herbal supplement saw palmetto. Which statement is the nurse's best response?
    1. "Use of saw palmetto is an old wives' tale."
    2. "This herb does help shrink the prostate tissue."
    3. "Have you noticed any itching or rashes?"
    4. "Saw palmetto has been known to cause cancer."

23. The client diagnosed with moderate benign prostatic hypertrophy (BPH) is being treated with the alpha–adrenergic agonist tamsulosin (Flomax). Which intervention should the nurse implement?
    1. Check the client's blood pressure.
    2. Send a urinalysis to the laboratory.
    3. Determine if the client has nocturia.
    4. Plan a scheduled voiding pattern.

24. The client diagnosed with benign prostatic hypertrophy has had a transurethral resection of the prostate. The client returns to the unit with a continuous bladder irrigation (Murphy drip) in place. The unlicensed assistive personnel records emptying the catheter bag of red drainage three times during the shift of 1500 mL, 2100 mL, and 1950 mL. The nurse records infusing 4100 mL of normal saline irrigation fluid. Which is the client's corrected urinary output for the shift?

    Answer _____

25. Which is the scientific rationale for administering the 5-alpha-reductase inhibitor dutasteride (AVODART) to a client diagnosed with benign prostatic hypertrophy (BPH)?
    1. The medication elevates male testosterone levels and decreases impotence.
    2. AVODART causes a rapid reduction in the size of the prostate and relief of symptoms.
    3. The medication decreases the mechanical obstruction of the urethra by the prostate.
    4. AVODART is as fast as surgery in reducing the obstructive symptoms of BPH.

26. The client who has had a transurethral resection of the prostate is complaining of bladder spasms. The HCP prescribed an opiate suppository, belladonna and opiate (B & O). Which is the first action the nurse should take when administering this medication?
    1. Obtain the correct dose of the medication.
    2. Lubricate the suppository with K-Y jelly.
    3. Wash hands and don nonsterile gloves.
    4. Check the client's armband for allergies.

27. The nurse is administering morning medications. Which combination of medications should the nurse question administering?
    1. Terazosin (Hytrin), an alpha$_1$-adrenergic agonist, and captopril (Capoten), an ACE inhibitor.
    2. Finasteride (Proscar), a 5-alpha–reductase inhibitor, and digoxin (Lanoxin), a cardiac glycoside.
    3. Tamsulosin (Flomax), an alpha$_1$-adrenergic agonist, and metformin (Glucophage), a biguanide.
    4. *Serenoa repens* (saw palmetto), an herbal preparation, and metoprolol (Toprol XL), a beta blocker.

28. Which intervention is priority for a pregnant nurse when administering dutasteride (AVODART) to a client diagnosed with benign prostatic hypertrophy (BPH)?
    1. Use goggles for personal eye protection.
    2. Protect the nurse's mucosa from contact with liquid.
    3. Ask a male nurse to administer the medication.
    4. Wear gloves while administering the medication.

29. The client diagnosed with benign prostatic hypertrophy has had a transurethral resection of the prostate (TURP). The client is complaining of lower abdominal pain. Which intervention should the nurse implement? Rank in order of performance.
    1. Administer the prescribed morphine by slow IVP.
    2. Check the urinary catheter for drainage and clots.
    3. Determine if the client has a hard, rigid abdomen.
    4. Adjust the saline irrigation to flush the bladder.
    5. Dilute the morphine with several milliliters of normal saline.

30. The client diagnosed with benign prostatic hypertrophy (BPH) and congestive heart failure (CHF) is receiving furosemide (Lasix), a loop diuretic, daily. Which information provided by the unlicensed assistive personnel (UAP) best indicates to the nurse that the medication is effective?
    1. The UAP recorded the intake as 350 mL and the output as 450 mL.
    2. The UAP stated that the client ambulated to the bathroom without dyspnea.
    3. The UAP emptied a moderate amount of urine from the bedside commode.
    4. The UAP reports that the client lost 1 pound of weight from the day before.

A Client with Renal Calculi

31. The client with renal calculi was prescribed allopurinol (Zyloprim) for uric acid stone calculi. Which medication teaching should the nurse discuss with the client?
    1. Inform the client to report chills, fever, and muscle aches to the HCP.
    2. Instruct the client to avoid driving or other activities that require alertness.
    3. Tell the client that the medication must be taken on an empty stomach.
    4. Explain the importance of not eating breads, cereals, and fruits.

32. The client with renal calculi was prescribed allopurinol (Zyloprim) for uric acid stone calculi. Which statement would warrant intervention by the nurse?
    1. "I had to take two Tylenol because of my headache."
    2. "I drink at least eight glasses of water a day."
    3. "My joints ache so I take a couple of aspirins."
    4. "I do not drink wine or any type of alcoholic drinks."

33. Which intervention should the nurse discuss with the client who has calcium/oxalate renal calculi and who has been prescribed a thiazide diuretic?
    1. Tell the client to decrease the intake of fluids.
    2. Explain the need to check the potassium level daily.
    3. Inform the client to check the blood pressure daily.
    4. Instruct the client to take the diuretic in the morning.

34. The client is admitted to the surgical department diagnosed with renal calculi. The HCP prescribes a morphine patient-controlled analgesia (PCA). Which intervention should the nurse implement?
    1. Instruct the client to push the control button as often as needed.
    2. Explain that the medication will ensure the client has no pain.
    3. Discuss that medication effectiveness is evaluated with the Wong-Baker FACES Pain Scale.
    4. Inform the client to ambulate very carefully to the bathroom and to strain urine.

35. The male client diagnosed with renal calculi is receiving pain medication via a morphine patient-controlled analgesia (PCA) pump. The HCP prescribed the non-steroidal anti-inflammatory drug (NSAID) indomethacin (Indocin) in a rectal suppository. Which action should the nurse take?
    1. Question and clarify the prescription with the health-care provider.
    2. Give the suppository to the client and allow the client to insert it into the rectum.
    3. Administer a Fleets enema to clear the bowel prior to administering the suppository.
    4. Have the client lie on the side and insert the rectal suppository with nonsterile gloves.

36. The client diagnosed with renal calculi is receiving pain medication via morphine patient-controlled analgesia (PCA). The client is still voicing excruciating pain and is requesting something else. Which intervention should the nurse implement first?
    1. Administer the rescue dose of morphine intravenous push.
    2. Check the client's urine for color, sediment, and output.
    3. Determine the last time the client received PCA morphine.
    4. Demonstrate how to perform guided imagery with the client.

37. The client with calcium renal calculi is prescribed cellulose sodium phosphate (Calcibind). The client asks the nurse, "How will this medication help prevent my stones from coming back?" Which statement is the nurse's best response?
    1. "Calcibind reduces the uric acid level in your bloodstream and the uric acid excreted in your urine."
    2. "This medication will decrease calcium levels in the bloodstream by increasing calcium excretion in the urine."
    3. "It binds calcium from food in the intestines, reducing the amount absorbed in the circulation."
    4. "The medication will help alkalinize the urine, which reduces the amount of cystine in the urine."

38. The client diagnosed with rule-out renal calculi is scheduled for an intravenous dye pyelogram (IVP). Which action should the nurse implement?
    1. Keep the client NPO.
    2. Check the serum creatinine level.
    3. Assess for antibiotic allergy.
    4. Insert an 18-gauge angiocatheter.

39. The client diagnosed with renal calculi is being scheduled for surgery. The client is having epidural anesthesia. Which intervention should the circulating nurse implement?
    1. Have the client lie on the side in the fetal position.
    2. Determine if the client has an advance directive.
    3. Assess the client's gag and swallowing reflex.
    4. Ensure that the head of the client's stretcher is elevated 30 degrees.

40. The client diagnosed with renal calculi has just had an intravenous pyelogram (IVP). Which task would be the most appropriate for the nurse to delegate to the unlicensed assistive personnel (UAP)?
    1. Hang a new bag of intravenous fluid.
    2. Discontinue the client's intravenous catheter.
    3. Assist the client outside to smoke a cigarette.
    4. Maintain the client's intake and output.

An Adolescent with a Sexually Transmitted Disease

41. The 16-year-old female client tells the public health nurse that she thinks her boyfriend gave her a sexually transmitted disease (STD). Which statement by the nurse would be the best response?
    1. "You will need parental permission to be seen in the clinic."
    2. "Be sure and get the proper medications so that you don't become pregnant."
    3. "How would you know that you have a sexually transmitted disease?"
    4. "You need to have tests so you can be started on medications now."

42. The teenage client has just delivered a 7-pound baby. The girl has not received any prenatal care. Which medication is administered to the neonate to prevent complications related to sexually transmitted diseases?
    1. Zidovudine (Retrovir), a nucleoside reverse transcriptase inhibitor (NRTI).
    2. Valacyclovir (Valtrex), an antiretroviral.
    3. Erythromycin ophthalmic ointment, an antibiotic.
    4. Metronidazole (Flagyl), a gastrointestinal anti-infective.

43. The 17-year-old client is prescribed metronidazole (Flagyl) and erythromycin (E Mycin) for a persistent *Chlamydia* infection. Which statement by the client indicates the need for further teaching?
    1. "I can have a beer or two while taking these medications."
    2. "My boyfriend will have to take the medications too."
    3. "I can develop more problems if I don't treat this disease."
    4. "My birth control pills may not work because of the medications."

44. The school nurse is teaching a class on sexually transmitted diseases to a group of high school students. Which statement provides accurate information regarding treatment of sexually transmitted diseases?
    1. Medications are available to cure STDs if the client is not allergic.
    2. Medications will not cure all sexually transmitted diseases.
    3. Medications that prevent pregnancy will prevent most STDs.
    4. Medications that treat STDs enhance sexual libido.

45. The 18-year-old male client is diagnosed with gonorrhea of the pharynx. The HCP has prescribed ceftriaxone (Rocephin), a cephalosporin. Which intervention should the nurse implement?
    1. Administer the medication intramuscularly in the gluteus muscle.
    2. Have the client drink a full glass of water with the pill.
    3. Use a tuberculin syringe to draw up the medication.
    4. Make sure the client has eaten before administering the drug.

46. Which is the preferred treatment for the diagnosis of primary syphilis in a teenage client?
    1. Doxycycline (Vibramycin), a tetracycline, po every 4 hours for 10 days.
    2. Benzathine penicillin G, an antibiotic, IM one time only.
    3. Miconazole (Monistat), an antifungal, topical daily for 1 week.
    4. Nitrofurantoin (Macrodantin), a macrolide, b.i.d. for 1 month.

47. The teenaged male client is diagnosed with herpes simplex 2 viral infection and is prescribed valacyclovir (Valtrex). Which information should the nurse teach?
    1. The medication will dry the lesions within a day or two.
    2. Valtrex may be taken once a week to control outbreaks.
    3. The use of condoms will increase the spread of the herpes.
    4. Even after the lesions have gone, it is still possible to transmit the virus.

48. The 16-year-old male client is diagnosed with pediculosis pubis and is prescribed permethrin (Nix), an ectoparasiticide cream rinse. Which data indicates the treatment has been effective?
    1. There are no scratches on the client's penis.
    2. The client shaved his head and his scalp is clear.
    3. The client reports that the intense itching has abated.
    4. The client has no visible lice or nits on his head.

49. The 18-year-old female client has been diagnosed with genital warts and has been treated with cryotherapy with liquid nitrogen, a freezing agent, on the external genitalia. Which discharge information should the nurse teach?
    1. Wipe the perineum from front to back to prevent cross-contamination of the area.
    2. Encourage the use of peripads during the client's menstrual cycle.
    3. Gently cleanse the perineum with a squirt bottle and tepid water after urinating.
    4. Administer daily Betadine douches until the area has healed completely.

50. The 19-year-old client diagnosed with a severe herpes simplex 2 viral infection is admitted to the medical floor. The HCP prescribes acyclovir (Zovirax), an antiretroviral medication, 10 mg/kg IVPB every 8 hours. The client weighs 220 pounds. How many milligrams will the nurse administer with each dose?

    Answer _____

A Client Experiencing Pregnancy

51. Which medication category is contraindicated in clients who are pregnant?
    1. Pregnancy category A
    2. Pregnancy category B
    3. Pregnancy category C
    4. Pregnancy category D

52. The client who is pregnant is prescribed ferrous sulfate (Feosol), an iron product. Which statement indicates to the nurse the client needs more teaching?
    1. "I should increase my fluid intake and fiber when taking this medication."
    2. "I will take a daily stool softener to prevent becoming constipated."
    3. "If I notice that my stool becomes black or dark, I will call my obstetrician."
    4. "I should take my iron tablet 2 hours after I eat."

53. The client who is 32 weeks pregnant and in preterm labor is prescribed terbutaline (Brethine), a beta-adrenergic agonist. Which data would warrant intervention by the nurse?
    1. The client's respiratory rate is 34.
    2. The fetus's heart rate is 150 bpm.
    3. The client's apical heart rate is 104.
    4. The client reports no contractions.

54. The nurse is preparing to administer medication in a labor and delivery unit. Which medication would the nurse question administering?
    1. The anticonvulsant magnesium sulfate to a client with preeclampsia.
    2. The synthetic prostaglandin dinoprostone (Cervidil) to a client with asthma.
    3. The corticosteroid betamethasone (Celestone) to a client who is 27 weeks pregnant.
    4. The tocolytic oxytocin (Pitocin) to a client with an incomplete abortion.

55. The nurse is preparing to administer a combination hydrocortisone and pramoxine (Proctofoam), a local anesthetic, to a client with a fourth-degree episiotomy. Which interventions would the nurse implement? List in order of performance.
    1. Position the client on the side with top leg up and forward.
    2. Wash hands and don nonsterile examination gloves.
    3. Check the client's MAR with the identification band.
    4. Ask the client if she is allergic to any "-caine" drugs.
    5. Apply the Proctofoam to the perineal area.

56. The client in labor has an epidural catheter in place for anesthesia. Which intervention is most important for the labor and delivery nurse?
    1. Assist the client with breathing exercise during contractions.
    2. Ensure the client's legs are correctly positioned in the stirrups.
    3. Have the significant other scrub for the delivery of the baby.
    4. Titrate the epidural medication to ensure analgesic effect.

57. Which assessment data would warrant immediate intervention for the client in labor who is receiving an oxytocin (Pitocin) drip, a tocolytic agent?
    1. The uterus periodically becomes hard and firm.
    2. The client complains of an urgency to void.
    3. The client denies the urge to push.
    4. The fetal heart rate does not return to baseline.

58. The client who is 38 weeks pregnant and diagnosed with preeclampsia is admitted to the labor and delivery area. The HCP has prescribed intravenous magnesium sulfate, an anticonvulsant. Which data indicates the medication is effective?
    1. The client's deep tendon reflexes are 4+.
    2. The client's blood pressure is 148/90.
    3. The client's deep tendon reflexes are 2 to 3+.
    4. The client's deep tendon reflexes are 0.

59. Which statement best indicates the scientific rationale for administering corticosteroid therapy to a client who is 30 weeks pregnant?
    1. Steroids are administered to decrease uterine contractions in preterm labor.
    2. Steroids will increase the analgesic effects of opioid narcotics.
    3. Steroids accelerate lung maturation, resulting in fetal surfactant development.
    4. Steroids will prevent the development of maternal antibodies to the fetus's blood.

60. The client is experiencing postpartum hemorrhage and has received an ergot alkaloid, methylergonovine (Methergine). Which intervention is priority when administering this medication?
    1. Check the client's hemoglobin and hematocrit levels.
    2. Monitor the client's peripad count frequently.
    3. Assess the client's vital signs every 2 hours.
    4. Determine the client's fundal height.

A Client Experiencing Infertility

61. The male client experiencing infertility problems tells the clinic nurse that he is taking St. John's wort for his depression. Which statement would be the nurse's best response?
    1. "This herb is useful for depression. I hope it will help."
    2. "Did you discuss taking this herb with your psychologist?"
    3. "This herb may cause more infertility problems."
    4. "Is your significant other taking any herbal medication?"

62. The female client is taking clomiphene (Clomid), an estrogen antagonist. Which statement indicates the client understands the risk of taking this medication?
    1. "The medication may cause my child to have Down syndrome."
    2. "There are very few risks associated with taking this medication."
    3. "I should stagger the times that I take this medication."
    4. "This medication may increase my chance of having twins."

63. The client who is infertile and diagnosed with endometriosis is prescribed leuprolide (Lupron), a GnRH medication. Which information should the nurse discuss with the client?
    1. Explain that this medication may take 3–6 months to work.
    2. Discuss that this medication will help regulate the client's menstrual cycle.
    3. Instruct to take the Lupron every night to help decrease menstrual pain.
    4. Teach to abstain from sexual intercourse 72 hours after taking the medication.

64. The client experiencing infertility is prescribed bromocriptine (Parlodel). The client calls the clinic nurse and reports that she thinks she may be pregnant. Which intervention should the clinic nurse implement first?
    1. Schedule the client for a pelvic sonogram.
    2. Instruct the client to quit taking the medication.
    3. Tell the client to make an appointment with the HCP.
    4. Encourage the client to confirm with a home pregnancy test.

65. The client experiencing infertility is receiving menotropin (Pergonal), an ovarian stimulant, and human chorionic gonadotropin. Which diagnostic test would indicate the medications are effective?
    1. A serum human chorionic gonadotropin level.
    2. A serum estrogen level.
    3. A negative urine pregnancy test.
    4. A hemoglobin A1c.

66. The female client has been taking infertility medications. Which signs or symptoms would indicate ovarian overstimulation syndrome?
    1. Abdominal bloating and vague gastrointestinal discomfort.
    2. Bright-red vaginal bleeding with golf ball–size clots.
    3. A positive fluid wave and lower abdominal wave.
    4. Burning and an increased frequency of urinating.

67. The nurse administers human chorionic gonadotropin (HCG) intramuscularly to the female client who is infertile. Which instruction should the nurse discuss with the couple regarding coitus?
    1. Explain the need to abstain from sexual intercourse for 14 days after receiving the medication.
    2. Instruct the male partner to wear boxer shorts while his female partner is taking human chorionic gonadotropin.
    3. Discuss taking the basal metabolic temperature and having sexual intercourse when it becomes elevated 2 degrees.
    4. Advise the couple to have intercourse on the eve of receiving medication and 3 days after receiving medication.

68. The nurse is preparing a client for in vitro fertilization (IVF). Which statement best describes the scientific rationale for administering supplemental progesterone to this client?
    1. To enhance the receptivity of the endometrium to implantation.
    2. To provide more hormone to the ovary for egg production.
    3. To help regulate the client's monthly menstrual cycle.
    4. To decrease galactorrhea in the client if fertilization occurs.

69. The nurse is discussing fertility issues. Which statement indicates the couple is knowledgeable of fertility issues?
    1. "My insurance should cover the cost of the medications completely."
    2. "A multifetal pregnancy can result in preterm labor and birth."
    3. "There is an excellent probability we will get pregnant the first time."
    4. "Most of the implanted zygotes will result in a live birth."

70. The male client who is infertile asks the clinic nurse, "Is there anything I can take to increase my chances of fathering a child?" Which statement is the nurse's best response?
    1. "I am sorry, but there are no medications to help men with infertility."
    2. "Are you concerned about not being able to father a child?"
    3. "Testosterone therapy may help increase your sperm count."
    4. "You can take Clomid and it will help your partner get pregnant."

A Client Using Birth Control

71. The couple has decided to use a spermicide for birth control. Which information should the nurse discuss with the female partner?
    1. Insert the foam prior to having sexual intercourse.
    2. Douche with vinegar and water immediately after sex.
    3. Apply spermicide to the male partner's penis.
    4. Use the spermicide immediately after having intercourse.

72. Which female client would the nurse recommend taking oral contraceptive pills for birth control?
    1. The client who smokes two packs of cigarettes a day.
    2. The client who is taking an angiotensin-converting enzyme medication.
    3. The client who is 65″ tall and weighs 100 kg.
    4. The client who has a family history of ovarian cancer.

73. Which instruction should the nurse discuss with the client who is prescribed oral contraceptives for birth control?
    1. Never take more than one birth control pill a day.
    2. If breakthrough bleeding occurs, discontinue the pill.
    3. Take a missed pill as soon as you realize you have missed it.
    4. Antibiotics will increase the ovulation suppression effect of the pill.

74. The nurse is providing discharge instructions for the postpartum client concerning birth control methods. Which question is most important for the nurse to ask the client?
    1. "Has your doctor discussed when to resume sexual activity?"
    2. "Have you decided if you will be breastfeeding your baby?"
    3. "Are you concerned about how this baby will change your life?"
    4. "Does your partner agree with the type of birth control you will use?"

75. The male adolescent who is sexually active tells the school nurse, "I am embarrassed, but I don't know who else to tell. Last night when I used a condom with my girlfriend I got a red itchy rash down there. I don't know what it is or what to do." Which statement would be the nurse's best response?
    1. "You should abstain from sex until you are older."
    2. "Use a condom made out of a lamb's intestines."
    3. "Do you think your girlfriend gave you an STD?"
    4. "Encourage your girlfriend to use a diaphragm."

76. Which statement indicates to the nurse that the client using a vaginal contraceptive ring understands the birth control teaching?
    1. "If the ring falls out during intercourse, I should get a new ring."
    2. "I should insert the ring 30 minutes before having intercourse."
    3. "I will remove the ring 3 weeks after I have inserted it."
    4. "I am so glad that I will not have a period when using the ring."

77. The client has been taking birth control pills for 5 weeks. Which statement from the client would warrant intervention by the clinic nurse?
    1. "I stay nauseated and my breasts are very tender."
    2. "I have not had a period since I started the pill."
    3. "I make my boyfriend use a condom even though I am on the pill."
    4. "I took the pills for 3 weeks then stopped for 1 week."

78. The client is prescribed a 28-day oral contraceptive pack. Which statement best describes the scientific rationale for this birth control product?
    1. This causes longer intervals between menses.
    2. A hormone pill daily decreases cramping during menses.
    3. It is not as expensive as other birth control products.
    4. This ensures that the client will take a pill every day.

79. The adolescent client is prescribed the birth control medication depot medroxyprogesterone (Depo-Provera). Which interventions should the clinic nurse implement? Select all that apply.
    1. Instruct the client to schedule an appointment every 3 months.
    2. Explain that infertility may occur up to 2 years after discontinuing.
    3. Demonstrate how to administer the medication subcutaneously in the abdomen.
    4. Discuss how to care for the intrauterine device inserted in her vagina.
    5. Tell the client that she will not have to take a pill every day.

80. The 14-year-old client is prescribed oral contraceptive medication for menstrual irregularity. Which assessment data indicates the medication is effective?
    1. The client has a period every 28 days.
    2. The client has a decrease in abdominal bloating.
    3. The client has a negative pregnancy test.
    4. The client reports a decrease in facial acne.

A Client with Chronic Renal Failure

1. 1. Epogen is a glycoprotein produced by the kidney that stimulates red blood cell production in response to hypoxia. A biologic response modifier, Epogen, is prescribed to treat the anemia that occurs in clients with chronic renal failure.
   2. Filgrastim (Neupogen) is the biologic response modifier that stimulates white blood cells and is not used in the treatment of chronic renal failure.
   3. Oprelvekin (Neumega) is the biologic response modifier that stimulates megakaryocyte and thrombocyte production, which stimulates platelet production to prevent thrombocytopenia in clients receiving chemotherapy.
   4. There is no medication that increases the production of urine. Diuretics increase the excretion of urine but do not affect the production of urine.

2. 1. Do not shake the vial because shaking may denature the glycoprotein, rendering it biologically inactive.
   2. The nurse should apply ice to numb the injection site, not a warm washcloth after administration.
   3. The nurse should only use the vial for one dose. The nurse should not reenter the vial and should discard any unused portion because the vial contains no preservatives.
   4. The medication should be stored in the refrigerator, not the freezer, and should be warmed to room temperature prior to its being administered.

3. 1. This is the scientific rationale for administering antacids to clients with peptic ulcer disease or gastritis, not clients with chronic renal failure.
   2. Clients in CRF experience an increase in serum phosphorus levels (hyperphosphatemia), and aluminum hydroxide binds with phosphorus to be excreted in the feces.
   3. Amphojel does not affect the calcium level.
   4. Aluminum hydroxide can cause constipation; it is not used to treat constipation.

4. 1. Calcitriol does not affect the availability of vitamin D.
   2. Calcitriol is used to treat hypoparathyroidism, but it does not stimulate excretion of calcium from the parathyroid gland.

3. The client in end-stage renal failure has hypocalcemia, not hypercalcemia.
   4. This is the scientific rationale for administering this medication to a client in chronic renal failure. Calcitriol increases serum calcium levels by promoting calcium absorption and thereby helps to manage hypocalcemia, which is a symptom of CRF.

5. 1. Nausea is a side effect of calcitriol and can also result from ESRD itself.
   2. Diarrhea is an expected side effect of the medication; therefore, it would not warrant intervention from the nurse.
   3. The client in ESRD would have an increased serum creatinine level; therefore, this would not warrant immediate intervention by the nurse.
   4. Hematuria is an adverse effect of calcitriol and the nurse should notify the health-care provider. This would warrant taking the client off the medication.

MEDICATION MEMORY JOGGER: Any time there is blood in the urine it is a cause for concern, and the nurse should intervene and investigate what is causing the hematuria.

6. 1. The client should not drink more than 4 ounces of water because water quickens the gastric emptying time.
   2. The client should drink some water to ensure the medication gets to the stomach.
   3. Liquid antacids should be taken with 2–4 ounces of water to ensure that the medication reaches the stomach.
   4. Antacids should be taken on an empty stomach and are effective for 30–60 minutes before passing into the duodenum.

7. 1. Kayexalate is a medication that is administered to decrease an elevated serum potassium level. Therefore, an elevated serum potassium (>5.5 mEq/L) would indicate the medication is not effective.
   2. Kayexalate is not used to alter the serum sodium level.
   3. Kayexalate is a medication that is administered to decrease an elevated serum potassium level. A potassium level within the normal range of 3.5–5.5 mEq/L indicates the medication is effective.
   4. Kayexalate is not used to alter the serum sodium level.

MEDICATION MEMORY JOGGER: The nurse determines the effectiveness of a medication by assessing for the symptoms, or lack

thereof, for which the medication was prescribed.

8. 1. The client in ESRD would have a less than normal urine output, so the nurse would not question giving the client a diuretic.
2. An elastic skin turgor indicates the client is well-hydrated; therefore, the nurse would not question administering this medication.
3. The medication is being administered to help decrease the sacral edema; therefore, the nurse would not question administering this diuretic.
4. Diuretics reduce circulating blood volume, which may cause orthostatic hypotension. Because the client's blood pressure is low, the nurse should question administering this medication.

MEDICATION MEMORY JOGGER: The nurse must be knowledgeable of accepted standards of practice for medication administration, including which client assessment data and laboratory data should be monitored prior to administering the medication.

9. 1. A decreased potassium level indicates the dialysis is effective but not that the medication is effective.
2. Fosrenol does not affect sodium level.
3. A decreased BUN level indicates the dialysis is effective but not the medication.
4. Fosrenol decreases phosphate absorption in the intestines and is excreted in the feces.

10. 1. Whole tablets of Fosrenol should not be swallowed. The medication must be chewed for absorption in the intestines.
2. Fosrenol may cause graft occlusion, not bleeding.
3. Fosrenol does not increase gastric acid secretion; therefore, the client would not need to take a proton-pump inhibitor.
4. Fosrenol may cause hypotension and the blood pressure must be checked, but it does not affect the pulse rate.

A Client with Urinary Tract Infection

11. 1. Cranberry juice is acidic and will change the pH of the urine, making it harder for bacteria to survive in the environment. It can be used prophylactically to prevent urinary tract infec-

tions. It does not treat an infection. The nurse can arrange with the dietitian to include this in the client's dietary plan.
2. This is a prescription medication that is used to treat chronic urinary tract infections, but the nurse could not order this medication.
3. In a long-term care facility, this over-the-counter vitamin would require an HCP order.
4. This is an herb used for urinary tract infections, but in a long-term care facility it would require an HCP order.

MEDICATION MEMORY JOGGER: Nurses do not order medications. Nurses do have latitude in deciding on components and consistency of the meals provided. The dietitian can include cranberry juice in any diet.

12. 1. The IV is important to initiate therapy, but the nurse should obtain a clean voided midstream urine for culture and sensitivity before initiating the treatment. If the culture is not obtained prior to initiating the antibiotic, the results of the laboratory test will be skewed.
2. This should definitely be done, but obtaining the culture is the first intervention.
3. **The nurse should obtain a clean voided midstream specimen for culture and sensitivity before initiating the antibiotics. This is the first intervention to implement.**
4. A diet order is not priority over getting the treatment started. Urinary tract infections in males are difficult to treat and can be life threatening.

MEDICATION MEMORY JOGGER: The first step in initiating antibiotic therapy is to obtain any ordered culture. Then the nurse must place a priority on initiating IV antibiotic therapy in a timely manner, within 1–2 hours after the order is written, depending on the facility's standard protocol.

13. 1. A urine specific gravity can indicate dehydration or water intoxication, but it will not provide information about a urinary tract infection.
2. A WBC of 35/hpf indicates a urinary tract infection—not that the antibiotic is effective. Normal is <5/hpf.

3. Normal urine pH is 5.0–9.0, but the pH does not evaluate a urinary tract infection.
4. **A negative urine leukocyte esterase indicates the antibiotic is effective in treating the infection. Leukocytes and nitrates are used to determine bacteriuria and other sources of urinary tract infections.**

14. 1. Rocephin is in the pregnancy risk category B. No research has shown harm to the fetus in humans or in animals. The nurse would not question this medication.
2. **A cross-sensitivity exists in some clients between penicillin and the cephalosporins. The nurse should assess the type of reaction that the client experienced when taking penicillin. If the client indicates any symptom of an anaphylactic reaction, the nurse would hold the medication and discuss the situation with the HCP.**
3. There is no reason for the nurse to question Bactrim for a client who has had prostate surgery.
4. There is no reason for the nurse to question Macrodantin for a client who has urinary stasis. Macrodantin is used to prevent or treat chronic urinary tract infections.

MEDICATION MEMORY JOGGER: The nurse must be knowledgeable of accepted standards of practice for disease processes and conditions. If the nurse administers a medication the health-care provider has prescribed and it harms the client, the nurse could be held accountable. Remember that the nurse is a client advocate.

15. 1. The urinary output should be measured frequently in a client who has had a transurethral resection of the prostate. The client will have bladder irrigation and the indwelling catheter bag will need to be emptied frequently. The nurse would not intervene to stop this action.
2. **A green–blue color indicates the client is taking bethanechol (Urecholine), a urinary stimulant used for clients with a neurogenic bladder. This is an expected color, and the UAP should not indicate that something is wrong with the client.**
3. The client should be encouraged to drink fluids. The nurse would not intervene to stop this action.
4. This action encourages bowel and urine continence and is part of a falls prevention

protocol. The nurse would not intervene to stop this action.

16. 1. The therapeutic range of vancomycin is 10–20 mg/dL. The nurse would not hold the medication because the client has not reached a therapeutic range.
2. Vancomycin is not in the penicillin family of medications. An allergy to penicillin would not prevent administering the vancomycin.
3. **Vancomycin is administered over a minimum of 1 hour. The nurse should obtain an infusion pump to regulate the speed of administration.**
4. Vancomycin is nephrotoxic. The nurse would monitor the BUN and creatinine levels, especially in children and the elderly, but there is no need to monitor cardiac enzymes.

17. 1. **This is a side effect of nitrofurantoin. The client should be warned that the urine might turn brown. This color will disappear when the client is no longer taking the medication. If the client is taking an oral suspension, the nurse should instruct to rinse the mouth after taking the medication to prevent staining of the teeth.**
2. This does not indicate cystitis.
3. The client should be instructed to take the medication with food to avoid GI upset.
4. This is a side effect of the medication and does not indicate another problem.

18. 1. Pyridium is not an antibiotic; it will not treat an infection.
2. Pyridium is a urinary analgesic, not a urinary stimulant. It will not increase bladder tone.
3. **Pyridium is a urinary analgesic. It is useful in treating the pain and burning associated with a urinary tract infection.**
4. Antimuscarinic/anticholinergic medications control an overactive bladder; urinary analgesic medications do not. Pyridium does help control urinary frequency associated with a urinary tract infection.

19. 1. The client voiding 300–400 mL with each voiding indicates the client is able not to void until the bladder is full. This indicates the client is responding to the antibiotic and the medication is effective.
2. **Urinary frequency and burning indicate a urinary tract infection and that the medication is not effective.**

3. The client is afebrile. This indicates the client is responding to the antibiotic and the medication is effective.

4. This is a normal finding and indicates the client is responding to the antibiotic and the medication is effective.

20. 1. This is not a priority; the tubing should be taped to the leg on the side of the bed the bag will be suspended from.

2. This could be asked, but it is not priority.

3. This could be asked, but it is not priority.

4. **Indwelling catheter kits come prepackaged with povidone iodine (Betadine) to use for cleansing the perineal skin before inserting the catheter. The nurse should assess for allergies to the medication before preparing to cleanse the perineum. Another type of skin cleanser may need to be used.**

A Client with Benign Prostatic Hypertrophy and Spinal Anesthesia

21. 1. The client's intake of water will not affect the medication. Drinking this much water each day until the medication has had an opportunity to shrink the enlarged prostate tissue could cause the client to have a difficult time emptying an uncomfortably full bladder.

2. The medication takes 6–12 months to have a full effect. There is no reason for the client to be seen in 1 week.

3. **Proscar decreases serum prostate-specific antigen (PSA) levels. The client should have a PSA level drawn before beginning Proscar and a level drawn after 6 months. If the PSA level does not drop, the client should be assessed for cancer of the prostate.**

4. Clients do not need to measure their urine outputs daily.

22. 1. There is documented evidence that this herb effectively treats BPH. Its use is not a folk remedy without a sound basis.

2. **Research has proved the efficacy of saw palmetto in treating BPH. The exact mechanism of action is unknown, but the herb does shrink prostate tissue, resulting in relief of urinary obstructive symptoms.**

3. The client reported that he has been taking the herb. The time to discuss allergies is before or shortly after initiation of a medication.

4. Research indicates that saw palmetto is as effective as finasteride (Proscar) but has fewer side effects. It is considered a safe and effective treatment for BPH. There is no evidence that the herb causes cancer.

23. 1. **The medications used to treat hyperplasia of the prostate were originally developed to treat high blood pressure. The client may develop hypotension when taking these medications. This side effect makes them useful for clients who are also hypertensive.**

2. The medication is not given for urinary tract infections; there is no need for a urinalysis to be done when administering this medication.

3. The client has symptoms of BPH, which could include nocturia, but this is not pertinent when administering the medication.

4. This is an intervention that assists clients who have incontinence, not BPH.

24. **1450 mL of corrected urinary output.** The drainage in the catheter bag equals 5550 mL of drainage. 1500 mL + 2100 mL + 1950 mL = 5550 mL of drainage emptied for the shift. Subtract the 4100 mL of normal saline irrigation fluid from the 5550 total drainage = 1450 mL of corrected urinary output.

25. 1. Testosterone is converted to dihydrotestosterone (DHT) in the prostate; the 5-alpha-reductase inhibitors reduce DHT but not testosterone. With a reduction in DHT, the prostate tissue shrinks. The 5-alpha-reductase inhibitors do not elevate testosterone, nor do they improve impotence problems.

2. The 5-alpha-reductase inhibitors require 6–12 months for therapeutic relief of symptoms of BPH to occur.

3. **The 5-alpha-reductase inhibitors work by reducing the size of the prostate gland, resulting in a relief of the obstructive symptoms of urgency, frequency, difficulty initiating a urine stream, and nocturia.**

4. Surgery provides faster relief of symptoms after recovery has taken place. AVODART requires a lengthy time period for therapeutic effects of the medications and may not provide adequate relief of symptoms if the client has severe BPH.

26. 1. B & O suppositories come in 15A (1/2 grain) and 16A (1 grain) formulations. When obtaining the medication from the narcotic cabinet the nurse should obtain the correct dose for the client. B & O suppositories are used to reduce bladder spasms for clients who have had bladder surgery.
    2. Lubricating the suppository is the last step before inserting the suppository.
    3. This is the third step of the steps listed in this question.
    4. The nurse should check the armband before opening the medication and preparing to administer it.

27. 1. The major adverse effect of Hytrin is hypotension. Most blood pressure–lowering medications can also cause hypotension. The nurse would question administering two medications that can cause the client to become dizzy upon standing, possibly resulting in a fall. The medications that shrink the prostate gland were originally developed to treat high blood pressure. This is a safety issue.
    2. Proscar does not cause hypotension and does not interact with digoxin. The nurse would not question administering these medications.
    3. Flomax is an alpha$_1$-adrenergic agonist but does not cause hypotension. Glucophage does not interact with Flomax. The nurse would not question administering these medications.
    4. Saw palmetto has fewer side effects than most prescription medications that treat BPH and it does not cause hypotension or interact with Toprol XL. The nurse would not question administering these medications.

    MEDICATION MEMORY JOGGER: If the test taker did not know these medications, an alpha blocker usually will have some effect on the cardiovascular system and an ACE inhibitor is used to treat high blood pressure. Most blood pressure medications can cause orthostatic hypotension. Two medications that can cause similar side effects would be questioned.

28. 1. The medication is manufactured in a pill form; the nurse does not need eye protection to prevent exposure.
    2. The nurse's mucosa should not be exposed to the medication because it comes only in pill form.
    3. The nurse can administer dutasteride safely using the appropriate personal protective equipment. The nurse should not ask for another nurse to administer the medication.
    4. Dutasteride is considered a category X medication and will cause harm to a developing fetus. The medication can be absorbed through the skin. The nurse should wear gloves when administering the medication. Men should not donate blood for at least 6 months after discontinuing the medication to avoid administration of the medication to a pregnant client through the transfusion.

    MEDICATION MEMORY JOGGER: The nurse must remember that some medications can cause harm when administering the medication. A nurse who is pregnant must be cautious.

29.   2, 4, 3, 5, 1
    2. The most obvious reason for a client post-TURP to be having lower abdominal pain is that the bladder has blood clots that need to be flushed out. Clots that are not flushed from the bladder result in bladder spasms. Assessing the urinary drainage would be the first step.
    4. The next step is to adjust the rate of the irrigation to ensure adequate drainage of blood and clots from the bladder.
    3. Before administering a narcotic analgesic the nurse should rule out complication. Assessing for peritonitis (hard, rigid abdomen) is the next step in this situation.
    5. Morphine and most other narcotic medications require a very slow intravenous rate, around 5 minutes, according to the manufacturer's recommendations. The morphine is dispensed in 1-mL tubex syringes or vials. It is difficult to maintain a steady, slow administration of the medication with only 1 mL over 5 minutes. If the medication is diluted to a total volume of 10 mL, then the nurse can administer the medication at a rate of 1 mL every 30 seconds. Dilution causes less

pain for the client and helps decrease
irritation to the vein.

1. The final step in this sequence is to
actually administer the analgesic.

30. 1. The client's intake and output measure-
ments are important, but even accurate
intake and output recordings cannot measure for insensible losses. An output of 100
mL over the intake may or may not be
considered adequate to determine effectiveness of a diuretic.

2. Ambulating to the bathroom without
dyspnea is an indicator that the client is
not experiencing pulmonary complications
related to excess fluid volume, but it is not
the best indicator of the effectiveness of a
diuretic.

3. Terminology such as small, moderate, and
large are not objective words. To quantify
the results the nurse should use objective
data—in this situation, numbers. This
would provide an accurate comparison of
data to determine the effectiveness of the
medication.

4. **The most reliable method of determining changes in fluid-volume status is to
weigh a client in the same type of
clothing at the same time each day.
One liter (1000 mL) is approximately
0.9 kg, or 2 pounds. This client has
lost approximately 500 mL more fluid
than was taken in.**

A Client with Renal Calculi

31. 1. The client should notify the HCP if a
skin rash or influenza symptoms (chills,
fever, muscle aches and pain, nausea or
vomiting) develop because these signs
and symptoms may indicate hypersen-
sitivity.

2. Allopurinol does not cause drowsiness, so
the nurse does not need to tell the client
to avoid activities that require alertness.

3. Allopurinol may be administered with milk
or meals to minimize gastric irritation.

4. The client with uric acid should be eating
a low-purine diet. A low-purine diet
includes breads, cereals, cream-style soups
made with low-fat milk, fruits, juices, low-
fat cheeses, nuts, peanut butter, coffee,
and tea.

**MEDICATION MEMORY JOGGER: If the
client verbalizes a complaint, if the nurse
assesses data, or if laboratory data indicates an adverse effect secondary to a**

medication, the nurse must intervene.
The nurse must implement an independent intervention or notify the health-care
provider because medications can result
in serious or even life-threatening complications.

32. 1. The client should take acetaminophen
(Tylenol), instead of aspirin (salicylic acid),
to reduce acidity of the urine. This statement does not warrant intervention by the
nurse.

2. The client should increase fluid intake
when taking allopurinol to prevent drug
accumulation and toxic effects and to
minimize the risk of kidney stone formation. Therefore, this statement does not
warrant intervention by the nurse.

3. **Salicylic acid (aspirin) increases the
acidity of the urine, and the urine
should be alkaline; therefore this
statement warrants intervention by
the nurse.**

4. The client should avoid high-purine foods
(wine, alcohol, organ meats, sardines,
salmon, gravy) to help keep the urine alkaline; therefore, this statement does not
warrant intervention by the nurse.

33. 1. The client should drink adequate fluids
or increase fluids when taking a thiazide
diuretic and to help prevent formation
of renal calculi.

2. Thiazide diuretics cause an increase in
potassium loss in the urine but not as
significant as loop diuretics. In any case,
the client would not check the potassium
level daily at home.

3. The thiazide diuretic is not being administered to decrease blood pressure; therefore, the blood pressure would not have to
be checked daily to ensure the effectiveness of the medication.

4. **Diuretics should be taken in the morning so that the client is not up all night
urinating. Thiazide diuretics are
prescribed because they decrease the
amount of calcium released by the
kidneys into the urine by favoring
calcium retention in the bone. Most
kidney stones (75% to 80%) are
calcium stones, composed of calcium.**

34. 1. The PCA pump automatically administers a specific amount and has a lock-
out interval time in which the PCA
pump cannot administer any morphine.
The client can push the control button

as often as needed and will not receive an overdose of pain medication.

2. The nurse should inform the client that the pain should be tolerable, not necessarily absent.

3. The Wong-Baker FACES Pain Scale is used for children; adult clients use the 1–10 pain scale with 0 being no pain and 10 being the worst pain.

4. The client receiving PCA morphine should be instructed not to ambulate without assistance, and the nurse strains the urine, not the client.

35. 1. This prescription would not need to be clarified with the HCP.

2. The client should not administer the suppository to himself or herself.

3. The client does not need to have a clean bowel to receive a suppository.

4. **This medication is prescribed because it may reduce the amount of narcotic analgesia required for acute renal colic.**

36. 1. Administering the rescue of morphine is an appropriate intervention, but it is not the nurse's first action.

2. **Assessing the client and ruling out any complications is the nurse's first intervention.**

3. The nurse should determine the last time the client received morphine and the amount of morphine the client has received, but it is not the first intervention.

4. Nonpharmacologic interventions are appropriate to address the client's pain, but they should not be implemented first for a client with renal calculi.

37. 1. This is the scientific rationale for administering allopurinol (Zyloprim) to help reduce the formation of uric stones.

2. This is the scientific rationale for administering a thiazide diuretic to help reduce the formation of calcium renal calculi. This medication will decrease calcium levels in the bloodstream by increasing calcium excretion in the urine.

3. **This is the scientific rationale for administering Calcibind to reduce the formation of calcium renal calculi.**

4. This is the scientific rationale for administering penicillamine to help prevent the formation of uric stones.

38. 1. The client does not need to be NPO for this procedure because it is used to diagnose renal abnormalities, not gastrointestinal abnormalities.

2. The client should not have this diagnostic test if the kidneys are not working properly. The intravenous dye could damage the kidneys if normal functioning is not present.

3. The nurse would assess for iodine allergy, not an antibiotic allergy. The nurse should ask if the client is allergic to Betadine or shellfish.

4. This diagnostic test does not require blood administration; therefore, the nurse should start a smaller gauge intravenous catheter such as a 22- or 20-gauge angiocatheter.

39. 1. **This is the correct position for the client when an epidural anesthesia is being inserted.**

2. The nurse would determine if the client's operative permit is signed. The admission nurse is responsible for determining if the client has an advance directive.

3. A client's gag and swallowing reflexes are assessed postoperatively for the client who has had general anesthesia.

4. The client's stretcher should be flat so that the client can lie on the side in the fetal position.

40. 1. Intravenous fluids are medications and the nurse cannot delegate medication administration to the UAP.

2. The UAP may be able to discontinue an IV, but the question asks which is the most appropriate task and the nurse should always delegate the least invasive and the simplest task.

3. The UAP should not be assigned to take a client outside to smoke. This is not in the job description of a hospital employee. After the nurse discourages the client from going downstairs to smoke, a family member or friend should escort the client outside.

4. **The UAP can document the client's oral intake and urinary output, but the UAP cannot evaluate if the urine output is adequate and appropriate for the IVP procedure.**

An Adolescent with a Sexually Transmitted Disease

41. 1. Sexually transmitted diseases are considered a public health hazard and the client can be treated without parental permission.

2. Pregnancy may be a concern, but the client is discussing sexually transmitted disease and the nurse should address the client's concerns.

3. This is a judgmental statement and the nurse should not impair communication with the client.

4. **There are many different STDs. The client needs to have tests run based on her presenting symptoms so that appropriate treatment can be initiated.**

42. 1. NRTI medications are prescribed for clients who are HIV positive during pregnancy to prevent maternal transmission of the virus to the fetus.

2. Valtrex is prescribed to treat herpes simplex 2 viral infections, but it is not administered routinely to neonates at birth.

3. **Erythromycin ophthalmic ointment is the medication of choice to prevent ophthalmia neonatorum (blindness caused by a gonorrhea infection acquired when passing through the birth canal or coming into contact with the mother's tissues). Because the client has had no prenatal care, this would be recommended procedure in case the infant has been exposed to gonorrhea.**

4. Metronidazole is administered for some STDs, but it is not routinely administered to neonates.

43. 1. **Consuming alcohol concurrently with Flagyl can cause a severe reaction. This statement indicates the need for more teaching.**

2. The sexual partners must be treated simultaneously to prevent a reinfection from occurring. This statement indicates the client understands the teaching.

3. Untreated STDs can lead to pelvic inflammatory disease, scarred fallopian tubes, and infertility. This statement indicates the client understands the teaching.

4. Antibiotics may interfere with the effectiveness of some birth control pills. The client should use a supplemental form of birth control when taking birth control pills. This statement indicates the client understands the teaching.

MEDICATION MEMORY JOGGER: The test taker should realize that consuming alcohol is contraindicated with most medications.

44. 1. There are no medications, whether the client is allergic or not, available to cure the herpes simplex 2 virus and the human immunodeficiency virus (HIV). This is a false statement but one that teenagers would like to believe because of their feelings of invincibility.

2. **There are no medications available to cure the herpes simplex 2 virus and the human immunodeficiency virus (HIV). There are many medications available to treat the problems associated with these STDs, and they provide hope for the client, but the students must be aware of the long-term ramifications of STDs.**

3. Birth control medications provide no protection against an STD. They may increase the chance of acquiring an STD because the fear of pregnancy is removed, making sexual activity more likely.

4. Antibiotics have side effects and the medications for HIV infections have especially strong associated side effects and adverse reactions. The side effects and adverse reactions are more likely to decrease libido than to enhance it.

45. 1. **Rocephin is administered IM or IV. There is no pill form of the medication. The medication burns when administered and should be administered in the large gluteus muscle.**

2. There is no pill form of Rocephin, so drinking water will not affect the medication.

3. Rocephin is administered IM or IV. A tuberculin syringe is used to administer medications by the subcutaneous or intradermal route.

4. There is no pill form of the medication, so eating will not affect the medication.

46. 1. Syphilis is treated with a penicillin antibiotic unless the client is allergic to penicillin. The dosing schedule of every 4 hours for 10 days would make it difficult to achieve compliance from an adult, much less an adolescent.

2. **A one-time injection of benzathine penicillin G is the usual treatment for primary syphilis infections.**

3. Syphilis is a bacterial infection, and an antifungal medication would not treat a bacterial infection. The antibiotic must be taken internally to treat syphilis.

4. Macrodantin is an antibiotic used primarily for chronic urinary tract infections, not syphilis.

47. 1. The time period for the lesions to heal depends on several factors, including the immune status of the infected individual and the amount of stress the individual is experiencing at the time. It usually requires several days to more than a week for an outbreak to be healed.
    2. Suppressive therapy with Valtrex is once daily, every day. This is an advantage of Valtrex over other antiretroviral agents, which require twice-a-day dosing.
    3. The use of condoms may prevent the spread of herpes infections; it does not increase the spread of the virus.
    4. **It is possible to transmit the virus to a sexual partner with no visible signs of a lesion being present. Valtrex will not absolutely prevent the spread of the virus. It will treat an outbreak and decrease the risk of transmission.**

48. 1. No scratch marks on the penis indicate the client has not scratched himself but does not indicate a lack of infestation in the pubic hair.
    2. Pediculosis pubis is pubic lice, not head lice; a clear scalp would not indicate a lack of a pubic infestation.
    3. **Pediculosis causes intense itching. A lack of itching indicates the treatment is effective. A 16-year-old client is unlikely to submit to a visual inspection of his pubic area by the nurse.**
    4. Pediculosis pubis is pubic lice, not head lice, so no visible lice or nits on the head would not indicate a lack of a pubic infestation.

    MEDICATION MEMORY JOGGER: The nurse determines the effectiveness of a medication by assessing for the symptoms, or lack thereof, for which the medication was prescribed.

49. 1. Wiping the perineum from front to back is encouraged to prevent a urinary tract infection from fecal contamination of the urethral meatus.
    2. The procedure should be planned immediately after the menstrual cycle has ended so that protection will not be needed until the client has had time to heal.

3. **The liquid nitrogen causes a chemical burn to form, destroying the genital wart. The client should be taught to cleanse the area carefully to decrease pain and risk of infection.**
4. Daily Betadine douches would increase pain and discomfort. Betadine is an iodine preparation and could cause the area to sting. The client should be encouraged to limit use of any soap or chemical preparation until released to do so by the HCP.

50. **1000 mg of medication will be administered with each dose.**
    The client weighs 220 pounds. Convert weight to kilograms by dividing by 2.2 (220 ÷ 2.2 = 100 kg). Multiply 100 times 10 mg equals 1000 mg per dose.

A Client Experiencing Pregnancy

51. 1. Category A medications have a remote risk of causing fetal harm and are prescribed for clients who are pregnant.
    2. Category B medications have a slightly higher risk of causing fetal abnormalities than do Category A medications, but they are often prescribed for clients who are pregnant.
    3. Category C medications pose a greater risk than category B medications and are cautiously prescribed for clients who are pregnant. Medications in this category have either not yet been the subject of research or may show a risk in animal studies.
    4. **Category D medications have a proven risk of fetal harm and are not prescribed for clients who are pregnant unless the mother's life is in danger. Category X medications have a definite risk of fetal abnormality or abortion.**

52. 1. Iron causes constipation; therefore, the client should increase fluid and fiber to help decrease the possibility of becoming constipated.
    2. Iron causes constipation; therefore, the client is instructed to take a daily stool softener to prevent constipation.
    3. **The iron preparation causes the stool to become black and tarry; therefore, the client would not need to notify the obstetrician.**

4. Iron should be taken between meals,
2 hours after a meal, because food
decreases absorption of the medication
by 50%–70%.

53. 1. Brethine causes bronchodilatation, and
if the client's respiratory rate is greater
than 30 or if there is a change in quality of lung sounds (wheezing, rales, or
coughing), the HCP should be notified.
2. The normal FHR is 110–160; therefore,
an FHR of 150 is within normal limits and
would not warrant intervention by the
nurse.
3. The client's apical heart rate is just above
normal (60–100) and would not warrant
intervention by the nurse.
4. Brethine is administered to prevent
contractions; therefore, the medication is
effective.

54. 1. The client with preeclampsia would be
receiving magnesium sulfate to help
prevent seizures; therefore, the nurse
would not question administering this
medication.
2. **Cervidil is contraindicated in clients
who have asthma because it can initiate
an asthmatic attack; therefore, the
nurse should question administering
this medication.**
3. Celestone is a medication used to increase
surfactant in fetal lungs and would be
administered to a client who is less than
36 weeks pregnant; therefore, the nurse
would not question administering this
medication.
4. Pitocin, a uterine stimulant, would be
administered after a client has experienced
an incomplete abortion to help the client
expel the fetal fragments; therefore, the
nurse would not question administering
this medication.

55.   3, 4, 2, 1, 5
3. The nurse must first determine if this
is the right client receiving the right
medication.
4. The nurse should always check about
allergies. With this medication,
"-caine" drugs are anesthetics and, if
the client is allergic to lidocaine (sutur-
ing lacerations) or Novacaine (dental
procedures), the client should not
receive this medication.
2. Once the nurse determines that this is
the right client receiving the right
medication and that the client has no

allergies, then the nurse must wash his
or her hands and use gloves to administer a medication to the perineal area.
1. This position allows maximum exposure to the area that should be
medicated.
5. After completing all of the previous
steps, the nurse can apply the
medication.

56. 1. Breathing exercises are important, but the
protection of the client's lower extremities
while under anesthesia should be priority
for the nurse.
2. **Because the legs are numb as a result
of the epidural, the nurse must ensure
the legs are in the stirrups correctly so
that the client will not experience
neurovascular compromise or any type
of injury to the legs when they are in
the stirrups.**
3. Preparing the significant other for the
delivery is important, but it is not priority
over the safety of the mother's lower
extremities.
4. The anesthesiologist or nurse anesthetist
would be responsible for administering
the anesthesia during the delivery.

57. 1. The uterus becoming hard and firm periodically indicates a contraction, which is
expected when administering a uterine
stimulant.
2. The client wanting to urinate would be
expected because the baby's head is push-
ing against the bladder.
3. Denying the urge to push indicates the
client is not in the last stages of labor.
4. **During a contraction the fetal heart
rate will decrease but should return to
the baseline FHR after the contraction.
If this does not occur, it indicates the
infant is in distress and this warrants
immediate intervention. This could
also be a sign of uterine rupture resulting from overstimulation of the uterus.**

58. 1. If the client's deep tendon reflexes are 4+,
this indicates the client may have a seizure
at any time, which, in turn, indicates the
medication is not effective.
2. Magnesium sulfate is not administered to
treat the client's blood pressure; therefore,
this data cannot be used to evaluate the
effectiveness of the medication.
3. **Magnesium sulfate is administered to
prevent seizure activity and is determined to be effective and in the thera-**

peutic range when the client's deep
tendon reflexes are normal, which is 2
to 3+ on a 0–4+ scale.

    4. A "0" deep tendon reflex indicates the
client has received too much magnesium
sulfate and would not indicate the medication is effective. The client is at risk for
respiratory depression.

59. 1. This is the scientific rationale for administering corticosteroids. A beta-adrenergic
agonist, not a corticosteroid, is given to
decrease uterine contractions in preterm
labor.

    2. This is not the reason why steroids are
administered; it is not the rationale for any
medication administered to the client who
is pregnant.

    **3. This is the scientific rationale for
administering corticosteroids. They are
administered to a client who is in
preterm labor because they accelerate
lung maturation, resulting in surfactant
development in the fetus.**

    4. Rho (D) immune globulin (RhoGAM) is
administered to a mother who has Rh-
negative blood and is pregnant with a Rh-
positive fetus to prevent the development
of maternal antibodies to the fetus's blood.
Corticosteroids are not given for this
reason.

60. 1. The client's H&H should be monitored,
but an ongoing assessment of how much
the client is bleeding is priority.

    **2. Monitoring the client's peripad count
will allow the nurse to directly assess
how much the client is bleeding, which
will help determine if the medication is
effective.**

    3. Vital signs should be monitored, but an
ongoing assessment of how much the
client is bleeding is priority.

    4. The client's fundal height should be
assessed, but it will not help determine
how much blood the client has lost.

A Client Experiencing Infertility

61. 1. This herb is taken to treat depression, but
it can cause more infertility problems;
therefore, the nurse should discuss this
with the client.

    2. The client should discuss taking herbs
with all health-care providers, but this is
not the nurse's best response.

    3. St. John's wort may cause effects on
sperm cells, decreased sperm motility,
and decreased viability; therefore, this
client should not take this herb.

    4. The significant other taking herbs should
not affect the client's fertility; therefore,
this is not an appropriate response.

62. 1. This is no increased risk of having a child
with Down syndrome when taking this
medication.

    2. There are many risks associated with
taking this fertility medication, including
multiple fetuses, pain, visual disturbances,
abnormal bleeding, and ovarian failure.

    3. This medication should be taken at the
same time every day to maintain a therapeutic drug level.

    **4. Clomid is an ovarian stimulant that
promotes follicle maturation and
ovulation. Many follicles can mature
simultaneously, resulting in the
increased possibility of multiple births.**

63. 1. **The client should be aware that it may
take 3–6 months for leuprolide therapy
to achieve maximum benefits; therefore, the nurse should discuss the long-
term possibility with the client.**

    2. Continuous use of this medication
may cause amenorrhea or menstrual
irregularities.

    3. This medication is either given intramus-
cularly once a month or it is an implant
that is given once every 12 months, but it
is not administered daily.

    4. This medication does not affect when the
client can have intercourse.

64. 1. A pelvic sonogram is used to determine
ovarian response to Parlodel, but because
the client thinks she is pregnant, performing a sonogram is not the first intervention.

    **2. The client must quit taking the
medication immediately because it can
cause a miscarriage of the fetus. Once
the client becomes pregnant, the
medication is not needed anymore.**

    3. The client needs to see the HCP, but it is
not the first intervention the nurse should
discuss with the client.

    4. The client can perform a home pregnancy
test, but it is not the first intervention the
nurse should discuss with the client.

**MEDICATION MEMORY JOGGER: The test
taker should question administering any
medication to a client who is pregnant.**

Many medications cross the placental barrier and could affect the fetus.

65. 1. This test determines how much medication has been administered, but it does not indicate that the medication is effective.
    2. **The serum estrogen level should increase three to four times the pretreatment baseline if the medications are effective and the client may be able to get pregnant.**
    3. A negative pregnancy test indicates the medications are not effective.
    4. This is the test that determines the 3-month average blood glucose level.

66. 1. Abdominal bloating and vague gastrointestinal discomfort are signs of ovarian cancer.
    2. This could indicate a miscarriage but does not support the diagnosis of ovarian hyperstimulation syndrome.
    3. **Ovarian hyperstimulation syndrome involves marked ovarian enlargement with exudation of fluid into the woman's peritoneal and pleural cavities. This syndrome can result in ovarian cysts that may rupture, causing pain.**
    4. These are signs and symptoms of urinary tract infection.

67. 1. HCG acts immediately to promote ovulation; therefore, the couple should not wait to have sexual intercourse.
    2. Wearing tight-fitting underwear causes the scrotum to be close to the body and the heat reduces the sperm count, which is why boxer shorts are recommended, but this has nothing to do with the HCG medication.
    3. Taking the basal metabolic temperature is a first-line intervention for clients experiencing infertility to determine when a woman is ovulating. HCG stimulates ovulation, which should occur within hours to a day or two of administration of the medication.
    4. **The couple should have sexual intercourse during this time because this is the probable period of ovulation.**

68. 1. **Progesterone enhances the receptivity of the endometrium to implantation—the function of progesterone in the body—and is the scientific rationale for administering supplemental progesterone to a client preparing for in vitro fertilization.**
    2. Providing more hormones to the ovary for egg production is not the scientific rationale for administering supplemental progesterone to a client preparing to undergo in vitro fertilization.
    3. Regulation of the menstrual cycle is not the scientific rationale for administering this medication.
    4. This is not the scientific rationale for administering this medication.

69. 1. Infertility therapy is extremely expensive and most insurances do not cover it at all or cover only a small portion.
    2. **Pregnancy with more than twins carries a substantially higher risk to the mother and the fetuses because of preterm labor and birth, placental insufficiency, and high demand on maternal body systems.**
    3. There is no guarantee of pregnancy on the first attempt.
    4. Most of the implanted zygotes do not result in live births.

70. 1. There is no documented drug regimen that helps men achieve sperm levels, except possibly testosterone medications or supplements.
    2. This is a therapeutic response and the client is asking for information; therefore, the nurse should provide the facts.
    3. **Administration of testosterone will improve hormonal levels, resulting in a potential for increased spermatogenesis.**
    4. Clomid is an ovarian stimulant and will not help a male client.

A Client Using Birth Control

71. 1. **Correct use of spermicide is required for contraceptive efficacy. The spermicide must be in place prior to intercourse, and the foam is immediately active. If a suppository or tablet is used, it must be inserted 10–15 minutes before intercourse to allow time for it to dissolve.**
    2. Douching is not allowed for at least 6 hours after intercourse; douching will remove the spermicide.
    3. The spermicide must be inserted into the female's vagina, not on the male's penis.
    4. The spermicide is not effective if it is inserted after intercourse.

72. 1. The client who smokes more than 15 cigarettes a day is at a greater risk for cardiovascular complications when taking oral contraceptives.
2. A client taking an ACE inhibitor would have cardiovascular problems. Oral contraceptives elevate blood pressure by increasing both angiotensin and aldosterone; therefore, this client should not take oral contraceptives.
3. A client who is obese is at risk for hypertension, hypercholesterolemia, and deep vein thrombosis and should not take oral contraceptives.
4. **Oral contraceptives decrease the risk for several disorders, including ovarian cancer, endometrial cancer, pelvic inflammatory disease, premenstrual syndrome, toxic shock, fibrocystic breast disease, ovarian cysts, and anemia. In addition to providing birth control for the client, the client gets a secondary benefit of decreasing her risk for ovarian cancer.**

73. 1. The client should be instructed to take any missed pill as soon as the omission is recognized; therefore, the client could and should take more than one pill in a day.
2. Breakthrough bleeding may mean the dosage of the oral contraceptive is not appropriate, but this is not a reason to discontinue taking the medication. The client should see the HCP.
3. **The client should be instructed to take any missed pill as soon as the omission is recognized. Therefore, the client could and should take more than one pill in a day. To maintain ovulation suppression the client must take the medication routinely.**
4. Antibiotics decrease the effectiveness of some oral contraceptives, and a secondary form of birth control should be used during antibiotic therapy.

74. 1. This is an appropriate question, but the timing of the sexual activity is not the important consideration for a new mother taking her baby home when discussing birth control.
2. **This is the most important question because if the mother has decided on breastfeeding, the nurse should discourage the use of birth control pills. Birth control pills enter breast milk and reduce milk production. Breastfeeding may delay ovulation but**

should not be used as a form of birth control.
3. This is a question that the nurse could ask, but it is not the most important when concerned about birth control.
4. This question could be asked, but the most important issue is protecting the baby if the mother chooses to breastfeed because anything the mother ingests may affect the baby. This includes the effects of the type of birth control if the mother chooses to breastfeed.

MEDICATION MEMORY JOGGER: The test taker should question administering any medication to a client who is breastfeeding. Many medications are transmitted to the baby via breast milk.

75. 1. This statement is judgmental, and because he is already sexually active, it is not going to protect him from fathering a child or getting a STD. The nurse should encourage the sexually active adolescent to use protection.
2. **The adolescent's comments should make the school nurse consider an allergic reaction to the condom, most of which are made of latex. Suggesting a type of condom made from lamb's intestines would prevent an allergic reaction.**
3. STDs require an incubation period, and the red rash area would not occur the next morning.
4. A diaphragm is a form of birth control, but most are made of latex, which may cause a reaction for the male adolescent.

76. 1. If the ring is expelled before 3 weeks have passed, it can be washed off in warm water and reinserted. A new one is reinserted only if the expelled ring cannot be used.
2. This statement is appropriate for using a diaphragm, not the ring.
3. **The vaginal contraceptive ring works on the same principle that oral contraceptives work. It provides 21 days of hormone suppression, followed by 7 days to allow for menses. The ring slowly releases hormones that penetrate the vaginal mucosa and are absorbed by the blood and distributed throughout the body. The contraception occurs from systemic effects, not local effects in the vagina.**
4. The client will have a period when using this form of birth control.

MEDICATION MEMORY JOGGER: Medications are not usually administered to stop normal body functions, especially with birth control medication because the uterus must be able to expel the lining that was prepared for an ovum that did not appear.

77. 1. If signs of estrogen excess are apparent (nausea, edema, or breast discomfort), a preparation with lower estrogen content is needed. This statement therefore warrants the nurse to intervene.
    2. Oral contraceptives may decrease or eliminate menstrual flow during the initial months of use; therefore, the nurse would not intervene based on this statement.
    3. This statement would warrant praise from the clinic nurse because birth control pills do not protect the client from STDs. Only condoms or abstinence can do that.
    4. The birth control pill suppresses ovulation for 3 weeks; then, when the pill is not taken, the client has her period. This statement indicates the client understands the teaching and does not warrant intervention.

78. 1. This is not a true statement. The client will have a normal 28-day cycle.
    2. Birth control pills will decrease cramping, but 7 days out of the month the pill the client takes does not contain hormones; it is a placebo.
    3. This product is not any more expensive or cheaper than a 21-day product.
    4. This 28-day pack contains 21 days of the hormone and 7 days of placebos. The client takes a pill every day. This eliminates the need for the woman to remember which day to restart taking the pill, as she would have to with a 21-day pack, with which the woman takes a pill for 21 days and then no pill for 7 days and then restarts a new pack.

79. 1. Depo-Provera is a safe, effective contraceptive that is effective for 3 months or longer and is administered via intramuscular injection every 3 months to provide for continuous protection.
    2. When injections are discontinued, an average of 12 months is required for fertility to return. Some women remain infertile for as long as 2 1/2 years.
    3. This medication is administered intramuscularly every 3 months.
    4. An intrauterine device is not necessary when using this medication. An IUD is inserted by the HCP, not by the client.
    5. The advantage to this medication is that it is only taken every 3 months, which is why it is recommended for adolescents or women who may not use other methods of birth control reliably.

80. 1. Because the client is receiving the medication for menstrual irregularity it is effective when the menstrual cycle is regular, which is every 28 days.
    2. A decrease in abdominal bloating may occur, but it does not indicate the medication is effective.
    3. This should occur but this is not why the client is taking the medication; therefore, it cannot be used to indicate the medication is effective.
    4. Birth control pills have a positive effect on acne, but this is not why the client is taking the medication; therefore, it cannot be used to indicate the medication's effectiveness.

MEDICATION MEMORY JOGGER: The nurse determines the effectiveness of a medication by assessing for the symptoms, or lack thereof, for which the medication was prescribed.

1. The client postbirth via C-section is receiving epidural morphine. The unlicensed assistive personnel (UAP) tells the primary nurse the client has a pulse of 84, respirations of 10, and a blood pressure of 102/78. Which action should the nurse implement first?
   1. Administer naloxone (Narcan), a central nervous system antagonist.
   2. Assess the client's pain using the numerical (1–10) pain scale.
   3. Check the client's respiratory rate and pulse oximeter reading.
   4. Complete a neurovascular assessment of the client's lower extremities.

2. Which male client would the nurse consider at risk for complications when taking sildenafil (Viagra), a sexual stimulant?
   1. A 56-year-old client with unstable angina.
   2. An 87-year-old client with glaucoma.
   3. A 44-year-old client with Type 2 diabetes.
   4. A 32-year-old client with an L-1 spinal cord injury.

3. The 33-year-old female client is being prescribed an antibiotic for a urinary tract infection (UTI). Which question is most important for the nurse to ask the client when discussing the medication?
   1. "How many UTIs have you had in the last year?"
   2. "What type of underwear do you wear usually?"
   3. "Which way do you clean after a bowel movement?"
   4. "Are you currently using any type of birth control?"

4. The client with gestational diabetes asks the nurse, "Why do I have to take shots? Why can't I take a pill?" Which statement is the nurse's best response?
   1. "The shots will help keep your blood glucose level down better."
   2. "Pills may hurt the development of the baby in your womb."
   3. "Insulin will help prevent you from having the baby too early."
   4. "Pills for diabetes may delay the baby's lung development."

5. The elderly male client is prescribed tolterodine (Detrol-LA), an anticholinergic, for urge incontinence. Which statement would warrant notifying the health-care provider?
   1. "I have to suck on sugarless candy because my mouth is so dry."
   2. "I am so glad I can go all day without having to go to the bathroom."
   3. "I really have problems swallowing the pills whole with water."
   4. "I hate I had to give up my grapefruit juice, but I know it is best."

6. The mother with preeclampsia is received magnesium sulfate, an anticonvulsant, during labor and delivery. Which intervention will the nursery nurse implement for the newborn?
   1. Assess the lungs for meconium aspiration.
   2. Prepare to administer naloxone (Narcan).
   3. Administer 2 ounces of glucose water.
   4. Stimulate the baby by tapping the feet.

7. The 56-year-old Asian female client tells the nurse that she is taking the herb *Angelica sinensis* (dong quai). Which data would indicate to the nurse that this medication is effective?
   1. The client has normal menstrual cycles.
   2. The client does not have abdominal bloating.
   3. The client reports fewer hot flashes.
   4. The client has a normal bone density test.

8. Which statement best indicates the scientific rationale for administering vitamin K (AquaMEPHYTON) to the newborn infant?
   1. It promotes blood clotting in the infant.
   2. It prevents conjunctivitis in the infant's eyes.
   3. It stimulates peristalsis in the small intestines.
   4. It helps the digestive process in the newborn.

9. The nurse is preparing to insert an 18-gauge indwelling urinary (Foley) catheter in a client who has a latex allergy. Which intervention is most important for the nurse to implement?
   1. Use latex-free gloves when performing this procedure.
   2. Insert a 16-gauge Foley catheter into the client.
   3. Obtain an appropriate Foley catheter for the client.
   4. Use povidone iodine solution to cleanse the perineal area.

10. The client is diagnosed with *Chlamydia trachomatis*, a sexually transmitted disease, and asks the nurse, "Why must I take an antibiotic when I don't have any itching or pain?" Which statement would be the nurse's best response?
    1. "The itching and pain will start within 2 or 3 days."
    2. "The antibiotics will prevent canker sores on your genitalia."
    3. "If you use a condom, then you don't have to take the antibiotic."
    4. "If it is not treated, you may never be able to have a baby."

11. The preterm infant is receiving synthetic surfactant. Which data indicates the medication is effective?
    1. The infant's heel stick capillary blood glucose level is 90 mg/dL.
    2. The infant's arterial blood gases are within normal limits.
    3. The positive end expiratory pressure (PEEP) on the ventilator is turned off.
    4. The infant's pulse oximeter reading fluctuates between 90% and 92%.

12. The 19-year-old client presents to the emergency department with trauma to the flank area resulting from a motor vehicle accident. The client's first urine specimen shows bright-red urine. Which intervention should the nurse implement first?
    1. Initiate an 18-gauge angiocath with normal saline.
    2. Send a sterile urine specimen to the laboratory.
    3. Type and crossmatch for 2 units of blood.
    4. Prepare the client for a CT scan of the abdomen.

13. The labor and delivery nurse is preparing the client for spinal anesthesia. Which intervention should the nurse expect the nurse anesthetist to implement?
    1. Administer 500 to 1000 mL of intravenous fluid before inserting the spinal catheter.
    2. Instruct the client to lie in the lithotomy position when inserting the catheter.
    3. Perform a complete neurovascular assessment on the lower extremities.
    4. Monitor blood pressure, pulse, and respirations immediately prior to insertion.

14. The client who was raped is admitted to the emergency department and tells the nurse, "I will kill myself if I get pregnant from this monster." Which statement is the nurse's best response?
    1. "Have you ever thought about killing yourself and do you have a plan?"
    2. "There are medications that must be taken within 72 hours to prevent pregnancy."
    3. "A vaginal spermicide can be prescribed that will prevent pregnancy."
    4. "You may have to have an elective abortion if you do become pregnant."

15. The client who is pregnant asks the nurse, "What does category A mean if the doctor orders that medication for me?" Which statement best describes the scientific rationale for the nurse's response?
    1. Category A is the safest medication a client can take when pregnant.
    2. Category A medications are safe as long as the client does not take them during the first trimester.
    3. Research has not determined if these medications are harmful to the fetus or not.
    4. This category is dangerous to the fetus but could be prescribed in emergencies.

16. The 17-year-old male athlete admits to the nurse that he has been taking anabolic steroids to increase his muscle strength. Which action should the nurse implement?
    1. Inform the client's parents about the illegal use of anabolic steroids.
    2. Ask the client where he has been obtaining these anabolic steroids.
    3. Assess the client for moon face, buffalo hump, and weight gain.
    4. Explain that long-term effects of steroids may cause him to never father a baby.

17. The client with chronic kidney disease is admitted to the medical floor for pneumonia. The admission orders include Zithromax, cyclosporine, and Mylanta. Which question should the nurse ask the client?
    1. "Are you allergic to iodine or any type of shellfish?"
    2. "When is the last time you had your dialysis treatment?"
    3. "Have you had any type of organ transplant?"
    4. "Why don't you take Amphojel instead of Mylanta?"

18. The woman who is Rh negative and a Jehovah's Witness delivers a baby who is Rh positive. The HCP prescribed RhoGAM for the mother. Which action should the nurse implement first?
    1. Administer the RhoGAM to the client within 72 hours.
    2. Obtain a signed permit for administering this medication.
    3. Confirm the infant's blood type with the laboratory.
    4. Explain to the client that RhoGAM is a blood product.

19. The nurse is administering medication to a client who has had a kidney transplant and is taking cyclosporine, an antirejection medication. Which medication would the nurse question administering?
    1. The ACE inhibitor captopril (Capoten).
    2. The antibiotic trimethoprim-sulfamethoxazole (Bactrim DS).
    3. The analgesic acetaminophen (Tylenol).
    4. The antiemetic prochlorperazine (Compazine).

20. The male client with a renal stone is admitted to the medical department. The nurse administers intravenous morphine over 5 minutes. Which intervention should the nurse implement first?
    1. Instruct the client to call for help before getting out of bed.
    2. Tell the client to urinate into the urinal at all times.
    3. Document the time in the MAR and the client's chart.
    4. Reevaluate the client's pain within 30 minutes.

1. 1. This is the antidote for morphine overdose, but the nurse would not administer the medication without first assessing the client because these data were provided by the UAP.
   2. The client's respiration is less than normal; therefore, the priority should be assessing the respiratory status, not the client's pain level.
   3. **Because the UAP provided the initial abnormal data, the nurse should first assess the client to determine and validate the client's respiratory status.**
   4. The client's neurovascular status should be assessed because of the epidural analgesia, but the client's respiratory status is priority.

2. 1. **Viagra should be used cautiously in clients with coronary heart disease because during sexual activity the client could have a myocardial infarction from the extra demands on the heart. Specifically, clients taking nitroglycerin or any nitrate medication should not take Viagra because the vasodilatation effect of Viagra may cause hypotension. A client with unstable angina would be taking a nitrate medication.**
   2. Viagra is not contraindicated for clients diagnosed with glaucoma.
   3. Viagra is not contraindicated for clients diagnosed with Type 2 diabetes and may help erectile dysfunction.
   4. Viagra is not contraindicated for clients with an SCI and may help erectile dysfunction.

3. 1. The number of UTIs is information the nurse would need to determine if the client is at risk for developing chronic urinary tract infections, but this is not the most important question when discussing antibiotic therapy.
   2. Wearing cotton underwear or underwear with a cotton crotch should be encouraged because cotton is a natural material that breathes and allows air to circulate to the area, decreasing the risk for UTIs. It is an appropriate question, but it is not the most important question when discussing antibiotic therapy.
   3. Cleaning from back to front after a bowel movement increases the risk of fecal contamination of the urinary meatus, but this is not the most important question when discussing antibiotic therapy.

   4. **Birth control pills and certain antibiotics may interact, making the birth control pills ineffective in preventing pregnancy. This is the most important question for the nurse to ask.**

   MEDICATION MEMORY JOGGER: Any time the client is of childbearing age the nurse should determine if there is a potential pregnancy or drug interaction with birth control methods.

4. 1. Insulin may better help control the blood glucose level, but that is not the reason why it is used during pregnancy.
   2. **Oral hypoglycemics are not used during pregnancy because they cross the placental barrier; they stimulate fetal insulin production and may be teratogenic.**
   3. Insulin has no effect on preterm labor.
   4. Oral hypoglycemics do not affect fetal lung development.

5. 1. Anticholinergic medications block the muscarinic receptors on the salivary glands and inhibit salivation, resulting in a dry mouth. This comment would not warrant notifying the HCP.
   2. **Inability to void all day long indicates an overdose of the medication and would require notifying the health-care provider to decrease the dosage.**
   3. The "LA" in the medication indicates this medication is long acting and should not be crushed. Because the client is swallowing the pill, the HCP would not need to be notified.
   4. Grapefruit juice increases the effect of Detrol; therefore, the client not drinking it would not warrant notifying the HCP.

   MEDICATION MEMORY JOGGER: Grapefruit juice can inhibit the metabolism of certain medications. Specifically, grapefruit juice inhibits cytochrome P450-3A4 found in the liver and the intestinal wall. The nurse should investigate any medications the client is taking if the client drinks grapefruit juice.

6. 1. There is no data in the stem that indicates that the baby is postmature; therefore, the nursery nurse would not assess for meconium aspiration.
   2. Glucose water is given to infants who are experiencing hypoglycemia. There is no indication that this infant is experiencing

hypoglycemia, the mother does not have diabetes, and hypoglycemia in the infant does not occur as a result of preeclampsia.

3. The antidote for magnesium sulfate overdosage is calcium gluconate. Narcan is an opioid agonist and might be needed if the mother took morphine during the labor and delivery.

4. **The baby is at risk for respiratory or neurological depression; therefore, the nurse should stimulate the baby until the effects of the magnesium sulfate have dissipated.**

7. 1. The nurse would expect that a 56-year-old client should not be having normal menstrual cycles.

2. Abdominal bloating is associated with premenstrual syndrome and the nurse would not expect that a 56-year-old client would be having normal menstrual cycles.

3. **Dong quai is used for menopausal symptoms and premenstrual syndrome, but because the client is 56 years old the nurse should consider the medication effective when there is a lack of menopausal symptoms.**

4. This herb does not affect bone density.

8. 1. **The newborn's gut is sterile and the liver cannot synthesize vitamin K from the food ingested until there are bacteria present in the gut.**

2. Ophthalmic ointment is administered to prevent eye infections.

3. Routine medications administered to the newborn do not include medications to stimulate the small intestines.

4. Routine medications administered to the newborn do not include medications to stimulate the digestive process.

9. 1. The nurse should use latex-free gloves when touching the client, but this is not the most important intervention because this is a very short-term exposure to the latex for the client.

2. A smaller catheter does not address the material the catheter is made out of.

3. **The most important intervention is for the client to have a latex-free Foley catheter because this will stay in the client for an extended period.**

4. The solution used to clean the client would not have a bearing on the latex allergy.

10. 1. *Chlamydia* is frequently asymptomatic and is diagnosed with an annual Pap smear.

2. *Chlamydia* does not cause canker sores; these sores are caused by syphilis.

3. *Chlamydia* is bacteria and must be treated with an antibiotic; condoms are used to prevent transmission to a partner.

4. **Untreated *Chlamydia* can lead to pelvic inflammatory disease and long-term effects, including chronic pain, increased risk for ectopic pregnancy, postpartum endometritis, and infertility.**

11. 1. Synthetic surfactant does not affect the infant's blood glucose level.

2. **Synthetic lung surfactant coats the alveoli and prevents collapse of the lung by reducing the surface tension of pulmonary fluids. Normal ABGs indicate the lungs are adequately oxygenating the body, which means the medication is effective.**

3. PEEP cannot be used on a newborn because it increases intrathoracic pressure and increases the risk for pneumothorax.

4. Pulse oximeter readings measure peripheral oxygenation and should be greater than 93%, which indicates the client's arterial oxygen level would be above 80. A 90% to 92% pulse oximeter reading indicates hypoxia and that the medication is not effective.

12. 1. **The nurse must first initiate steps to prevent the client from developing hypovolemic shock; therefore, the nurse should start a large-bore IV to infuse isotonic normal saline to maintain blood pressure. The nurse should anticipate the client receiving a blood transfusion, which supports the need for an 18-gauge catheter.**

2. A urine specimen should be sent to the laboratory, but the client's safety and prevention of shock are the nurse's first priority.

3. Ordering blood is a priority but not a priority over caring for the client who may be going into hypovolemic shock.

4. Determining the source of bleeding is important, but caring for the client is priority.

MEDICATION MEMORY JOGGER: The nurse's first priority is always caring for the client, not a laboratory or diagnostic test.

13. 1. **Spinal anesthesia has been shown to be well-tolerated by a healthy fetus when a maternal intravenous fluid preload in excess of 500 to 1000 mL precedes the administration of the spinal.**
2. The client will be in the sidelying or fetal position; the lithotomy position has the client supine with the feet in the stirrups.
3. This assessment would be performed after the spinal anesthesia to determine the effectiveness of the anesthesia.
4. Baseline vital signs can be obtained 30 minutes to 1 hour prior to spinal anesthesia; postprocedure vital signs are monitored every 1–2 minutes for the first 10 minutes and then every 5–10 minutes throughout the delivery.

14. 1. The client is understandably distressed and is in a crisis situation. The suicide threat is not imminent in the emergency department and she would not know if she were pregnant for several weeks.
2. **There are three emergency contraception options available: (1) Yuzpe regimen, which is a combination of estrogen and progesterone pills administered within 72 hours and a second dose 12 hours later that will initiate the onset of menstrual bleeding within 21 days; (2) the administration of mifepristone (RU 486) plus misoprostol (Cytotec), which will prevent pregnancy; and (3) the insertion of a copper IUD within 5 days of unprotected intercourse, which can prevent pregnancy (99% effective).**
3. Spermicide after intercourse is not effective to prevent pregnancy.
4. If the client is adamant about not carrying a baby to term, then the nurse should discuss other available options to prevent the pregnancy.

15. 1. **Category A medications have a remote risk of causing fetal harm and are prescribed for clients who are pregnant.**
2. Category B medications are associated with a slightly higher risk than are category A medications and are often prescribed for clients who are pregnant. These medications should not be taken during the first 3 months of pregnancy.
3. Category C medications pose a greater risk than category B medications and are cautiously prescribed for clients who are pregnant. Research on medications in this category has not been done or may show risk in animal studies.
4. Category D medications have a proven risk of fetal harm and are not prescribed for clients who are pregnant unless the mother's life is in danger. Category X medications have a definite risk of fetal abnormality or abortion.

16. 1. This action would break the nurse–client relationship. The nurse should encourage the client to tell his parents.
2. The nurse should not be concerned with where the medications are being obtained. The nurse should strongly discourage use of anabolic steroids because of the long-term effects, including psychological changes.
3. These are side effects of glucocorticosteroids, not of anabolic steroids.
4. **Anabolic steroids have serious side effects including low sperm counts and impotence in men, along with permanent liver damage and aggressive behavior. The use of anabolic steroids to improve athletic performance is illegal and strongly discouraged by HCPs and athletic associations.**

17. 1. Questions about allergies to iodine or shellfish would be appropriate for a client undergoing a test with contrast dye.
2. The nurse should realize that a client taking cyclosporine has had some type of organ transplant because it is a major immune suppressant drug.
3. **Cyclosporine would not be an expected medication for a client diagnosed with pneumonia or chronic kidney disease unless the client has had a kidney transplant; therefore, asking this question is appropriate.**
4. Because the client has functioning kidneys there is no need to take the Amphojel, which is a phosphate binder.

18. 1. The RhoGAM prevents the formation of antibodies to the fetus's Rh-positive blood in the mother, but this cannot be done first because the client is a Jehovah's Witness.
2. The mother must sign a permit when taking this medication, but this is not the nurse's first intervention because the client is a Jehovah's Witness.
3. The nurse can confirm the newborn's blood type, but this is not the first intervention because the client is a Jehovah's Witness.

4. The RhoGAM is derived from blood products; therefore, the nurse must explain this to the client whose faith prohibits the administration of blood or blood products.

19. 1. ACE inhibitors would not be questioned in clients with kidney transplants or taking cyclosporine.
    2. **Bactrim reduces cyclosporine levels, which can lead to organ rejection; therefore, the nurse should question administering this medication.**
    3. Tylenol is not contraindicated in clients with kidney transplants; it is contraindicated in clients with liver disorders.
    4. Compazine is not contraindicated in clients with kidney transplants; it is contraindicated in clients with a liver disorder.

MEDICATION MEMORY JOGGER: The nurse must be knowledgeable of accepted standards of practice for disease processes and conditions. If the nurse administers a medication the health-care provider has prescribed and it harms the client, the nurse could be held accountable. Remember that the nurse is a client advocate.

20. 1. Safety of the client is priority.
    2. This is an appropriate intervention, but it is not priority over safety.
    3. The nurse must document the medication in the MAR and the chart because it is a PRN medication, but it is not the first intervention after administering the medication.
    4. The nurse must evaluate the client's pain to determine the effectiveness of the medication, but this is not the first intervention.

Musculoskeletal System

"Never regard study as a duty, but as the enviable opportunity to learn to know the liberating influence of beauty in the realm of the spirit for your own personal joy and to the profit of the community your later work belongs."

—Albert Einstein

PRACTICE QUESTIONS

A Client with Low Back Pain

1. The client is diagnosed with low back pain and is prescribed the muscle relaxant cyclobenzaprine (Flexeril). Which instructions should the clinic nurse teach the client?
   1. Take the medication just before leaving home for work each day.
   2. Drink a full glass of water with each dose of medication.
   3. The medication can cause drowsiness that may make driving unsafe.
   4. Divide the dose of medication between early morning and bedtime.

2. The charge nurse on an orthopedic unit is transcribing orders for a client diagnosed with back pain. Which HCP order should the charge nurse question?
   1. Physical therapy for hot packs and massage.
   2. CBC and CMP (complete metabolic panel).
   3. Hydrocodone (Vicodin), an opioid analgesic, PRN.
   4. Carisoprodol (Soma), a muscle relaxant, po, b.i.d.

3. The nurse is administering medications to clients on an orthopedic unit. Which medication should the nurse question?
   1. Ibuprofen (Motrin), an NSAID, to a client with back pain and a history of ulcers.
   2. Morphine, an opioid analgesic, to a client with back pain rated as "6."
   3. Methocarbamol (Robaxin), a muscle relaxant, to a client with chronic back pain.
   4. Propoxyphene (Darvon N), a narcotic agonist, to a client with mild back pain.

4. The client diagnosed with low back pain is prescribed morphine sulfate, an opioid analgesic. Which interventions should the nurse implement? Select all that apply.
   1. Discuss with the HCP starting the client on a stool softener.
   2. Teach the client about rating the pain on a numeric pain scale.
   3. Inform the client to rise quickly from a supine position.
   4. Administer anticonvulsant medications around the clock.
   5. Tell the client to call for assistance when getting out of bed.

5. The client diagnosed with low back pain is scheduled to have a steroid injection into the intrathecal space. Which statement by the client indicates that the client understands the procedure?
   1. "I will have to curl up like a Halloween cat."
   2. "This procedure will cure my back pain."
   3. "I will have an injection in each of my hips."
   4. "There is no risk with this procedure."

6. The nurse is completing the preoperative checklist for a client diagnosed with a herniated disc. Which information is priority for the nurse to notify the operating room staff?
   1. The client is complaining of a headache.
   2. The client is allergic to iodine and aspirin.
   3. The client has not had anything to drink.
   4. The client's hematocrit is 43%.

7. The client presents to the outpatient clinic complaining of back pain. Which assessment question should the nurse ask first?
   1. "What activity did you do to hurt your back?"
   2. "Which over-the-counter medications have you taken?"
   3. "Have you used illegal drugs to treat the back pain?"
   4. "Did you miss any work time because of this pain?"

8. The client with chronic low back pain has been taking baclofen (Lioresal), a muscle relaxant. Which instructions should the nurse review with the client?
   1. The medication can cause gastric ulcer formation.
   2. The client may consume no more than one glass of wine per day.
   3. The medication must be tapered off when discontinued.
   4. The client should not take the medication before bedtime.

9. The nurse is administering 0900 medications to clients on a medical unit. Which medication should be administered first?
   1. MS Contin, a narcotic analgesic, to a client with low back pain.
   2. Chlorzoxazone (Parafon Forte), a muscle relaxant, to a client on bed rest.
   3. Acetaminophen (Tylenol), an analgesic, to a client with a headache.
   4. Diazepam (Valium), a benzodiazepine, to a client with muscle spasms.

10. The client is admitted with severe low back pain and prescribed the muscle relaxant methocarbamol (Robaxin), IVPB every 8 hours. Which nursing intervention has priority when administering this medication?
    1. Ask the client to lie flat for 15 minutes following the IV infusion.
    2. Infuse at a rapid rate of 200–250 mL/hour via an infusion pump.
    3. Assess the IV site for extravasation after the infusion is complete.
    4. Monitor liver function laboratory tests daily.

A Client with Osteoarthritis

11. The client with osteoarthritis is prescribed the COX-2 inhibitor celecoxib (Celebrex), a nonsteroidal anti-inflammatory drug (NSAID). Which statement by the client would warrant intervention by the nurse?
    1. "I take aspirin daily to help prevent heart disease."
    2. "I am allergic to penicillin and aminoglycosides."
    3. "I know I am overweight and need to lose 50 pounds."
    4. "I walk 30 minutes at least three times a week."

12. The client with severe osteoarthritis of the left knee is receiving sodium hyaluronate (Hyalgan) injected directly into the left knee. Which information should be discussed with the client?
    1. Explain that this medication will cause some bleeding into the joint.
    2. Instruct the client to avoid any strenuous activity for 48 hours after injection.
    3. Discuss that the medication will be injected daily for 7 days.
    4. Tell the client that strict bed rest is required for 24 hours after the injection.

13. The nurse is preparing to administer the following medications. Which medication would the nurse question administering?
    1. Ibuprofen (Motrin), an NSAID, to a client receiving furosemide (Lasix).
    2. Nabumetone (Relafen), a COX-2 inhibitor, to a client receiving digoxin (Lanoxin).
    3. Acetylsalicylic acid (ASA), a salicylate, to a client receiving warfarin (Coumadin).
    4. Ketorolac (Toradol), an NSAID, intramuscularly to a client on a morphine PCA.

14. The client is taking acetylsalicylic acid (ASA) four to five times a day for severe osteoarthritic pain. Which teaching interventions should the nurse discuss with the client? Select all that apply.
    1. Do not drink any type of alcoholic beverages.
    2. Keep the ASA bottle out of the reach of children.
    3. Inform the dentist of taking high doses of ASA.
    4. Maintain a serum salicylate level between 15 and 30 mg/dL.
    5. Explain that ringing in the ears is a common side effect.

15. At 0900 the charge nurse observes the primary nurse crushing an enteric-coated aspirin in the medication room. Which action should the charge nurse implement?
    1. Take no action because this is an acceptable standard of practice.
    2. Correct the primary nurse's behavior in the medication room.
    3. Explain that enteric-coated medication should not be crushed.
    4. Complete an adverse occurrence report on the primary nurse.

16. The client with osteoarthritis of the hands is prescribed capsaicin (Capsin) cream, a nonopioid topical analgesic. Which intervention should the nurse discuss with the client concerning this medication?
    1. Wash the hands immediately after applying the cream.
    2. Remove cream immediately if burning of the skin occurs.
    3. Apply a heating pad to the affected area after applying the cream.
    4. Do not remove the cream for at least 30 minutes after application.

17. The elderly client in the hospital is complaining of arthritic pain. Which action should the nurse implement?
    1. Administer meloxicam (Mobic), an NSAID COX-2 inhibitor.
    2. Administer acetylsalicylic acid (ASA), a salicylate.
    3. Administer acetaminophen (Tylenol), a nonnarcotic analgesic.
    4. Administer morphine intravenous push, a narcotic analgesic.

18. The female client with osteoarthritis tells the clinic nurse that she started taking the herb ginkgo. Which action should the nurse take?
    1. Determine what medications the client is currently taking.
    2. Praise the client because this herb helps decrease inflammation.
    3. Notify the health-care provider that the client is taking ginkgo.
    4. Examine why the client thought she needed to take herbs.

19. The HCP is administering an intraarticular corticosteroid mixed with lidocaine to a client with severe osteoarthritis in the right knee. Which statement by the client would warrant intervention by the nurse?
    1. "I have taken off work tomorrow so I can rest my knee."
    2. "I am attending physical therapy once a week."
    3. "I alternate heat and ice on my knee when I am having pain."
    4. "I had one of these just last month and it really helped the pain."

20. The client with osteoarthritis who is taking the COX-2 inhibitor celecoxib (Celebrex), a nonsteroidal anti-inflammatory drug (NSAID), calls the clinic and reports having black, tarry stools. Which action should the clinic nurse take?
    1. Ask if the client is taking any type of iron preparation.
    2. Tell the client to not take any more of the Celebrex.
    3. Instruct the client to bring a stool specimen to the clinic.
    4. Explain that this is a side effect of the medication.

A Client with Osteoporosis

21. The postmenopausal client is prescribed alendronate (Fosamax), a bisphosphonate, to help prevent osteoporosis. Which information should the nurse discuss with the client?
    1. Chew the tablet thoroughly before swallowing.
    2. Eat a meal prior to taking the medication.
    3. Take the medication at night before going to sleep.
    4. Remain upright 30 minutes after taking the medication.

22. The client with postmenopausal osteoporosis is prescribed calcitonin (Calcimar) intranasal. Which instructions should the nurse discuss with the client?
    1. Notify the health-care provider if nausea and vomiting occur.
    2. Decrease calcium and vitamin D intake during drug therapy.
    3. Remove the nasal spray from the refrigerator immediately before using.
    4. Expect to experience rhinitis when taking the medication.

23. The client is prescribed raloxifene (Evista), a selective estrogen receptor modulator (SERM). Which information should the nurse discuss with the client?
    1. Instruct the client to walk for 10 minutes every hour when traveling in a car.
    2. Encourage the client to decrease smoking cigarettes and drinking alcohol.
    3. Explain that Evista will decrease the hot flashes experienced with menopause.
    4. Discuss the importance of performing non-weightbearing activities.

24. The long-term care nurse is preparing to administer calcium gluconate (Kalcinate) to a client with osteoporosis. Which data would warrant the nurse questioning administering this medication?
    1. The client asks the nurse for a walker to ambulate.
    2. The client's oral intake is 850 mL and urinary output is 1250 mL.
    3. The client is lethargic, is drowsy, and has increasing weakness.
    4. The client has abnormal bleeding when brushing the teeth.

25. Which statement best describes the scientific rationale for administering calcitonin (Calcimar) to a client diagnosed with osteoporosis?
    1. It blocks estrogen receptors in the uterus and breast.
    2. It inhibits bone reabsorption by suppressing osteoclast activity.
    3. It increases bone density and reduces the risk of vertebral fractures.
    4. It increases the progesterone and estrogen levels in the blood.

26. The nurse is discussing ways to prevent osteoporosis to a group of elderly women. A woman in the audience asks, "Why aren't doctors prescribing hormone replacement therapy?" Which statement by the nurse would be most appropriate?
    1. "There are many other, better ways to treat osteoporosis than HRT."
    2. "HRT treatment is very expensive and many insurances will not pay."
    3. "There is an increased risk of cancer and deep vein thrombosis associated with HRT."
    4. "Research has shown that it is not effective in treating osteoporosis."

27. Which assessment data best indicate to the nurse that the medication therapy for a client with osteoporosis has been effective?
    1. The client's serum calcium level is 7.5 mg/dL.
    2. The client does not experience any pathologic fractures.
    3. The client has adequate urinary output.
    4. The client loses less than 1 inch in height.

28. The client with osteoporosis is prescribed sodium fluoride, a mineral. Which information should the nurse discuss with the client?
    1. Monitor serum fluoride levels daily.
    2. Have bone mineral density studies monthly.
    3. Maintain an adequate calcium intake.
    4. Sprinkle medication on food.

29. Which statement indicates the 30-year-old client does not understand the teaching concerning how to prevent osteoporosis?
    1. "I need to take at least 1500 mg of calcium daily."
    2. "Milk and dairy products are good sources of vitamin D."
    3. "I must get shots weekly to increase my calcium level."
    4. "I should take steps to prevent osteoporosis now."

30. Which statement indicates the postmenopausal client with osteoporosis understands the medication teaching concerning the bisphosphonate alendronate (Fosamax)?
    1. "I do not use sunscreen when working outside in my yard."
    2. "I take the medication with 6–8 ounces of tap water."
    3. "I drink orange juice when I take the medication at breakfast."
    4. "I may experience some heartburn when taking this medication."

A Client Undergoing an Orthopedic Surgery

31. The client who had surgery for a hip fracture is complaining of severe pain 45 minutes after the nurse administered morphine IVP. Which intervention should the nurse implement first?
    1. Administer another dose of morphine.
    2. Turn on the television to distract the client.
    3. Assess the client's affected leg for alignment.
    4. Notify the health-care provider of the problem.

32. The client postoperative from hip surgery is scheduled to ambulate with the physical therapist. Which intervention should the nurse implement to assist the client to be able to perform the therapy?
    1. Assist the client to the bedside chair with the therapist's help.
    2. Administer pain medication 30 minutes before the therapy.
    3. Ask the unlicensed assistive personnel to brush the client's hair.
    4. Allow the client to delay the therapy until late in the day.

33. The 84-year-old female client with a fractured knee is unable to rate her pain on a numeric pain scale. Which intervention should the nurse implement?
    1. Have the client use a pediatric faces scale.
    2. Don't try to get the client to rate the pain.
    3. The nurse should decide the amount of pain.
    4. Check the pulse and blood pressure for elevation.

34. The male client who has had bilateral knee replacement surgery calls the nurse's desk and reports that he noticed bruises on both sides of his abdomen while taking his bath. The client's MAR notes Ancef, an antibiotic; morphine, a narcotic analgesic; and Lovenox, a low molecular weight heparin. Which is the nurse's best response to the client?
    1. "This is a reaction to the antibiotic you are receiving and it will need to be changed."
    2. "This is caused by straining when trying to have a bowel movement."
    3. "This occurs because of the positioning during the surgical procedure."
    4. "This happened because of the medication used to prevent complications."

35. The client who has had a total knee surgery returns to the room with an autotransfusion drainage system (cell saver) device inserted into the wound. Which interventions should the nurse implement? Select all that apply.
    1. Monitor the drainage in the collection chamber every 30–45 minutes.
    2. Take the drainage to the blood bank when it reaches 200 mL.
    3. Attach a filter to the drainage before administering.
    4. Have a second nurse verify the client's ID band.
    5. Monitor vital signs every 5–15 minutes when transfusing the blood.

36. The 78-year-old client who had hip surgery is to receive a unit of packed red blood cells (PRBC). The nurse's assessment reveals bilateral crackles in the lungs and 2+ edema of the sacrum. The PRBCs contain 250 mL of cells and 60 mL of preservative solution. At what rate will the nurse set the IV infusion pump after the initial 15 minutes?

    Answer _____

37. A 10-year-old child sustained a compound fracture of the left forearm and has returned to the unit after an open reduction and internal fixation (ORIF). Which interventions should the nurse implement?
    1. Assess the child's ability to rate the pain on a pain scale.
    2. Ask the parent to determine when the child needs pain medication.
    3. Apply a heat pack to the cast until the cast is completely dry.
    4. Check the child's fingertips for warmth and color every 4 hours.

38. The nurse is administering medications at 2100. Which medication should the nurse question?
    1. An NSAID to a 24-year-old female client recovering from an arthroscopy.
    2. An opioid analgesic to a 50-year-old male client with a fractured femur.
    3. A sedative hypnotic to a 65-year-old female client with a total knee replacement.
    4. A muscarinic antagonist to an 89-year-old male client with a hip fracture.

39. The client is postoperative for a cervical laminectomy and is prescribed meperidine (Demerol), a narcotic analgesic, by patient-controlled analgesia (PCA) pump. Which instruction regarding pain control should the nurse teach the client?
    1. Notify the nurse when needing pain medication.
    2. Press the button on the pump when the client feels pain.
    3. Have the significant other push the button on the pump frequently.
    4. Use the pain medication sparingly to prevent narcotic addiction.

40. The nurse and unlicensed assistive personnel (UAP) are caring for clients on an orthopedic unit. Which action by the UAP requires immediate intervention?
    1. The UAP obtains a fracture pan for a client with a laminectomy to use.
    2. The UAP attempts to ambulate an elderly client immediately after receiving pain medication.
    3. Prior to bedtime, the UAP provides a back rub to a client with low back pain.
    4. The UAP places moisture barrier cream on a client's perineal area.

A Client with Low Back Pain

1. 1. Taking the medication before leaving the house could be a danger to the client and others because this medication can cause drowsiness. The client should not be driving or operating equipment until the client has determined the effect of the medication on his or her body.
   2. There is no need to drink a full glass of water when taking Flexeril.
   3. **The medication acts on the central nervous system and can cause drowsiness. The client should be warned not to drive until the client understands the effects on his or her body. Driving could be dangerous for the client and others.**
   4. This is prescribing. The HCP will prescribe how frequently the dose should be administered.

2. 1. Physical therapy for heat and massage is standard therapy for back pain. There is no reason to question this order.
   2. Many medications can affect the kidneys or the liver and the blood counts. Baseline data should be obtained. There is no reason to question this order.
   3. **This medication order is incomplete. The nurse should contact the HCP for a time limitation.**
   4. Soma comes in one strength so this order is complete. There is no reason to question this order.

   MEDICATION MEMORY JOGGER: All medication orders must be complete, and the nurse is responsible for determining all the parameters before administering a medication.

3. 1. **NSAIDs decrease prostaglandin production in the stomach, increasing the client's risk of developing ulcers. This client has a known risk of peptic ulcer disease. The nurse should question the medication and discuss this with the HCP.**
   2. Opioid analgesics are administered for pain. The client is in the moderate to severe pain range. The nurse would administer this medication.
   3. Muscle relaxant medications are administered to clients with back pain to relax the muscles and decrease the pain. The nurse would administer this medication.
   4. Darvon N is a pain medication. The nurse would administer this medication.

4. 1. Narcotic pain medications slow peristalsis in the small and large intestines, increasing the risk for constipation and fecal impaction. The nurse should discuss a bowel regimen with the HCP.
   2. **The nurse should attempt to have the client quantify the pain so that the effectiveness of interventions can be evaluated. The numeric pain scale is one method of objectifying the pain.**
   3. Rising quickly from a flat-on-the-back (supine) position could increase the client's pain. Some of the medications administered for back pain can cause orthostatic hypotension. The nurse should teach the client to turn on the side and push up on the elbow slowly when getting out of bed.
   4. The client may be taking antispasmodic and pain medications, but there is no reason for anticonvulsant medications.
   5. **This is a safety issue. The client should call for assistance to prevent falls.**

5. 1. **Intrathecal indicates into the central nervous system via a lumbar puncture. The client will be positioned with the back arched, much like a Halloween cat, for the HCP to be able to insert the needle between the vertebrae.**
   2. The procedure provides temporary relief of inflammation of affected nerves.
   3. The injections are into the intravertebral space, not into the hips. An injection in the hips indicates an intramuscular injection.
   4. There is risk with any procedure. In this procedure, nerve damage is the greatest risk.

6. 1. The client's complaint of a headache occurs frequently when clients have not been able to eat or drink, especially caffeine drinks. This is not a priority at this time.
   2. **The standard surgical scrub is a povidone–iodine (Betadine) antiseptic skin preparation. This should be brought to the attention of the surgical nurse who will be preparing the surgical site so that a substitute can be used.**
   3. Clients going to surgery should be NPO for several hours to prevent aspiration during anesthesia.
   4. This is a normal hematocrit.

7. 1. This is important, but it is not priority during the initial assessment. The nurse should determine how the client has been treating the injury. This would be the second query, not the first.

2. The priority at this time is to determine what medications have been tried in order to assess the full extent of the injury. This is the first intervention. Adult clients will frequently only seek the HCP's advice and treatment when over-the-counter remedies have failed.
3. This is an accusatory statement and most likely will make the client mistrust the nurse's objectives. This should not be asked at this time.
4. This is the third query the nurse could ask. Missed work time is important, but to treat the client, the HCP must be aware of the attempted treatments.

8. 1. This medication is not known to increase the risk of ulcers.
   2. The client should be warned not to consume any alcohol while taking baclofen. Baclofen is a central nervous system depressant, as is alcohol. The combination of alcohol and baclofen could intensify the depressant effects.
   3. **Baclofen must be tapered off when being discontinued. Abrupt withdrawal after prolonged use can cause anxiety, agitated behavior, hallucinations, severe tachycardia, acute spasticity, and seizures.**
   4. The medication can cause drowsiness, which might assist the client to rest. Administration at bedtime is preferred if this is so.

MEDICATION MEMORY JOGGER: There is rarely any medication for which the client will be told that concurrent administration with alcohol is appropriate.

9. 1. MS Contin is a sustained-release tablet. This medication is to provide relief of chronic pain over the course of the day. It does not need to be the first medication administered.
   2. The client prescribed bed rest usually takes a muscle relaxant as a routine medication; it does not need to be administered first.
   3. A headache that is to be treated with Tylenol (for mild pain) would not be the first medication for the nurse to administer.
   4. **A client having muscle spasms is a priority for the nurse. Muscle spasms can be extremely painful. This medication should be administered first.**

10. 1. The client should be kept recumbent during and for at least 15 minutes following the administration of Robaxin IV to reduce the risk of orthostatic hypotension.
    2. The medication must be administered slowly at a rate of no greater than 300 mg per minute, not by rapid infusion.
    3. The IV site should be assessed prior to the initiation of the medication to prevent complications from extravasation of the medication into the tissues.
    4. Robaxin is detoxified by the kidneys, not the liver.

A Client with Osteoarthritis

11. 1. **The client should not take aspirin with an NSAID because it can increase the risk of gastrointestinal upset and possible gastrointestinal bleeding.**
    2. Allergies to antibiotics are not a contraindication to the use of NSAIDs.
    3. Obesity is not contraindicated in clients taking NSAIDs.
    4. Exercising is recommended for clients with osteoarthritis unless it causes pain; therefore, this activity would not warrant the client not taking Celebrex.

12. 1. Any bleeding into the joint is a complication. Bleeding into a joint would not be the expected benefit of any type of medication.
    2. **After the injection the client can walk and perform routine daily activities, but running, bicycling, or strenuous activity should be avoided. Hyalgan is a preparation of a chemical normally found in high amounts in the synovial fluid. The injection replaces or supplements the body's natural hyaluronic acid that deteriorates as a result of the inflammation of osteoarthritis.**
    3. The treatment includes three to five injections; the client receives one injection every week.
    4. This injection is done in an HCP's office, and the client will be able to walk out of the clinic after the injection.

MEDICATION MEMORY JOGGER: The nurse should realize that the joint must have time for the medication to be effective and injecting daily would not allow this. The nurse should realize that a medication should not cause an abnor-

mal body function, such as bleeding into the joint.

13. 1. NSAIDs do not interfere with the effectiveness of loop diuretics; therefore, the nurse would not question administering the Motrin.
2. COX-2 inhibitors do not interfere with the effectiveness of cardiac glycosides; therefore, the nurse would not question administering the Relafen.
3. **Aspirin displaces warfarin from protein-binding sites and will increase the client's bleeding; therefore, the nurse should question administering the aspirin.**
4. Toradol is often administered around the clock to a client in pain, along with a narcotic analgesic. Toradol decreases the inflammation to help decrease the pain.

14. 1. Alcohol displaces warfarin from protein-binding sites and will increase the client's bleeding; therefore, the nurse should instruct the client not to drink alcohol.
2. **ASA poisoning can kill children, and all medications, prescription or nonprescription, should be kept out of the reach of children.**
3. **High doses of ASA can cause bleeding; therefore, the dentist should be made aware of the client's medication use.**
4. **Aspirin toxicity can occur when the client is taking ASA four to five times a day; therefore, the serum level should be kept within normal limits (15–30 mg/dL). Mild toxicity occurs with serum levels above 30 mg/dL and severe toxicity occurs above 50 mg/dL.**
5. **Tinnitus (ringing in the ears) is a sign of aspirin toxicity and should be reported to the health-care provider.**

15. 1. Enteric-coated aspirin should not be crushed.
2. The charge nurse should not correct the primary nurse in front of other staff and, at 0900 in the morning, there would be other nurses in the medication room.
3. **The charge nurse should explain to the primary nurse that enteric-coated ASA should not be crushed because the coating that ensures the ASA will dissolve in the small intestine is destroyed. The aspirin will be absorbed in the stomach if the coating is crushed.**

4. Because the client did not receive the crushed enteric-coated ASA, no adverse occurrence report needs to be completed. This form is completed if the client's condition has been compromised in some way.

16. 1. This medication is being administered for the hands; therefore, the client should not wash off the medication immediately after application.
2. The client should know that transient burning occurs with the application.
3. The client should not apply heat because this will increase the burning of the skin secondary to the cream application. Burning is increased by heat, sweating, bathing in warm water, humidity, and clothing.
4. **The topical cream should be kept in place at least 30 minutes after application because it is being administered for osteoarthritis of the hands. If not being applied for hands, the cream should be washed off immediately.**

17. 1. These medications are administered around the clock and are not specifically for acute pain.
2. Aspirin has side effects, such as gastrointestinal discomfort, and is not the drug of choice for elderly clients.
3. **Acetaminophen is generally preferred for use in older clients because it has fewer toxic side effects.**
4. Morphine is a narcotic, is not used to treat chronic arthritis pain, and should be used cautiously in elderly clients.

18. 1. **The first intervention the nurse should implement is to determine if the client is taking any medication that will interact with the herb. Ginkgo, along with dong quai, feverfew, and garlic, when taken with NSAIDs may cause bleeding.**
2. Gingko is used to treat allergic rhinitis, Alzheimer's disease, anxiety or stress, dementia, tinnitus, vertigo, and poor circulation. It is not known to decrease inflammation.
3. The nurse should determine what medications the client is currently taking and if gingko interacts with them prior to notifying the HCP.
4. The nurse does not need to know why the client thought he or she needed to take the herb; this is an accusatory intervention.

The nurse should support alternative-type medicine if it does not interfere with other medications the client is currently taking.

MEDICATION MEMORY JOGGER: Some herbal preparations are effective, some are not, and a few can be harmful or even deadly. If a client is taking an herbal supplement and a conventional medicine, the nurse should investigate to determine if the combination will cause harm to the client. The nurse should always be the client's advocate.

19. 1. Resting the knee after the injection is an appropriate action for the client to take. It would not warrant intervention by the nurse.
    2. Physical therapy for range-of-motion exercises is an acceptable conservative treatment for osteoarthritis. The client should inform the physical therapist of the treatment, but this statement does not warrant immediate intervention by the nurse.
    3. Alternating ice and heat is an acceptable conservative treatment for easing the pain secondary to osteoarthritis. This statement would not warrant intervention by the nurse.
    4. **This procedure does provide marked pain relief, but it should not be done more than every 4–6 months because it can hasten the rate of cartilage breakdown. This statement should be reported to the HCP. Clients often go to more than one HCP.**

20. 1. Iron preparations can cause black, tarry stool, but because the client is taking an NSAID the nurse should realize tarry stools are a sign of gastrointestinal distress, which is a complication of NSAID medications.
    2. **NSAIDs are notorious for causing gastrointestinal upset and peptic ulcer disease. Black, tarry stool indicates GI bleeding; therefore, the client should stop taking the medication.**
    3. A specimen is not sent to the laboratory when the stool is black and tarry. The nurse should know these are signs of GI bleeding.
    4. This is not an expected side effect of the medication, and the NSAID should be discontinued immediately.

MEDICATION MEMORY JOGGER: If the client verbalizes a complaint, if the nurse

assesses data, or if laboratory data indicates an adverse effect secondary to a medication, the nurse must intervene. The nurse must implement an independent intervention or notify the health-care provider because medications can result in serious or even life-threatening complications.

A Client with Osteoporosis

21. 1. The client should swallow the medication. The client should not crush, chew, or suck on the medication.
    2. The medication should be taken on an empty stomach at least 30 minutes before eating or drinking any liquid. Foods and beverages greatly decrease the effect of Fosamax.
    3. The medication will irritate the stomach and esophagus if the client lies down; therefore, the medication should be taken when the client can remain upright for at least 30 minutes.
    4. **This client must remain upright to facilitate the passage of the medication to the stomach and minimize the risk of esophageal irritation.**

22. 1. Nausea and vomiting occur during the initial therapy and will disappear as the treatment continues; therefore, the client does not need to notify the HCP.
    2. The client should consume an adequate amount of calcium and vitamin D while taking this medication.
    3. The nasal spray should be room temperature before using. The nasal spray is not kept in the refrigerator.
    4. **Rhinitis, a runny nose, is the most common side effect with calcitonin nasal spray, but the client should not quit taking the medication if this occurs.**

23. 1. **Evista increases the risk of venous thrombosis; therefore, the client should avoid prolonged immobilization including driving long distances in a car.**
    2. The client should not just decrease smoking and alcohol. The client needs to stop both of these activities because they interact with the medication.
    3. Evista will not reduce hot flashes or flushes associated with estrogen deficiency and may cause hot flashes.

4. The nurse should emphasize the importance of regular weightbearing exercise to help increase bone density.

24. 1. Safety is priority for clients diagnosed with osteoporosis; therefore, the client requesting a walker would not warrant the nurse questioning administering this medication.
    2. This indicates the client's kidneys are functioning adequately. The nurse would question administering the calcium if the client had signs of renal deficiency.
    3. **The nurse must monitor for signs of hypercalcemia, which include drowsiness, lethargy, weakness, headache, anorexia, nausea or vomiting, increased urination, and thirst.**
    4. Abnormal bleeding is a cause for the nurse to investigate, but it would not warrant questioning this medication because this is not an expected side effect or adverse effect of this medication.

MEDICATION MEMORY JOGGER: The nurse must be knowledgeable of accepted standards of practice for medication administration, including which client assessment data and laboratory data should be monitored prior to administering the medication.

25. 1. Blocking estrogen receptors is the scientific rationale for administering selective estrogen receptor modulators (SERMS) to clients with osteoporosis.
    2. Inhibiting bone reabsorption by suppressing osteoclast activity is the scientific rationale for administering bisphosphonates to clients with osteoporosis.
    3. **Calcimar is a natural product obtained from salmon and is approved for treatment of osteoporosis in women who are more than 5 years postmenopause. It increases bone density and reduces the risk of vertebral fractures.**
    4. The scientific rationale for administering hormone replacement therapy is to increase progesterone and estrogen levels.

26. 1. There are medications to treat and prevent osteoporosis that are safer than HRT and do not result in the serious complications that occur with HRT. HRT is better than some medications in treating osteoporosis, but because of possible complications HRT is not recommended for this purpose.
    2. Expense should not be an issue when treating chronic illnesses.

3. Until recently, HRT with estrogen was one of the most common treatments for osteoporosis in postmenopausal women, but research has shown that serious complications can occur from HRT use; therefore, it is no longer recommended.
4. HRT was one of the most common treatments for osteoporosis, but as a result of complications associated with its use, it is no longer recommended.

27. 1. The normal serum calcium level is 8.5–11.5 mg/dL; a low calcium level indicates the medication therapy is not effective.
    2. **As a result of decreased bone density, a client with osteoporosis is at risk for pathological fractures. If the client does not experience these types of fractures, it indicates that the medication therapy is effective.**
    3. The client must have normal renal function to take these medications, but this does not indicate the medication is effective.
    4. Any loss of height indicates the medication is not effective. The loss of height occurs as a result of collapse of the vertebral bodies.

MEDICATION MEMORY JOGGER: The nurse determines the effectiveness of a medication by assessing for the symptoms, or lack thereof, for which the medication was prescribed.

28. 1. Serum fluoride levels are monitored every 3 months, not daily.
    2. Bone mineral density studies are usually conducted every 6 months to document progress in bone growth.
    3. **When taking fluoride, a relatively new but promising treatment for osteoporosis, the client should maintain an adequate calcium intake. Because the main risk factor for developing osteoporosis is low calcium level, the client should keep taking calcium no matter what medication is prescribed to help prevent or treat osteoporosis.**
    4. The sodium fluoride tablets should be taken after meals and the client should avoid milk or dairy products because they cause a reduction in gastrointestinal absorption of the sodium fluoride.

MEDICATION MEMORY JOGGER: Few (electrolyte, hormone) levels are monitored daily, one being glucose levels.

29. 1. A woman who does not take estrogen needs about 1500 mg of calcium daily to minimize the risk of developing osteoporosis. The client understands the teaching.
   2. The best dietary sources of vitamin D are milk and other dairy products, including yogurt, which indicates the client understands the teaching.
   3. **Calcium is not available in injections; therefore, the client does not understand the teaching. Dietary treatment, sunshine, or calcium supplements are recommended to maintain adequate serum calcium levels.**
   4. Osteoporosis is usually diagnosed in older clients, but the prevention starts when the client is young. Steps must be taken to maintain bone density and prevent bone demineralization. The client understands this.

30. 1. The client should use sunscreen and protective clothing to prevent a photosensitivity reaction that is caused by this medication.
   2. **The medication must be taken with a full glass of water to ensure proper swallowing of the medication and reduce the risk of mouth or throat irritation.**
   3. The client should not take the medication with orange juice, mineral water, coffee, or other beverages (other than water) because it will greatly decrease the absorption of the medication.
   4. Taking the medication incorrectly may result in mouth or throat irritation or esophageal irritation. Therefore, if the client experiences pain or difficulty swallowing, retrosternal pain, or heartburn, the client should notify the HCP.

A Client Undergoing an Orthopedic Surgery

31. 1. The nurse will be given time limit parameters for the administration of PRN medication, usually a longer time interval than 45 minutes. Because the client has received no relief of pain the nurse needs to determine the reason for the continued pain.
   2. Distraction may be needed if the nurse determines that a complication is not occurring.

3. **The client is not receiving pain relief from the morphine. The client should have better relief than "severe" 45 minutes after an IVP. One cause of unrelieved pain would be dislocation of the affected joint. The nurse should assess the situation to determine further action.**
   4. The nurse should assess the client before notifying the HCP.

32. 1. The client should be allowed to rest until the therapist is ready to have the client ambulate. Ambulating is not sitting in a bedside chair.
   2. **The client will be more able to work with the therapist if not experiencing pain. The nurse should anticipate the need for pain control and administer the medication before the therapist arrives to start the therapy.**
   3. Brushing the client's hair will not assist the therapist in gaining the cooperation of the client with therapy.
   4. The client should be encouraged to work with the therapist when the therapy is scheduled. The client may be too tired to perform therapy if waiting until late in the day.

33. 1. **The nurse should attempt to use another method of rating pain because the client is cognitively unable to use the numeric scale. Young children are able to point at a face and tell the nurse how they feel. This scale should be presented to the client for use.**
   2. Pain is a subjective symptom; the nurse should attempt to get the client to describe her pain.
   3. Pain is a subjective symptom; the nurse should attempt to get the client to describe her pain. The nurse is not experiencing the pain.
   4. Acute pain does cause an elevated pulse and blood pressure, but many other reasons could cause these same elevations. The nurse should attempt to have the client rate her own pain.

34. 1. Antibiotics might cause a rash on the trunk of the body but not this phenomenon.
   2. Straining to have a bowel movement would not cause external bruising on the abdomen.
   3. The client is not positioned on the abdomen for a knee replacement, and

great care is taken in the operating room to prevent any injury to the client. The nurse should never suggest that the client was not positioned correctly.

4. **Lovenox is a low molecular weight heparin and is administered in the "love handles" or upper anterior lateral abdominal walls. Small "bruises" or hematomas in this area suggest a non–life-threatening side effect of this medication's administration.**

35. 1. **An autotransfusion drainage system is used to collect the client's own blood after a particularly bloody surgery. The surgeon is unable to cauterize or suture bones to prevent bleeding. The collections should be monitored frequently and the blood should be reinfused when the amount of drainage is approximately 200 mL. Any blood in the system longer than 4 hours is discarded.**
2. The drainage is not stored for future use. If not used in the immediate postoperative period, it is discarded.
3. There could be fat globules, tiny bone fragments, and clots in the drainage; a filter must be attached before infusing the product back into the client.
4. A second nurse is not required to attach the drainage from the client back to the client.
5. The client should be monitored every 5–15 minutes during the initial reinfusion as per all blood protocols.

36. **78 mL per hour.** A total of 310 mL of blood product is to be infused (250 mL + 60 mL) over a 4-hour period. 310 mL ÷ 4 = 77.5 mL, or 78 mL/hour. Blood cannot hang any longer than 4 hours to prevent an infection and contaminated blood. The client has symptoms of congestive heart failure (bilateral cackles and edema of the sacrum), and the nurse should plan to administer the blood over the entire 4-hour time period to prevent any further fluid volume overload.

37. 1. **Children should be included in their care at the level that they can understand and participate. A 10 year old should be able to describe his or her own pain and rate it on a pain scale. The nurse should determine the child's ability and work from there.**

2. The parents may not want the child to receive pain medication because of a fear of narcotics, or they may want the child medicated when the child is not in pain. Pain is a subjective symptom and the child should request his or her own medication.
3. A heat pack would not be applied to the cast. An ice pack is sometimes ordered to reduce swelling and pain.
4. The child's neurovascular status should be monitored every 15 minutes when first returning to the floor and then every 2 hours.

38. 1. NSAID medications should provide pain relief for the pain resulting from an arthroscopy.
2. Opioid analgesics are frequently used to provide pain relief for all types of surgeries.
3. A sedative hypnotic (sleeping pill) would not be questioned for a client with a total knee replacement.
4. **An 89-year-old male client who is not able to stand to void could develop bladder retention when taking muscarinic antagonists. Muscarinic antagonists relax the bladder muscles by blocking involuntary bladder contractions and are used to treat urge incontinence.**

MEDICATION MEMORY JOGGER: The nurse must be knowledgeable of accepted standards of practice for disease processes and conditions. If the nurse administers a medication the health-care provider has prescribed and it harms the client, the nurse could be held accountable. Remember that the nurse is a client advocate.

39. 1. The PCA pump was developed for clients to be able to control their own pain. The nurse should assess the amount of relief the client is obtaining and any complications, but it is not necessary for the client to notify the nurse when needing pain medication.
2. The client can push the button on the PCA pump whenever the client feels pain. There is a 4-hour lock out programmed into the machine to prevent overdose.
3. No one but the client should push the button for the client to receive medication. The antidote for pain is narcotic medication. If the client is resting and

does not have pain, continuous administration of medication could result in an overdose.

4. The client should not be concerned with narcotic addiction. The medication should be discontinued prior to this becoming a problem.

40. 1. A fracture pan is preferred for clients who have back pain or surgeries because the pan has a smaller rim and will displace the back less. The nurse would not need to intervene.

2. **The UAP should be instructed not to get the client out of bed immediately after taking pain medication. The client may be drowsy and could fall.**

3. A back rub prior to bedtime would assist the client to rest. The nurse would not need to intervene.

4. UAPs are allowed to apply barrier protectant creams as part of their duties when changing a client who has soiled himself or herself. The nurse would not need to intervene.

1. The client is 4 hours postamputation. The nurse notes a large amount of bright red blood on the dressing and notifies the surgeon. The client's prothrombin time (PT) result is 22.5. Which action would the nurse implement based on the PT results?
   1. Prepare to administer warfarin (Coumadin).
   2. Prepare to administer vitamin K (AquaMEPHYTON).
   3. Apply direct pressure to the residual limb.
   4. Prepare to administer protamine sulfate.

2. The day surgery nurse is caring for a client scheduled for an arthrocentesis. Which information would warrant notifying the surgeon?
   1. The client reports an allergy to prednisone, a glucocorticoid.
   2. The client is allergic to ibuprofen, an NSAID.
   3. The client has a history of peptic ulcer disease (PUD).
   4. The client informs the nurse of getting a rash with soaps.

3. The client is 2 days postoperative right total hip replacement and is receiving the low molecular weight heparin (Lovenox) subcutaneously. Which laboratory data should the nurse monitor?
   1. The prothrombin time (PT).
   2. The International Normalized Ratio (INR).
   3. There is no laboratory data to monitor.
   4. The partial thromboplastin time (PTT).

4. Which medication would the nurse prepare to administer to a client with a right long leg cast who is complaining of severe itching under the cast?
   1. The topical anti-itch medication Caladryl.
   2. The antiallergy medication pseudoephedrine (Sudafed).
   3. The intravenous antihistamine diphenhydramine (Benadryl).
   4. The oral antihistamine hydroxyzine (Vistaril).

5. The client with a fractured femur has an external fixation device. The nurse assesses reddened, inflamed skin around the insertion site. Which action should the nurse implement?
   1. Cleanse the insertion site with alcohol swabs.
   2. Put a sterile, nonadhesive dressing on the site.
   3. Readjust the clamps on the external fixator frame.
   4. Apply topical Neosporin antibiotic ointment.

6. The female client comes to the clinic with an injured right ankle and has an abnormally large amount of ecchymotic tissue. Which question would be most appropriate for the nurse to ask the client concerning the ecchymotic tissue?
   1. "Is there any chance you could be pregnant?"
   2. "Are you currently taking aspirin routinely?"
   3. "How long did you apply ice to the ankle?"
   4. "Do you take any antihypertensive medications?"

7. The client in pelvic traction on strict bed rest has a red, edematous, tender left calf. Which medication would the nurse prepare to administer?
   1. The intravenous anticoagulant heparin.
   2. The oral anticoagulant warfarin (Coumadin).
   3. The subcutaneous antiplatelet clopidogrel (Plavix).
   4. The oral antiplatelet acetylsalicylic acid (aspirin).

8. The elderly client with a fractured hip in Buck's traction has a stage I pressure ulcer on the lateral ankle over the bony prominence. Which action should the nurse implement?
   1. Massage the reddened area gently.
   2. Rub moisture barrier cream into the area.
   3. Apply a Duoderm dressing to the area.
   4. Put a hydrophilic foam dressing on the area.

9. The client diagnosed with osteomyelitis of the right trochanter is receiving the aminoglycoside antibiotic vancomycin intravenously. The HCP has ordered a peak and trough on the third dose. Which interventions should the nurse implement when administering the third dose? Rank in order of performance.
   1. Administer the medication via an IV pump.
   2. Check the client's identification band.
   3. Have the laboratory draw the trough level.
   4. Request the laboratory to draw the peak level.
   5. Determine the client's trough level.

10. The client with low back pain syndrome is prescribed chlorzoxazone (Parafon Forte), a skeletal muscle relaxant. Which statement by the client would warrant intervention by the nurse?
    1. "I have had this flu since I started taking the medication."
    2. "I am always drowsy after taking this medication."
    3. "I do not drive my car when I take my back pain medicine."
    4. "If I miss a dose, I wait until the next dose time to take a pill."

11. Which risk factor would the nurse assess for the client diagnosed with osteomalacia?
    1. A vitamin C deficiency.
    2. A vitamin D deficiency.
    3. An increase in uric acid production.
    4. An increase in calcium intake.

12. The male client tells the clinic nurse that he takes glucosamine and chondroitin for joint aches. Which statement best describes the scientific rationale for the efficacy of these over-the-counter medications?
    1. This medication will help reduce the inflammation in the joints to decrease pain.
    2. They will help prevent joint deformity and improve mobility for the client.
    3. This medication will increase the production of synovial fluid in the joint.
    4. They improve tissue function and retard the breakdown of cartilage in the joint.

13. The elderly female client diagnosed with osteoporosis is prescribed risedronate (Actonel), a bone resorption inhibitor. Which statement best describes the therapeutic goal of this therapy?
    1. This medication helps the client regain lost height.
    2. It strengthens the bone and prevents fractures.
    3. It increases the absorption of calcium by the body.
    4. This medication improves the movement of the joint.

14. Which test would be most useful to determine the efficacy of the pharmacological therapy for the client diagnosed with osteoporosis?
    1. A dual energy x-ray absorptiometry (DEXA).
    2. A serum calcium level.
    3. An arthrography.
    4. A bone scan.

15. The client with osteoarthritis asks the nurse, "I saw on the television that a medication called Celebrex was good for osteoarthritis. What do you think about it?" Which statement is the nurse's best response?
    1. "This medication is very good at reducing the pain and stiffness of osteoarthritis."
    2. "This medication does not have the gastrointestinal side effects of other NSAIDs."
    3. "There are some concerns about that medication. You should talk to your doctor."
    4. "You should be cautious about information that you see on the television."

16. The client taking the combination medication hydrocodone and acetaminophen (Vicodin), a narcotic analgesic, calls the clinic and tells the nurse, "I have not had a bowel movement in more than 3 days." Which statement is the nurse's best response?
    1. "This medication causes constipation. You need to increase your fluid intake."
    2. "Have you been taking the stool softeners that I told you to take along with Vicodin?"
    3. "You should go to the emergency department so that you can see a doctor."
    4. "You should take a laxative, and if you do not have a BM within 24 hours, call me."

17. The nurse is preparing to administer medications to clients on an orthopedic floor. Which medication would the nurse question administering?
    1. An NSAID to the client diagnosed with tendonitis that has a history of duodenal ulcer.
    2. A PRN narcotic to a client with an open reduction and internal fixation of the left tibia.
    3. A COX 2-inhibitor to a client who is diagnosed with osteoarthritis and has joint stiffness.
    4. A cephalosporin antibiotic to a client with osteomyelitis and an allergy to sulfa drugs.

18. The client has a callus on the bony protuberance of the left fifth metatarsal. The client asks the clinic nurse, "My grandmother told me to dissolve an aspirin to put on my corn. Is that all right to use?" Which statement would be the nurse's best response?
    1. "I would recommend using a pumice stone to rub it off, but not the aspirin."
    2. "Yes, but make sure you do not get the dissolved aspirin on the surrounding skin."
    3. "There are OTC preparations using salicylic acid that will help remove the corn."
    4. "This is an old wives' tale and you should not pay attention to these remedies."

19. The client 4 hours postoperative bunionectomy (removal of hallux valgus) is prescribed hydromorphone (Dilaudid), a narcotic analgesic. The client is complaining of pain "9" on the 1–10 pain scale. Which action should the nurse implement?
    1. Request the HCP to prescribe a less potent analgesic.
    2. Administer the pain medication as prescribed.
    3. Encourage the client to use distraction techniques.
    4. Give the client an NSAID with one full glass of water.

20. The client with a Morton's neuroma in the right foot is being injected with bupivacaine (Marcaine), a local anesthetic, along with hydrocortisone, a steroid. Which discharge instruction should the nurse discuss with the client?
    1. Instruct the client to put inner soles in the shoe.
    2. Tell the client to soak the foot in warm water.
    3. Teach the client to exercise the foot daily.
    4. Apply ice and elevate the foot for 24 hours.

1. 1. Warfarin is an anticoagulant that would cause increased bleeding; therefore, the nurse would not prepare to administer this medication.
   2. **Vitamin K increases clotting; therefore, the surgeon would order this medication to decrease the prolonged PT. (A normal PT is 12.9 seconds.)**
   3. Applying direct pressure will help decrease bleeding but will not correct a prolonged PT.
   4. Protamine sulfate is the antidote for heparin and the postoperative client would not be taking heparin, an anticoagulant.

2. 1. **An arthrocentesis is an aspiration of synovial fluid and an injection of pain medication and anti-inflammatory medication, which would be a steroid; if the client were allergic to the steroid prednisone, the nurse should notify the surgeon.**
   2. The client would not be receiving any type of NSAID during this procedure; therefore, this information would not warrant notifying the surgeon.
   3. A history of PUD would be pertinent if the client was receiving oral steroids, not intra-articular steroids. Therefore, this information would not warrant notifying the surgeon.
   4. This information would not be pertinent to this procedure; therefore, this information would not warrant notifying the surgeon.

MEDICATION MEMORY JOGGER: If the client verbalizes a complaint, if the nurse assesses data, or if laboratory data indicates an adverse effect secondary to a medication, the nurse must intervene. The nurse must implement an independent intervention or notify the health-care provider because medications can result in serious or even life-threatening complications.

3. 1. The PT is monitored when the client is receiving oral anticoagulant therapy.
   2. The INR is monitored when the client is receiving oral anticoagulant therapy.
   3. **This anticoagulant is administered prophylactically to prevent deep vein thrombosis, but it will not achieve a therapeutic value because of its short half-life; therefore, no bleeding studies are monitored.**
   4. The PTT is monitored when the client is receiving continuous intravenous anticoagulant therapy.

MEDICATION MEMORY JOGGER: The nurse must be knowledgeable about diagnostic tests and surgical procedures.

4. 1. Nothing should be put down the cast; therefore, a topical medication would not be appropriate for this client.
   2. This medication is prescribed for allergy or colds and would not be appropriate for this client.
   3. The intravenous route for administering an antihistamine is appropriate to prevent or reduce the severity of an anaphylactic reaction. It is not used to treat itching.
   4. **Vistaril is effective in reducing itching; therefore, this would be an expected order.**

5. 1. Alcohol swabs may cause burning and they have a drying effect on the skin; therefore, they are not used to cleanse the area. A sterile normal saline swab should be used to cleanse the area.
   2. The insertion sites are left open to air because of the external fixator frame. A reddened, inflamed area must be treated, not covered up.
   3. The nurse never adjusts the clamps; only the HCP adjusts the clamps.
   4. **A topical antibiotic ointment is used to help prevent infection at the insertion sites.**

6. 1. This would be an appropriate question prior to x-raying the ankle to determine if there is a fracture, but it has nothing to do with the ecchymotic area.
   2. **Ecchymosis (bruising) is secondary to bleeding in the tissue, an abnormal amount of bruising may indicate a bleeding problem, and taking aspirin daily would increase the bleeding.**
   3. Applying ice would not increase bruising to the right ankle.
   4. Antihypertensive medication would not affect the ecchymotic area.

7. 1. **The drug of choice for acute deep vein thrombosis is intravenous heparin, an anticoagulant. These signs and symptoms should indicate DVT to the nurse.**
   2. Oral anticoagulants are prescribed for a resolving DVT to a client prior to discharge from the hospital.
   3. Antiplatelets are for arterial blood disorders, and they are not administered subcutaneously.
   4. Aspirin is prescribed as an antiplatelet for arterial disorders, not venous disorders.

MEDICATION MEMORY JOGGER:
Remember that antiplatelet medications are prescribed for arterial blood disorders, such as arteriosclerosis, whereas anticoagulant medications are prescribed for venous blood disorders, such as DVTs.

8. 1. A stage I pressure ulcer should not be massaged because it may cause further tissue breakdown and damage.
   2. The moisture barrier cream would prevent the protective dressing from adhering, and rubbing the area may cause further tissue breakdown and damage.
   3. **A Duoderm dressing provides a barrier and cushion for the reddened area and is used to prevent further breakdown of the reddened area.**
   4. This dressing is used to absorb moisture and exudate from an open wound. A stage I is a reddened area that does not resolve after 30 minutes without pressure; it is not an open wound.

9.   **3, 5, 2, 1, 4**
   3. **The nurse should first have the trough level drawn to determine how much medication is remaining in the blood after the drug has been metabolized and excreted.**
   5. **If the facility has the capability, the nurse should obtain the trough results prior to administering the medication. This medication is nephrotoxic and ototoxic. If the trough level is above therapeutic range, the nurse should hold the medication.**
   2. **Prior to administering any medication, the nurse must determine if it is the right client.**
   1. **After the trough level is drawn and evaluated and the ID band is checked, then the nurse can administer the medication to the client.**
   4. **After the medication has infused over 1 hour, the peak level is drawn 30 minutes to an hour later, depending on hospital policy.**

10. 1. **This medication causes agranulocytosis; the flulike symptoms are indicative of this reaction and warrant intervention by the nurse.**
   2. Drowsiness is an expected side effect of the medication and would not warrant intervention by the nurse. The nurse should discuss the expected drowsiness with the client.

3. The client's not driving the car is an expected comment because this medication causes drowsiness. The comment would not require intervention.
4. Missed doses should be taken within 1 hour of the normal dosing schedule time or the dose should be omitted until the next normal dosing schedule time. Do not double dose. This comment would not warrant intervention.

11. 1. A vitamin C deficiency would result in an increased susceptibility to infection, but not osteomalacia.
   2. **Osteomalacia, adult rickets, is a metabolic bone disorder characterized by inadequate or delayed mineralization of bone. The major risk factors are a diet low in vitamin D, decreased endogenous production of vitamin D because of inadequate sun exposure, impaired intestinal absorption of fats (vitamin D is fat soluble), and disorders that interfere with the metabolism of vitamin D to its active form.**
   3. An increase in uric acid production causes gout.
   4. An increase in calcium intake decreases the risk for osteomalacia, or adult rickets.

12. 1. NSAIDs are used to help decrease the inflammation in the joints.
   2. These medications do not treat rheumatoid arthritis (joint deformities), which this client does not have.
   3. These medications do not affect the production of synovial fluid.
   4. **These OTC medications are recommended to clients with osteoarthritis to help build up and reduce the destruction of cartilage in the joints.**

13. 1. The height lost in a client with osteoporosis is the result of fractures of the vertebrae and is permanent.
   2. **This medication inhibits bone resorption and reduces bone turnover; it normalizes serum alkaline phosphatase and reverses the progression of osteoporosis.**
   3. This medication works by reducing bone loss, not by increasing calcium reabsorption.
   4. This medication improves the bone structure, not the joint flexibility.

14. 1. **A DEXA is a painless test that determines the bone density at the waist, hip, or spine to estimate the extent of**

osteoporosis or to monitor the client's response to treatment.

2. This test determines how much calcium there is in the blood, not the strength of the bone.

3. This test is used to visualize the joint cavity and identify acute or chronic tears in a joint capsule.

4. A bone scan is performed to detect metastatic or primary bone tumors, osteo-myelitis, and aseptic necrosis.

15. 1. This is a true statement, but the nurse should refer the client to the HCP because of the potential adverse effects of the medication.

2. COX-2 inhibitors do not inhibit the isoform of COX that protects the stom-ach; therefore, there is a lower incidence of gastroduodenal ulcers, but there are potential life-threatening adverse effects associated with COX-2 inhibitors. Therefore, this is not the nurse's best response.

3. **Celecoxib (Celebrex), a COX-2 inhibitor, is used to treat osteoarthritis, but more data is needed to determine how safe the medication is for certain clients. Research shows an increase in heart attacks and strokes, and the drug is contraindicated in clients with liver and renal disease. The nurse should refer the client to the HCP.**

4. The client should be cautious about what is advertised on the television about medication and ask the nurse or HCP for further clarification prior to taking the medication.

16. 1. The client should increase the fluid intake because Vicodin slows peristalsis and creates a risk for constipation, but the client is already constipated so this is not the nurse's best response.

2. The client should be taking stool softeners because Vicodin slows peristalsis and creates a risk for constipation, but the client is already constipated so this is not the nurse's best response.

3. The client does not need to go to the emergency department yet; the client needs a stimulant laxative to attempt to evacuate the bowel.

4. **The nurse can recommend an over-the-counter stimulant laxative to help evacuate the bowel because the nurse is aware that constipation is a side**

effect of Vicodin. Giving the client a 24-hour deadline for having a bowel movement is a safeguard.

17. 1. **An NSAID decreases prostaglandin production, a protective mechanism to prevent ulcers. The nurse should question administering this medication to a client with a history of ulcers.**

2. A client with an ORIF of the left tibia would be expected to have pain and the nurse would not question administering a PRN pain medication.

3. A COX-2 inhibitor is prescribed for a client with osteoarthritis and joint stiff-ness; therefore, the nurse would not question administering this medication.

4. Cephalosporins are second- or third-generation penicillins, but they do not have cross-sensitivity to sulfa drugs. The nurse would not question administering this medication.

18. 1. The client cannot use the pumice stone until the callus or corn is softened; there-fore, this is not the best answer.

2. Dissolved aspirin may help erode the corn over time, but it will also erode good skin. This is not the best answer because it would be very difficult to keep the aspirin on the corn only.

3. **Medicated disks impregnated with sali-cylic acid are available OTC to help dissolve calluses and corns. The sali-cylic acid softens the callus, which can then be removed with a pumice stone.**

4. Folk remedies often are based on fact and should not be immediately discounted.

19. 1. The surgery causes extreme pain, and potent narcotics are frequently prescribed for this client.

2. **A hallux valgus is a deformity in which the great toe deviates laterally. The surgery to correct this deformity may cause an intense throbbing pain at the operative site that requires liberal amounts of potent analgesics.**

3. This surgery causes intense throbbing pain, and distraction techniques could be used in conjunction with narcotics, but they could not be used alone.

4. An NSAID medication is not the drug of choice for a client with intense throbbing pain secondary to a surgical procedure.

20. 1. This is considered conservative treatment designed to balance the metatarsal pads,

spread the metatarsal heads, and balance foot posture for Morton's neuroma. This does not address the injection procedure.

2. Warm water would not do anything for the injection procedure; therefore, the nurse should not recommend this action.

3. The Morton's neuroma results in ischemia of the nerve, and exercise will not help the pathological changes nor the injection procedure.

4. **Morton's neuroma is a plantar digital neuroma of the third branch of the median plantar nerve on the foot resulting in a burning pain of the foot. The injection relieves the burning and pain, but it does cause edema and pain at the injection site. Elevating the foot and applying ice will address the acute discomfort associated with the injection.**

Integumentary System

"I was gratified to be able to answer promptly. I said, 'I don't know.'"

—Mark Twain

A Client with Burns

1. The client with a partial-thickness burn to the right arm is prescribed mafenide acetate (Sulfamylon), a topical antimicrobial. Which intervention should the emergency department nurse implement when applying this medication?
   1. Do not administer if the serum sodium level is decreased.
   2. Assess the client's urine for any increased concentration.
   3. Determine the amount of burned skin using the Rules of Nine.
   4. Premedicate the client prior to administering the medication.

2. The nurse is discussing the application of silver nitrate, an antimicrobial agent, to a client with a partial-thickness burn to the left leg. Which information should the nurse teach the client when discussing how to apply this medication after discharge?
   1. Administer the silver nitrate ointment directly to the burned area twice a day.
   2. Notify the HCP if a black discoloration occurs on the burned area.
   3. Apply the silver nitrate solution to the wound dressing every 2 hours.
   4. Do not allow anyone except the HCP to change the wound dressing.

3. The client with a full-thickness burn over 38% of the body is admitted to the burn unit 4 hours after the fire. The HCP writes an order for Ringer's lactate 450 mL/hour. Which action should the nurse implement?
   1. Question the health-care provider's orders.
   2. Administer the intravenous fluid on a pump.
   3. Do not administer more than 200 mL an hour.
   4. Verify the order with another nurse in the burn unit.

4. The client experienced an electrical burn that resulted in full-thickness burns to the right and left hand. The HCP ordered the fluid resuscitation rates. Which data indicates the fluid resuscitation is effective?
   1. The client's urine output is less than 30 mL/hour.
   2. The client's urine output is at least 50 mL/hour.
   3. The client's urine output is 75 to 100 mL/hour.
   4. The client's urine output is greater than 200 mL/hour.

5. The client is admitted to the emergency department with a partial- and full-thickness burn to the left leg. Which question is most important for the nurse to ask the client?
   1. "When was your last tetanus shot?"
   2. "Can you tell me how this burn happened?"
   3. "Will you need any help when you go home?"
   4. "Have you taken any antibiotics in the last week?"

6. The client with a partial-thickness burn to the entire right leg who is being treated with silver sulfadiazine (Silvadene), a sulfonamide antibacterial agent, develops leukopenia. Which action would the nurse suspect that the HCP would prescribe?
   1. Discontinue the Silvadene ointment immediately.
   2. Continue administering the Silvadene ointment.
   3. Administer aminoglycoside antibiotics intravenously.
   4. Administer a hydrocortisone cream to the burned area.

7. For which client would the nurse use caution when applying mafenide acetate (Sulfamylon), a topical antimicrobial agent, to a burned area?
   1. A client with a creatinine level of 0.8 mg/dL.
   2. A client with chronic obstructive pulmonary disease.
   3. A client with a pulse oximeter reading of 95%.
   4. A client with Type 2 diabetes who is taking insulin.

8. The client with partial- and full-thickness burns to 35% of the body is admitted to the burn department. The HCP has prescribed famotidine (Pepcid), a histamine$_2$ antagonist. Which statement best describes the scientific rationale for administering this medication?
   1. Pepcid acts on the cell wall to prevent bacterial growth.
   2. Pepcid will help control the client's pain.
   3. Pepcid will help decrease the client's nausea and vomiting.
   4. Pepcid will help decrease gastric acid production.

9. The HCP prescribed morphine 2–5 mg IM every 2 hours for the client with full-thickness burns to the chest and abdominal area. The client reports pain of "10" on the 1 to 10 scale. Which intervention should the nurse implement?
   1. Administer 5 mg of morphine IM to the client immediately.
   2. Contact the HCP to request an increase in the medication.
   3. Request a patient-controlled analgesia (PCA) pump for the client.
   4. Assess the client for complications and then administer the medication.

10. The client is prescribed silver sulfadiazine (Silvadene), a topical antimicrobial agent, for a partial-thickness burn to the back. Which information should the nurse discuss concerning this medication?
    1. Encourage the client to drink 3000 mL of water.
    2. Discuss the need to eat foods high in protein.
    3. Teach the client how to test the urine for ketones.
    4. Instruct to change the dressing twice a day.

A Client with Pressure Ulcers

11. The nurse is using the antimicrobial binding dressing Actisorb Silver 222 for a Stage 3 pressure ulcer on the left hip area. The dressing is a combination of silver and activated charcoal. Which intervention should the nurse implement?
    1. Perform the sterile dressing change twice a day.
    2. Avoid cutting the dressing when applying it to the wound.
    3. Premedicate the client with a narcotic analgesic.
    4. Do not use tape to hold the secondary dressing in place.

12. The male client with a Stage 4 pressure ulcer on the coccyx area is being treated with an autolytic medication for debridement and an occlusive dressing. The wife of the client asks the nurse, "Why isn't someone doing something about that foul odor my husband has?" Which statement is the nurse's best response?
    1. "I will contact your husband's doctor when he makes rounds."
    2. "The odor is secondary to an infection and he is taking antibiotics."
    3. "The odor is an expected reaction to the pressure dressing."
    4. "I am sorry the odor bothers you. We will bathe your husband."

13. The nurse is changing a hydrocolloid antimicrobial barrier dressing with silver for a client with a Stage 4 pressure ulcer. Which intervention should the nurse implement first?
    1. Rinse the wound with physiologically normal saline.
    2. Remove the old dressing and assess the pressure ulcer.
    3. Hold the dressing in place for 5 seconds after applying.
    4. Apply sterile gloves when performing the procedure.

14. The nurse is caring for a client with a Stage 3 pressure ulcer. The client has a CombiDerm nonadhesive, sterile, hydrocolloidal dressing. Which data indicates the dressing is ready to be removed?
    1. The exudate begins to pool on the wound surface.
    2. The color of the drainage changes from brown to a yellow–gray.
    3. The health-care provider must write an order to remove the dressing.
    4. The softened area is approaching the edge of the dressing.

15. The client with a Stage 2 pressure ulcer is prescribed a hydrogel dressing. Which statement indicates the client understands the teaching about the hydrogel dressing?
    1. "The hydrogel dressing is soothing and reduces pain."
    2. "It must be used because my pressure ulcer drains a lot."
    3. "This dressing can only be used if my wound is not infected."
    4. "This dressing is very difficult to apply and remove from the wound."

16. While giving the elderly client a bath, the nurse notices a reddened area over the coccyx area but the skin is intact. Which action should the nurse implement?
    1. Notify the wound care nurse to assess the wound.
    2. Apply a bio-occlusive transparent dressing to the area.
    3. Contact the HCP to request a systemic antibiotic.
    4. Place the client in the prone position every 1 hour.

17. For which client with a Stage 2 pressure ulcer would the nurse question the use of Iodosorb gel, a wound filler?
    1. The client with an adverse reaction to bovine products.
    2. The gel can be used on any client.
    3. The client who has a pressure ulcer that is infected.
    4. The client who has a known sensitivity to iodine.

18. The nurse is applying Accuzyme papain-urea, a debriding agent, to a client who has a Stage 3 pressure ulcer. Which intervention should the nurse implement?
    1. Cleanse the wound with hydrogen peroxide solution.
    2. Rub the papain cream directly into the wound.
    3. Apply 1/8-inch papain ointment to the pressure ulcer.
    4. Be sure that no medication is applied on viable tissue.

19. The client has a Stage 4 pressure ulcer with tunneling. Which intervention should the nurse implement when instructed to apply a medicated roped dressing to the wound?
    1. Question inserting any medicated dressing into the tunnel.
    2. Apply a topical anesthetic to the wound before entering the tunnel.
    3. Use a sterile cotton swab and insert the dressing into the tunnel.
    4. Insert sterile normal saline into the tunnel after inserting dressing.

20. The nurse is applying a DermaDress dressing to a client with a Stage 2 pressure ulcer on the coccyx. Which interventions should the nurse implement? Rank in the order of performance.
    1. Secure the edges of the dressing with gentle pressure.
    2. Remove one side of the backing of the dressing.
    3. Clean the wound with DermaKlenz wound cleaner.
    4. Place the dressing gently over the wound.
    5. Remove the remaining backing to cover the wound.

A Client with a Skin Disorder

21. The client is prescribed methotrexate (Rheumatrex), an antineoplastic agent, for psoriasis. Which data should the nurse monitor?
    1. The glomerular filtration rate.
    2. The BUN and creatinine.
    3. The complete blood count.
    4. The iron-binding capacity.

22. The client diagnosed with tinea pedis complains of intense itching. Which intervention should the nurse recommend?
    1. Shampoo the hair two to three times with a selenium sulfide shampoo.
    2. Soak the feet in vinegar and water twice a day until better.
    3. Take the prescribed Sporanox for 1 week a month for 3 months.
    4. Apply a petroleum-based ointment to the feet daily.

23. The nurse is administering medications. Which intervention or medication would the nurse question?
    1. Balneotherapy with medicated tar to a client when the exhaust fan is broken.
    2. A colloidal oatmeal (Aveeno) bath to a client with itching from poison ivy.
    3. Sprinkling zinc oxide powder on a client on continuous bed rest.
    4. Using Desitin topical ointment on a client who has an excoriated perianal area.

24. Which medication should the nurse administer first?
    1. Griseofulvin (Fulvicin), an antifungal, to a client with tinea corporis.
    2. Hydroxyzine (Atarax), an antihistamine, to a client who is itching.
    3. Acyclovir (Zovirax), an antiviral, to a client with herpes zoster.
    4. Doxycycline (Vibramycin), an antibiotic, to a client with acne.

25. The HCP ordered lindane (Kwell), a scabicide, to be administered to the client from an extended care facility who is diagnosed with scabies. Which intervention should the nurse implement?
    1. Apply the ointment by thoroughly massaging it into the scalp.
    2. Bathe the client, and then apply the lotion to the patient from the neck down.
    3. Scrape the scabies lesions with a sterile needle.
    4. Shampoo the head with the Kwell and comb with a fine-toothed comb.

26. The nurse is discussing skin care with a teenaged client who has mild acne. Which medication or treatment should the nurse discuss with the client?
    1. Injections of *Clostridium botulinum* into the acne lesions.
    2. Applying vitamin E oil directly to the acne pimples to keep them moist.
    3. Taking isotretinoin (Accutane) by mouth daily.
    4. Washing the face and neck morning and night with benzoyl peroxide.

27. The nurse in a plastic surgeon's office is discharging a client who had Botox injections. Which discharge instructions should the nurse provide?
    1. The client can expect permanent paralysis of the muscles.
    2. The client should notify the HCP if edema is noted.
    3. The results will develop slowly over 3–10 days.
    4. The only side effect is a localized reaction at the injection site.

28. The client diagnosed with atopic dermatitis (eczema) is prescribed tacrolimus ointment (Protopic). Which interventions should the nurse implement? Select all that apply.
    1. Avoid sunlight getting to the treated areas.
    2. Stop using the medication if redness or itching occurs.
    3. Apply a thin layer to the skin twice a day.
    4. Cover the area with an occlusive dressing.
    5. Take a bath in tepid water before each application.

29. The female client calls the clinic to report that she has a painful sunburn. Which information should the nurse discuss with the client?
    1. Rub the inside of the aloe plant leaves on the sunburn.
    2. Apply calamine lotion to the most severely burned areas.
    3. Apply *Echinacea* to the sunburn to take away the pain.
    4. Use a cool compress of baking soda to help the sunburn heal.

30. The occupational health nurse is presenting information regarding prevention of skin cancer to a group of workers in an industrial plant. Which information should the nurse include in the program?
    1. Sunscreen is ineffective in blocking UV rays.
    2. Many antibiotics lose efficacy if the client is exposed to sunlight.
    3. Use a sunscreen of at least 30 SPF when in the sun.
    4. Tanning beds do not have the same damaging rays as the sun.

A Client with Burns

1. 1. The serum sodium level is not affected by mafenide acetate (Sulfamylon); it is affected when administering silver nitrate, a topical antimicrobial that is also used to treat burns.
   2. Urine concentration may be affected by silver sulfadiazine (Silvadene), a topical antimicrobial that is used to treat burns, but Sulfamylon does not affect urine concentration.
   3. This should have been done prior to the emergency room physician prescribing this medication; therefore, this would not be an appropriate intervention.
   4. **The medication causes pain or a burning sensation following its application; therefore, the client should be premedicated.**

2. 1. This is the incorrect way to apply silver nitrate.
   2. Silver nitrate solution causes a black discoloration on all skin surfaces and dressings with which it comes into contact; therefore, the client would not need to notify the HCP.
   3. **Sliver nitrate is used as a 0.5% solution in distilled water and should be applied to the bulky gauze dressing every 2 hours, and the dressing should be changed twice a day.**
   4. The bulky wound dressing must be changed twice a day; therefore, the nurse must teach the client to change the dressing. A dressing change does not have to be done only by the HCP.

3. 1. The nurse should administer this intravenous fluid as ordered.
   2. **There are formulas that are used to determine the client's fluid-volume resuscitation. The formulas specify the total amount of fluid that must be infused in 24 hours—50% in the first 8 hours, followed by the other 50% over the next 16 hours. This is a large amount of fluid, but its administration is not uncommon in clients with full-thickness burns over more than 20% of their total body surface.**
   3. This is not an unusual amount of fluid to be infused. There is no absolute amount of fluid that a client may require during fluid resuscitation.
   4. There is no reason to verify this order with another nurse in the burn unit.

4. 1. A urine output of less than 30 mL/hour would not indicate the fluid resuscitation is effective.
   2. This would indicate effective fluid resuscitation for a client with a thermal burn but not for a client with an electrical burn.
   3. **The client with an electrical burn should have a urine output of 75 to 100 mL/hour for the fluid resuscitation to be effective.**
   4. An output of greater than 100 mL/hour would indicate the client is losing too much fluid and that the fluid resuscitation is not effective.

5. 1. **A tetanus toxoid is administered intramuscularly early in the acute phase of burn care to prevent *Clostridium tetani* infection. If the client has not had a tetanus shot within the last 10 years or if the time is in doubt, a booster of tetanus toxoid should be administered.**
   2. This may be an appropriate question, but it is not the most important question.
   3. This is an appropriate question, but it is not the most important question.
   4. This question would not be pertinent to the client's burn and medical care in the emergency department.

6. 1. Leukopenia improves over the course of the treatment with Silvadene and does not warrant discontinuing the medication.
   2. **Many clients develop marked leukopenia in response to Silvadene. The leukopenia will improve spontaneously over the course of treatment. Leukopenia does not contraindicate use of this medication.**
   3. Leukopenia secondary to Silvadene therapy does not warrant the administration of aminoglycoside antibiotics.
   4. Hydrocortisone cream does not treat leukopenia secondary to Silvadene.

7. 1. Sulfamylon affects the acid–base balance in the body and should not be administered to clients with renal disease. A 0.8 mg/dL serum creatinine level is within normal range of 0.5 to 1.5 mg/dL; therefore, the nurse would not need to use caution with this client.
   2. **Sulfamylon impairs the renal mechanism involved in the buffering of the blood, thereby increasing the excretion of bicarbonate in the urine. When this occurs, the pulmonary system effects a**

compensatory hyperventilatory status to maintain normal acid–base balance. If this compensation cannot take place as a result of pulmonary disease, the client develops metabolic acidosis.

3. This client has adequate respiratory status; therefore, the nurse would not need to use caution with this client.

4. There is no reason a client with diabetes could not be prescribed mafenide acetate.

8. 1. Silver sulfadiazine (Silvadene), not Pepcid, acts on the cell membrane and cell wall of susceptible bacteria and binds to cellular DNA.

2. Intravenous opioid medications, not Silvadene, will help decrease the client's pain.

3. Antiemetics, not Silvadene, will help prevent the client's nausea and vomiting.

4. **Curling's ulcer (stress ulcer) is an acute ulceration of the stomach or duodenum that forms following a burn injury. Histamine$_2$ antagonists like Pepcid are administered to decrease gastric acid secretion in the acute phase of burn care.**

9. 1. The client should receive intravenous (IV) medication, not intramuscular (IM) medication.

2. The client should receive IV medication, not IM medication; therefore, the nurse should be a client advocate and notify the health-care provider for a change in the route of the morphine.

3. **The client should have intravenous pain medication until hemodynamic stability and unimpaired tissue perfusion return. The PCA pump provides an intravenous route, and the client can control the amount of medication administered with the PCA, ensuring safe limits of pain medication.**

4. The client should receive IV medication, not IM medication; therefore, the nurse should not administer this medication after assessing the client.

10. 1. **The client should drink large amounts of fluids to prevent sulfa crystals from forming in the urine.**

2. The client should eat foods high in protein for healing purposes, but this does not specifically concern this medication.

3. Ketones are a byproduct of fat breakdown and would not be specific for teaching about Silvadene.

4. The client should change the dressing twice a day, but this is not part of teaching about the medication Silvadene.

A Client with Pressure Ulcers

11. 1. The dressing may be left in place for up to 7 days or may be changed every 24 hours, but it would not be changed twice a day. This does not allow the dressing adequate time to increase healing of the wound.

2. **The nurse should avoid cutting the dressing because particles of activated charcoal may get into the wound and cause discoloration.**

3. The dressing change does not warrant administering a narcotic analgesic to the client.

4. Tape should be used to hold the secondary dressing in place or the antimicrobial binding dressing will not remain in the pressure ulcer.

12. 1. There is no reason to contact the HCP because this is an expected reaction to the pressure dressing.

2. The client may have an infection and is taking antibiotics, but this is not causing the foul odor.

3. **This is an expected reaction to the pressure dressing. The foul odor is produced by the breakdown of cellular debris and does not indicate that the wound is infected.**

4. Bathing the husband will not help the odor; therefore, this response is not appropriate.

13. 1. The nurse should rinse the wound with physiologically normal saline, but this is not the first intervention.

2. **Removing the old dressing and assessing the pressure ulcer for healing is the first intervention.**

3. This dressing must be held in place for 5 seconds after applying it to the pressure ulcer.

4. The dressing change is performed with nonsterile gloves using aseptic technique; therefore, this is not an appropriate intervention.

14. 1. This would indicate when an alginate dressing, not a hydrocolloidal dressing, is ready to be removed.
    2. The Iodosorb gel, not the CombiDerm dressing, should be changed when the color changes from brown to a yellow–gray.
    3. The nurse does not need a written order from the health-care provider to change the dressing.
    4. **This dressing is an absorbent hydro-colloidal dressing that provides a moist environment, absorbs exudates, and is nondamaging to the skin. When the softened area approaches the edge of the dressing, it must be removed and a new one must be applied.**

15. 1. **Hydrogels help maintain a moist healing environment, granulation, and epithelialization, and they facilitate autolytic debridement. One advantage of a hydrogel dressing is that it is soothing and reduces pain.**
    2. One of the disadvantages of hydrogel dressings is that they are not recommended for wounds with heavy exudate.
    3. An advantage of using hydrogel dressings is that they can be used when infection is present.
    4. An advantage of using hydrogel dressings is that they are easily applied and removed from the wound.

16. 1. The wound care nurse is usually not contacted until the pressure ulcer is at a Stage 2.
    2. **Bio-occlusive transparent dressing is a semiocclusive bacterial and viral barrier that protects skin from exogenous fluid and contaminants. It is used for areas where the skin is intact.**
    3. A Stage 1 pressure ulcer does not require systemic antibiotic therapy because the skin remains intact.
    4. The nurse does not place clients with Stage 1 pressure ulcers in the prone position (on the stomach). The nurse would turn the client from side to side.

17. 1. A Catrix wound dressing, which is a topically applied powder made from bovine tracheal cartilage, not an Iodosorb dressing, would be contraindicated in a client with a pressure ulcer who has an adverse reaction to bovine products.
    2. The nurse would question use of Iodosorb in certain clients because there are some contraindications to its use.
    3. Iodosorb gel cleanses the wound by absorbing; the nurse would not question the use of this gel for the client with an infection.
    4. **Iodosorb gel, cadexomer iodine, is an iodine-based wound filler. If the client has a known sensitivity to iodine, the nurse would not use this dressing.**

MEDICATION MEMORY JOGGER: If the test taker has no idea what the answer to the question is, then the test taker should look at the name of the medication. In this question, the medication has "iodo" in the name. This should make the nurse thinks about iodine and select option "4."

18. 1. Hydrogen peroxide solution should not be used because it may inactivate the papain.
    2. Cream should not be rubbed into the wound because it will cause further tissue damage.
    3. **This ointment is made from the proteolytic enzyme from the fruit of *Carica papaya* and is a debriding product. After cleansing the pressure ulcer, the nurse should apply 1/8-inch thickness of ointment.**
    4. Accuzyme papain-urea is a potent digestant of nonviable protein matter, but it is harmless to viable tissue.

19. 1. Inserting the medicated dressing is an appropriate intervention; therefore, the nurse should not question this order.
    2. Topical anesthetic is not used to dress a Stage 4 pressure ulcer.
    3. **The nurse must insert the roped dressing into the tunnel to ensure wound healing. Using a sterile cotton swab will allow the dressing to be inserted into the tunnel and will not cause damage to the tissue.**
    4. The wound should be cleansed with normal saline or some type of sterile solution before dressing the wound, not after dressing the wound.

20.   3, 2, 4, 5, 1
    3. **The wound needs to be cleaned with some type of solution. Even if the test taker were not familiar with DermaKlenz, he or she should select this option as the first intervention.**

2. **DermaDress is a multilayered water-proof sterile dressing, and the nurse must remove one side of the backing before applying to the wound.**
4. **After the backing is removed, the nurse should apply the dressing to the wound.**
5. **The nurse should then remove the remaining back and cover the wound.**
1. **The nurse should then secure the dressing in place.**

A Client with a Skin Disorder

21. 1. The glomerular filtration rate (GFR) monitors for renal function. Methotrexate is not toxic to the kidneys so monitoring of GFR would not be needed.
2. The BUN and creatinine tests monitor for renal problems. Methotrexate is not toxic to the kidneys.
3. **Methotrexate causes hematopoietic depression. The nurse should monitor for leukopenia, thrombocytopenia, and anemia. The CBC provides information in all these areas.**
4. Methotrexate does not interfere with the iron-binding capacity.

22. 1. Tinea pedis is athlete's foot. Shampooing with a selenium sulfide shampoo is recommended for children with tinea capitis (ringworm).
2. **Tinea pedis is athlete's foot. The nurse should recommend that the client soak the feet twice a day in a vinegar and water solution. If this is not successful in treating the problem, then the client should contact an HCP for a prescription antifungal agent.**
3. Sporanox is the treatment for tinea unguium, a toenail infection. The HCP would have to prescribe this treatment.
4. Petroleum-based products are not used to treat fungal foot infections.

23. 1. **Balneotherapy involves therapeutic baths with or without medications. Tar baths are recommended for clients with severe psoriasis or eczema. Because tars are volatile, the bath area should be well-ventilated. The nurse would question this medication at this time.**
2. Oatmeal baths are useful in relieving the itching associated with poison ivy rashes.

The nurse would not question this medication.
3. Although the therapeutic duration of relief from powders is brief, powders act as a hygroscopic agent to retain and absorb moisture from the air and reduce friction between skin surfaces and clothing or bedding. The nurse would not question this medication.
4. Desitin ointment is a zinc oxide–based preparation used to treat erythema and excoriated areas of the perineum or around the anus (perianal). The nurse would not question this medication.

24. 1. This client has a fungal infection of the body that is not life threatening, and the option did not state the client was uncomfortable. The client with a comfort problem (itching) should receive the medication first.
2. **Atarax is prescribed to relieve itching. Pruritus is an uncomfortable sensation. This client should receive the medication first.**
3. Zovirax is administered several times a day for herpes infections. The viral infection is not life threatening. The client who is uncomfortable should receive the medication first.
4. Vibramycin is an antibiotic that is administered orally for acne, but acne is not life threatening, and the client who is uncomfortable should receive medication first.

25. 1. The medication is a cream, not an ointment, and scabies infestations occur on the body, usually between the fingers or toes, wrists, elbows, and waistline. When Kwell is used on the scalp, it is used to treat lice and it is shampooed in.
2. **All creams, lotions, powders, and the like should be removed before applying a cream to the body, so the client should be bathed prior to the application of the cream. The nurse then applies a thin layer of cream over the entire body starting at the neck, avoiding the face and urethral meatus, and including the soles of the feet. The skin is allowed to dry and cool after the application. The medication is removed after 8–12 hours by a bath or shower.**
3. The nurse does not scrape the lesions. Scabies mites burrow under the client's skin and the medication is applied to the

entire body surface area, excluding the face and urethral meatus.

4. This is how to apply Kwell for head lice, not for scabies.

26. 1. *Clostridium botulinum* is Botox, which is used to decrease the appearance of wrinkles. It is not used to treat acne.

2. Clients with acne have too much oil production. Applying vitamin E oil would increase the client's problem.

3. Accutane has serious side effects, and its use is restricted to only those with severe, disfiguring acne.

4. **Benzoyl peroxide is used for mild acne to suppress the growth of *P. acnes* and promote keratolysis (peeling of the horny layer of epidermis).**

27. 1. This not a true statement. The paralysis of the facial muscles lasts from 3–6 months.

2. Facial edema is expected after the procedure. The nurse should teach the client to apply ice to the site and avoid using alcohol or NSAID products for a week prior to the procedure.

3. **The results are neither instantaneous nor permanent. Results develop over 3–10 days.**

4. In addition to mild edema, there can be more side effects to Botox injections. Excessive dosing can cause facial paralysis, and clients can lose the ability to smile, frown, raise the eyebrows, or squint.

28. 1. **Tacrolimus increases the risk of skin cancer when the client is exposed to UV light. The clients should be told to avoid direct sunlight or use of tanning beds.**

2. Common side effects of Protopic are erythema, pruritus, and a burning sensation at the site of application. These reactions lessen as the skin heals. The client should not stop using the medication.

3. **This is the normal dosing schedule.**

4. The skin should be left uncovered.

5. The client does not have to take a bath before each application. The first application will have absorbed into the skin prior to the next dose.

29. 1. **The juice from the aloe plant is used topically to treat minor burns, insect bites, and sunburn. This is an appropriate suggestion by the nurse.**

2. Calamine is used to decrease the itching associated with poison ivy, oak, or sumac. It would not help a sunburn.

3. Echinacea is used topically to treat canker sores or fungal infections, not sunburn.

4. Baking soda paste is helpful in treating insect bites, not sunburn.

30. 1. Sunscreen is very useful in preventing sun damage to the skin. An SPF of at least 30 should be used.

2. Sunlight does not affect the efficacy of antibiotics taken internally; some antibiotics might cause the client to be more susceptible to photosensitivity, but efficacy of the antibiotics would not be affected.

3. **Clients should be told to use a sunscreen of at least SPF 30 when in the sun. The higher the number, the better the blocking of the sun's UV rays occurs.**

4. Tanning beds use UV rays and may be more damaging than the sun because of the concentrated time clients stay under the tanning bed lamps.

1. The client has a Stage 4 pressure ulcer and is being treated with enzymatic debriding agent and occlusive dressing. The nurse notices a foul odor. Which action should the nurse take?
   1. Notify the wound care nurse that there is a foul odor.
   2. Explain to the client that this odor is expected.
   3. Assess the client's oral temperature.
   4. Request an order for an antibiotic from the HCP.

2. The client with poison ivy is prescribed a dose pack of the steroid prednisone. Which statement best describes the scientific rationale for prescribing the dose pack?
   1. The steroid will help decrease the inflammation secondary to poison ivy.
   2. The dose pack will ensure that the medication is tapered as needed.
   3. The dose pack will gradually increase the dose of the steroid taken daily.
   4. The steroid will reduce the amount of redness that is on the client's skin.

3. The child with pediculosis capitis is prescribed lindane (Kwell), a pediculocide. Which information should the nurse discuss with the parents?
   1. Wash the hair with an antimicrobial shampoo prior to using lindane.
   2. Scrub the head and wash the hair for 2 minutes and then remove the lindane.
   3. Apply the shampoo to dry hair and use a small amount of water to lather.
   4. Use the Kwell shampoo daily before going to bed for 1 week.

4. Which information should the nurse discuss with the client who has seborrheic dermatitis of the scalp?
   1. Use a fine-toothed comb to comb out the hair after shampooing.
   2. Dry the hair using the high heat setting for at least 5 minutes.
   3. Apply an oil-based cream after the shampoo and do not rinse.
   4. Rotate two or three different types of shampoos daily.

5. The client with a verruca vulgaris (wart) on the left ring finger below the knuckle is prescribed a colloidal acid solution. Which information should the nurse discuss with the client?
   1. Apply the solution to the wart every 12 hours.
   2. Expect the wart to disappear within 1 week.
   3. Be careful because the wart may spread easily.
   4. Do not wear any rings on the left hand.

6. The nurse is discussing the System to Manage Accutane-Related Teratogenicity (SMART) with a client who has severe acne. Which statement by the female client would cause the HCP to not prescribe Accutane?
   1. "The only contraception I use is birth control pills."
   2. "My menstrual cycles have been regular and heavy."
   3. "I hope this works because I am so tired of being ugly."
   4. "I will have to come in every month for a pregnancy test."

7. The female client diagnosed with acne is prescribed tetracycline. Which intervention should the nurse include in the medication teaching?
   1. Take the medication with milk or milk products.
   2. Explain that this medication may cause the teeth to discolor.
   3. Tell the client to use sunscreen and protective clothing when outside.
   4. Advise the client to take birth control pills.

8. Which information should the nurse discuss with the 16-year-old female client diagnosed with acne who is prescribed estrogen, a dominant oral contraceptive compound, to treat her acne?
   1. This medication will prevent the client from getting pregnant.
   2. Do not take this medication on an empty stomach.
   3. The medication will turn the urine and body fluids orange.
   4. Take the medication daily for 3 weeks, then stop for 1 week.

9. The child has impetigo on the hands. The HCP prescribes topical mupirocin (Bactroban), an antibiotic. Which intervention should the nurse demonstrate to the parents when discussing this medication?
   1. Apply the ointment with sterile gloves.
   2. Scrape the lesions prior to applying ointment.
   3. Soak the hands in soapy water.
   4. Cleanse the impetigo with hydrogen peroxide.

10. The client with cellulitis of the left arm is seen in the clinic. Which intervention would the nurse expect the HCP to prescribe when discharging the client home?
   1. Apply topical corticosteroid ointment to the affected area.
   2. Take a 7–10-day regimen of systemic antibiotics.
   3. Apply cold, dry compresses to the reddened, inflamed skin.
   4. Continue activity as needed with no specific restrictions.

11. Which procedure should the nurse teach the client who is scheduled for a chemical face peel?
   1. Do not wear any type of makeup for 1 week prior to the scheduled procedure.
   2. Apply a heat lamp to the face for 10 minutes three times a day.
   3. Take all the prescribed antibiotics for 5 days prior to the procedure.
   4. Clean the face and hair with hexachlorophene for 3 days prior to the procedure.

12. The client has second- and third-degree burns to 40% of the body. The HCP writes an order for 9000 mL of fluid to be infused over the next 24 hours. The order reads that 1/2 of the total amount should be administered in the first 8 hours with the other 1/2 being infused over the remaining 16 hours. What rate would the nurse set the intravenous pump for the first 8 hours?

   Answer _____

13. The client with acute herpes zoster is prescribed oral acyclovir (Zovirax), an antiviral medication. Which statement by the client indicates the client needs more medication teaching?
   1. "I am so glad this medication will cure my shingles."
   2. "I will have to take the pill five times a day."
   3. "I should take this medication for 7–10 days."
   4. "If the shingles gets near my eyes, I will call my HCP."

14. The client with male pattern baldness is prescribed finasteride (Propecia), a hair growth stimulant. When should the nurse evaluate for effectiveness of the medication?
   1. After the client has been taking the medication for 1 month.
   2. When the client states there are no hair strands in the comb.
   3. At the time the client's hair changes texture and color.
   4. One year after taking the hair growth stimulant medication daily.

15. The client with psoriasis who is being treated with a tar preparation (Estar) calls the clinic nurse and reports an odor and staining of the client's shirt. Which action should the nurse implement?
   1. Have the client come to the clinic immediately.
   2. Tell the client that the odor and staining are expected.
   3. Discontinue the tar preparation immediately.
   4. Apply a diluted bleach solution to the affected area.

16. The nurse and the unlicensed assistive personnel (UAP) are treating the client with pruritus. Which task can be delegated to the UAP?
   1. Cut the client's fingernails to prevent scratching.
   2. Administer the antihistamine diphenhydramine (Benadryl).
   3. Remove all caffeine-containing products from the room.
   4. Apply a moisturizing lotion to the client's skin.

17. The client has been applying a topical hydrocortisone cream to dry rough skin for more than 2 years. Which data should the nurse assess for in the client?
    1. Check for signs or symptoms of adrenal insufficiency.
    2. Assess for a buffalo hump and a moon face.
    3. Assess for thin, fragile skin in the area near the dry, rough skin.
    4. Monitor the client's serum blood glucose level.

18. The parents of a 2-year-old child with measles call the pediatric clinic and tell the nurse the child is very uncomfortable, irritable, and fretful. Which recommendation should the nurse discuss with the parents?
    1. Alternate Motrin with children's aspirin every 4 hours.
    2. Apply diphenhydramine (Benadryl) cream to the rash.
    3. Administer acetaminophen (Tylenol) elixir to the child.
    4. Tell the parents that there is no medication for the child.

19. The client is complaining of inability to sleep because of pruritus secondary to a skin irritation on the lower extremities. Which information should the nurse discuss with the client?
    1. Take the antihistamine hydroxyzine (Atarax) at bedtime.
    2. Apply antibacterial ointment to the skin irritation.
    3. Soak the lower extremities in warm, soapy water.
    4. Place an occlusive dressing over the irritated skin.

20. Which statement describes the advantage for the client with acute herpes infection taking valacyclovir (Valtrex) over acyclovir (Zovirax)?
    1. Valtrex does not cost as much as the acyclovir.
    2. Valtrex only requires taking medication three times a day.
    3. Acyclovir has to be taken for a longer period of time.
    4. Acyclovir must be taken on an empty stomach.

1. 1. This odor does not indicate that the wound is infected; therefore, the nurse should not notify the wound care nurse who is usually responsible for treating a Stage 4 pressure ulcer.
   2. **When an enzymatic debriding agent is used under a occlusive dressing, a foul odor is produced by the breakdown of cellular debris. The nurse should explain to the client that the odor is expected.**
   3. This odor does not indicate that the wound is infected; therefore, the nurse would not need to assess the client's temperature to determine if there is an elevation.
   4. This odor does not indicate that the wound is infected; therefore, the client would not need to be receiving antibiotic therapy.

2. 1. Decreasing inflammation is the scientific rationale for prescribing the steroid, but it is not the specific rationale for prescribing the dose pack.
   2. **Steroids must be tapered to prevent adrenal insufficiency. The dose pack is prescribed to ensure that the client takes the correct amount of medication daily.**
   3. The steroid dose pack is gradually decreased, not increased.
   4. This is the scientific rationale for prescribing the steroid, not the rationale for prescribing the dose pack.

3. 1. The hair does not need to be shampooed with an antimicrobial solution prior to applying lindane.
   2. The head must be scrubbed for 4 minutes before rinsing the shampoo.
   3. **This child has head lice and the treatment of choice is shampooing the hair with Kwell. It should be applied to dry hair with a small amount of water so that the medication is not washed off the hair but is rubbed into the hair to kill the lice.**
   4. The Kwell shampoo may be repeated in a week to kill newly hatched lice, but it should not be used daily nor does it matter the time of day the shampoo is used. Daily shampooing with Kwell may cause central nervous system toxicity, especially in children.

4. 1. A fine-toothed comb is used to remove nits in clients with head lice; it is not used to treat seborrheic dermatitis (dandruff).
   2. Using the hair dryer at the high heat setting will further dry out the scalp and increase dandruff production.
   3. This information is not appropriate for a client with dandruff.
   4. **Two or three different types of shampoos should be used in rotation to prevent the seborrhea from becoming resistant to a specific shampoo. This treatment for dandruff is used initially; then, as the condition is improved, the treatment can be less frequent.**

5. 1. **Acid therapy (of 16% salicylic acid and 16% lactic acid) is a common way to remove warts. It should be applied every 12–24 hours for 2–3 weeks.**
   2. The wart should disappear in 2–3 weeks.
   3. The acid therapy will not cause the wart to spread.
   4. There is no reason the client cannot wear rings on the left hand while applying acid therapy to the wart.

6. 1. **The client must be using two forms of birth control when taking Accutane because Accutane is extremely damaging to the fetus. The SMART protocol has been instituted to ensure that no female clients are or become pregnant while taking this medication.**
   2. Accutane is extremely damaging to the fetus, and because the client is having regular and heavy menses the HCP could prescribe this medication knowing that the client is not pregnant.
   3. Accutane is prescribed for acne; therefore, this statement would not cause the HCP not to prescribe Accutane.
   4. One of the requirements of the SMART protocol is a pregnancy test monthly because Accutane is extremely damaging to the fetus.

7. 1. The tetracycline should not be taken with milk or milk products because those products prevent the absorption of the medication in the stomach.
   2. Tetracycline may cause discoloration or a yellow–brown color of the teeth in children younger than 8 years old or in the fetus of a client who is pregnant. This client is not pregnant and is an adult; therefore, this intervention is not appropriate.
   3. **Photosensitivity (sun reaction) may occur in persons taking tetracycline; therefore, the client should be taught to use safety precautions when in the sunlight.**

4. The female client should use a nonhormonal method of contraception because birth control pills interact with the tetracycline and the client will be unprotected from pregnancy.

8. 1. The medication is not being prescribed for birth control; it is being prescribed for acne. The client is 16 years old, and if she is sexually active, a condom should be worn to prevent sexually transmitted disease.
   2. Birth control pills can be taken on an empty stomach or with food.
   3. Birth control pills do not turn body fluids orange.
   4. **This medication may be used as a birth control pill, but it is also used to treat acne by suppressing sebum production and reducing skin oiling. The client must take the medication exactly as prescribed.**

9. 1. The parents should wash their hands prior to administering the medication and can use nonsterile gloves or a tongue depressor when applying the medication. They do not need to use sterile gloves, but they should not touch the affected area.
   2. Scraping the lesions would hurt the child and cause bleeding, which results in a scab, which, in turn, must be removed prior to applying ointment. Do not scrape the lesions.
   3. **The soapy water will help to remove the central site of bacterial growth, giving the topical antibiotic the opportunity to reach the infected site.**
   4. Hydrogen peroxide is not used to cleanse impetigo. A 1:20 Burow's solution may be used to put compresses on the impetigo.

10. 1. Cellulitis is not a topical infection and is not treated with topical ointments.
    2. **Systemic antibiotic therapy is the treatment of choice for cellulitis, an inflammation of the skin and subcutaneous tissue.**
    3. The HCP would prescribe hot, moist compresses, not cold, dry compresses, to the area to help decrease pain and redness.
    4. The HCP would prescribe rest with immobilization of the extremity.

11. 1. There is no reason the client cannot wear makeup prior to the procedure, especially for 1 week. Makeup is not allowed for a few weeks after the procedure.

2. Use of a heat lamp is not prescribed prior to having a chemical face peel.
3. A chemical face peel does not necessitate antibiotic therapy before the procedure, but the client may be prescribed antibiotics after the procedure.
4. **Cleaning the face and hair with hexachlorophene will decrease the risk of infection during and after the procedure.**

12. **563/hr.** Because half of the total dose of 9000 mL should be administered in the first 8 hours, the nurse should determine how many milliliters should be given in the first 8 hours. 9000 ÷ 2 = 4500 mL. Then, the 4500 must be divided by 8 to determine the rate per hour. 4500 ÷ 8 = 562.5, or rounded off to 563. There are formulas that are used to determine the client's fluid-volume resuscitation. The formulas specify the total amount of fluid that must be infused in 24 hours, 50% in the first 8 hours followed by the other 50% over the other 16 hours. This is a large amount of fluid, but it is not uncommon in clients with full-thickness burns over more than 20% total body surface area burned.

13. 1. **The client must understand that no medication will cure a herpes viral infection. Zovirax shortens the time of symptoms and speeds healing, but it does not cure the shingles. The client needs more medication teaching.**
    2. This medication is prescribed for five times a day dosing because of the short half-life of the medication.
    3. The medication is prescribed for 7–10 days when the client has an acute exacerbation of a herpes virus.
    4. If the herpes zoster occurs near or in the eyes, it could cause blindness and is considered an ophthalmic emergency.

14. 1. The medication must be taken for at least 1 year before determining adequate response to the medication.
    2. Not finding any hair in the comb does not indicate the medication is stimulating hair growth.
    3. The hair texture and color have nothing to do with determining the effectiveness of the medication.
    4. **Only 50% of clients regrow hair, and it may require up to 1 year of daily treatment to determine if the medication is effective.**

15. 1. This is an expected action of the tar preparation, and the client does not need to come to the clinic.
2. **Preparations made of coal tar are messy, they cause staining, and they have an unpleasant odor, but they are an effective form of treatment for psoriasis.**
3. Psoriasis is extremely difficult to treat, and tar preparations are an effective form of treatment and should not be discontinued because of expected effects.
4. Bleach will not treat the stains on the skin and will dry out the skin.

16. 1. The nurse should not delegate cutting the fingernails to a UAP because the length of the client's fingernails is an individual preference.
2. The nurse cannot delegate the administration of medication.
3. Caffeine will keep the client awake and should be discouraged, but this task cannot be delegated because the nurse must teach this rationale to the client.
4. **The UAP can put a moisturizing lotion on the client. This is not considered a medication.**

17. 1. The client would not experience signs of systemic withdrawal because of a steroid being applied topically.
2. The client would not experience signs of prednisone toxicity because topical steroids are used.
3. **After prolonged use of topical steroids, the dermis and epidermis will atrophy, resulting in thinning of the skin, striae, and purpura; therefore, the nurse should assess for this data.**
4. The client would not have elevated blood glucose levels because the medication is a topical cream.

18. 1. A child should not take aspirin because it may cause Reye's syndrome.
2. Benadryl ointment should not be applied to the rash area.
3. **Tylenol elixir is the drug of choice for children to decrease irritability and any discomfort.**
4. There is no treatment for the measles; it must run its course, but a mild nonnarcotic analgesic such as Tylenol can decrease irritability and discomfort.

19. 1. **Atarax is an antihistamine medication that decreases itching and is also prescribed as a sedative at bedtime because it is effective in producing a restful and comfortable sleep.**
2. Antibacterial ointment will not help the client sleep; therefore, it is not information the nurse should discuss with the client.
3. Warm soapy water will not help decrease the itching and may increase the skin irritation.
4. An occlusive dressing will not help decrease the client's complaints of itching.

20. 1. Valtrex costs more than acyclovir; therefore, the cost is not an advantage.
2. **Acyclovir requires the client to take medication five times a day and Valtrex is only taken three times a day. Fewer dosing times increase compliance with the medication and are an advantage of Valtrex.**
3. Both antiviral medications are taken for the same period of time; therefore, there is not an advantage of taking Valtrex.
4. Both medications can be taken with or without food; therefore, this is not an advantage to taking Valtrex.

Immune Inflammatory System

10

"*The new gold standard system of checking used by nurses is called the '6 Rights'—the right client, right medication, right dose, right route, right time, and the sixth is right documentation.*"

—Helen Harkreader and Mary Ann Hogan

PRACTICE QUESTIONS

A Client with an Autoimmune Disease

1. The nurse is administering medications to the clients on a medical unit. Which medication would the nurse question administering?
   1. Atropine, an antimuscarinic, to a client with myasthenia gravis.
   2. Chloroquine, an antimalarial, to a client with a butterfly rash.
   3. Prednisone, a corticosteroid, to a client with polymyalgia rheumatica.
   4. Mestinon, a cholinesterase inhibitor, to a client in a cholinergic crisis.

2. The client diagnosed with systemic lupus erythematosus (SLE) is experiencing an acute exacerbation and the HCP has ordered high doses of glucocorticoid medications. Which statement supports the goal of this therapy?
   1. To provide a permanent cure for lupus.
   2. To allow a peaceful, dignified death.
   3. To help enable the client to maintain weight.
   4. To prevent permanent damage to the organs.

3. The female client diagnosed with systemic lupus erythematosus (SLE) complains to the nurse that she has pain; she is stiff when she gets up in the morning; and she takes ibuprofen, an NSAID, to help ease the pain and stiffness. Which question is most important for the nurse to ask the client?
   1. "How often do you have to take the ibuprofen?"
   2. "Do you take the medication on an empty stomach?"
   3. "Does the medication help with menstrual cramping too?"
   4. "Have you noticed an improvement in the pain and stiffness?"

4. The client diagnosed with multiple sclerosis (MS) is prescribed the intravenous glucocorticoid hydrocortisone (Solu-Cortef). The client has a saline lock. Which procedures should the nurse follow when administering the medication? Rank in order of performance.
   1. Administer the diluted medication intravenously over 1–2 minutes.
   2. Aspirate the syringe to obtain a blood return.
   3. Flush the saline lock with 2 mL of sterile normal saline.
   4. Flush the saline lock again with 2 mL of normal saline.
   5. Check the client's identification bands against the MAR.

5. The client diagnosed with multiple sclerosis is prescribed baclofen (Lioresal), an antispasmodic. Which data is most important for the nurse to assess?
   1. The client's serum baclofen levels.
   2. The client's urinary output.
   3. The client's pain, muscle rigidity, and range of motion.
   4. The client's BUN and creatinine levels.

6. The nurse is administering 0800 medications on a medical floor. Which medication should the nurse administer first?
   1. Prostigmin, a cholinesterase inhibitor, to a client diagnosed with myasthenia gravis.
   2. Methylprednisolone, a glucocorticoid, to a client diagnosed with lupus erythematosus.
   3. Morphine, a narcotic analgesic, to a client diagnosed with Guillain-Barré syndrome.
   4. Etanercept, a biologic response modifier, to a client with rheumatoid arthritis.

7. The nurse administered edrophonium (Tensilon), a cholinesterase inhibitor, to a client diagnosed with rule-out myasthenia gravis (MG). Which response by the client indicates the client has myasthenia gravis?
   1. The client loses the ability to breathe without mechanical support.
   2. The client's strength improves briefly without signs of fasciculations.
   3. The client cannot gaze at the ceiling for 2 minutes without fatigue.
   4. The client's paroxysmal atrial tachycardia converts to normal sinus rhythm.

8. The client diagnosed with an acute gout attack is prescribed allopurinol (Zyloprim). Which data indicates the medication is effective?
   1. The client has been symptom-free for several days.
   2. The client has developed an aversion reaction to alcohol.
   3. The serum uric acid levels are within normal limits.
   4. The client develops tophi in the joints of the feet.

9. The female client diagnosed with myasthenia gravis complains that the anticholinesterase medication makes her nauseated. Which information should the nurse teach the client?
   1. Decrease the dose of the medication.
   2. Hold the medication and notify the HCP.
   3. Take the medication with milk and crackers.
   4. Take an over-the-counter proton-pump inhibitor.

10. The male client diagnosed with paranoid schizophrenia has been taking the antipsychotic medication chlorpromazine (Thorazine). The client tells the psychiatric clinic nurse that he has frequent joint pain and stiffness and gets a rash when in the sun. Which statement is the nurse's best response?
    1. "This is part of your illness and will go away if you don't pay attention."
    2. "What have your voices said about the aches and pains and rash?"
    3. "Don't take your medication today, and come in to see the HCP."
    4. "This is a reaction to medications and you can no longer take medications."

A Client with Acquired Immunodeficiency Syndrome

11. The clinic nurse is discussing medication compliance with a client diagnosed with acquired immunodeficiency syndrome (AIDS). Which information should the nurse discuss with the client?
    1. The availability of insurance to pay for the medications.
    2. Whether the client wants to try to manage the disease without medications.
    3. Include over-the-counter herbs in the medication regimen.
    4. The importance of taking multiple vitamins at least twice a day.

12. The nurse received a needle stick with a "dirty" needle from a client diagnosed with acquired immunodeficiency syndrome (AIDS). Which medications should the nurse begin within hours of the needle stick?
    1. A combination of antiviral and antifungal medications with an antibiotic.
    2. A combination of a protease inhibitor and nucleoside reverse transcriptase inhibitors.
    3. Single-agent therapy with a non-nucleoside transcriptase inhibitor.
    4. No medications are recommended to prevent the conversion to HIV positive.

13. The pregnant client's HIV test is positive. Which medication should the client take to prevent transmission of the virus to the fetus?
    1. Efavirenz (Sustiva), a non-nucleoside reverse transcriptase inhibitor.
    2. Lopinavir (Kaletra), a protease inhibitor.
    3. Zidovudine (AZT), a nucleoside reverse transcriptase inhibitor.
    4. Ganciclovir (Cytovene), an antiviral.

14. The nurse is caring for clients diagnosed with acquired immunodeficiency syndrome (AIDS). Which action by the unlicensed assistive personnel (UAP) warrants immediate action by the nurse?
    1. The UAP uses nonsterile gloves to empty the client's urinal.
    2. The UAP is taking a glass of grapefruit juice to the client.
    3. The UAP provides a tube of moisture barrier cream to a client.
    4. The UAP fills the client's water pitcher with ice and water.

15. The client diagnosed with acquired immunodeficiency syndrome (AIDS) is prescribed a combination of a protease inhibitor, a non-nucleoside reverse transcriptase inhibitor, and two nucleoside reverse transcriptase inhibitors. Which statement best describes the scientific rationale for combining these medications?
    1. The combination prevents or delays the client's complications from HIV infection.
    2. Multiple medications are needed to eradicate all of the HIV infection.
    3. The combination of medications is less expensive than hospitalization for HIV.
    4. Protease inhibitors counteract the side effects of the other medications.

16. The home health nurse is caring for a client diagnosed with HIV infection. Which data suggest the need for prophylaxis with trimethoprim sulfa (Bactrim)?
    1. The client has a positive HIV viral load.
    2. The client's white blood cell count is 5000/mm^3.
    3. The client has a hacking cough and dyspnea.
    4. The client's CD4 count is less than 300/mm^3.

17. The client diagnosed with AIDS is to receive an initial dose of amphotericin B (Fungizone), an antifungal agent. Which intervention should the nurse implement first?
    1. Administer IVPB in 500 mL of D$_5$W over 6 hours.
    2. Administer Demerol 25 mg IVP over 5 minutes.
    3. Administer a test dose of 1 mg over 20 minutes.
    4. Administer acetaminophen (Tylenol) 650 mg orally.

18. The client diagnosed with AIDS and cytomegalovirus retinitis is prescribed the antiviral agent ganciclovir (Cytovene). Which information about the medication should the home health nurse discuss with the client?
    1. The client will have to take the medication for the rest of his or her life.
    2. The client will take the medication for 1 week each month.
    3. The medication should infuse over 1 hour every day.
    4. The medication can run simultaneously with the client's TPN.

19. The client diagnosed with AIDS has a positive skin test for tuberculosis. Which medication order would the nurse anticipate?
    1. Fluconazole (Diflucan), an antifungal.
    2. Ethambutol (Myambutol), an anti-infective.
    3. Acyclovir (Zovirax), an antiviral.
    4. Enfuvirtide (Fuzeon), an HIV fusion inhibitor.

20. The intensive care nurse is preparing to administer trimetrexate (Neutrexin) to a client diagnosed with AIDS and *Pneumocystis carinii* pneumonia (PCP). Which intervention is the most important safety consideration for the nurse?
    1. Administer IV via gravity infusion.
    2. Administer concurrently with leucovorin.
    3. Monitor the client's complete blood count.
    4. Monitor the client's liver enzymes.

A Client with Allergies

21. The client with allergies is prescribed diphenhydramine (Benadryl), an antihistamine. Which statement indicates the client understands the teaching concerning this medication?
    1. "If I get any ringing in my ears, I should notify my HCP."
    2. "I will probably get drowsy when I take this medication."
    3. "It is not uncommon to get a buffalo hump or moon face."
    4. "I will have to taper off the medications when I quit taking them."

22. The client has a severe anaphylactic reaction to insect bites. Which priority discharge intervention should the nurse discuss with the client?
    1. Wear an insect repellent on exposed skin.
    2. Keep prescribed antihistamines on their person.
    3. Have an "EpiPen" available at all times.
    4. Wear a MedicAlert identification bracelet.

23. The client with seasonal allergic rhinitis is prescribed fluticasone (Flonase), an intranasal glucocorticosteroid. Which intervention should the nurse implement first?
    1. Instruct the client not to eat licorice.
    2. Explain that this is for short-term use.
    3. Instruct not to use other nasal decongestants.
    4. Assess the nares for excoriation or bleeding.

24. Which client should the nurse question administering the H_1 receptor antagonist fexofenadine (Allegra)?
    1. The client who smokes two packs of cigarettes daily.
    2. The athlete who runs 2 miles every day.
    3. The client diagnosed with an antibiotic allergy.
    4. The client experiencing nasal congestion and sneezing.

25. The client is prescribed clemastine (Tavist), an H_1 receptor antagonist, prophylactically for allergies. Which statement indicates the client needs more teaching concerning this medication?
    1. "I will suck on hard candy if I have a dry mouth."
    2. "I will notify my HCP if I take an over-the-counter medication."
    3. "I will experience some blurred vision when taking Tavist."
    4. "I need to maintain adequate fluid intake when taking this medication."

26. The clinic nurse is discussing over-the-counter (OTC) oxymetazoline (Afrin 12 Hour Nasal Spray), a sympathomimetic, with a client experiencing nasal congestion. Which information should the nurse discuss with the client?
    1. Do not use the Afrin spray any longer than 3–5 days.
    2. Clear the nose immediately after using the nasal spray.
    3. Immediately swallow the postnasal medication residue.
    4. Take additional nasal sprays if congestion is not relieved.

27. The male client taking a nasal glucocorticoid spray calls the clinic nurse and reports that the medication is not helping his condition. Which question should the nurse ask the client first?
    1. "Are you sure you are taking the spray correctly?"
    2. "Did you shake the bottle before taking the spray?"
    3. "What time of the day are you taking the medication?"
    4. "How long have you been using the spray?"

28. Which interventions should the nurse implement for the elderly client receiving antihistamine therapy? Select all that apply.
    1. Auscultate the client's breath sounds.
    2. Assess the client's level of consciousness.
    3. Evaluate the client's intake and output.
    4. Encourage the client to ambulate.
    5. Provide an acid-ash diet for the client.

29. The health-care provider has prescribed the topical steroid hydrocortisone for a client experiencing allergic dermatitis. Which instruction should the nurse discuss with the client?
    1. Wash the inflamed area with soap and water.
    2. Apply an adherent dressing after applying the medication.
    3. Rub the cream into the irritated and inflamed area.
    4. Wash the hands before applying the topical steroid.

30. The nurse administers a dose of an intravenous antibiotic to the client. Twenty minutes later the client is complaining of shortness of breath, itching, and difficulty swallowing. Which action should the nurse implement first?
    1. Prepare to administer subcutaneous epinephrine.
    2. Discontinue the client's intravenous antibiotic.
    3. Assess the client's apical pulse and blood pressure.
    4. Administer 10 liters of oxygen via nasal cannula.

A Client with Rheumatoid Arthritis

31. The client with rheumatoid arthritis is prescribed hydroxychloroquine sulfate (Plaquenil), a disease-modifying antirheumatic drug (DMARD). Which statement indicates the client needs more teaching concerning the medication?
    1. "I will get my eyes checked every 6 months."
    2. "I should not drink alcohol while taking this drug."
    3. "It is important to take this medication with milk."
    4. "I will call my HCP if the pain is not relieved in 2 weeks."

32. The client diagnosed with rheumatoid arthritis is taking the disease-modifying antirheumatic drug (DMARD) leflunomide (Arava). Which comment by the client would warrant intervention by the nurse?
    1. "I have noticed that I am starting to lose my hair."
    2. "I sometimes get dizzy and drowsy."
    3. "My spouse and I are trying to start a family."
    4. "I will not get any vaccines while taking this medication."

33. Which instruction should the nurse discuss with the client diagnosed with rheumatoid arthritis who is prescribed methotrexate, a disease-modifying antirheumatic drug (DMARD)?
    1. Use a soft-bristled toothbrush when brushing teeth.
    2. Wear warm clothes when it is less than 40°F.
    3. Gargle with mouthwash at least four times a day.
    4. Use a sunscreen with an SPF 15 or lower when outside.

34. The client with rheumatoid arthritis is taking phenylbutazone (Butazolidin), a pyrazoline nonsteroidal anti-inflammatory drug (NSAID). Which statement would make the nurse question administering this medication?
    1. "I have had a sore throat and fever the last few days."
    2. "I have not had a bowel movement in more than 3 days."
    3. "I can't believe I have gained 3 pounds in the last month."
    4. "I have been having trouble sleeping at night."

35. The client with rheumatoid arthritis has been taking methotrexate, a disease-modifying antirheumatic drug (DMARD), for 2 weeks. Which laboratory data would warrant intervention by the nurse?
    1. A serum creatinine level of 0.9 mg/dL.
    2. A red blood cell count of 2.5 million/mm.
    3. A white blood cell count of 9000 mm.
    4. A hemoglobin of 14.5 g/dL and hematocrit of 43%.

36. Which assessment data would the nurse expect for the client with rheumatoid arthritis who is taking sulfasalazine (Azulfidine), an antirheumatic medication?
    1. Orange or yellowish discoloration of the urine.
    2. Ulcers and irritation of the mouth.
    3. Ecchymosis of the lower extremities.
    4. A red, raised skin rash over the back.

37. The client recently diagnosed with rheumatoid arthritis is prescribed 4 grams of aspirin daily. Which statement indicates the client needs more teaching concerning the medication?
    1. "I will decrease my dose for a few days if my ears start ringing."
    2. "I should take my aspirin with meals, food, milk, or antacids."
    3. "I need to take the entire aspirin dose at night before going to bed."
    4. "If I have any stomach upset, I will take enteric-coated aspirin."

38. The client with rheumatoid arthritis is prescribed prednisone, a glucocorticoid, for an acute episode of pain. The client asks the nurse, "Why can't I be on this forever since it helps the pain so much?" Which statement would be the nurse's best response?
    1. "The medication will cause you to have a buffalo hump or moon face."
    2. "The medication has long-term side effects, such as osteoporosis."
    3. "If you continue taking the medication, it may cause an Addisonian crisis."
    4. "There are other medications that can be prescribed to help the pain."

39. The client with rheumatoid arthritis is prescribed capsaicin (Zostrix), a topical analgesic. Which information should the nurse discuss with the client?
    1. Apply the cream as needed for severe arthritic pain.
    2. Notify the HCP if burning of the skin occurs after application.
    3. It may take up to 3 months for the medication to become effective.
    4. Rub the cream into skin until no cream is left on the surface.

40. The client with rheumatoid arthritis is taking etodolac (Lodine), a nonsteroidal anti-inflammatory drug (NSAID). The client is complaining of a headache. Which action should the nurse implement?
    1. Administer two aspirins to the client.
    2. Administer an additional dose of Lodine.
    3. Administer one oral narcotic analgesic.
    4. Administer two acetaminophen (Tylenol).

A Child Receiving Immunizations

41. The nurse in the pediatrician's office is recording a child's immunizations. Which information is the nurse required to document?
    1. The vaccinations that the client should have received.
    2. Centers for Disease Control Guidelines for the client.
    3. The vaccination type, manufacturer, and lot number.
    4. The date the next required vaccination should be administered.

42. The mother of a child scheduled to receive a measles, mumps, and rubella vaccination asks the nurse, "What could happen to my child if I don't let you give the vaccination?" Which statement is the nurse's best response?
    1. "If your child gets one of the diseases, it could lead to serious complications."
    2. "Your child will not be allowed to attend any public school in the country."
    3. "Nothing can happen to you or the child if you don't get the vaccination."
    4. "You sound worried. Have you heard of problems associated with the shot?"

43. The parent of a child who received an immunization for varicella earlier in the day calls the clinic and tells the nurse that the child now has chickenpox because the child has a fever of 101°F. Which statement is the nurse's best response?
    1. "You signed a permit knowing this might happen as a result."
    2. "You need to take the child to the emergency department now."
    3. "Has the child been exposed to any illness recently?"
    4. "This is a reaction to the injection, but it is not chickenpox."

44. To which client would the nurse question administering a live virus vaccine?
    1. The child who is afraid of needles and health-care personnel.
    2. The child who lives with a grandparent undergoing chemotherapy.
    3. The child who has not received an immunization previously.
    4. The child whose parent's religion is Jehovah's Witness.

45. The nurse is preparing to administer measles, mumps, and rubella vaccinations to a 15-month-old child. Which description is the correct administration procedure?
    1. Inject the medication into the dorsogluteal muscle.
    2. Use the deltoid muscle for the injection.
    3. Administer the medication into the vastus lateralis muscle.
    4. Give subcutaneously in the abdomen.

46. At which age is it considered safe to administer the hepatitis B vaccine?
    1. At birth.
    2. At age 12 months.
    3. At age 6 years.
    4. At age 18 years.

47. The clinic nurse is discussing immunizations with the parent of a male child diagnosed with Type 1 diabetes mellitus. Which information should the nurse teach the client?
    1. The child should not receive immunizations because of the diabetes.
    2. The child is at greater risk of complications from immunizations.
    3. The child will not mind the injections because he is used to them.
    4. The child should receive a flu vaccination every year.

48. The 14-year-old adolescent has not received the varicella vaccine, and the HCP cannot determine that the teen has ever had chickenpox. Which statement indicates the correct administration procedures?
    1. Administer the single-dose injection as soon as possible.
    2. Administer two injections at least 4 weeks apart.
    3. Administer a series of three injections over 6 months.
    4. Do not administer the vaccine because by age 13 the client is considered immune to varicella.

49. The parent of a child about to receive the intramuscular polio vaccine, inactivated poliovirus vaccine (IPV), asks the nurse "Why can't my child get the oral vaccine like I took when I was a child?" Which statement by the nurse is the best explanation to give the client?
    1. "I don't know why, but the manufacturer has stopped making the oral drug."
    2. "There were some cases of polio that developed from the oral vaccine."
    3. "I will check with your health-care provider and see about changing the order."
    4. "The intramuscular route is more effective in preventing polio than the oral route."

50. The clinic nurse has administered several recommended vaccinations to a 2-month-old infant. Which discharge instructions should the nurse give to the parents?
    1. Notify the health-care provider if the infant develops a low-grade fever.
    2. Use a humidifier in the infant's room to reduce congestion.
    3. Give the infant the prescribed amount of acetaminophen for comfort.
    4. Keep the infant in the parents' room at night for a few days.

A Client with an Autoimmune Disease

1. 1. Atropine works in an opposite manner from the cholinesterase inhibitors administered to treat myasthenia gravis, but atropine in small doses is prescribed to reduce the gastrointestinal side effects of the cholinesterase inhibitor. The nurse would not question this medication.
   2. The antimalarial medications are prescribed to treat cutaneous lupus erythematosus. The nurse would not question this medication.
   3. The client diagnosed with polymyalgia rheumatica must take the prescribed steroid medication or he or she can become blind. The nurse would not question this medication.
   4. **Mestinon is prescribed to increase the available amount of acetylcholine for muscle movement. A client in a cholinergic crisis has too much medication on board. The nurse would question administering this medication until the crisis is resolved.**

2. 1. There is no cure for SLE. The goal of treatment is to prevent or minimize damage to the internal organs.
   2. The goal is not death, but to assist the client to live as full a life as possible.
   3. The medication may have a side effect of weight gain, but this is not the desired result.
   4. **The goal of high-dose steroids during an exacerbation is to decrease the inflammatory response in the internal organs and prevent permanent damage.**

3. 1. This may be asked, but it is not the most important question.
   2. **This is the most important question. The client reports the pain and stiffness on awakening in the morning. Taking NSAIDs then places the client at risk for developing peptic ulcer disease. The client should be taught to take these medications with food.**
   3. NSAID medications are frequently taken by female clients to relieve menstrual cramps. This is not the most important question.
   4. This is the reason the client is taking the medication. NSAIDs are used to treat the pain and stiffness, but they are also helpful in decreasing the inflammation associated with SLE and in allowing a reduction in the dosage of steroids.

4. 5, 2, 3, 1, 4
   5. The nurse must determine that the "right" medication is being administered to the "right" client. This is the first step.
   2. The nurse should assess the intravenous catheter placement prior to administering the medication. If there is a blood return, the catheter is in the vein.
   3. The nurse should flush the saline lock with 2 mL of sterile saline before administering the medication to make sure that any previously administered medication is flushed from the line to avoid inadvertent mixing of medications.
   1. Solu-Cortef can be administered safely over 1–2 minutes.
   4. The final step is to flush the saline lock to make sure the client receives all the prescribed medication.

5. 1. There is no serum baclofen level.
   2. Baclofen can cause urinary urgency, but the client does not have to monitor urinary output.
   3. **Baclofen is administered to treat the spasticity associated with MS. The nurse should assess for muscle spasticity, rigidity, movement, and pain to determine the effectiveness of the medication.**
   4. The medication can affect the liver, but it does not damage the kidneys.

6. 1. **This medication must be administered exactly on time to maintain muscle movement and ability to swallow in clients diagnosed with MG. This is the priority medication.**
   2. This medication can be administered within the 30-minute acceptable time frame.
   3. A pain medication is a priority but not over prevention of aspiration and maintaining the client's ability to use the muscles of respiration.
   4. Etanercept (Enbrel) can be administered within the 30-minute acceptable time frame.

7. 1. Tensilon is used to help diagnose MG and to determine if a client diagnosed with MG is in a cholinergic versus a myasthenic crisis. A client losing the ability to breathe without mechanical support when given Tensilon is in a cholinergic crisis in which too much medication is in the body.
   2. **This response is the response that is diagnostic of myasthenia gravis.**

3. This is a nonpharmacologic test that can be performed to assess for MG. This is a positive finding, but it does not apply to edrophonium.

4. An unlabeled use for edrophonium is to terminate paroxysmal atrial tachycardia, but this does not diagnose MG.

8. 1. There are four phases of gout. Phase 1 is asymptomatic hyperuricemia; phase 2 is acute gouty arthritis; phase 3 is intercritical gout; and phase 4 is chronic tophaceous gout. Being asymptomatic after an acute attack indicates the client is in phase 3, intercritical gout; it does not indicate that the medication is effective.

2. Zyloprim does not cause an aversion reaction to alcohol. The client should be instructed not to consume alcoholic beverages because alcohol can induce an attack.

3. **The main problem in gout is hyperuricemia. A normal value indicates a suppression of the production of uric acid by the body and that the medication is effective.**

4. Tophi are accumulations of sodium urate crystals, which are deposited in peripheral areas of the body. The presence of tophi indicates the medication is not effective.

MEDICATION MEMORY JOGGER: The nurse determines the effectiveness of a medication by assessing for the symptoms, or lack thereof, for which the medication was prescribed.

9. 1. The nurse should not tell the client to decrease the dose of medication. Achieving the correct dose is extremely difficult and may require frequent modification, especially when the client is under stress or has an illness. Only the HCP should advise the client about the correct dose.

2. Holding the medication could result in respiratory compromise. The nurse should teach the client how to minimize the side effects of the medication.

3. **The nurse should teach the client how to minimize the side effects of the medication. Taking the medication with milk or crackers will reduce the gastrointestinal effects. The HCP can prescribe small doses of atropine to counteract the side effects if this suggestion is not successful, but the client must take the medication.**

4. The client does not need an over-the-counter medication to counteract the side effect of nausea.

10. 1. These symptoms are not part of schizophrenia and should be investigated.

2. The hallucinations the client has are not part of actual physical symptoms. Further investigation is needed to determine if the client is having a reaction to the medication.

3. **This is the best response by the nurse. These are symptoms of drug-induced systemic lupus erythematosus. The nurse should make sure the client is seen by the HCP.**

4. The nurse should not tell the client that he or she would no longer be able to take medications to control the symptoms of schizophrenia. The Thorazine may need to be changed to a different medication. Medication compliance in clients with psychiatric illnesses can be poor. This statement would give the client a reason not to take any medication.

A Client with Acquired Immunodeficiency Syndrome

11. 1. If the client does not have insurance to help pay for the medications, the client may have trouble complying with the regimen. The current regimens include four or more daily medications costing upwards of $6000 per drug per year.

2. Currently AIDS cannot be managed without the use of medications. With the medications, it is possible to reduce the viral load to undetectable in serum samples.

3. Many over-the-counter medications and herbs interact with the medications used to treat AIDS. The nurse should assess each over-the-counter preparation taken by the client but should not encourage their use.

4. One multiple vitamin is usually sufficient. The body excretes any water-soluble vitamin that is not needed.

MEDICATION MEMORY JOGGER: Some herbal preparations are effective, some are not, and a few can be harmful or even deadly. If a client is taking an herbal supplement and a conventional medicine, the nurse should investigate to determine

if the combination will cause harm to the client. The nurse should always be the client's advocate.

12. 1. These medications treat actual infections and are sometimes administered prophylactically, but they will not prevent conversion to HIV-positive status.
    2. **The combination of specific medications depends on the health-care facility's protocol, but most include a combination of two nucleoside reverse transcriptase inhibitors and a protease inhibitor. The Centers for Disease Control and Prevention has a hotline that can be accessed for specific recommendations (800-458-5231 or www.cdc.gov).**
    3. Single-agent therapy is not recommended because of the speed at which the virus can mutate.
    4. There are medications that can possibly prevent conversion to HIV-positive status.

13. 1. Sustiva is not approved for prevention of transmission of HIV in pregnant women.
    2. Kaletra is not approved for prevention of transmission of HIV to the fetus.
    3. **Although AZT is a pregnancy category C drug, research has proved that taking the drug during pregnancy reduces the risk of maternal-to-fetal transmission of the HIV virus by almost 70%. This is the only medication approved for this purpose.**
    4. Ganciclovir is not approved for prevention of transmission of HIV to the fetus.

14. 1. This is standard precaution and does not require intervention by the nurse.
    2. **Many of the protease inhibitors used to treat AIDS interact with grapefruit juice. The nurse should stop the UAP until the nurse can determine if the client is receiving a medication that would interact with the grapefruit juice.**
    3. The client can apply his or her own moisture barrier protection cream. This does not warrant immediate intervention by the nurse.
    4. This is a comfort measure and does not warrant intervention by the nurse.

MEDICATION MEMORY JOGGER: Grapefruit juice can inhibit the metabolism of certain medications. Specifically, grapefruit juice inhibits cytochrome P450-3A4 found in the liver and the intestinal wall.

The nurse should investigate any medications the client is taking if the client drinks grapefruit juice.

15. 1. **The current treatment is a combination of HAART (highly active antiretroviral therapy) medications. These medications can decrease HIV detectable levels with current technology. They are not a cure, are expensive, and have serious side effects, but the mortality rate from AIDS has decreased 70% with this therapy.**
    2. The problem with a retrovirus is that it does not die until the host dies. The medications delay the onset of problems. There is no cure for an HIV infection.
    3. The medications can cost $24,000–$30,000 per year, and hospitalization would be more expensive, but this is not the reason for the medications to be prescribed.
    4. Protease inhibitors have their own side effects and can complicate the side effects from the other medications.

16. 1. The client who is HIV positive could be expected to have a positive viral load. This is a reason to institute HAART (highly active antiretroviral therapy) but not Bactrim.
    2. This is a normal WBC count and is not a reason to start a prophylactic antibiotic.
    3. This client is showing symptoms of *Pneumocystis carinii* pneumonia (PCP); any treatment now would not be prophylactic.
    4. **The client with a CD4 count of less than 300/mm³ is at risk for developing *Pneumocystis carinii* pneumonia (PCP). Bactrim is prophylaxis for PCP. Normal levels for CD4 are 450–1400/mm³.**

17. 1. The medication should be administered daily over 6 hours but not before the nurse knows the client will not have a reaction to the medication. Amphotericin B is compatible only with D_5W.
    2. Demerol is used as a premedication to prevent an extrapyramidal reaction.
    3. **The first action by the nurse is to administer a small test dose of Fungizone to assess for the client's potential response.**
    4. This is done to prevent a febrile reaction to the medication.

18. 1. Before HAART (highly active antiretroviral therapy), the client would have had to continue taking ganciclovir for the rest of

his or her life to prevent blindness; now with HAART, however, the CD4 counts are able to rebound and the client usually only needs to take the medication for 3–6 months.

2. This is not the regimen for ganciclovir. It is administered daily.

3. **Initial therapy is intravenous and care must be taken not to infuse the medication too rapidly. The infusion should be administered on a pump over 1 hour.**

4. The medication is incompatible with TPN.

MEDICATION MEMORY JOGGER: Nothing should run in the same line as TPN. This is an infection-control issue.

19. 1. Diflucan treats fungal infections, and Mycobacterium avium complex (tuberculosis) is a bacterium.

2. **Ethambutol is a treatment for tuberculosis.**

3. Zovirax treats viral infections, and the causative agent for tuberculosis is a bacterium.

4. This is the newest classification of drugs used to treat HIV viral infections, but it is effective against viruses, not bacteria.

20. 1. The medication should infuse over 60–90 minutes, and for best control, the infusion should be placed on an infusion pump.

2. **Leucovorin is the "rescue factor" to prevent an adverse reaction to the Neutrexin. The nurse should have both medications infusing simultaneously.**

3. The medication can cause myelosuppression and the CBC should be monitored, but this is not the most important consideration for the nurse.

4. The medication can cause a transient elevation in the client's liver enzymes, but this is not the most important consideration for the nurse.

A Client with Allergies

21. 1. Tinnitus (ringing in the ears) is not a side effect of antihistamines; tinnitus usually occurs with aspirin toxicity.

2. **Antihistamines cause drowsiness; therefore, the client should avoid driving or engaging in hazardous activities.**

3. A buffalo hump and moon face are side effects of glucocorticoids, not of antihistamines.

4. Benadryl does not require tapering when discontinuing the medication.

22. 1. Wearing insect repellent is an appropriate intervention, but if the client has an insect bite, the repellent will not help prevent anaphylaxis. Therefore, this is not the priority intervention.

2. Antihistamines are used in clients with anaphylaxis, but it takes at least 30 minutes for the medication to work, and if the client has an insect bite, it is not the priority medication.

3. **Clients with documented severe anaphylaxis should carry an EpiPen, which is a prescribed injectable device containing epinephrine that the client can administer to himself or herself in case of an insect bite. This will save the client's life; therefore, this is the priority intervention.**

4. The client should wear an identification bracelet stating the allergy, but it will not help the client if he or she is bitten by an insect; therefore, it is not the priority intervention.

23. 1. Glucocorticoid intranasal spray should be used with caution in clients taking herbal supplements such as licorice, which may potentiate the effects of glucocorticoids, but this is not the first intervention the nurse should implement.

2. Therapy usually begins with two sprays in each nostril twice a day and then decreases to one dose per day for a specific period. The nurse should educate the client, but this is not the first intervention.

3. Concomitant use of a local nasal decongestant spray may increase the risk of nasal irritation or bleeding. Both sprays may be used together for a client with chronic rhinitis but not for seasonal allergies. The nurse should educate the client, but this is not the first intervention.

4. **The nurse must first assess the client's nares because broken mucous membranes allow direct access to the bloodstream, increasing the likelihood of systemic effects of the drug. Therefore, this is the first intervention the nurse should implement. The HCP may not prescribe the medication if nasal excoriation or bleeding is present.**

MEDICATION MEMORY JOGGER: Some herbal preparations are effective, some are not, and a few can be harmful or even

deadly. If a client is taking an herbal supplement and a conventional medicine, the nurse should investigate to determine if the combination will cause harm to the client. The nurse should always be the client's advocate.

24. 1. **Allegra is contraindicated in clients with asthma and in clients who use nicotine because of its anticholinergic effects on the respiratory system.**
2. There are no contraindications for use of H$_1$ receptor antagonist in clients who run daily; therefore, the nurse would not question administering this medication.
3. There are no contraindications for H$_1$ receptor antagonist in clients with antibiotic allergies; therefore, the nurse would not question administering this medication.
4. Allegra is prescribed prophylactically in clients with nasal sneezing and tearing of the eye; therefore, the nurse would not question administering this medication.

25. 1. This medication has anticholinergic effects; therefore, a dry mouth is an expected side effect and sucking on hard candy will help relieve the dry mouth. This statement indicates the client understands the teaching.
2. The client is at risk for anticholinergic crisis and should notify the HCP or pharmacist of taking an H$_1$ receptor antagonist. This statement indicates the client understands the teaching.
3. **The client should be aware of signs or symptoms of an anticholinergic crisis such as blurred vision, confusion, difficulty swallowing, and fever or flushing. This statement indicates the client needs more teaching concerning this medication.**
4. This medication has anticholinergic effects and the client should maintain adequate fluid intake to help prevent dehydration. This statement indicates the client understands the teaching.

26. 1. **Prolonged use of sympathomimetic nasal sprays causes hypersecretion of mucus and nasal congestion to worsen once the drug effects wear off. This sometimes leads to a cycle of increased drug use, as the condition worsens. This rebound congestion is why it should not be used for more than 3–5 days.**
2. The client should avoid clearing the nose immediately after spraying so that the medication can stay in the nares.
3. The postnasal medication should be spit out, not swallowed.
4. The medication should be administered exactly as prescribed; additional dosing will not speed relief of the nasal congestion.

27. 1. This is an appropriate question, but it is not the first question the nurse should ask the client.
2. The spray bottle should be shaken thoroughly, but this is not the first question the nurse should ask the client.
3. The client should take the medication as prescribed, but this is not the first question the nurse should ask the client.
4. **The medication may take 2 to 4 weeks to be effective. Therefore, the nurse should first determine how long the client has been taking the medication.**

28. 1. **Anticholinergic effects of antihistamines may trigger bronchospasms; therefore, the nurse should assess for wheezing or difficulty breathing.**
2. **Elderly clients are at an increased risk of increased sedation and other anticholinergic effects; therefore, the nurse should assess the level of consciousness.**
3. **Antihistamines promote urinary retention, and the nurse should ensure adequate intake and output.**
4. Antihistamines cause drowsiness; therefore, the nurse should institute safety and fall precautions and not encourage the client to ambulate without assistance.
5. There are no dietary precautions for clients taking antihistamines.

29. 1. The area should be washed with warm water before applying the cream; instruct the client not to use soap, which could further irritate the area.
2. The area should be left open after the medication is applied. An adherent dressing may stick to the area and cause further irritation of the affected area.
3. The cream should be applied gently to the inflamed area; it should not be rubbed into the area.
4. **The client should have clean hands before applying the cream to the affected area to help prevent infection.**

30. 1. The drug of choice for an anaphylactic reaction is epinephrine (Adrenalin) administered subcutaneously, but it is not the first intervention.
   2. **The nurse should realize that the client is having an allergic reaction to the intravenous antibiotic and immediately discontinue the medication. This is the nurse's first intervention.**
   3. The nurse should not take time to assess the client when it is apparent the client is having an allergic reaction to the antibiotic.
   4. Oxygen should be applied, but it is not the nurse's first intervention in this situation. The antibiotic that is causing the anaphylactic reaction should be discontinued first.

A Client with Rheumatoid Arthritis

31. 1. Plaquenil can cause pigmentary retinitis and vision loss so the client should have a thorough vision examination every 6 months. The client does not need more teaching.
   2. Plaquenil may increase the risk of liver toxicity when administered with hepatotoxic drugs; therefore, alcohol use should be eliminated during therapy. The client does not need more teaching.
   3. The medication should be taken with milk to decrease gastrointestinal upset. The client does not need more teaching.
   4. **The medication takes 3–6 months to achieve the desired response, and many clients do not experience significant benefits.**

   MEDICATION MEMORY JOGGER: Drinking alcohol is always discouraged when taking any prescribed or over-the-counter medication because of potential adverse interactions. The nurse should encourage the client not to drink alcoholic beverages.

32. 1. Alopecia is a common side effect of Arava. This should be discussed with the client before starting the medication, and methods of coping with hair loss should be explored. This comment would not warrant intervention by the nurse.
   2. This medication causes dizziness; therefore, this comment would not warrant intervention by the nurse.
   3. **This medication is teratogenic. Women must undergo the drug-elimination**

procedure and men must take 8 grams of cholestyramine three times daily for 11 days to minimize any possible risk of harm to the fetus his partner is carrying.
   4. The client should avoid vaccinations with live vaccines during and following therapy; therefore, this comment does not require nursing intervention.

33. 1. **Methotrexate causes bone marrow depression, which may lead to abnormal bleeding. Therefore, the client should use a soft-bristled toothbrush.**
   2. Methotrexate has no effect on the client's response to cold weather.
   3. The client is at risk for mouth ulcers and should not use any type of commercially available mouthwash. The client should rinse the mouth with water after eating and drinking.
   4. Methotrexate may increase the sensitivity of the skin to sunlight. The client should use a sunscreen of SPF 30 or higher and wear protective clothing when exposure to the sun is unavoidable.

34. 1. **The most dangerous adverse reaction to this classification of medication is blood dyscrasias, which are manifested in the client by flulike symptoms.**
   2. Constipation is not a side effect of Butazolidin. The nurse would not question administering the medication.
   3. Weight gain is not a side effect of Butazolidin. The nurse would not question administering the medication.
   4. Insomnia is not a side effect of Butazolidin. The nurse would not question administering the medication.

   MEDICATION MEMORY JOGGER: Usually if a client is prescribed a new medication and has flulike symptoms within 24 hours of taking the first dose, the client should contact the HCP. These are signs of agranulocytosis, which indicates the medication has caused a sudden drop in the white blood cell count, leaving the body defenseless against bacterial invasion.

35. 1. This is within the normal range of 0.5 to 1.5 mg/dL for serum creatinine
   2. **This RBC count indicates thrombocytopenia, which would warrant intervention by the nurse. The normal RBC is 4.6 to 6.0 million/mm for men and 4.0 to 5.0 million/mm for women.**

3. The white blood cell count is within the normal range of 4500/mm to 10,000/mm.
4. These are within the normal range—hemoglobin (Hgb) 13.5 to 18 g/dL in males and 12 to 16 g/dL in females, and hematocrit (Hct) 40% to 54% in males and 36% to 46% in females.

36. 1. **Azulfidine may cause an orange or yellowish discoloration of urine and the skin; this is expected and is not significant.**
2. Stomatitis is not an expected side effect of Azulfidine, and the HCP should be notified.
3. Ecchymosis (unexplained bleeding) is not an expected side effect of Azulfidine, and the HCP should be notified.
4. A rash is not an expected side effect, and the HCP should be notified.

37. 1. This dose of aspirin is just less than the toxic dose that produces tinnitus and hearing loss, but this is the dose needed to treat RA. The client should reduce the dose by two to three tablets per day until the tinnitus resolves. This statement indicates the client does not need more teaching.
2. Gastrointestinal side effects are common with aspirin therapy; therefore, the client should take aspirin with food. This statement indicates the client does not need more teaching.
3. **The aspirin should be taken in divided doses (three to four 325-mg tablets four times a day). This statement indicates the client needs more teaching.**
4. Enteric-coated aspirin produces less gastric distress than plain buffered aspirin. The client's statement does not need more teaching.

38. 1. A buffalo hump and moon face are expected side effects, are not life threatening, and would not be a problem if the client took the medication forever. These side effects affect body image, but most individuals in severe pain would rather have body-image problems than pain.
2. **Prednisone has serious long-term side effects that can lead to possible life-threatening complications. Therefore, the client cannot take prednisone forever.**
3. An Addisonian crisis (adrenal insufficiency) is a complication that may occur

when the patient stops the medication abruptly but not if it is tapered off.
4. This response does not answer the client's question; therefore, it is not the best response.

39. 1. Pain relief lasts only as long as the topical analgesic is applied regularly, not as needed (PRN).
2. Transient burning may occur with application if applied fewer than three to four times daily; burning usually disappears after a few days but may continue for 2–4 weeks or longer.
3. If the pain persists longer than 1 month, the client should discontinue the cream and notify the HCP.
4. **The cream should be rubbed into the skin until little or no cream is left on the surface of the skin. The hands should be washed immediately after the cream is applied to the skin.**

40. 1. The client should not take aspirin, an NSAID, while taking another NSAID.
2. The client should not receive an additional dose of a routine medication that is being administered for treatment of rheumatoid arthritis.
3. The nurse should administer a nonnarcotic analgesic for a headache, not a narcotic.
4. **Acetaminophen, a nonnarcotic analgesic, would be the most appropriate medication to give the client who is experiencing a headache and is taking an NSAID.**

A Child Receiving Immunizations

41. 1. This may be important information to give to the parent, but it is not the legal requirement for documentation of immunizations.
2. This may be important information to give to the parent, but it is not the legal requirement for documentation of immunizations.
3. **The National Childhood Vaccine Act of 1986 requires that a permanent record of the vaccinations a child receives be maintained. The required information is date of the vaccination; route and site of the vaccination; vaccine type, manufacturer, lot number, and expiration date; and the**

name, address, and title of the person administering the vaccination.

   4. This may be important information to give to the parent, but it is not the legal requirement for documentation of immunizations.

42. 1. **Potential complications of measles include blindness and deafness. Potential complications of mumps include aseptic meningitis; for adolescent and adult males, orchitis is another complication. Potential complications for rubella include arthritis in women and birth defects or miscarriage for pregnant women.**
   2. The public school system encourages all children to be immunized according to the Centers for Disease Control and Prevention guidelines, but there are exceptions. The nurse should know the requirements for the state where the nurse is practicing.
   3. Immunizations prevent many illnesses.
   4. This parent is asking for information, not a therapeutic conversation.

MEDICATION MEMORY JOGGER: The nurse must be knowledgeable of accepted standards of practice for disease processes and conditions. If the nurse administers a medication the health-care provider has prescribed and it harms the client, the nurse could be held accountable. The nurse is a client advocate and should provide honest information to the client.

43. 1. The parent may have allowed the immunization to take place, but a specific signed permission is not needed.
   2. The nurse should teach the parent how to care for the child, not send the child to the emergency department.
   3. The problem is probably related to the immunization, not a secondary infection.
   4. **The varicella vaccine can cause a fever spike to 102°F, a mild rash with a few lesions, and pain and redness at the injection site. The nurse should tell the parents how to care for the child.**

44. 1. Most children are afraid of being hurt by the injections, but this is not a reason to question administering the injection.
   2. **The child will shed the vaccine in the urine and feces. The grandparent is immunocompromised as a result of the chemotherapy and could become ill. This child should receive an inactivated**

vaccine. The nurse should question this vaccine.

   3. This is a reason to give the vaccine, not question it.
   4. Jehovah's Witnesses do not refuse vaccinations because of religious beliefs.

45. 1. This is not a safe administration site for a 15-month-old child.
   2. This is not the best site for a toddler.
   3. **Infants and toddlers should receive intramuscular injections in the vastus lateralis muscle, the large muscle of the thigh. This muscle is large and away from any nerves that could be damaged by the injection.**
   4. The immunizations are given intramuscularly, not subcutaneously.

46. 1. **Infants born to mothers who are positive for hepatitis B surface antigen (HBsAg) should receive hepatitis B immunization within 12 hours of birth. All infants should receive the vaccine prior to discharge, but they may receive the first dose at any time before 2 months old.**
   2. The injection series should be started by age 2 months.
   3. The injection series should be started by age 2 months.
   4. The injection series should be started by age 2 months.

47. 1. The child has a chronic disease, and it is very important for the child to receive all immunizations.
   2. The child is at greater risk of complications of the illnesses the immunizations prevent because of the diabetes. The child should receive all recommended immunizations.
   3. The child does not "get used" to the needles, and the child likely will mind the injections.
   4. **Children with chronic illnesses are encouraged to receive a yearly flu vaccine.**

48. 1. The injection should be administered, but a single injection is not sufficient for this age child.
   2. **The correct procedure for a child age 13 or older is to administer two injections at least 4 weeks apart.**
   3. Two injections are recommended. Three injections are the recommended schedule for hepatitis B.
   4. Adults can become ill with varicella.

49. 1. The nurse should be aware of important information regarding the medications being administered so that the nurse can inform the clients.
2. **The manufacture of the oral vaccine has been discontinued because several children developed polio from the live virus. The intramuscular vaccine is the only vaccine available. It is an inactivated form of the virus.**
3. There is no reason to ask the HCP for a change of order.
4. Both vaccines prevented polio, but the oral route also caused polio in some children.

50. 1. The nurse should inform the parents to expect a fever as a side effect of the vaccination; the nurse should not have the parents call the HCP.
2. Vaccinations should not cause congestion; therefore, a humidifier is not needed.
3. **Acetaminophen is the treatment to manage the side effects of sore injection site and fever.**
4. The parents do not have to keep the infant in their room.

1. The client presents to the clinic reporting that his girlfriend was diagnosed with hepatitis B yesterday. The client asks the nurse, "Can you give me something so that I won't get hepatitis?" Which statement is the nurse's best response?
   1. "You should take 500 mg of over-the-counter vitamin C every day."
   2. "You need to have the hepatitis B vaccine injections starting today."
   3. "At this time, there is no treatment to make sure you don't get hepatitis."
   4. "You need to receive an injection of gamma globulin IM today."

2. The male 4-year-child is prescribed prednisolone (Pediapred), a glucocorticoid, for juvenile arthritis. Which statement by the child's mother would warrant immediate intervention?
   1. "My child is current with all the required immunizations."
   2. "I can crush the tablet and put it in some of his favorite pudding."
   3. "My 2-year-old daughter is at home with chickenpox."
   4. "I need to notify my HCP if my son's temperature is higher than 100°F."

3. The client diagnosed with AIDS is receiving intravenous acyclovir (Cytogenesis), an antiviral medication. Which intervention should the home health-care nurse implement when administering this medication?
   1. Restrict all visitors when administering this medication.
   2. Arrange for IV tubing and bag to be incinerated
   3. Store reconstituted solutions at room temperature.
   4. Have the pharmacy mix the medication for 1 week at a time.

4. The client diagnosed with AIDS has a pruritic rash with pinkish–red macules. Which medication would the nurse suspect is causing the rash?
   1. The antibiotic trimethoprim–sulfamethoxazole (Bactrim).
   2. The antiretroviral medication nelfinavir (Viracept).
   3. The non-nucleoside reverse transcriptase inhibitor efavirenz (Sustiva).
   4. The nucleoside analog reverse transcriptase inhibitor zidovudine (AZT).

5. The home health-care nurse is reviewing the list of daily medications the client diagnosed with AIDS is prescribed. For which medication would the nurse need further clarification?
   1. The glucocorticoid prednisone (Deltasone).
   2. The selective serotonin reuptake inhibitor fluoxetine (Prozac).
   3. The antiretroviral medication saquinavir (Invirase).
   4. The non-nucleoside reverse transcriptase inhibitor nevirapine (Viramune).

6. The client diagnosed with Guillain-Barré syndrome is complaining of pain. The client has an order for morphine 2 mg IVP. Which interventions should the nurse implement? Rank in order of performance.
   1. Administer the morphine diluted over 5 minutes.
   2. Assess the client's respiratory status.
   3. Check the two identifiers against the MAR.
   4. Sign out the medication as per hospital policy.
   5. Check the last time the morphine was administered.

7. The wife of the client diagnosed with Guillain-Barré (GB) syndrome asks the nurse, "Don't you have something that will cure this disease?" Which statement is the nurse's best response?
   1. "Long-term steroid therapy will help reverse the paralysis."
   2. "High doses of intravenous antibiotics may help cure GB."
   3. "There is no medication known that will cure this disease."
   4. "A medication called Amevive has side effects, but it can cure GB."

8. The client with multiple sclerosis is being treated with the biologic response modifier interferon beta-1a (Avonex). Which diagnostic test would the nurse monitor to determine the effectiveness of the medication?
   1. The cerebrospinal fluid white blood cell count.
   2. The magnetic resonance imaging (MRI) scan.
   3. An electromyogram (EMG).
   4. An electroencephalogram (EEG).

9. The female client diagnosed with multiple sclerosis (MS) tells the nurse, "I am having problems having regular bowel movements." Which statement by the client indicates the client needs more medication teaching?
   1. "I am taking a Dulcolax tablet every day."
   2. "I am taking a fiber laxative daily."
   3. "I take the stool softener Colace at bedtime."
   4. "I keep a glass of water with me at all times."

10. The client has systemic lupus erythematosus and is prescribed azathioprine (Imuran). Which medication teaching should the nurse discuss with the client?
    1. Instruct the client on how to use a glucometer.
    2. Tell the client to come to the office for lab tests.
    3. Explain that low-grade fevers are expected initially.
    4. Discuss the need for recording an accurate urinary output.

11. The client diagnosed with systemic lupus erythematosus is experiencing an acute exacerbation and is prescribed a high dose of intravenous steroid. Which statement by the client indicates the need for further teaching?
    1. "I must take this medication even though I hate the side effects."
    2. "My glucose levels may go up while I am on this medication."
    3. "I will not allow you to administer this medication to me today."
    4. "My appetite increases whenever I am taking steroids."

12. The client diagnosed with rheumatoid arthritis is undergoing long-term therapy with hydroxychloroquine (Plaquenil). Which action by the client indicates compliance with the medication teaching?
    1. The client takes the medication on an empty stomach.
    2. The client drinks at least 3000 mL of water daily.
    3. The client has not had any unexplained weight loss.
    4. The client sees the ophthalmologist every 6 months.

13. The client with rheumatoid arthritis is prescribed the disease-modifying antirheumatic drug (DMARD) methotrexate (Rheumatrex). After 3 days, the client reports that the medication is not working. Which statement is the clinic nurse's best response?
    1. "I will make you an appointment with the health-care provider immediately."
    2. "You are concerned that this medication is not going to work like the other ones."
    3. "Have you lost any more range of motion in your upper extremities?"
    4. "That is normal because it takes 3–6 weeks for the medication to work."

14. The clinic nurse is scheduling the follow-up appointment for the client diagnosed with rheumatoid arthritis who received the initial IM injection of gold salts. When should the nurse schedule the next appointment?
    1. In 7 days.
    2. In 2 weeks.
    3. In 1 month.
    4. In 3 months.

15. The hospital nurse has developed a latex allergy. Which action should the hospital nurse implement?
    1. Investigate working for a home health-care agency.
    2. Wash hands thoroughly instead of wearing gloves.
    3. Request a box of nonlatex gloves from the hospital.
    4. File workers' compensation with the employee health nurse.

16. The mother of an 8-year-old boy brings her son to the clinic, where the child is diagnosed with poison ivy. She is worried about him attending school. Which medication should the nurse recommend to help decrease pruritus while in school?
    1. Aveeno, an oatmeal bath.
    2. Caladryl, a topical antihistamine.
    3. Oral diphenhydramine (Benadryl), an H_1 antagonist.
    4. Polymyxin, an antibiotic ointment.

17. The 16-year-old female who is sexually active is being seen in the clinic for a Pap test. She has requested to receive Gardasil, a vaccine for human papillomavirus. Which information should the nurse discuss with the client?
    1. "You must ask your parents if you can take this medication."
    2. "The medication is administered in a series of injections."
    3. "Gardasil will guarantee you won't get cervical cancer."
    4. "This medication must be taken for the rest of your life."

18. The nurse is preparing to administer the morning medications to the client who is 1-day postoperative total knee replacement. Which medication would the nurse question administering?
    1. Ceftriaxone (Rocephin), a broad-spectrum antibiotic.
    2. Enoxaparin (Lovenox), a low molecular weight heparin.
    3. Cyclosporine (Neoral), an immunosuppressant.
    4. Morphine PCA, a narcotic analgesic.

19. The client post–kidney transplant is prescribed cyclosporine (Gengraf), an immunosuppressant. The HCP prescribes 9 mg/kg daily. The client weighs 220 pounds. The hospital has 100-mg tablets on hand. How many tablets would the nurse administer?

    Answer _____

20. The nurse is preparing to administer morning medications. Which medication should the nurse administer first?
    1. Hydrocodone (Vicodin), a narcotic analgesic, to the client with pain "7" on the 1–10 scale.
    2. Furosemide (Lasix), a loop diuretic, IVP to a client with 2+ pitting edema.
    3. Metformin (Glucophage), a biguanide, po to a client diagnosed with Type 2 diabetes.
    4. Neostigmine (Prostigmin), a anticholinesterase, orally to the client diagnosed with myasthenia gravis.

1. 1. Vitamin C will increase the efficiency of the immune system, but it will not prevent the client from getting hepatitis B.
   2. Vaccines provide immunity when administered prior to exposure to hepatitis B, but they are not effective in preventing hepatitis B after exposure.
   3. This is a false statement because there is a treatment available.
   4. **Gamma globulin may be administered to a client exposed to hepatitis B within 24 hours to 7 days of exposure to the virus. This will provide passive immunity to the client.**

2. 1. While the child is receiving prednisolone, immunizations should not be administered. If a child is immunocompromised, then only attenuated vaccines can be administered.
   2. This medication can be crushed because it is not a sustained-release formulation or enteric coated.
   3. **Children taking prednisolone are more prone to infection and should avoid exposure to measles or chickenpox while taking prednisolone.**
   4. Steroid medication suppresses the immune system; therefore, an elevated temperature should be reported the HCP.

3. 1. There is no reason to restrict visitors during the administration of the medication. The client is immunocompromised, which may require restriction of visitors with known infections.
   2. **Ganciclovir is teratogenic and carcinogenic; therefore, it must be disposed in a manner that protects the environment. It should be burned at a high temperature to prevent the chemical from reaching the environment.**
   3. The reconstituted solutions must be stored in the refrigerator to protect their efficacy.
   4. The medication is only viable for 24 hours after mixing the solution. Therefore, the pharmacy cannot mix a week at a time.

4. 1. **A sulfa allergy with this type of rash develops in up to 60% of clients diagnosed with AIDS.**
   2. Common side effects of Viracept are hyperglycemia and diarrhea but not allergic rashes.
   3. Common side effects of Sustiva are central nervous system symptoms but not allergic rashes.
   4. Gastrointestinal intolerance and bone marrow suppression are common side

effects of Invirase, but allergic rashes are not.

MEDICATION MEMORY JOGGER: Whenever a client develops a rash and is receiving an antibiotic, the nurse should suspect that the antibiotic is the cause of the rash.

5. 1. **The nurse would need further clarification for a steroid because the client is already immunosuppressed, and this medication would further suppress the immune system.**
   2. The nurse must realize that depression is common in clients with chronic illnesses; therefore, a prescription for Prozac would not need further clarification.
   3. Antiviral medications are commonly prescribed for clients with AIDS to suppress the replication of the AIDS virus.
   4. Non-nucleoside reverse transcriptase inhibitors are commonly prescribed for clients with AIDS to suppress the replication of the AIDS virus.

6.   **5, 4, 2, 3, 1**
   5. One of the five rights is the right time, and the nurse must check PRN medications to make sure it is within the prescribed time frame.
   4. Narcotics are locked up and must be signed out and accounted for prior to administering.
   2. If the client's respiratory rate is less than 12 breaths a minute, the medication should be questioned.
   3. The Joint Commission has mandated that the nurse must identify the client with two identifiers prior to administering the medication.
   1. The nurse should dilute the medication to help prevent pain during administration, to increase the longevity of the vein, and to allow administration of the medication over the 5-minute period.

7. 1. There is no medication that can cure GB.
   2. There is no medication that can cure GB.
   3. **At this time, the medical treatment for GB is supportive until the Guillain-Barré resolves on its own.**
   4. Amevive is a medication used to treat psoriasis.

8. 1. WBCs in the CSF indicate an infection such as meningitis, not multiple sclerosis.
   2. **Interferon can reduce the frequency of relapse by 30% and decrease the appearance of new lesions on the MRI by 80%.**

The decrease in the appearance of new lesions indicates the medication is effective.

3. The EMG would not help determine if the medication was effective because the results will be skewed from previous damage.

4. The EEG would not help determine if the medication was effective because it measures the brain activity, not appearance of plaque.

MEDICATION MEMORY JOGGER: The nurse must be knowledgeable of accepted standards of practice for medication administration, including which client assessment data, laboratory data, or diagnostic test should be monitored to determine the effectiveness of a medication.

9. 1. **Dulcolax is a stimulant laxative and should not be taken every day because it will cause a decrease in the bowel tone. A client with MS already has difficulty with bowel tone.**

2. The client with MS is at risk for constipation, fecal incontinence, and fecal impaction because of decreased bowel tone. A fiber laxative increases the bulk of the stool and helps prevent constipation; therefore, the medication teaching is effective.

3. The client with MS is at risk for constipation, fecal incontinence, and fecal impaction because of decreased bowel tone. A stool softener will help prevent constipation and can be taken at any time of the day; therefore, the medication teaching is effective.

4. Increasing the fluid intake will help the bulk laxative to work and will help soften the stool; therefore, the client understands the medication teaching.

10. 1. The client's blood glucose level is not affected by Imuran; therefore, there is no need to monitor the glucose level.

2. **Bone marrow depression may occur when taking Imuran. The client must have a CBC and platelet counts every week the first month of therapy, then biweekly for 2–3 months, and monthly thereafter.**

3. Low-grade fever is not expected and is a sign of infection and must be reported to the HCP.

4. Kidney function is monitored through laboratory tests, not the client's urine output.

11. 1. The medication is prescribed to prevent organ damage and the client must receive it, even though it has side effects.

2. Steroids interfere with glucose metabolism, and blood glucose levels should be monitored. The client understands the medication teaching.

3. **The client needs the medication to prevent permanent organ damage. The medication should not be abruptly discontinued. It should be tapered off. The client needs more teaching about the medication to get the client to take the medication.**

4. Steroids do increase the client's appetite. The client understands the medication teaching.

12. 1. The client should take the medication with meals or milk to reduce gastrointestinal distress.

2. Constipation is not a side effect of this medication; therefore, the client does not need to increase fluid intake. Diarrhea is a side effect.

3. Weight gain or loss would not be an indicator of medication compliance.

4. **Plaquenil can cause retinopathy, blurred vision, and difficulty focusing; therefore, the client should have periodic eye examinations.**

13. 1. Rheumatrex takes up to 6 weeks to be therapeutic; therefore, this is not an appropriate response.

2. This is a therapeutic response used to encourage the client to ventilate feelings, but it is not the best response because the client needs factual information.

3. This comment does not address the client's concern that the medication is not working.

4. **Methotrexate is the most rapid-acting DMARD, but therapeutic effects may not develop for 3–6 weeks.**

14. 1. **After the initial gold salt injection, the next injection is scheduled for 7 days later, the next is 14 days later, and then it is weekly until a cumulative dose of 1 gram of gold salt has been administered.**

2. Two weeks would be the second follow-up visit.

3. This is not correct.

4. This is not correct.

15. 1. All nurses must wear gloves when exposed to blood and body fluids, regardless of work setting.
    2. According to Standard Precautions, the nurse must wear gloves when exposed to blood and body fluids.
    3. **The hospital must provide the nurse with nonlatex gloves and the nurse must keep them available for use when the nurse may be exposed to blood and body fluids.**
    4. This is not a workers' compensation issue. The nurse has not been injured.

16. 1. Baths cannot be given at school.
    2. **Caladryl is calamine lotion and Benadryl combined. The lotion dries the lesions, and the topical Benadryl decreases the itching. This medication can be administered at school.**
    3. Oral Benadryl could have the systemic effect of drowsiness, which would interfere with the child's ability to function.
    4. Polymyxin is a combination antibiotic, but it is not administered for a topical dermatitis.

17. 1. A 16-year-old female who is sexually active does not have to have parental permission to be treated for sexually transmitted diseases or to receive a vaccine designed to prevent an STD.
    2. **This is the first vaccine developed to prevent HPV infections and is administered in a series of injections. The nurse must discuss this with the patient to ensure that she will return for the entire series.**
    3. The Gardasil vaccine can prevent infection from HPV types 6, 11, 16, and 18 but not from every type of HPV.
    4. The Gardasil vaccine is given in a series of injections; it is not an oral medication to be taken for life.

18. 1. The nurse would not question administering a broad-spectrum antibiotic. The client has had surgery, and antibiotics are prescribed prophylactically.
    2. Lovenox is prescribed to prevent deep vein thrombosis, and the nurse would not question administering this medication.
    3. **Cyclosporine is not an expected medication to be prescribed for a client with total knee replacement. The nurse should determine why the client is receiving this medication. The client taking cyclosporine has had some type of organ transplant.**
    4. The nurse would expect the postoperative client to receive pain medication.

19. **9 tablets** To determine how many tablets should be administered the nurse should first determine that the client weighs 100 kg (220 ÷ 2.2 = 100). Then, the nurse multiplies 9 mg times 100 kg, which equals 900 mg a day. 900 mg divided by 100 mg = 9. The nurse would administer 9 tablets.

20. 1. Pain medication is priority but not over a medication that will prevent a potentially life-threatening event.
    2. Lasix would be administered to treat the edema, but it is not priority for someone with 2+ edema.
    3. Glucophage is not given for a life-threatening condition; therefore, it can be administered after the Prostigmin.
    4. **A client with MG must take medications on time to ensure muscle function while eating or performing ADLs. Prostigmin is one of the few medications that must be administered exactly on time.**

Cancer Treatments

11

"Few things are of more concern to patients at end of life and to their family than that pain will be well controlled."

—Nessa Coyle and Mary Layman-Goldstein

PRACTICE QUESTIONS

A Client Receiving Chemotherapy

1. The client has received chemotherapy 2 days a week every 3 weeks for the last 8 months. The client's current lab values are Hgb and Hct 10.3 and 31, WBC 5.2, neutrophils 50, and platelets 89. Based on the laboratory results, which information should the nurse teach the client?
   1. Avoid individuals with colds or other infections.
   2. Maintain nutritional status with supplements.
   3. Plan for periods of rest to prevent fatigue.
   4. Use a soft-bristled toothbrush and an electric razor.

2. The nurse is preparing to administer 0900 medications on an oncology floor. Which medication should the nurse administer first?
   1. An analgesic to a female client with a headache of "3" on the pain scale.
   2. An antiemetic to a female client who thinks she might become nauseated.
   3. A mucosal barrier agent to a male client who has peptic ulcer disease.
   4. A biologic response modifier to a male client with low red blood cell counts.

3. The male client receiving plant alkaloid antineoplastic medications for cancer complains to the clinic nurse that he has been "so clumsy lately that I can't even pick up a dime." Which statement is the nurse's best response?
   1. "This is normal and will resolve when your therapy is complete."
   2. "There is no reason to worry about a minor side effect of the drugs."
   3. "Have you also noticed a difference in your bowel movements?"
   4. "Are you also weak and dizzy when you try to stand up?"

4. The client has received the second dose of chemotherapy and is ready for discharge. Which information should the nurse teach the client?
   1. Tell the client to notify the HCP of a temperature of 100°F.
   2. Have the client drink dietary supplements three times a day.
   3. Encourage the client to stay away from all people outside of the home.
   4. Apply a continuous ice pack to the intravenous site.

5. The nurse is reviewing the laboratory data of a male client receiving chemotherapy. Based on the laboratory results, which action should the nurse implement?

Client:	Account Number: 1 234 56	Date: Today
Laboratory Data	**Client Values**	**Normal Values**
WBC	2.4	4.5–11.0 (10^3)
RBC	4.0	M: 4.7–6.1 (10^6) F: 4.2–5.4 (10^6)
Hemoglobin	11.6	M: 13.5–17.5 g/dL F: 11.5–15.5 g/dL
Hematocrit	34.2	M: 40%–52% F: 36%–48%
MCV	83	81–96 μg/m^3
MCHC	31	33–36 g/dL
RDW	12	11%–14.5%
Reticulocyte	1.4	0.5%–1.5%
Platelets	110	150–400 (10^3)
Differential		
Neutrophils	40	40%–75% (2500–7500/mm^3)
Lymphocytes	50	20%–50% (1500-5500/mm^3)
Monocytes	2	1%–10% (100–800/mm^3)
Eosinophils	6	0%–6% (0–440/mm^3)
Basophils	20	%–2% (0–200/mm^3)

1. Assess for an infection.
2. Assess for bleeding.
3. Assess for shortness of breath.
4. Assess for pallor.

6. At 1000 the client diagnosed with cancer and receiving chemotherapy is complaining of unrelieved nausea. Based on the following MAR which action should the nurse take?

Medication Administration Record				
Client:	Account #: 1 234 56		Date: Today	
Height: 67 inches	Weight: 209 lbs		Allergies: NKA	
Date	Medication	2301–0700	0701–1500	1501–2300
	Ondansetron (Zofran) 4 mg IVP every 4 hours PRN	0100 NN 0500 NN	0900 DN	
	Morphine 2 mg IVP every 2–3 hours PRN	0315 NN		
	Prochlorperazine Spansule (Compazine) 5 mg po T.I.D. PRN	0630 NN		
Nurse Signature/Initials	Day Nurse RN/DN		Night Nurse RN/NN	

1. Administer another Compazine Spansule.
2. Discuss the nausea medications with the HCP.
3. Teach the client how to control nausea at home.
4. Turn the client on his or her side to prevent aspiration.

7. The client diagnosed with cancer has developed diarrhea after the third round of chemotherapy. Which intervention should the clinic nurse implement?
1. Have the client take up to 12 Imodium 2-mg tablets per day.
2. Place the client on a clear liquid diet.
3. Medicate the client with Phenergan suppositories.
4. Discuss adding a fiber supplement to the client's diet.

8. The client has received five treatments of combination chemotherapy for cancer of the lung. Which data indicates the medications are effective?
1. The client's hair has begun to grow back in again.
2. The client only has nausea during the treatments.
3. The client reports being able to ambulate around the block.
4. The client's lung sounds are clear.

9. Which statement by the client receiving adjunct chemotherapy for breast cancer warrants immediate intervention by the nurse?
1. The client complains of numbness and tingling in her feet.
2. The client complains that she feels unattractive without hair.
3. The client says she is unable to eat for 2 days after a treatment.
4. The client tells the nurse she has lost 2 pounds since the last treatment.

10. The client receiving intravenous chemotherapy was nauseated and vomited twice the day before. Which action should the nurse implement?
1. Ask the dietary department to provide full liquids.
2. Hold all meal trays until the client is not nauseated.
3. Premedicate the client before each meal.
4. Have the client suck on ice chips frequently.

A Client Receiving a Biologic Response Modifier

11. Which instructions should the nurse teach the client receiving oprelvekin (Neumega), a hematopoietic growth factor?
    1. Report any edema of arms, legs, or both.
    2. Take the pill with food to prevent gastric distress.
    3. Monitor the blood glucose levels daily.
    4. See the ophthalmologist if vision becomes blurred.

12. The client diagnosed with chronic kidney disease is prescribed erythropoietin (Procrit). Which intervention should the nurse implement? Select all that apply.
    1. Administer it intramuscularly in the deltoid.
    2. Have the client take Tylenol, an analgesic, for pain.
    3. Monitor the client's complete blood count.
    4. Teach the client to pace activities.
    5. Inform the client not to drive for 90 days.

13. Which statement is the scientific rationale for administering the biologic response modifier interferon (Intron A) to a client diagnosed with hepatitis C?
    1. Intron A suppresses cell proliferation in proliferative diseases.
    2. Intron A decreases the production of cytotoxic macrophages.
    3. Intron A increases the production of suppressor genes.
    4. Intron A reprograms virus-infected cells to inhibit virus replication.

14. The client diagnosed with cancer has received several treatments of combination chemotherapy and has a WBC of 2.2 and neutrophil count of 79. Which hematopoietic growth factor should the nurse administer?
    1. Darbepoetin, Aranesp.
    2. Oprelvekin, Neumega.
    3. Filgrastim, Neupogen.
    4. Erythropoietin, Epogen.

15. The nurse on an oncology floor is administering morning medications. Which medication would the nurse question?
    1. Cyanocobalamin (vitamin B_{12}) to a client with pernicious anemia.
    2. Erythropoietin (Epogen) to a client with chronic lymphocytic leukemia.
    3. Filgrastim (Neupogen) to a client with a solid tissue tumor.
    4. Heparin intravenously to a client with disseminated intravascular coagulation.

16. The nurse is preparing to administer pegfilgrastim (Neulasta). Which procedure indicates the correct administration of this medication?
    1. Use a 3-mL syringe with a $1^{1}/_{2}$ inch needle and administer in the hip.
    2. Mix the powder with sterile normal saline and administer within 1 hour.
    3. Check the client's blood pressure and pulse prior to administration.
    4. Hold the medication 24 hours before or after chemotherapy.

17. The client who received the hematopoietic growth factor darbepoetin (Aranesp) calls the clinic nurse and reports aching in the back and legs. Which statement is the nurse's best response?
    1. "This is unrelated to the medication. You may be getting the flu."
    2. "You should come to the clinic immediately to see the HCP."
    3. "This is an expected side effect of the medication and can be treated."
    4. "Have you taken your blood pressure medication today?"

18. Which client would the nurse question receiving the hematopoietic growth factor erythropoietin (Epogen)?
    1. The client diagnosed with end-stage renal disease.
    2. The client diagnosed with essential hypertension.
    3. The client diagnosed with lung cancer and metastasis.
    4. The client diagnosed with anemia and leukopenia.

19. The client on the medical unit is a Jehovah's Witness and has anemia, and the HCP orders erythropoietin (Procrit). Which intervention should the nurse implement?
    1. Question the order on religious grounds.
    2. Have the client sign an informed consent.
    3. Ask the laboratory to confirm the RBC.
    4. Administer the medication subcutaneously.

20. The client is scheduled to receive anakinra (Kineret), an immunomodulator. Which data would make the nurse question administering the medication?
    1. The client has joint deformities of the hands.
    2. The client has a temperature of 100.4°F.
    3. The client received a dose 2 days ago at the same time.
    4. The client took Tylenol for a headache 2 hours ago.

A Client Receiving Hormone Therapy

21. The 45-year-old female client with a family history of breast cancer asks the nurse, "Is there anything I can do to improve my chances of not getting breast cancer like my sister and mother?" Which statement is the nurse's best response?
    1. "There are medications and lifestyle changes to reduce the risk."
    2. "No. Clients that have a strong family history just have to hope they don't get it."
    3. "You sound worried. Would you like to talk about how you feel?"
    4. "Do any other relatives have breast or other female cancers?"

22. The male client diagnosed with prostate cancer is prescribed hormone suppression therapy. Which statement is the scientific rationale for administering this medication?
    1. Statement suppression therapy will increase the client's libido and the ability to maintain an erection.
    2. Hormone suppression therapy shrinks the prostate tissue by destroying tumor cells during replication.
    3. Hormone suppression therapy will cause the client to experience menopausal-like symptoms.
    4. Hormone suppression therapy changes the internal host environment to decrease cell growth.

23. The male client diagnosed with prostate cancer is receiving leuprolide (Lupron LA), a GnRH agonist, implant. Which procedure is the correct method of administration?
    1. Use a tuberculin syringe and administer subcutaneously.
    2. Insert the 16-gauge needle at a 30-degree angle into the abdomen.
    3. Place the medication into the rectal vault using a nonsterile glove.
    4. Administer with an antacid to prevent peptic ulcer disease.

24. The postmenopausal client with breast cancer is placed on the aromatase inhibitor anastrozole (Arimidex). Which data indicates the medication is effective?
    1. The client reports a positive body image.
    2. The client is able to discuss her feelings openly.
    3. The client's bone and lung scans are negative.
    4. The client's DNA ploidy tests show diploid cells.

25. The male client diagnosed with acquired immunodeficiency syndrome (AIDS) is prescribed megestrol (Megace), an antineoplastic hormone. Which data indicates the medication is effective?
    1. The Kaposi's lesions have become light brown.
    2. The client ate 90% of the meals served him.
    3. The client experiences a decrease in nausea.
    4. The client is able to complete activities of daily living.

26. The client diagnosed with a brain tumor is prescribed dexamethasone (Decadron), a glucocorticoid hormone. Which instructions should the nurse teach?
    1. Take on an empty stomach for better absorption.
    2. The medication may decrease the appetite.
    3. Do not abruptly stop taking the medication.
    4. Decadron may cause a headache.

27. The nurse is discharging the male client diagnosed with cancer of the prostate with a prescription for diethylstilbestrol (DES), an estrogen. Which information should the nurse teach the client?
    1. The client should not father any children while taking the medication.
    2. The client may experience hot flashes and breast enlargement.
    3. The client should decrease calcium intake while taking DES.
    4. The client's body hair will grow at a faster rate and will be coarse.

28. The 45-year-old female client has had a left breast biopsy that revealed carcinoma of the breast and the following laboratory report regarding estrogen and progesterone influence on the tumor. Which medications should the nurse discuss with the client?

Client: F/45	Account #: 2 345 67	Date: Yesterday
Cytochemical Report		
Estrogen receptor assay: Greater than 45% of the cell nuclei stained Progesterone receptor assay: Greater than 20% of the cell nuclei stained		

    1. Supplemental estrogen and progesterone hormone.
    2. Glucocorticoid and mineral corticoid hormones.
    3. Gonadotropin-releasing hormone agonists (GnRH).
    4. Antiestrogen/progesterone hormone medications.

29. The 60-year-old female client has taken hormone replacement therapy for control of menopausal symptoms for the last 9 years. Which statement by the nurse indicates the client's risk for developing breast cancer?
    1. "The risk of getting cancer decreases each year that the client takes hormones."
    2. "The risk is the same as for women who do not take hormone replacement."
    3. "The risk increases each year the client is taking hormone replacement therapy."
    4. "The risk is only slightly greater while taking hormone replacement."

30. The 39-year-old client diagnosed with breast cancer is prescribed the antiestrogen hormone tamoxifen (Nolvadex). Which information is most important for the nurse to teach the client?
    1. The medication will cause menopause symptoms.
    2. Nolvadex may cause vaginal discharge and nausea.
    3. Tamoxifen will slow the growth of estrogen-positive tumors.
    4. It is important to see the gynecologist regularly.

A Client Receiving an Investigational Protocol

31. The client is scheduled to receive an investigational medication for the treatment of cancer. Which intervention is the nurse's first action?
    1. Explain the risks and benefits of the medication to the client.
    2. Administer the medication per the protocol.
    3. Contact the pharmacy to deliver the medication to the unit.
    4. Find information on administration procedures and side effects.

32. Which statement is the primary reason to enroll a client in an investigational proto-
    col for the treatment of cancer?
    1. The HCP feels that the investigational drug has the best chance of a cure.
    2. The client has failed conventional treatment and there is a poor prognosis.
    3. The HCP can provide care at a reduced rate because of subsidies.
    4. The client does not like the standard treatment regimen for his or her disease.

33. The nurse is caring for clients on an oncology unit. Which task is an inappropriate
    delegation or assignment by the nurse?
    1. Have the licensed practical nurse administer the IV investigational medication.
    2. Request the unlicensed assistive personnel measure and record the client output.
    3. Assign a new graduate nurse to care for a client receiving packed red blood
       cells.
    4. Delegate care of a client who is seriously ill and taking an investigational drug to
       a registered nurse.

34. The nurse is working in a clinic that uses investigational protocols to determine the
    effectiveness of new medications. Which information regarding the use of placebo
    medications should the nurse teach the clients?
    1. Placebos are not used in investigational protocols because of ethical consid-
       erations.
    2. The placebo will contain the active ingredient under study in the protocol.
    3. Clients in the control group will receive a medication that does not help the
       disease.
    4. Clients should insist in not being placed in the group that gets the placebo pill.

35. The nurse working in an outpatient clinic is screening clients for inclusion in an
    investigational medication protocol for rheumatoid arthritis. Which screening ques-
    tions should the nurse include? Select all that apply.
    1. Which medications has the client been prescribed for arthritis?
    2. Which herbs and over-the-counter medications has the client taken?
    3. Is the client allergic to any soaps or clothing dyes?
    4. Does the client have any other immune system disease?
    5. Does the client have insurance to pay for the medication?

36. The male client participating in an investigational protocol calls the clinic and tells
    the nurse that the medications have made him "sick to my stomach all night." Which
    statement is the nurse's best response?
    1. "You should consider whether or not you want to be in the study."
    2. "This must be uncomfortable for you. Let's talk about your feelings."
    3. "Come to the clinic to see the HCP. You may be reacting to the drug."
    4. "This is a temporary problem and will go away with future doses."

37. The client receiving an investigational medication protocol must be hydrated with at
    least 1000 mL of IV fluid in the immediate 4 hours before the infusion of the investi-
    gational medication. At which rate would the nurse set the pump?

    Answer _____

38. The nurse is administering medications on a medical unit. Which medication should
    the nurse administer first?
    1. The investigational medication to a client who wants to go home now.
    2. The investigational medication to the client who has not signed a permit.
    3. The investigational medication that must be administered at a specific time.
    4. The investigational medication that must infuse over 24 hours.

39. Which statement is the scientific rationale for a control group of participants in an investigational protocol?
    1. A control group is used to compare the responses to the medication group for efficacy of the medication.
    2. The control group is used to prove that the side effects of the medication are not caused by anything else.
    3. The researcher cannot determine effectiveness of the medication unless there is a control group.
    4. The researcher uses the control group to gauge the amount of medication needed to treat the disease.

40. The nurse on an oncology unit is administering morning medications. Which medication should the nurse question administering? The investigational protocol medication to the client who states:
    1. "I am sure I am getting better every day."
    2. "I'm not sure I want to continue this treatment."
    3. "The doctor told me there were no guarantees."
    4. "Can you explain the side effects of the medication?"

A Client Undergoing Surgery for Cancer

41. The client has had an implanted port placed to receive chemotherapy. When the nurse attempts to access the device, there is no backflow of blood and the nurse meets resistance when flushing. Which action should the nurse take to access the implanted port?
    1. Forcefully insert 3 mL of heparin into the port.
    2. Flush the implanted port with 5–10 mL of normal saline.
    3. Instill a prescribed amount of urokinase into the port.
    4. Schedule the client for a newly implanted port placement.

42. The nurse is accessing a newly implanted port intravenous line. Which interventions should the nurse implement? Rank in order of performance.
    1. Set up the sterile field and don sterile gloves.
    2. Cleanse the skin with antiseptic skin prep.
    3. Palpate the rim of the port with two fingers.
    4. Insert a noncoring needle between the fingers.
    5. Explain the procedure to the client and wash hands.

43. The client diagnosed with cancer of the head of the pancreas has had a Whipple procedure (pancreatoduodenectomy). Which discharge instructions should the nurse teach the client?
    1. Administer insulin subcutaneously.
    2. Take acetaminophen for an elevated temperature.
    3. Change the surgical dressing weekly.
    4. Increase the calories and protein in the diet.

44. The nurse assesses excoriated skin surrounding the colostomy stoma of a client diagnosed with cancer of the colon. Which intervention should the nurse implement first?
    1. Request a consult from a wound ostomy continence nurse.
    2. Apply a skin barrier protectant paste around the stoma.
    3. Gently cleanse the area with mild soap and water.
    4. Replace the pouch with one that is 1/3 inch larger than the stoma.

45. The client diagnosed with metastatic brain tumors has an Ommaya reservoir placed for delivery of chemotherapy. Which statement is the scientific rationale for the placement of this device?
    1. Use of this device bypasses the blood–brain barrier to deliver the medication.
    2. The implanted port provides venous access for the client receiving chemotherapy.
    3. There is less nausea and vomiting associated with the use of an Ommaya access.
    4. Ommaya reservoirs are used to deliver sustained-release medications over time.

46. The client diagnosed with cancer of the prostate has had prostate surgery using spinal anesthesia. Which safety precaution should the postanesthesia care nurse use?
    1. Cover the client with a heating device to avoid hypothermia.
    2. Keep the head of the bed elevated until the feeling returns to the legs.
    3. Medicate the client with intravenous narcotic analgesics for pain.
    4. Hold pressure on the epidural insertion site for at least 5 minutes.

47. The client with an implanted port has completed the chemotherapy medications and is ready for discharge. Which action should the nurse take to prepare the client for discharge?
    1. Teach the client how to manage the port at home.
    2. Insert a sterile, noncoring needle into the port.
    3. Flush the port with saline followed by heparin.
    4. Scrub the port access with povidone-iodine (Betadine).

48. The client diagnosed with cancer of the ovary had an extensive resection of the bowel and is receiving total parenteral nutrition (TPN). Which laboratory data would the nurse monitor daily?
    1. Blood urea nitrogen and creatinine levels.
    2. Sodium, potassium, and glucose levels.
    3. Urine and serum osmolality levels.
    4. CA-125 and carcinoembryonic antigen (CEA).

49. The client who had a right upper lobectomy for cancer of the lung returns to the intensive care unit with a patient-controlled analgesia (PCA) pump for pain control. Which action should the nurse implement first?
    1. Show the client how to use the PCA pump.
    2. Obtain a new cartridge of medication.
    3. Determine the level of pain relief obtained.
    4. Check the HCP orders against the settings.

50. The client who had a Whipple resection (pancreatoduodenectomy) for cancer of the pancreas has arterial blood gases of pH 7.29, PCO_2 40, HCO_3 18, and PaO_2 100. Which medication should the nurse prepare to administer?
    1. Intravenous normal saline at a keep-open rate.
    2. Intravenous insulin by continuous infusion.
    3. Sodium bicarbonate intravenously.
    4. Sliding-scale Humulin N subcutaneous.

A Client with Chronic Pain

51. The client diagnosed with terminal cancer is experiencing significant pain. Which information is most important for the hospice nurse to teach the client and significant other?
    1. If the pain medications are not working, try to divert the client's attention.
    2. Take the pain medications at the onset of pain before it becomes severe.
    3. Do not allow family or friends to visit when the client is in pain.
    4. Too much narcotic pain medication will cause the client to be addicted.

52. The client calls the nursing station and requests pain medication. When the nurse enters the room with the narcotic medication, the nurse finds the client laughing and talking with visitors. Which action should the nurse take?
    1. Administer the client's prescribed pain medication.
    2. Confront the client's narcotic-seeking behavior.
    3. Wait until the visitors leave to administer any medication.
    4. Check the MAR to see if there is a nonnarcotic medication ordered.

53. Which discharge instructions should the nurse provide for the client diagnosed with cancer who is taking hydrocodone with acetaminophen (Vicodin) PRN for pain?
    1. Take the medication only when the pain is severe.
    2. Use Tylenol for any pain unrelieved by the Vicodin.
    3. Notify the HCP if the medication relieves the pain.
    4. Increase the intake of fluids and roughage in the diet.

54. The client diagnosed with cancer notifies the nurse of pain of an "11" on the pain scale but is unable to localize the pain to a specific area or tell when the pain began. Which action should the nurse implement?
    1. Discuss the importance of knowing where the pain is located.
    2. Prepare to administer the prescribed narcotic pain medication.
    3. Refer the client to a chaplain or social worker for counseling.
    4. Ask the client to use the faces pain scale to rate the pain.

55. The terminally ill client complains that despite hourly intravenous narcotic pain medication administered in increasingly higher doses, the pain is getting progressively worse. Which intervention should the nurse implement?
    1. Request an increase in the dosage of medication from the HCP.
    2. Ask the significant other to try to distract the client.
    3. Use therapeutic communication to discuss the client's concerns.
    4. Teach the client nonpharmacologic pain control measures.

56. The male client diagnosed with cancer tells the nurse that he hates feeling "doped up" during the day but needs pain medication to be able to rest at night. Which statement is the nurse's best response?
    1. "Sometimes it is necessary to just take as much medication as you can to get to sleep. Ask the HCP for stronger medications."
    2. "I am sure that this must be uncomfortable for you. You need to talk about how you are feeling."
    3. "We could try to balance your pain medications with sleeping medications to help you get comfortable at night."
    4. "Too much pain medication will cause you to have many other complications and should be avoided."

57. The nurse administered a narcotic pain medication to a client diagnosed with cancer. Thirty minutes after administering the medication, which data indicates the medication was effective?
    1. The client keeps his or her eyes closed and the drapes drawn.
    2. The client uses guided imagery to help with pain control.
    3. The client states that the pain has gone down 5 points on the scale.
    4. The client is lying as still as possible in the bed.

58. The client admitted with intractable pain from osteosarcoma is being discharged. Which information should the nurse emphasize with the client?
    1. The client will need to accept some pain as part of the disease process.
    2. Most pharmacies will be able to fill the medication whenever it is needed.
    3. Be sure to have an adequate supply of medication on weekends and holidays.
    4. The client should return to the hospital if the pain returns.

59. The nurse is caring for a client diagnosed with cancer. At 1000 the client is complaining of pain and nausea. Based on the medication administration record, which action should the nurse implement?

Medication Administration Record

Client:		Account #: 1 234 56		Date: Today
Height: 64 inches		Weight: 156 lbs		Allergies: NKA

Date	Medication	2301–0700	0701–1500	1501–2300
	Ondansetron (Zofran) 4 mg IVP every 4 hours PRN		0900 DN	
	Morphine 2 mg IVP every 2–3 hours PRN	0575 NN	0800 DN	
	Liquid morphine (Roxanol) 10 mg po every 1 hour PRN	0100 NN		
	Prochlorperazine Spansule (Compazine) 5 mg po T.I.D. PRN		0730 DN	
	Prochlorperazine 5–10 mg IVP every 2 hours PRN			
Nurse Signature/Initials		Day Nurse RN/DN		Night Nurse RN/NN

1. Administer Roxanol 10 mg orally and hold any antiemetic medication.
2. Administer the Compazine and morphine but use separate syringes.
3. Administer the Roxanol now and the Zofran in 3 hours.
4. Administer 2 mg of morphine combined with 10 mg of Compazine IV.

60. The client with chronic pain is prescribed both MS Contin and liquid morphine (Roxanol), narcotic analgesics. How should the nurse administer the medications?
    1. Administer the MS Contin at prescribed intervals and the Roxanol PRN.
    2. Administer both medications PRN for the client's chronic pain.
    3. Administer the Roxanol every 4 hours and the MS Contin PRN pain.
    4. Administer the MS Contin for breakthrough pain and hold the Roxanol.

A Client Receiving Chemotherapy

1. 1. This is good information to teach, but it is not based on the laboratory values. The client's WBC and absolute neutrophil counts are within normal range.
   2. This is good information to teach, but it is not based on the laboratory values. The client may develop mouth ulcers as a result of chemotherapy administration, and the nurse should discuss methods of maintaining nutrition for this reason but not because of the laboratory values.
   3. This is good information to teach, but it is not based on the laboratory values. Fatigue related to cancer and its treatment is real and should be addressed, and an Hgb and Hct of around 8 and 24 could cause fatigue, but the client's levels do not indicate this.
   4. **A platelet count of less than 100,000 is the definition of thrombocytopenia. The nurse should teach measures to prevent bleeding.**

2. 1. A "3" is considered mild pain and could wait until the more emergent client is medicated.
   2. **Anticipatory nausea and vomiting are very difficult to control. It is important for the nurse to medicate the client to prevent the nausea from occurring. This client should be medicated first.**
   3. At 0900 the breakfast tray should have already been consumed. Administering a mucosal barrier agent after a meal places medication in the stomach that will coat the food, not the stomach lining. This medication should be retimed for 0730 and not administered until later in the morning after the breakfast meal has had a chance to leave the stomach.
   4. This medication stimulates the bone marrow to produce red blood cells; the full effect of the medication will not be seen for 30–90 days. It could be administered after the antiemetic and the analgesic.

3. 1. This is not normal and could indicate that the client is developing a neuropathy from the medications. The danger is that the innervation to the small bowel may be compromised as well. It will not go away when the therapy is complete.
   2. This is not a minor side effect of the medication; it may indicate that the client must be changed to a different antineoplastic agent.
   3. This may indicate a potential life-altering complication of the chemotherapy. The client may have nerve damage caused by the plant alkaloid medications. The nerves of the intestines may also be compromised, causing decreased peristalsis. The nurse should assess the situation and notify the HCP.
   4. Plant alkaloid medications do not cause orthostatic hypotension.

4. 1. **The client should be given information regarding potential complications of therapy and when to notify the HCP. A temperature of 100°F or greater should be immediately brought to the attention of the HCP. The client could be developing an infection and must be treated as soon as possible.**
   2. The client may or may not need dietary supplements at this time. The client should be referred to a dietitian for a consultation regarding nutritional status, but dietary supplements three times a day would not allow the client to enjoy normal foods. This would be recommended if the client were not tolerating any normal dietary intake.
   3. Clients should not isolate themselves from enjoying the extended family. They should be told to avoid clients with known contagious illness.
   4. If the client has a tender vein that has been assessed by the HCP and found not to be an extravasation of the medication, the client can apply intermittent warm packs. Ice packs restrict blood flow to the area.

MEDICATION MEMORY JOGGER: Usual discharge instructions include teaching the client to notify the HCP in case of a fever. The test taker might choose this option based on standard procedure.

5. 1. **The client has a low white blood cell count, which is 2.4 times 10^3, or 2400 actual white blood cells counted. Of this amount only 40% are mature neutrophils capable of fighting a bacterial invasion. Multiply 2400 times 40% (0.4) and determine that the absolute neutrophil count is 960. This count, far below the normal of 2500–7500, puts the client at risk for an infection. The nurse should assess the client for infection.**
   2. The client's platelet count is less than normal (150,000 to 400,000), but it is still greater than 100,000. Less than 100,000 is

thrombocytopenia. Critical values begin at 50,000.

3. The client's hemoglobin is less than normal but not critically low. This client might fatigue easily because of oxygen demands on the body but should not be short of breath with this hemoglobin.

4. This hemoglobin and hematocrit are below normal in values but not enough for the client to become pale as a result.

MEDICATION MEMORY JOGGER: The nurse must be aware of which laboratory values should be monitored for specific medication administration.

6. 1. Compazine Spansules are used before meals to assist in control of nausea so the client can eat. This did not take care of the nausea; the nurse should discuss the situation with the HCP.

2. **The client is having unrelieved nausea and the night nurse has already tried to control the nausea with all the medication the HCP has ordered. It is time to notify the HCP to discuss alternative medications or increasing the dose of Zofran.**

3. Clients who are experiencing discomfort are not ready to be taught anything. This client needs to know that control of the nausea is possible in the hospital before the client will be ready to learn how to control it at home.

4. The stem of the question did not say the client was sedated. There is no reason to position the client on the side.

7. 1. The maximum dose of Imodium per day is 16 mg; this would exceed the recommended dose per day.

2. Clear liquids will not provide the needed bulk to the stools and will not provide sufficient calories to prevent malnutrition.

3. Phenergan is an antiemetic, not an antidiarrheal, and any medication administered by the rectal route would probably be expelled before absorbing into the client's system.

4. **Clients with diarrhea need to add bulk to the diet in the form of fiber supplements or dietary intake to decrease the liquid nature of the stools.**

8. 1. The client's hair will grow back when treatments are discontinued and sometimes during the treatments, but this does not indicate the medications are killing cancer cells.

2. Nausea during or after the treatments is not a measure of cell kill.

3. The client being able to tolerate activity indicates the client has adequate lung capacity. This indicates the lung cancer has not enveloped the entire lung fields and the medications are effective. Lung cancer has a poor prognosis, and the treatment goal is to improve or maintain quality of life.

4. The client's lung fields being clear do not indicate quality of life or cell kill.

9. 1. This client may have metastasis to the spinal column, and this information should be immediately reported to the HCP for emergency evaluation or the client could become paralyzed.

2. Body image suffers when a client has alopecia (hair loss) from the antineoplastic agents, but it is not life threatening or permanent.

3. Being able to resume nutritional intake after 2 days is not a cause for immediate intervention by the nurse.

4. Treatments are scheduled every 3–4 weeks, and a 2-pound weight loss is not significant in this time period.

10. 1. The client should receive whatever the client wishes to eat within the prescribed diet. The nurse should not autocratically decide the client should eat full liquids.

2. The client may wish to attempt to eat; the nurse should not autocratically decide the client should not eat.

3. **The client may be able to tolerate meals if the client receives an antiemetic medication 30 minutes before each meal. The nurse can administer a PRN medication prior to each meal or request a routine medication order from the HCP.**

4. The client will not become dehydrated while receiving intravenous fluids with the antineoplastic medications. Ice chips will not prevent nausea.

A Client Receiving a Biologic Response Modifier

11. 1. Neumega is a biologic response modifier that acts on the bone marrow to increase the production of platelets. It can also cause cardiovascular stimulation, tachycardia, vasodilation, palpitations, dysrhythmias, and edema. The client should report any of these symp-

toms and shortness of breath or blurred vision immediately.

2. Neumega is administered by subcutaneous injection.

3. Neumega does not affect blood glucose levels.

4. The client should notify the oncologist or HCP who ordered the Neumega immediately so the medication can be discontinued; the ophthalmologist need not be notified. The medication is causing the blurred vision.

12. 1. The medication is administered subcutaneously.

2. **The medication stimulates the bone marrow to produce red blood cells. The bone marrow is located inside the bones. The client may experience aches and pains of the bony areas as a result. Tylenol usually will remedy this side effect.**

3. **Epogen stimulates the production of red blood cells, and the CBC should be monitored at regular intervals.**

4. **This should be done for any client with anemia to prevent fatigue. The medication is ordered to treat anemia.**

5. **Because the potential for seizures exists during periods of rapid hematocrit increase, the client should be warned not to drive or operate any heavy equipment for a period of 90 days until the hematocrit has stabilized.**

13. 1. Intron A is useful for several disease processes because of its different mechanisms of action. Suppression of cell proliferation is the action that is desired in clients diagnosed with leukemia.

2. Intron A does not affect macrophages.

3. Intron A does not increase tumor suppressor genes.

4. Intron A reprograms virus-infected cells to inhibit viral replication. This is the reason that it is useful in treating hepatitis.

14. 1. Aranesp stimulates the production of red blood cells. The question does not give the client's RBC count. (The advantage of Aranesp over Procrit or Epogen, which also stimulate the production of RBCs, is that it is administered once a week, instead of daily.)

2. Neumega stimulates the production of platelets. The question does not refer to the client's platelet count.

3. **Neupogen stimulates the production of white blood cells, and this client has a low white blood cell count and thus is at risk for an infection. The client's absolute neutrophil count is only 1738 (2.2 times 1000 equals 2200, then multiply this number times 0.79 equals 1738). Clients with an absolute neutrophil count below 2500 are at risk for infection.**

4. Epogen stimulates the production of red blood cells.

15. 1. Cyanocobalamin is the treatment for pernicious anemia. The nurse would not question administering this medication.

2. **Erythropoietin stimulates the bone marrow to produce more cells. Stimulation of the bone marrow is questioned when the cancer is in the bone marrow.**

3. Stimulation of the bone marrow is not questioned in clients with solid tissue tumors. The nurse would not question administering this medication.

4. Heparin is part of the standard treatment regimen for disseminated intravascular coagulation (DIC).

16. 1. The medication is administered subcutaneously or IV, not intramuscularly.

2. The medication comes in a vial 10-mg per mL already prepared. If mixed for an IV infusion, D_5W is used.

3. The client receiving a red blood stimulant (Epogen, Procrit, Aranesp) should have the blood pressure monitored because rapid increases in the hematocrit will also increase the blood pressure, but this does not happen with Neulasta, which stimulates white blood cell production.

4. **Neulasta stimulates the production of white blood cells. Cytotoxic chemotherapy acts on the bone marrow to decrease the production of white blood cells, an opposite response. The nurse should hold the medication and resume it 24 hours after the administration of the chemotherapy.**

17. 1. The aching in the back and legs is probably caused by hyperstimulation of the bone marrow to produce red blood cells, not by the flu.

2. The HCP does not need to see the client immediately. Tylenol will usually treat the problem. The HCP only needs to see

the client if over-the-counter analgesic medications do not relieve the pain.

3. Hyperstimulation of the bone marrow is the probable cause of the aches and should be treated with over-the-counter pain medications.

4. The client's blood pressure should be monitored during the administration of medications that increase the hematocrit, but not taking blood pressure medication would not cause aches in the bones.

MEDICATION MEMORY JOGGER: The nurse must be aware of the safety precautions when administering medications.

18. 1. Epogen is frequently administered to clients in end-stage kidney disease to stimulate their bodies to produce red blood cells. The kidneys naturally produce erythropoietin to stimulate red blood cell production, but clients with renal disease may not be able to produce the cytokine erythropoietin.

2. **A rapid increase in hematocrit, which may occur with Epogen, can result in uncontrolled hypertension. The client must have the hypertension well-controlled for Epogen to be administered safely. The nurse would question this medication for this client.**

3. The client diagnosed with lung cancer and metastasis would be a candidate for Epogen. The nurse would not question this medication.

4. Epogen is given to clients with anemia. Leukopenia will not be increased or decreased by the medication.

19. 1. Members of the Jehovah's Witness church refuse to allow blood and blood products. Procrit is not a blood product. There is no reason to question the medication on religious grounds.

2. The client in the hospital signs a permit to treat when admitted. There is no need for another consent form.

3. The laboratory does not need to confirm the data.

4. **The nurse should administer the medication. Procrit is administered subcutaneously.**

20. 1. Deformities of the hands indicate rheumatoid arthritis. Anakinra (Interleukin 1) is used to treat rheumatoid arthritis in clients who have failed other treatments.

2. **This medication suppresses the immune system and should not be** administered to anyone with an infection. A temperature greater than 100°F indicates an infection.

3. The normal dosing schedule is every 2 days at the same time.

4. Tylenol does not interfere with Anakinra, and a headache would not indicate an infection.

A Client Receiving Hormone Therapy

21. 1. Tamoxifen and raloxifene have been researched in the Study of Tamoxifen and Raloxifene (STAR) trial and have proven efficacy in reducing the risk of breast cancer in women who have primary relatives with breast cancer. Lifestyle modifications such as consuming a low-fat diet and avoiding obesity are also recommended to reduce the risk of breast cancer.

2. There are lifestyle modifications and hormone-suppressing medications that can reduce the risk of developing breast cancer.

3. The client is asking for information and the nurse should provide the factual information.

4. This statement does not address the client's question.

22. 1. Hormone suppression therapy in a male client would decrease the client's libido and decrease the ability to sustain an erection.

2. Hormone suppression therapy does not destroy cancer cells; it works by changing the hormonal environment of the host and depriving the cancer of the hormones that stimulate its growth.

3. This is a true statement, but it is not the rationale for how the medications work in the body.

4. **Gender-specific cancers may replicate better in the presence of the hormones specific to that sex. Suppressing the androgens produced in the testes results in a reduction in the growth rate of the tumor.**

23. 1. The medication is an implant that slowly dissolves over a month's time. The drug is formulated in a pellet that is dispensed through a 16-gauge needle.

2. Lupron LA is an implant that slowly dissolves over a month's time. The

drug is formulated in a pellet that is dispensed through a 16-gauge needle under the skin of the abdomen.

   3. This is not a suppository.

   4. The medication does not cause peptic ulcer disease and is not administered orally.

24. 1. Aromatase inhibitors block the production of estrogen and androgen precursors, but they do not have any positive effect on body image. The client may experience a negative effect on body image if she develops facial hair (hirsutism).

   2. Aromatase inhibitors are not antidepressants and would not affect the client's ability to express her feelings.

   3. Aromatase inhibitors are used to treat postmenopausal breast cancer. Two prime metastasis sites for breast cancer are the lungs and bones. Negative findings in these areas indicate the medication is effective.

   4. DNA ploidy tests are conducted on the tumor cells at the beginning of treatment to determine the prognosis of the disease. The test is not used to monitor the progress of therapy.

25. 1. Kaposi's lesions are normally light brown to a purple color; this does not indicate effectiveness of the medication.

   2. Megace is an antineoplastic hormone used to treat metastatic cancer of the breast and endometrium. Side effects of the medication include an increased appetite. It is prescribed in an unlabeled use for increasing the appetite in clients diagnosed with AIDS or under the name of Appetrol.

   3. Megace does not treat nausea.

   4. Megace would not affect the ability to perform activities of daily living, except indirectly by increasing the client's nutritional intake.

MEDICATION MEMORY JOGGER: The nurse must be aware that some medications are used for other than the original purpose. Megace is one of those medications.

26. 1. All steroids can cause gastric upset; the client should take the medication with food.

   2. Steroids usually increase the appetite, increasing the client's weight gain.

   3. Decadron is a steroid, and when discontinuing a steroid, the client

should be informed about tapering the medication. Decadron is the steroid of choice for disease processes occurring in the skull.

   4. The client may have a headache because of increased intracranial pressure from the tumor growth. Decadron decreases the edema surrounding the tumor and would help to prevent a headache.

27. 1. DES is a pregnancy category X drug, meaning that definite harm can occur to the fetus. Females exposed to DES in utero are at high risk for developing cervical cancer, but DES should not affect the sperm.

   2. DES suppresses the male androgens and the client may experience hot flashes and gynecomastia (breast development in men).

   3. DES can cause osteoporosis; therefore, the client should increase his intake of calcium.

   4. DES will not cause the client's hair to grow faster or change texture.

28. 1. This lab data indicates that the client's tumors grow best in the presence of estrogen and progesterone. Supplemental estrogen and progesterone would encourage tumor growth.

   2. The adrenal hormones are not indicated by this lab data.

   3. GnRH medications are used to suppress male androgens in clients diagnosed with prostate cancer.

   4. Estrogen and progesterone receptor assays are interpreted as follows: greater than 20% is favorable to the growth of the tumor; 11%–20% is borderline; and less than 10% is unfavorable. A favorable finding indicates that the client's tumor responds well to the presence of estrogen and progesterone. Suppressing or removing the ability to produce these hormones slows the tumor growth. Antiestrogen/ progesterone hormone medications would accomplish this.

29. 1. This is a false statement; the risk increases with prolonged use.

   2. This is a false statement; evidence indicates that the risk increases for women who take HRT.

   3. The risk of developing breast cancer increases each year the client takes hormone replacement therapy. Current research also implicates hormone

replacement therapy in the development of cardiovascular disease.
4. This is a false statement; the risk increases with prolonged use.

30. 1. Nolvadex will cause menopausal symptoms, but this is not the most important consideration to teach the client.
2. Nolvadex may cause vaginal discharge and nausea, but this is not the most important consideration to teach the client.
3. The fact that Nolvadex slows the growth of estrogen-positive tumors is the scientific rationale for administering this medication, but it is not the most important consideration to teach the client.
4. Tamoxifen increases the client's risk of developing endometrial cancer. Tamoxifen acts as an estrogen agonist at receptors in the uterus, causing proliferation of endometrial tissue that may result in endometrial cancer. For this reason, it is important that the client see the gynecologist regularly. This is the most important information to teach the client.

A Client Receiving an Investigational Protocol

31. 1. Explaining the risks and benefits of the medication to the client is the HCP's responsibility, not the nurse's.
2. The nurse should administer the medication per the protocol but not until the nurse knows what the mechanism of action and potential side effects are.
3. The nurse cannot administer the medication until it is available, but this is not the first action.
4. The nurse must know what the drug is, how it works in the body, and the potential side effects to assess for before administering any medication, especially an investigational medication.

MEDICATION MEMORY JOGGER: If the test taker placed the options in order of performance, then the test taker could eliminate options 2 and 3.

32. 1. The HCP will enroll clients that fit the protocol requirements. An investigational protocol is one that is being tried to determine the efficacy of the treatment, weighing the risks and benefits to the client. The investigation part is to determine what the

risks and benefits are. It is not necessarily the best chance for a cure.
2. Ethically, oncology clients will not be enrolled in a protocol if the standard therapy regimens have a good chance of providing an extension of life or quality of life for the client. If the client has received conventional therapy and has not responded well, then the HCP may suggest an investigational protocol. Usually this means the client has a poor prognosis before an investigational protocol is discussed.
3. Investigational protocol medication- and treatment-related expenses are provided at no cost to the client, but this is not the primary reason to place the client in a study.
4. This may be a reason the client chooses to participate in a study, but it is not the primary reason for enrolling the client in an investigational study.

33. 1. An experienced oncology nurse familiar with the investigational protocol should care for this client; a licensed practical nurse should not.
2. Measuring and recording client output is an appropriate delegation.
3. A new graduate nurse can care for a client receiving packed red blood cells. This is an appropriate assignment.
4. Care of a client who is seriously ill and taking an investigational drug can be assigned to a registered nurse.

34. 1. Placebos are not unethical as long as the clients have been informed of the possibility of receiving a placebo and of being randomly placed in a control group.
2. A placebo is an inactive substance resembling a medication that may be given experimentally or for its psychological effect.
3. Clients in investigational studies are informed that there are control groups that receive an inert medication for comparison to the medication group to determine the statistical effectiveness of the medication in treating the disease being studied.
4. Clients are not allowed to request this; no client wants to "not be treated." In a true investigational protocol, the clients are randomly selected for the medication group and the control group.

35. 1. The nurse should ask what has been prescribed for the client and how the client responded to the medications.
2. Herbs and over-the-counter medications may affect the client's response to proposed medication; therefore, this is an appropriate question to ask the client.
3. Soaps and clothing dyes should not affect the administration of a systemic medication for arthritis.
4. The client's response to the investigational medication for an immune system disease (rheumatoid arthritis) could be affected by a comorbid immune system disease. The nurse should assess this.
5. Medications, required laboratory tests, and HCP visits are free to the client in an investigational protocol. The ability to pay for the medication is not an issue.

36. 1. This is not for the nurse to determine. The client should be assessed by the HCP to decide if the side effect of nausea can be controlled.
2. The client has a real physiological problem, not a psychological one that requires a therapeutic conversation.
3. The client should be assessed by the HCP to determine if the side effect of nausea can be controlled. In any event, the side effects experienced by the client must be documented by the HCP. This is the nurse's best response.
4. This is a misleading and possibly false statement.

37.   250 mL
Intravenous infusion pumps are set at an hourly rate. The nurse is to infuse 1000 mL in 4 hours. 1000 ÷ 4 = 250 mL/hour.

38. 1. The client may want to leave "now," but this does not make the client the priority to receive their medication.
2. The nurse cannot administer the medication until the client has signed the protocol permit. This is not the first client to receive the medication.
3. Any medication that requires specific timing should be administered at the time required. This medication has priority.
4. A medication that is to be infused over 24 hours could wait to be administered until after the timed medication.

39. 1. Investigational studies use control groups for comparison to the medication group to determine statistical effectiveness of the medication in treating the disease being studied.
2. The control group should not develop the side effects produced by the medication being studied. A control group could not prove that a side effect of the study medication is not being caused by "anything" else. There are too many variables.
3. The researcher determines effectiveness by several means. The researcher may use a control group but will also use laboratory and radiologic data and client report of symptoms.
4. The researcher uses the study group and previous trials to determine the amount of medication required to treat the disease.

40. 1. The client is expressing a hope in the treatment; this is not a reason to question administering the medication.
2. **This client is having doubts about continuing the treatment. Until the client decides that he or she wishes to continue the treatment, the nurse should hold the medication and have the HCP discuss the client's concerns. The nurse would question administering this medication. The client has the right to withdraw from a protocol at any time.**
3. The HCP should never guarantee a positive response for any treatment. The nurse would not question administering the medication.
4. The nurse should explain the side effects of the medication to the client. Unless the client has concerns after the nurse teaches the client about the side effects, the nurse would administer the medication.

A Client Undergoing Surgery for Cancer

41. 1. Forcefully instilling anything into the port will push a clot into the client's body, and heparin is an anticoagulant, not a thrombolytic. It will not dissolve a clot. Anticoagulants prevent clot formation.
2. Flushing anything will infuse a clot into the client's body, possibly resulting in a stroke, pulmonary embolus, or myocardial infarction.

3. Urokinase is a thrombolytic. Instilling a small amount into the lumen of the implanted port and allowing the medication to sit in the catheter may dissolve the clot. The procedure may need to be repeated more than once to dissolve the entire clot.

4. The HCP is the person who determines if a new port should be placed and then schedules the procedure with the surgical staff.

MEDICATION MEMORY JOGGER: The nurse should learn medication by specific classifications. Anticoagulants do not dissolve clots; only thrombolytics dissolve clots. The "ase" ending in urokinase should clue the test taker to choose this option because thrombolytics are enzymes and enzymes usually end in "ase."

42. 5, 1, 2, 3, 4

5. The nurse should always inform the client of procedures prior to beginning to attempt to complete the procedure. The nurse should wash hands on entering the room.

1. The next step is to prepare the equipment and sterile field for the procedure to begin. Central line dressing kits contain sterile gloves for the nurse to use when performing the procedure.

2. Central line dressing kits include antiseptic solutions to be used to cleanse the skin. The nurse should know and follow the facility's procedure for accessing central line intravenous catheters.

3. Implanted ports can be palpated through the skin to determine where the diaphragm of the port is. The nurse then places a finger on each side of the diaphragm to maintain the correct placement target.

4. The diaphragm of the implanted port is designed to be punctured repeatedly over months to years. A noncoring needle (Huber) is used to prevent damage to the diaphragm. The nurse places the needle between the fingers and inserts it until the needle strikes the back of the reservoir.

43. 1. The Whipple procedure removes the islet cells of the pancreas, thus creating diabetes. The client must be knowledgeable about how to treat diabetes and administer insulin.

2. The client should be instructed to notify the HCP of an elevated temperature, not mask the symptoms of an infection.

3. The client should be taught to change the dressing daily. Waiting until once a week to change the dressing could result in the client having an undiscovered wound infection.

4. The client will now have diabetes and should follow a calorie-controlled diet.

44. 1. This should be done, but the nurse cannot wait until the wound care nurse arrives to implement skin protection for the client.

2. The nurse should apply a skin barrier paste to protect the skin around the stoma after cleansing the stoma and surrounding skin with a mild soap and water.

3. The skin barrier paste will not adhere to fecal-contaminated skin. The nurse should first gently cleanse the skin. Mild soap acts as an abrasive to remove feces and old barrier paste.

4. The pouch is replaced after the skin has been cleaned and protected.

45. 1. An Ommaya reservoir is similar to an implanted venous access device except that it is implanted directly into the ventricles of the brain. Medications can then be administered to the brain without the problem of being blocked by the blood–brain barrier.

2. An Ommaya reservoir is implanted into the ventricle of the brain, not into a vein.

3. Direct instillation of chemotherapy into the brain can cause more nausea.

4. Sustained-release medications are usually oral preparations; medications instilled into the Ommaya reservoir are liquid and are used immediately by the body.

46. 1. The client may need a warmed blanket in the PACU, but not a heating device.

2. If the anesthetic agent reaches the upper thoracic and cervical spinal cord, the client's respiratory muscles may be temporarily paralyzed. Keeping the head of the bed slightly elevated will prevent paralysis from occurring.

3. This would not be a safety measure; it is a pain control measure.

4. The anesthesiologist or nurse anesthetist is responsible for removing the catheter, not the PACU nurse.

47. 1. The advantage of implanted ports is that the client does not have to care for the port at home. The port should be flushed

monthly at the time of the therapy sessions. The skin forms a natural barrier from infection.

2. This is done when the client is being prepared to receive the chemotherapy, not when the client is being discharged.

3. **The nurse should make sure that all the chemotherapy is infused into the client by flushing the port with normal saline. Instilling heparin into the port, reservoir, and catheter will help to prevent clot formation in the catheter.**

4. This is done when the client is being prepared to receive the chemotherapy, not when the client is being discharged.

48. 1. These lab tests monitor kidney function and are not needed to monitor TPN.

2. **TPN solution contains high concentrations of glucose, proteins, lipids, and electrolytes. The nurse should monitor this lab data.**

3. Urine and serum osmolality levels are monitored for diabetes insipidus, not TPN.

4. CA-125 and carcinoembryonic antigen (CEA) levels may be monitored to follow the progress of the disease, but they are not daily tests and are not used for TPN.

49. 1. This should be done before the nurse leaves the client with the nurse call light access button, but it is not the first action.

2. This is done when a new cartridge is needed. The client should have a new cartridge in the pump because the pump came with the client from the operating room.

3. Determining the level of pain relief obtained is necessary but not until the nurse determines that the medication is being administered correctly.

4. **The nurse is still responsible for determining that the client is receiving the right dose of the right medication at the right time. The nurse should compare the settings to the HCP orders before the other steps.**

50. 1. This blood gas indicates metabolic acidosis. Normal saline at a keep-open rate would not treat metabolic acidosis.

2. **Clients who have had the islet cells removed are at risk for complications of diabetes mellitus. The blood gas results indicate metabolic ketoacidosis, and the treatment is continuous infusion of regular insulin.**

3. Bicarbonate infusion to correct acidosis is avoided because it can precipitate a sudden (and potentially fatal) decrease in serum potassium.

4. Humulin N insulin is not administered by sliding scale, and for acidosis the treatment is the more rapid-acting Humulin R insulin.

A Client with Chronic Pain

51. 1. The nurse should tell the client to notify the hospice staff if the client is not receiving adequate pain relief.

2. **The nurse should teach the client to take the pain medications as soon as the client begins to feel uncomfortable. Waiting to take the medication can make it difficult to get the pain under control.**

3. This would isolate the client unnecessarily. The client may always need medications to control the pain. The visitors should be sensitive to the client, and if the client becomes drowsy from the medication, then they should sit quietly near the client.

4. The client is terminally ill; addiction is not an issue.

52. 1. **Chronic pain is difficult to describe to persons not experiencing the pain. It is demoralizing and can result in clinical depression. Clients have to adjust to living with the pain and try to be as normal as possible. This is a classic picture of chronic pain. Pain is whatever the client says it is and occurs whenever the client says it does. The nurse should not judge the client; the nurse should administer the pain medication.**

2. The nurse should not confront the client's behavior. If the nurse is concerned that the client is exhibiting narcotic-seeking behavior, the nurse should discuss this with the HCP.

3. The client is in pain now; the nurse should not wait to administer the medication.

4. The nurse should administer the pain medication, not substitute a different medication.

MEDICATION MEMORY JOGGER: The nurse should remember basic tenets of nursing, such as that pain is whatever the

client says it is. Then, the answer to this question is obvious.

53. 1. The nurse should teach the client to take the pain medications as soon as the client begins to feel uncomfortable. Waiting to take the medication can make it difficult to get the pain under control.
2. The nurse should instruct the client to avoid using other forms of acetaminophen (Tylenol). The maximum daily adult dose is 4 grams. Each Vicodin tablet contains 500 mg of Tylenol, and Vicodin HP contains 660 mg.
3. The client only needs to notify the HCP if the pain is unrelieved.
4. **Hydrocodone slows peristalsis; the client should increase fluids and roughage in the diet to prevent constipation.**

54. 1. The client in chronic pain is often unable to localize the pain and may describe it as "all over" or "taking over my whole body." This is not important.
2. **The nurse should administer the pain medication without further delay.**
3. The client does not need a referral based on the information given.
4. There is no need to use a different scale; the client has rated the pain for the nurse.

55. 1. The client is receiving increasing amounts of narcotic without relief. The nurse should determine if there is some spiritual distress affecting the client's perception of the pain. An increased dose schedule has been tried without success.
2. Distraction techniques would not be successful with this level of pain.
3. **The nurse should determine if there is some spiritual distress affecting the client's perception of the pain. Increasing the client's pain medications has been tried without success. Therapeutic communication techniques are designed to allow the client to ventilate feelings.**
4. The client will not be willing or able to cooperate with any teaching until the pain has been controlled.

56. 1. Stronger medications would only make the client feel drowsier. The nurse should discuss ways of helping the client get the rest needed at night.
2. The client is not discussing feelings. The client is talking about not getting rest at night.

3. Sleeping medication (sedatives or hypnotics) are better options to induce the sleep the client needs at night. A combination of pain relief and sleep medication might be needed to allow the client to rest.
4. The nurse should not discourage the client from taking the medication needed to improve the quality of life. The nurse should teach the client how to cope with the side effects of all medications.

MEDICATION MEMORY JOGGER: The test taker should know the medications by the specific classifications. Medications in the same classification usually share the same side effects and adverse effects and the same interventions are needed to administer the medications safely.

57. 1. Keeping the eyes closed and drapes drawn would not indicate the pain medication is effective. These actions may be the client's way of dealing with the pain.
2. Using guided imagery is an excellent method to assist with the control of pain, but it does not indicate effectiveness of the medication.
3. **Because pain is whatever the client says it is and occurs whenever the client says it does, a client report of reduced pain indicates the medication is effective.**
4. This action may be the client's way of dealing with the pain, but it does not indicate the medication is effective.

58. 1. The client should be told that there are many different methods of relieving pain, and all of the available methods would have to have failed for this to be true.
2. This is not true, but it is what many clients believe to be true. Neighborhood pharmacies are usually willing to provide the medications their clientele require, but they may need advanced notice to obtain the amount of narcotic needed to fill a prescription for a client with cancer.
3. **Narcotic prescriptions need triplicate forms and are only good for 24 hours at a time. The client should try to anticipate when the medication needs to be refilled or he or she may run out over a weekend or holiday. Hospice will arrange to obtain any medication at any time for clients receiving their service.**

4. The client's pain has not been cured; it has only been controlled. The client will have pain if he or she does not take the medications as prescribed. The client should only notify the HCP if the pain becomes uncontrollable again on the prescribed pain control regimen.

59. 1. The client is nauseated. Roxanol can be taken orally or sublingually, but this could increase the nausea and cause vomiting. MS can be combined with an antiemetic to provide pain and nausea relief.
   2. Compazine and morphine are compatible in the same syringe. Using two syringes is not cost effective and would take more time to administer the medications.
   3. The Zofran has not relieved the client's nausea. The nurse should try IV Compazine. The client is nauseated. Roxanol can be taken orally or sublingually, but this could increase the nausea and cause vomiting.
   4. Compazine and morphine are compatible in the same syringe. Morphine (for the pain) should be administered over 5 minutes; Compazine (for the nausea) should be administered at a rate of 5 mg per minute. The nurse could administer both medications in one syringe over 5 minutes safely.

60. 1. MS Contin is a sustained-release formulation and is administered routinely every 6–8 hours to control chronic pain. Roxanol is administered sublingually to treat breakthrough pain. This is the correct administration procedure.
   2. MS Contin is not a PRN medication for pain.
   3. MS Contin is not a PRN medication for pain and Roxanol is absorbed very quickly through the veins under the tongue. The dosing for Roxanol is more frequently than every 4 hours.
   4. MS Contin will not control breakthrough pain because of its sustained-release formulation. The Roxanol should not be held.

1. The client who is postchemotherapy calls the clinic nurse and reports mouth ulcers that make it difficult for the client to eat. Which statement is the nurse's best reply?
   1. "It is fine if you are not able to eat for a while. Just be sure to drink."
   2. "Try swishing a teaspoon of antacid in your mouth before meals."
   3. "You must force yourself to get some nourishment, even if it hurts."
   4. "This is expected and will go away in a week to 10 days."

2. The client about to receive chemotherapy is complaining of nausea and nervousness. Based on the MAR, which of the PRN medications should the nurse administer?

Medication Administration Record				
Client:		**Account #: 1 234 56**	**Date:** Today	
Height: 64 inches		**Weight:** 156 lbs	**Allergies:** NKA	
Date	**Medication**	2301–0700	0701–1500	1501–2300
	Ondansetron (Zofran) 4 mg IVP every 4 hours PRN			
	Morphine 2 mg IVP every 2–3 hours PRN			
	Lorazepam (Ativan) 2 mg IVP every 2 hours PRN			
	Prochlorperazine Spansule (Compazine) 5 mg po T.I.D. PRN			
	Prochlorperazine 5–10 mg IVP every 2 hours PRN			
Nurse Signature/Initials		**Day Nurse RN/DN**		

   1. Ondansetron (Zofran) IVP.
   2. Morphine IVP.
   3. Lorazepam (Ativan) IVP.
   4. Prochlorperazine (Compazine) IVP.

3. The client is participating in a Phase III clinical trial for a new antineoplastic agent. Which scientific rationale is the purpose of this phase of the pharmacology trials?
   1. Determine optimum dosing, scheduling, and toxicity of the medication.
   2. Determine effectiveness against specific tumor types.
   3. Compare the new medication with the standard treatment procedures.
   4. Further investigate to determine if the medication may have other uses.

4. The client diagnosed with cancer complains of frequent nausea. Which information is most important for the nurse to discuss with the client?
   1. Teach the client to take an antiemetic 30 minutes before meals.
   2. Have the client keep a record of the nausea to discuss with the HCP.
   3. Notify the health-care provider if the client becomes dehydrated.
   4. The significant other should provide the client with his or her favorite foods.

5. The nurse is reviewing the laboratory report of a client diagnosed with cancer. Which biologic response modifier medication would the nurse question?

Client:	Account Number: 1 234 56	Date: Today
Laboratory Data	Client Values	Normal Values
WBC	10.2	4.5–11.0 (10^3)
RBC	3.56	M: 4.7–6.1 (10^6) F: 4.2–5.4 (10^6)
Hemoglobin	8.4	M: 13.5–17.5 g/dL F: 11.5–15.5 g/dL
Hematocrit	25.1	M: 40%–52% F: 36%–48%
MCV	72	81-96 μg/m³
MCHC	26	33–36 g/dL
RDW	9.2	11%–14.5%
Reticulocyte	1.5	0.5%–1.5%
Platelets	79	150–400 (10^3)
Differential		
Neutrophils	83	40%–75% (2500–7500/mm³)
Lymphocytes	17	20%–50% (1500–5500/mm³)
Monocytes	0	1%–10% (100–800/mm³)
Eosinophils	0	0%–6% (0–440/mm³)
Basophils	0	0% 2% (0–200.mm³)

1. Erythropoietin (Procrit).
2. Oprelvekin (Neumega).
3. Interferon (Intron A).
4. Filgrastim (Neupogen).

6. The client diagnosed with a solid tissue tumor scheduled to receive chemotherapy has a white blood cell count of 5.9 (10^3) with 12% neutrophils. Which intervention should the nurse implement first?
   1. Administer the chemotherapy as ordered.
   2. Assess the client's temperature and lung sounds.
   3. Provide the client with a soft-bristled toothbrush.
   4. Premedicate the client with an aminoglycoside antibiotic.

7. The nurse is preparing to administer a vesicant antineoplastic medication through a peripheral IV catheter. Which intervention is the priority intervention?
   1. Have the medication mixed in a large volume of IV fluid.
   2. Tell the client to let the nurse know if the IV site becomes red.
   3. Place the infusion on an intravenous infusion pump.
   4. Start a new intravenous access before beginning the administration.

8. The client receiving chemotherapy for non-Hodgkin's lymphoma asks the nurse, "Why do I need to take steroids? I've heard they can cause problems." Which statement is the nurse's best response?
   1. "Steroids suppress replication of lymphoid tissue and cause cell death."
   2. "Steroids will decrease the inflammation caused by the tumor cells."
   3. "The problems caused by the steroids are nothing compared to cancer."
   4. "It is possible to have the HCP order different medications for the cancer."

9. The client receiving doxorubicin (Adriamycin), an antineoplastic antibiotic, for cancer of the breast has developed alopecia. Which information is most helpful for the nurse to provide the client?
   1. Have the client shave the entire head as a comfort measure.
   2. Encourage the client to purchase a wig that matches her own hair.
   3. Try to get the client to discuss her feelings about the alopecia.
   4. Discuss measures to prevent sunburn of the scalp.

10. The client taking chemotherapy has developed a white, patchy area on the tongue and buccal mucosa. Which medication would best treat this condition?
   1. Ketoconazole (Nizoral), an anti-infective, to swish and swallow.
   2. Metronidazole (Flagyl), a GI anti-infective, by mouth.
   3. Miconazole (Monistat), an anti-infective, topically.
   4. Doxycycline (Vibramycin), an antibiotic, orally.

11. Today's laboratory report for a client receiving chemotherapy is H and H 11.2 and 34.0, WBC 4.8 (10^3), neutrophils 72, and platelets 13 (10^3). Which interventions should the nurse implement?
   1. Have the lab draw a type and cross-match.
   2. Request an order for antibiotics from the HCP.
   3. Prepare to transfuse 10 units of platelets.
   4. Place the client on neutropenic precautions.

12. The nurse is assessing the client prior to initiating the seventh round of chemotherapy. Which question is most important for the nurse to ask the client before beginning the treatment?
   1. "Has your insurance company precertified you to receive more than six treatments?"
   2. "How have you dealt with the fatigue that occurs with the cancer treatments?"
   3. "Did you take all of the prescription for antinausea medications?"
   4. "Have you experienced any difficulty swallowing or had a temperature?"

13. The client diagnosed with cancer tells the clinic nurse, "I am so afraid that I will die a horribly painful death." Which statement is the nurse's best response?
   1. "That is a concern. Let's sit down and discuss your concerns. I am here to talk if you need to."
   2. "Pain does not occur for everyone, but if it does, your HCP can prescribe medications to control it."
   3. "This does happen sometimes and it is a valid concern. I hope this does not happen to you."
   4. "There are medications that can be prescribed to control the pain, but they can cause you to become addicted."

14. The nurse is caring for clients on an oncology unit. Which medication should the nurse administer first?
    1. The scheduled dose of leucovorin (folinic acid), a rescue factor.
    2. The narcotic pain medication for a client with pain of "10" on the pain scale.
    3. The antiemetic to a client complaining of nausea and an emesis of 200 mL.
    4. The third dose of an aminoglycoside antibiotic to a client who has a fever.

15. The HCP has ordered two units of packed red blood cells (PRBC) for the client diagnosed with cancer and anemia. Which interventions should the nurse implement? Rank in order of performance.
    1. Initiate the transfusion at 10 mL per hour.
    2. Assess the client's lung sounds.
    3. Place the blood on an infusion pump.
    4. Run the transfusion at a 4-hour rate.
    5. Check the blood with another nurse.

16. The client diagnosed with a solid tissue tumor is prescribed darbepoetin (Aranesp), a hematopoietic growth factor. Which data should the nurse monitor?
    1. The white blood cell counts.
    2. The client's lung capacity.
    3. The client's blood pressure.
    4. The platelet counts.

17. The client diagnosed with cancer is being prepared for surgery. Which information should the outpatient surgery nurse convey to the surgeon immediately?
    1. The client takes digoxin (Lanoxin) for heart problems.
    2. The client stopped taking acetylsalicylic acid (aspirin) last week.
    3. The client has been taking clopidogrel (Plavix) every day.
    4. The client becomes nauseated after receiving anesthesia.

18. The nurse is preparing a client for discharge with intractable pain and a home infusion pump with a narcotic medication. Which information should the nurse include? Select all that apply.
    1. Teach the client signs of phlebitis or infection.
    2. Have the client sign out the medication.
    3. Remind the client to document the pain for the HCP.
    4. Refer the client to a home health agency.
    5. Discuss the use of the infusion pump.

19. Which intervention should the nurse in an oncology physician's office delegate to the unlicensed assistive personnel (UAP)?
    1. Administer the premedications for the chemotherapy.
    2. Provide discharge instructions to the client.
    3. Document the antineoplastic agents the client received.
    4. Apply A+D ointment to the head of a client who has alopecia.

20. The client receiving chemotherapy has developed stomatitis. Which referral should the nurse implement?
    1. Refer to a social worker.
    2. Refer to a dietitian.
    3. Refer to a hospice nurse.
    4. Refer to a physical therapist.

1. 1. It is not fine for the client to not be able to eat. The client needs a positive nitrogen balance if the client is to respond well to the treatment.
    2. **This is a suggestion to alleviate the pain caused by mouth ulcerations resulting from chemotherapy. The antacid coats the tender mucosal lining. If this does not work, then there are numbing medications that the HCP can prescribe.**
    3. This will cause pain and result in the client's dreading mealtime. There are interventions that can help the client with the problem.
    4. This may be expected as a result of the chemotherapy and it will go away when the client's immune system has a chance to recover from the insult caused by the chemotherapy, but it not the best response. The nurse should try to help the client deal with the mouth ulcers.

2. 1. Ondansetron will help the nausea, but it will not have any effect on the client's nervousness.
    2. Morphine is capable of producing analgesia and has bronchodilating effects, but it will not treat nausea or nervousness.
    3. **Lorazepam is a sedative hypnotic that has antiemetic and antianxiety properties. The nurse should administer this medication to treat both of the client's complaints.**
    4. Prochlorperazine will treat the nausea but not the nervousness. This is not the best medication for the nurse to administer.

    MEDICATION MEMORY JOGGER: The test taker should know the medications by the specific classifications. Medications in the same classification usually share the same side effects and adverse effects, and the same interventions are needed to administer the medications safely.

3. 1. Determining optimum dosing, scheduling, and toxicity of a medication is the purpose of a Phase I clinical trial. Clients participating in Phase I and II trials are not placed in the trials unless their cancers have failed to respond to standard treatment procedures.
    2. Determining the effectiveness of a medication against specific tumor types is the purpose of a Phase II clinical trial.
    3. **Comparing a new medication with the standard treatment procedures is the purpose of a Phase III clinical trial.**
    4. Further investigation to determine if a medication may have other uses is the purpose of a Phase IV clinical trial.

4. 1. **To prevent nausea the client should take an antiemetic 30 minutes before attempting to eat. Maintaining the client's nutritional status is the most important information for the nurse to discuss.**
    2. There is no reason for the client to keep a record of the nausea. If the nausea is not controlled, the client should report it to the HCP.
    3. Reporting to the HCP that a client has become dehydrated is important, but if the nurse is able to assist with interventions to maintain the client's nutritional status, the client will also be able to maintain his or her hydration status.
    4. The client should not try to eat favorite foods when nauseated. Doing so may create an aversion to the foods, and then the favorite foods will not be useful if dealing with anorexia.

5. 1. Procrit is administered to increase the production of red blood cells. The client's levels are below normal. The nurse would not question administering this medication.
    2. Neumega is administered to increase the production of platelets. The client's levels are below normal. The nurse would not question administering this medication.
    3. Interferon would not be questioned on the basis of information provided by a complete blood count.
    4. **Neupogen is administered to increase the production of white blood cells. It is discontinued when the WBC is 10,200, or 10.2×10^3. The nurse should hold this medication and notify the HCP of the client's laboratory values.**

6. 1. The client is neutropenic despite the number of white blood cells. The absolute neutrophil count is only 708 ($5900 \times 0.12 = 708$); normal is greater than 2500. This client is at great risk of developing an infection. The nurse would hold the chemotherapy and discuss the absolute neutrophil count with the HCP.
    2. **This client's laboratory data indicates a great risk for infection. The nurse should assess the client for any sign of an infection.**
    3. This is an intervention for thrombocytopenia, not neutropenia.

4. The client may need to be prescribed antibiotic therapy, but aminoglycoside antibiotics are used mainly for methicillin-resistant staphylococcus infections (MRSA).

7. 1. The medication is usually mixed in small volumes of fluid because the nurse should not leave the client during the administration of a vesicant.
2. The nurse should not leave the client; the nurse can observe this complication directly.
3. Infusion pumps are controversial because the pump could force the vesicant medication into the client's tissue and cause more extensive damage.
4. **When administering a vesicant medication into a peripheral intravenous line, the nurse must know that the vein is patent and that there is little likelihood of a leak-back phenomenon occurring—that is, a leaking of minute amounts of the medication into the tissue because the catheter has been in the vein too long and an enlarging of the insertion site has occurred. The nurse should start a new IV site.**

8. 1. **Steroid medications are particularly useful in the treatment of lymphomas because they exert direct toxicity on lymphoid tissue by suppressing mitosis of the cancer cells and dissolution of lymphocytes.**
2. Steroids do suppress inflammation, but this is not the reason to administer these medications to clients with a lymphoma.
3. This is a belittling statement and does not address the client's concerns.
4. Other medications that are prescribed have side effects also; the nurse should not undermine the HCP by suggesting this.

9. 1. Shaving the entire head would not create comfort. Hair keeps heat in the body and is aesthetic.
2. **Wearing a wig that matches the client's hair color and style will allow the client to appear in public without having comments made about her loss of hair.**
3. This is assuming that the client wants to discuss feelings about her body image.
4. The nurse should warn the client about being in the sun without covering her head, but it is not the most helpful information.

10. 1. **Ketoconazole is an anti-infective medication that treats yeast infections. White, patchy areas in the mouth indicate oral candidiasis, a yeast infection. The correct administration procedure is to have the client swish the medication around in the mouth and then swallow the medication to treat areas in the esophagus as well.**
2. Metronidazole treats intestinal amoebae, vaginal trichomonas, and anaerobic bacteria, not yeast infections.
3. Miconazole is used to treat yeast infections, but applying a topical cream to the oral mucosa would cause pain and would not adhere to the mucosal lining.
4. Doxycycline would further destroy the good bacteria needed to keep the yeast in check. This would increase the client's problem.

11. 1. Clients are not transfused unless the hemoglobin is less than 8 and the hematocrit is less than 24. There is no reason to type and cross-match the client.
2. The client's absolute neutrophil count—3456— is higher than 2500, indicating that the client has adequate circulating neutrophils to protect against infection.
3. **Thrombocytopenia is defined as a platelet count of less than 100,000. If it is less than 50,000, the client is at risk for bleeding; if it is less than 20,000, the client is at great risk for hemorrhage. This client's platelet count is 13,000. The nurse should prepare to infuse platelets to prevent hemorrhage.**
4. The client's absolute neutrophil count is higher than 2500 so the client has adequate circulating neutrophils to protect against infection. The client does not need to be placed in reverse isolation (neutropenic precautions).

12. 1. This may be an important question for the business manager to ask, but this is not the nurse's responsibility. The nurse should be concerned with administering the medications safely.
2. How the client deals with fatigue is not important when deciding if it is safe to administer the chemotherapy.
3. Using up a prescription is not the most important question when assessing the client for side effects or adverse effects of chemotherapy.

4. The medications' full effect will not occur until between the treatments. Nadir counts of white blood cells and other clinical manifestations relating to the chemotherapy should be assessed. The nurse should assess for stomatitis, infections, and nutritional status. A fever would indicate an infection, and difficulty swallowing could indicate mouth inflammation (stomatitis) or ulcerations.

13. 1. The nurse should address the client's concern with information. The client did say "I am afraid," but accurate information can alleviate the fear. This is not the best response.
   2. **The nurse should inform the client about pain control options; after the client has accurate information, the nurse can address the fear, if it still exists.**
   3. This does not give the client the information the client is seeking.
   4. Addiction should not be a concern of the client. Although it is a remote possibility, usually the client will taper the dose of the medication if it is too high. This client is worried about dying in pain, and addiction need not be a concern for a client who is terminally ill.

14. 1. **Rescue medications are specifically timed to prevent life-threatening complications. The nurse should administer this medication first.**
   2. Pain is a priority, but it is not life threatening if the client has to wait for a few minutes to receive the pain medication.
   3. An antiemetic medication is a priority, but it is not life threatening if the client has to wait for a few minutes to receive the antiemetic medication.
   4. The client has already had two doses of the medication. This is not the priority medication to administer.

   MEDICATION MEMORY JOGGER: The classification of "rescue factor" should provide the test taker with a clue about priority.

15.   2, 5, 3, 1, 4
   2. **The first step should be to assess the client for signs of fluid volume overload. Crackles in the lungs would indicate to the nurse to infuse the PRBCs as slowly as possible.**

5. Blood products require two nurses to verify that the correct product is being administered. This is the second step.
3. Administering infusions is safer when the nurse uses a pump. Infusion devices prevent inadvertent rapid administration of fluids, and pumps also prevent the transfusion from slowing down (blood is very thick) and not infusing within the time period.
1. Blood should initially be transfused at a very slow rate. The most common time for a life-threatening complication to occur is within the first 15 minutes of the transfusion. The nurse should not leave the client being given the transfusion for 15 minutes and should perform vital signs every 5 minutes. If at the end of the 15 minutes the client has not experienced any difficulty with the blood product, then the nurse should adjust the infusion rate to transfuse the PRBCs within 4 hours.
4. Setting the transfusion to infuse within the time period is the final step before the nurse leaves the client's room.

16. 1. Darbepoetin stimulates red blood cell production. Monitoring the white blood cell count would be appropriate for clients receiving Neupogen and Neulasta, both of which stimulate white blood cell production.
   2. Darbepoetin will not affect the client's lung capacity.
   3. **Darbepoetin stimulates red blood cell production. When the hematocrit rises, it can result in an increase in blood pressure. The nurse should monitor the client's blood pressure.**
   4. Darbepoetin stimulates red blood cell production. Monitoring platelet counts would be appropriate for a client receiving Neumega, which stimulates platelet production.

17. 1. Many clients take digoxin and do fine during surgery. The HCP should be aware of the client's cardiac status when he or she performed the history and physical. The nurse does not have to notify the surgeon about this medication.
   2. The client stopped taking the aspirin last week. The nurse does not have to notify the surgeon about this medication.

3. Clopidogrel is an antiplatelet medication the client has been taking. It should be discontinued at least 7 days before surgery. The nurse should notify the surgeon because the surgery will need to be rescheduled.
4. Many clients become nauseated following anesthesia. The nurse would not have to notify the surgeon.

18. 1. Because this client will be monitoring the intravenous injection site, the nurse should teach the client about signs of phlebitis (for a peripheral IV) or an infection and what to do if they occur.
2. The client will not receive the medication from the hospital pharmacy; the client will obtain the medication from a neighborhood pharmacy or from a home health-care agency pharmacy.
3. There is no need for the client to self-document the pain.
4. Arrangements for follow-up care should be made with a home care agency.
5. The medications will be administered using a pump designed for this purpose. The nurse should make sure the client is able to operate the pump.

19. 1. The nurse cannot delegate administration of medications in this setting and cannot delegate this particular type of medication in any setting.
2. The nurse cannot delegate teaching to a UAP.
3. The nurse must document what he or she does. This cannot be delegated.
4. The UAP could apply a topical over-the-counter preparation.

20. 1. Stomatitis is an inflammation of the buccal mucosa. A social worker would not be able to help with this client.
2. Stomatitis is an inflammation of the buccal mucosa. A dietitian can help the client by providing foods the client can swallow without too much chewing and at the same time receive adequate nutrition. The nurse should refer the client to the dietitian.
3. Stomatitis is not a terminal process. Hospice nurses care for the terminally ill.
4. Stomatitis is an inflammation of the buccal mucosa. A physical therapist would not be able to help with this client.

MEDICATION MEMORY JOGGER: The test taker must know medical terminology.

Mental Health Disorders

12

"Psychotropic medications are not intended to 'cure' the mental illness . . . they relieve physical and behavior symptoms. They do not resolve emotional problems."

—Mary Townsend

PRACTICE QUESTIONS

A Client with a Major Depressive Disorder

1. The client with a major depressive disorder taking the selective serotonin reuptake inhibitor (SSRI) fluoxetine (Prozac) calls the psychiatric clinic and reports feeling confused and restless and having an elevated temperature. Which action should the psychiatric nurse take?
   1. Determine if the client has flulike symptoms.
   2. Instruct the client to stop taking the SSRI.
   3. Recommend the client take the medication at night.
   4. Explain that these are expected side effects.

2. The client diagnosed with a major depressive disorder asks the nurse, "Why did my psychiatrist prescribe an SSRI medication rather than one of the other types of antidepressants?" Which statement by the nurse would be most appropriate?
   1. "Probably it is the medication that your insurance will pay for."
   2. "You should ask your psychiatrist why the SSRI was ordered."
   3. "SSRIs have fewer side effects than the other classifications."
   4. "The SSRI medications work faster than the other medications."

3. The client diagnosed with pneumonia is admitted to the medical unit. The nurse notes the client is taking an antidepressant medication. Which data best indicate the anti-depressant therapy is effective?
   1. The client reports a "2" on a 1–10 scale, with 10 being very depressed.
   2. The client reports not feeling very depressed today.
   3. The client gets out of bed and completes activities of daily living.
   4. The client eats 90% of all meals that are served during the shift.

4. The client diagnosed with depression is prescribed phenelzine (Nardil), a monoamine oxidase (MAO) inhibitor. Which statement by the client indicates to the nurse the medication teaching is effective?
   1. "I am taking the herb ginseng to help my attention span."
   2. "I drink extra fluids, especially coffee and iced tea."
   3. "I am eating three well-balanced meals a day."
   4. "At a family cookout I had chicken instead of a hotdog."

5. The client with major depressive disorder is suicidal. The client was prescribed the tricyclic antidepressant imipramine (Tofranil) 3 weeks ago. Which priority intervention should the nurse implement?
    1. Determine if the client has a plan to commit suicide.
    2. Assess if the client is sleeping better at night.
    3. Ask the family if the client still wants to kill himself or herself.
    4. Observe the client for signs of wanting to commit suicide.

6. The client with major depressive disorder has been taking amitriptyline (Elavil), a tricyclic antidepressant, for more than 1 year. The client tells the psychiatric clinic nurse that the client wants to quit taking the antidepressant. Which intervention is most important for the nurse to discuss with the client?
    1. Ask questions to determine if the client is still depressed.
    2. Ask the client why he or she wants to stop taking the medication.
    3. Tell the client to notify the HCP before stopping medication.
    4. Explain the importance of tapering off the medication.

7. The client with major depressive disorder is prescribed nefazodone (Serzone), an atypical antidepressant. The client tells the nurse, "I am going to take my medication at night instead of in the morning." Which statement would be the nurse's best response?
    1. "You really should take the medication in the morning for the best results."
    2. "It is all right to take the medication at night. It may help you sleep at night."
    3. "The medication should be taken with food so you should not take it at night."
    4. "Have you discussed taking the medication at night with your psychiatrist?"

8. The client admitted to the psychiatric unit for major depressive disorder with an attempted suicide is prescribed an antidepressant medication. Which interventions should the psychiatric nurse implement? Select all that apply.
    1. Assess the client's apical pulse and blood pressure.
    2. Check the client's serum antidepressant level.
    3. Monitor the client's liver function status.
    4. Provide for and ensure the client's safety.
    5. Evaluate the effectiveness of the medication.

9. The client diagnosed with major depression who attempted suicide is being discharged from the psychiatric facility after a 2-week stay. Which discharge intervention is most important for the nurse to implement?
    1. Provide the family with the phone number to call if the client needs assistance.
    2. Encourage the client to keep all follow-up appointments with the psychiatric clinic.
    3. Ensure the client has no more than a 7-day supply of antidepressants.
    4. Instruct the client not to take any over-the-counter medications without consulting with the HCP.

10. The client prescribed an antidepressant 1 week ago tells the psychiatric clinic nurse, "I really don't think this medication is helping me." Which statement by the psychiatric nurse would be most appropriate?
    1. "Why do you think the medication is not helping you?"
    2. "You think your medication is not helping you."
    3. "You need to come to the clinic so we can discuss this."
    4. "It takes about 3 weeks for your medication to work."

A Client with Bipolar Disorder

11. Which statement indicates the client diagnosed with bipolar disorder who is taking lithium (Eskalith), an antimania medication, understands the medication teaching?
    1. "I will monitor my daily lithium level."
    2. "I will make sure I do not get dehydrated."
    3. "I need to taper the dose if I quit taking it."
    4. "I need to take the medication on an empty stomach."

12. The nurse is preparing to administer lithium (Eskalith), an antimania medication, to a client diagnosed with bipolar disorder. The lithium level is 1.4 mEq/L. Which action should the nurse implement?
    1. Administer the medication.
    2. Hold the medication.
    3. Notify the health-care provider.
    4. Verify the lithium level.

13. To which client would the nurse question administering lithium (Eskalith), an antimania medication?
    1. The 54-year-old client on a 4-g sodium diet.
    2. The 23-year-old client taking an antidepressant medication.
    3. The 42-year-old client taking a loop diuretic.
    4. The 30-year-old client with a urine output of 40 mL/hour.

14. The 24-year-old female client with bipolar disorder is prescribed valproic acid (Depakote), an anticonvulsant medication. Which question should the nurse ask the client?
    1. "Have you ever had a migraine headache?"
    2. "Are you taking any type of birth control?"
    3. "When was the last time you had a seizure?"
    4. "How long since you have had a manic episode?"

15. The client diagnosed with bipolar disorder is taking lithium (Eskalith), an antimania medication. Which statement by the client warrants further clarification by the nurse?
    1. "I will limit the amount of caffeine I drink."
    2. "I really enjoy playing soccer on weekends."
    3. "I will drink at least 2000 mL of water a day."
    4. "I need to call my HCP if I develop diarrhea."

16. The client with bipolar disorder who is taking lithium (Eskalith), an antimania medication, has a lithium level of 3.1 mEq/L. Which treatment would the nurse expect the health-care provider to prescribe?
    1. No treatment because this is within the therapeutic range.
    2. Intravenous therapy with an 18-gauge angiocath.
    3. Preparation for immediate hemodialysis.
    4. The antidote for lithium toxicity.

17. The client with bipolar disorder is prescribed carbamazepine (Tegretol), an anticonvulsant. Which data indicates the medication is effective?
    1. The client is able to control extremes between mania and depression.
    2. The client's serum Tegretol level is within the therapeutic range.
    3. The client reports a "3" on a depression scale of 1–10, with 10 indicating severely depressed.
    4. The client has a decrease in delusional thoughts and hallucinations.

18. The client with bipolar disorder who is prescribed lithium (Eskalith), an antimania medication, is admitted to the psychiatric unit in an acute manic state. Which intervention should the nurse implement first?
    1. Determine the client's serum lithium level.
    2. Assess why the client quit taking the lithium.
    3. Implement care for the client's physiological needs.
    4. Administer a stat dose of lithium to the client.

19. Which information should the nurse discuss with the client diagnosed with bipolar disorder who is taking the anticonvulsant carbamazepine (Tegretol)?
    1. Instruct the client to use a soft-bristled toothbrush.
    2. Encourage the client to get ophthalmic examinations annually.
    3. Teach the client to monitor the blood pressure daily.
    4. Tell the client to avoid hazardous activities.

20. The client diagnosed with bipolar disorder is prescribed lithium (Eskalith), an anti-mania medication. Which interventions should the nurse discuss with the client? Select all that apply.
    1. Monitor serum therapeutic levels.
    2. Maintain an adequate fluid intake.
    3. Decrease sodium intake in diet.
    4. Do not take medication if the radial pulse is <60.
    5. Explain ways to prevent orthostatic hypotension.

A Client with Schizophrenia

21. The client admitted to the psychiatric unit diagnosed with schizophrenia is prescribed clozapine (Clozaril), an atypical antipsychotic. Which laboratory data should the nurse evaluate?
    1. The client's clozapine therapeutic level.
    2. The client's white blood cell count.
    3. The client's red blood cell count.
    4. The client's arterial blood gases.

22. The client admitted to the psychiatric unit experiencing hallucinations and delusions is prescribed risperidone (Risperdal), an atypical antipsychotic. Which intervention should the nurse implement?
    1. Provide the client with a low tyramine diet.
    2. Assess the client's respiration for 1 full minute.
    3. Instruct the client to change positions slowly.
    4. Monitor the client's intake and output.

23. The male client diagnosed with schizophrenia is prescribed ziprasidone (Geodon), an atypical antipsychotic. Which statement to the nurse indicates the client understands the medication teaching?
    1. "I need to keep taking this medication even if I become impotent."
    2. "I should not go out in the sun without wearing protective clothing."
    3. "This medication may cause my breast size to increase."
    4. "I may have trouble sleeping when I take this medication."

24. The client diagnosed with schizophrenia is prescribed clozapine (Clozaril), an atypical antipsychotic. Which information should the nurse discuss with the client concerning this medication?
    1. Discuss the need for regular exercise.
    2. Instruct the client to monitor for weight loss.
    3. Tell the client to take the medication with food.
    4. Explain to the client the need to decrease alcohol intake.

25. The client with paranoid schizophrenia is prescribed aripiprazole (Abilify), a dopamine system stabilizer (DDS). Which statement best describes the scientific rationale for administering this medication?
    1. It decreases the anxiety associated with hallucinations and delusions.
    2. It increases the dopamine secretion in the brain tissue to improve speech.
    3. It reduces positive symptoms of schizophrenia and improves negative symptoms.
    4. It blocks the cholinergic receptor sites in the diseased brain tissue.

26. Which information should the nurse discuss with the client diagnosed with schizophrenia who is prescribed an antipsychotic medication?
    1. Drink decaffeinated coffee and tea.
    2. Decrease the dietary intake of salt.
    3. Eat six small, high-protein meals a day.
    4. Limit alcohol intake to one glass of wine a day.

27. The nurse is discussing the prescribed antipsychotic medication with a family member of a client diagnosed with schizophrenia. Which information should the nurse discuss with the family member?
    1. Explain the need for the family member to give the client the medication.
    2. Encourage the family member to learn cardiopulmonary resuscitation (CPR).
    3. Discuss the need for the client to participate in a community support group.
    4. Teach the family member what to do in case the client has a seizure.

28. Which assessment data indicates the atypical antipsychotic quetiapine (Seroquel) is effective for the client diagnosed with paranoid schizophrenia?
    1. The client does not exhibit any tremors or rigidity.
    2. The client reports a "2" on an anxiety scale of 1–10.
    3. The family reports the client is sleeping all night.
    4. The client denies having auditory hallucinations.

29. The client diagnosed with paranoid schizophrenia has been taking haloperidol (Haldol), a conventional antipsychotic, for several years. Which statement indicates the client needs additional teaching concerning this medication?
    1. "I know that if I have any rigidity or tremors I must call my HCP."
    2. "I eat high-fiber foods and drink extra water during the day."
    3. "I am more susceptible to colds and the flu when taking this medication."
    4. "This medication will make my hallucinations and delusions go away."

30. The 43-year-old female client diagnosed with schizophrenia has been taking the conventional antipsychotic medication chlorpromazine (Thorazine) for 20 years. Which assessment data would warrant discontinuing the medication?
    1. The client has had menstrual irregularities for the last year.
    2. The client has to get up very slowly from a sitting position.
    3. The client complains of having a dry mouth and blurred vision.
    4. The client has fine, wormlike movements of the tongue.

A Client with an Anxiety Disorder

31. The client diagnosed with a general anxiety disorder is prescribed alprazolam (Xanax), a benzodiazepine. Which information should the clinic nurse discuss with the client?
    1. Explain to the client that this medication is for short-term use.
    2. Inform the client that rage and excitement are expected side effects.
    3. Tell the client to avoid foods that are high in vitamin K.
    4. Instruct the client to take the medication with at least 8 ounces of water.

32. The female client taking lorazepam (Ativan), a benzodiazepine, for panic attacks tells the clinic nurse that she is trying to get pregnant. Which action should the nurse take first?
    1. Tell the client to inform the obstetrician of taking Ativan.
    2. Instruct the client to quit taking the medication.
    3. Determine how long the client has been taking the medication.
    4. Encourage the client to stop taking Ativan prior to getting pregnant.

33. The nurse is preparing to administer the benzodiazepine alprazolam (Xanax) to a client who has a generalized anxiety disorder. Which intervention should the nurse implement prior to administering the medication?
    1. Assess the client's apical pulse.
    2. Assess the client's respiratory rate.
    3. Assess the client's anxiety level.
    4. Assess the client's blood pressure.

34. The client diagnosed with obsessive–compulsive disorder is prescribed the selective serotonin reuptake inhibitor (SSRI) sertraline (Zoloft). Which statement indicates the client understands the medication teaching?
    1. "If I get a headache or become nauseated, I will notify my HCP."
    2. "It will take a couple of months before I see a change in my behavior."
    3. "I need to be careful because SSRIs may cause physical addiction."
    4. "I am glad I do not need to go to my psychologist's appointments."

35. The client who returned from the war 1 month ago is diagnosed with posttraumatic stress disorder (PTSD) and prescribed paroxetine (Paxil), an SSRI. The client asks the nurse, "Will this medication really help me? I don't like feeling this way." Which statement is the nurse's best response?
    1. "The medication will make you feel better within a couple of days."
    2. "Why do you think the medication won't help you feel better?"
    3. "Nothing really helps PTSD unless you go to counseling weekly."
    4. "Because the traumatic event was within 1 month, the Paxil should be helpful."

36. The elderly client diagnosed with a panic attack disorder is in the busy day room of a long-term care facility and appears anxious, is starting to hyperventilate, is trembling, and is sweating. Which action should the nurse implement first?
    1. Administer the benzodiazepine alprazolam (Xanax).
    2. Assess the client's vital signs.
    3. Remove the client from the day room.
    4. Administer the selective serotonin reuptake inhibitor (SSRI) sertraline (Zoloft).

37. The client with an anxiety disorder is prescribed the anxiolytic alprazolam (Xanax). The client calls the clinic and reports a dizzy, weak feeling when getting out of the chair. Which action should the nurse take?
    1. Instruct the client to quit taking the medication.
    2. Make an appointment for the client to come to the clinic.
    3. Determine if the client is drinking enough fluids.
    4. Discuss ways to prevent orthostatic hypotension.

38. The conscious client was admitted to the emergency department with an overdose of the anxiolytic alprazolam (Xanax). Which intervention should the nurse implement first?
    1. Prepare to administer an emetic with activated charcoal.
    2. Request a mental health consultation for the client.
    3. Prepare to administer the antidote flumazenil (Romazicon) IV.
    4. Determine why the client chose to overdose on the medication.

39. The client is receiving the anxiolytic alprazolam (Xanax) for a generalized anxiety disorder. Which assessment data best indicates the medication is effective?
    1. The client reports not feeling anxious.
    2. The client's pulse is not greater than 100.
    3. The client's respiratory rate is not greater than 22.
    4. The client reports a "1" on a 1–10 anxiety scale.

40. The client is having a CT scan and starts having a severe anxiety attack. The HCP prescribed the anxiolytic diazepam (Valium), intravenous push. Which action should the nurse implement?
    1. Dilute the Valium with normal saline and administer IVP.
    2. Do not dilute the Valium and inject in a port closest to the client.
    3. Inject the Valium into a 50-mL normal saline bag and infuse.
    4. Question the order because Valium should not be administered IV.

A Child with Attention Deficit–Hyperactivity Disorder

41. The 10-year-old child diagnosed with attention deficit–hyperactivity disorder (ADHD) is taking methylphenidate (Ritalin), a central nervous stimulant. Which assessment data would warrant intervention from the pediatric clinic nurse?
1. The child has gained 3 kg in the last month.
2. The child's pulse is 98 and B/P is 100/70.
3. The child has multiple bruises on the arm.
4. The child sits quietly in the examination room.

42. The 7-year-old child newly diagnosed with attention deficit–hyperactivity disorder (ADHD) is prescribed methylphenidate (Ritalin), a central nervous stimulant. Which information should the nurse discuss with the parents?
1. Take the medication on an empty stomach.
2. Weigh your child daily in the morning.
3. Administer the medication at night.
4. Keep a behavior diary on your child.

43. The 6-year-old child with attention deficit–hyperactivity disorder (ADHD) is admitted to the pediatric department after having an emergency appendectomy. Which intervention should the nurse implement when administering methylphenidate (Ritalin), a central nervous stimulant to the child?
1. Check the child's glucose level.
2. Administer with a full glass of water.
3. Monitor the child's vital signs.
4. Assess the child's incisional wound.

44. The 14-year-old adolescent with attention deficit–hyperactivity disorder (ADHD) is taking methylphenidate (Ritalin), a central nervous stimulant. Which statement indicates to the nurse that the adolescent understands the medication teaching?
1. "I can carry my medication in a personal pill container with me at school."
2. "I hate that I have to go to the school nurse to take my medication."
3. "I just take my medication on days that I have important tests."
4. "A friend of mine has ADHD and I gave him one of my pills."

45. The mother of a male child with attention deficit–hyperactivity disorder (ADHD) tells the school nurse she does not want her son to take Ritalin and wants to know if there is any other medication her son could take. Which statement is the nurse's best response?
1. "There are no other medications that work as well as Ritalin."
2. "Why are you worried about your child taking Ritalin?"
3. "There is a nonstimulant medication called Strattera that your child could take."
4. "I think that is something you should discuss with your child's doctor."

46. The mother of a 7-year-old child taking methylphenidate (Ritalin), a central nervous stimulant, for attention deficit–hyperactivity disorder (ADHD) calls the pediatric clinic and tells the nurse her daughter has lost 4 pounds in the last 2 weeks. Which action should the nurse implement?
1. Make an appointment for the child to see the HCP.
2. Instruct the mother to discontinue the Ritalin.
3. Explain that this is normal response to the medication.
4. Tell the mother to increase the child's caloric intake.

47. Which assessment data indicate the central nervous stimulant methylphenidate (Ritalin) has been effective for the 8-year-old child diagnosed with attention deficit–hyperactivity disorder (ADHD)?
1. The child has two notes from the school for inappropriate behavior in 1 week.
2. The child sleeps 8 hours a night and falls asleep during the day.
3. The child is able to sit and play a game for 30 minutes with a friend.
4. The child has difficulty following verbal instructions from the teacher.

48. The 8-year-old child newly diagnosed with attention deficit–hyperactivity disorder (ADHD) is prescribed methylphenidate (Ritalin), a central nervous stimulant. Which statement by the mother indicates the medication teaching has not been effective?
    1. "I will keep the medication in a safe place."
    2. "I will schedule regular drug holidays for my child."
    3. "It may cause my child to have growth restriction."
    4. "My child will probably experience insomnia."

49. Which diagnostic test would the nurse expect the HCP to monitor for the child diagnosed with attention deficit–hyperactivity disorder (ADHD) who is prescribed methylphenidate (Ritalin), a central nervous stimulant?
    1. Complete blood cell count (CBC).
    2. Serum potassium and sodium levels.
    3. An annual bone density test.
    4. Serum methylphenidate level.

50. The 8-year-old child is newly diagnosed with attention deficit–hyperactivity disorder (ADHD) and is prescribed methylphenidate (Ritalin), a central nervous stimulant. Which assessment data should the nurse anticipate the HCP obtaining prior to the child starting the medication?
    1. A x-ray of the epiphyseal plate.
    2. The child's height and weight.
    3. An electrocardiogram (EKG).
    4. The child's head circumference.

A Client with a Sleep Disorder

51. The male client diagnosed with chronic obstructive pulmonary disease (COPD) is admitted to the medical unit. During the admission process the client tells the nurse that he cannot sleep without Valium, a benzodiazepine, every night. Which action should the nurse take?
    1. Inform the client that clients with COPD should not take Valium.
    2. Ask the client when was the last time he had any seizure activity.
    3. Determine what effect the Valium has on the client when he takes it.
    4. Ask the health-care provider for an order for Valium.

52. The elderly client being prepared for major abdominal surgery has been taking alprazolam (Xanax), a benzodiazepine, PRN for many years for nerves. Which information should the nurse discuss with the HCP?
    1. Discuss prescribing another benzodiazepine medication postoperatively.
    2. Make sure that the alprazolam (Xanax) is ordered after surgery.
    3. Taper the medication to prevent complications.
    4. Change the alprazolam (Xanax) to a medication for sleep.

53. The client diagnosed with insomnia is scheduled for sleep studies. Which medication should the nurse instruct the client not to take?
    1. The ACE inhibitor captopril.
    2. The antihistamine diphenhydramine.
    3. The loop diuretic furosemide.
    4. The thyroid medication levothyroxine.

54. The health-care provider has prescribed lorazepam (Ativan), a benzodiazepine, for a female client receiving chemotherapy who complains of inability to sleep. Which information should the nurse teach the client?
    1. Do not attempt to become pregnant while taking Ativan.
    2. Avoid consuming too much alcohol while taking Ativan.
    3. Try exercising to tire yourself just before bedtime.
    4. Do not take the medication too long to avoid addiction.

55. The day shift nurse finds an elderly client difficult to arouse during the initial morning shift assessment. The nurse reviews the client's medication record for the last 24 hours. Which action should the nurse implement first?

Medication Administration Record

Date: Yesterday

Client: J. Smith Sex: female	Account Number: 345555	Allergies: Penicillin	
Height: 64 inches	Weight: 50 kg	Date of Birth: 01-19-XX Age: 74	

Date	Medication	0701–1500	1501–2300	2301–0700
	Furosemide (Lasix) 40 mg po daily	0900 DN K+ 3.8		
	Digoxin (Lanoxin) 0.125 mg po daily	0900 DN AP 93 Dig level 1.4		
	Acetaminophen (Tylenol) 650 mg po Q 4–6 hours PRN		2115 EN	
	Promethazine (Phenergan) 12.5 mg IVP Q 3–4 hours PRN nausea			0425 NN
	Temazepam (Restoril) 15 mg po Q HS PRN		2115 EN	

Signature and Title/Initials	Day Nurse RN/DN	Night Nurse RN/NN
	Evening Nurse RN/EN	

1. Notify the health-care provider of the client's current status.
2. Make sure the client has a call light within reach.
3. Call a code and initiate cardiopulmonary resuscitation.
4. Reassess the client in 1 hour.

56. The client being admitted to the medical unit gives the nurse a list of medications being taken at home. Which question should the nurse ask the client?

John D. Medication List

Medication	Time Taken
Synthroid 0.75 mcg	Before breakfast
Prilosec OTC	Before breakfast
Capoten	Before breakfast
Melatonin	At night

1. "Why do you take the Synthroid?"
2. "Does your emesis have red or dark-brown flecks in it?"
3. "What was your blood pressure before starting taking Capoten?"
4. "Do you have difficulty sleeping at night?"

57. The client diagnosed with narcolepsy is prescribed methylphenidate (Ritalin), an amphetamine. Which information should the nurse teach the client?
    1. Take the medication early in the day.
    2. The medication should be taken at bedtime.
    3. Keep the medication in a locked cabinet.
    4. Notify the HCP if there is a decrease in appetite.

58. The male client is diagnosed with narcolepsy. Which over-the-counter preparations should the nurse teach the client about?
    1. Caffeinated beverages and diphenhydramine (Benadryl),
    2. Flavored water and beta carotene.
    3. Milk with added vitamin D and saw palmetto.
    4. Carbonated sodas and black cohosh.

59. The 10-year-old client has begun to sleepwalk, a parasomnia disorder. Which information should the nurse provide the parents of the child? Select all that apply.
    1. Give the child a mild sedative 2 hours before bedtime.
    2. Place a lock on the outer door out of the child's reach.
    3. Make the child wake up when an episode occurs.
    4. Have the child practice guided imagery before bedtime.
    5. Administer atomoxetine (Strattera) every morning.

60. The client has Pickwickian syndrome and falls asleep at inappropriate times. Which medication should the nurse prepare to administer?
    1. Maximum Strength NoDoz, a caffeine drug.
    2. An inhaled steroid in a bi-pap machine for nighttime sleep.
    3. Modafinil (Provigil), a central nervous system stimulant.
    4. Amitriptyline (Elavil), a tricyclic antidepressant.

A Client with Substance Abuse

61. The client who is a chronic alcoholic is admitted to the medical unit for pneumonia. Which medication would the nurse expect the health-care provider to prescribe to prevent delirium tremens?
    1. Chlordiazepoxide (Librium), a benzodiazepine.
    2. Thiamine (vitamin B_1), a vitamin.
    3. Disulfiram (Antabuse), an abstinence medication.
    4. Fluoxetine (Prozac), an antidepressant.

62. For which client would the nurse expect the health-care provider to prescribe methadone, an abstinence medication?
    1. A client addicted to cocaine.
    2. A client addicted to heroin.
    3. A client addicted to amphetamines.
    4. A client addicted to hallucinogens.

63. The client is discussing wanting to quit smoking cigarettes with the clinic nurse. Which intervention is most successful in helping the client to quit smoking cigarettes?
    1. Encourage the client to attend a smoking cessation support group.
    2. Discuss tapering the number of cigarettes smoked daily.
    3. Instruct the client to use nicotine replacement therapy, such as a patch.
    4. Explain that clonidine can be taken daily to help decrease withdrawal symptoms.

64. The client is prescribed methadone, an opiate agonist. Which intervention should the nurse discuss with the client?
    1. Take the medication on an empty stomach.
    2. Decrease the fiber in the diet while taking the medication.
    3. Do not take methadone if the radial pulse is less than 60.
    4. Learn how to prevent orthostatic hypotension.

65. The client has been taking alprazolam (Xanax), a benzodiazepine, daily for the last 2 years. Which signs or symptoms would warrant intervention by the nurse?
    1. Nausea, vomiting, and agitation.
    2. Yawning, rhinorrhea, and cramps.
    3. Disorientation, lethargy, and craving.
    4. Ataxia, hyperpyrexia, and respiratory distress.

66. To which client would it be most appropriate to prescribe disulfiram (Antabuse), an abstinence medication?
    1. A client with chronic alcoholism admitted to the medical unit.
    2. A highly motivated client who wants to quit drinking alcohol.
    3. A client who has been taking amphetamines for more than 1 year.
    4. A highly motivated client who wants to quit taking heroin.

67. A client in the medical unit has been NPO for 3 days and is complaining of a headache. Which question should the nurse ask the client in regard to determining the reason for the headache?
    1. "Do you eat a diet high in glucose?"
    2. "How often do you drink alcohol?"
    3. "Do you take sleeping pills regularly?"
    4. "How often do you drink caffeinated beverages?"

68. The male client with chronic alcoholism comes to the emergency department (ED) reporting he has not had an alcoholic drink in more than 1 week. Which action should the ED nurse implement first?
    1. Implement seizure precautions according to hospital policy.
    2. Rehydrate the client with large amounts of intravenous fluids.
    3. Discuss withdrawal treatment in a hospital environment.
    4. Administer thiamine (vitamin B$_1$) through an intravenous route.

69. The client with a staggering gait is brought to the emergency department by a friend. The client is short of breath and has an oral temperature of 104°F. Which question should the nurse ask the client's friend?
    1. "How many alcoholic drinks has your friend had today?"
    2. "When was the last time your friend took amphetamines?"
    3. "Has your friend been inhaling any type of paint thinner?"
    4. "Through which route and at what time did your friend take cocaine?"

70. Which pharmacologic intervention should the nurse discuss with the client who is requesting help to quit smoking marijuana?
    1. Explain that there is no specific pharmacologic intervention.
    2. Instruct the client to use a nicotine patch or chew nicotine gum.
    3. Encourage the client to have the HCP prescribe an antianxiety medication.
    4. Discuss tapering dronabinol (Marinol) over a 2-week time period.

A Client with a Major Depressive Disorder

1. 1. Confusion and restlessness would not indicate the flu. The elevated temperature should make the nurse suspect a possible serious complication of SSRIs.
   2. Serotonin syndrome is a serious complication of SSRIs that produces mental changes (confusion, anxiety, and restlessness), hypertension, tremors, sweating, hyperpyrexia (elevated temperature), and ataxia. Conservative treatment includes stopping the SSRI and supportive treatment. If untreated, ESE can lead to death.
   3. Taking the medication at night will not treat serotonin syndrome.
   4. These are not expected side effects. They require nursing intervention.

2. 1. The cost of the medication or the type of insurance should not be a reason why one medication is prescribed over another.
   2. This is passing the buck, and the psychiatric nurse should be knowledgeable about medications.
   3. SSRIs have the same efficacy as MAO inhibitors and tricyclics, but SSRIs are safer because they do not have the sympathomimetic effects (tachycardia and hypertension) and anticholinergic effects (dry mouth, blurred vision, urinary retention, and constipation) of the MAO inhibitors and tricyclics.
   4. All antidepressant medications take at least 14 to 21 days to become effective.

3. 1. Depression is subjective and the nurse does not know this client; therefore, asking the client to rate the depression on a scale best indicates the effectiveness of the medication. Any subjective data can be put on a scale to make it objective.
   2. This is a very vague statement and it is not objective; therefore, it is not the best indicator of effectiveness of the medication.
   3. Completing ADLs indicates the client is not severely depressed, but it does not objectively support that the client's antidepressant medication is effective.
   4. Consuming 90% of the food may indicate the client is not depressed, but the nurse does not know how the client eats when severely depressed. Therefore, it is not the best indicator of the medication's effectiveness.

MEDICATION MEMORY JOGGER: The nurse determines the effectiveness of a medication by assessing for the symptoms, or lack thereof, for which the medication was prescribed.

4. 1. The client should use herbs cautiously because ginseng causes headaches, tremors, mania, insomnia, irritability, and visual hallucinations.
   2. The client should refrain from drinking too many beverages containing caffeine.
   3. Eating three balanced meals a day is not information that the nurse would teach about MAO inhibitors.
   4. Taking MAO inhibitors requires adherence to strict dietary restrictions concerning tyramine-containing foods, such as processed meat (hot dogs, bologna, and salami), yeast products, beer, and red wines. Eating these foods can cause a life-threatening hypertensive crisis.

MEDICATION MEMORY JOGGER: Some herbal preparations are effective, some are not, and a few can be harmful or even deadly. If a client is taking an herbal supplement and a conventional medicine, the nurse should investigate to determine if the combination will cause harm to the client. The nurse should always be the client's advocate.

5. 1. The nurse should ask if the client has a plan to commit suicide. As the client begins to recover from both psychological and physical depression, the client's energy level increases, making the client more prone to commit suicide during this time. It takes 2–6 weeks for therapeutic effects of tricyclic antidepressants to be effective.
   2. As the depression gets better, the client will start sleeping better, which indicates the medication is effective, but this is not a priority intervention because the client is suicidal.
   3. The family is an excellent resource to determine how the client is tolerating the medication and if it is effective, but the nurse should ask the client directly, not the family members, if he or she has thoughts of suicide.
   4. If the client seriously wants to commit suicide, usually the client will not show objective signs of wanting to kill themselves. The nurse must directly ask the client if he or she has a plan to commit suicide.

6. 1. The nurse should discuss what behavior led to the client being prescribed antidepressants and determine if the client is still depressed, but the most important thing to discuss with the client is that the antidepressant medication should not be discontinued abruptly.

2. The nurse should discuss why the client wants to stop taking the medication, but the most important intervention is to teach the client that the medication must be tapered. The client could quit taking medication without telling an HCP; therefore, teaching safety is priority.

3. The client should notify the HCP before stopping the medication, but the most important intervention is to keep the client safe and inform the client to taper off the medication.

4. **The client must first know the importance of needing to taper off the medication because rebound dysphoria, irritability, or sleepiness may occur if the medication is discontinued abruptly. Then the client should see the HCP to determine what action should be taken because the client doesn't want to take the medication.**

7. 1. This medication does not need to be taken in the morning to be more effective.

2. **Antidepressants may cause central nervous depression, which causes drowsiness. Therefore, taking the medication at night may help the client sleep at night and relieve daytime sedation. This is the nurse's best response.**

3. Antidepressants do not need to be taken with food because they do not cause gastrointestinal distress.

4. The nurse can provide factual information to the client without contacting the HCP. Taking antidepressants at night is not contraindicated; therefore, the nurse can share this information with the client.

8. 1. Antidepressant medications may cause orthostatic hypotension, and the nurse should question administering the medication if the blood pressure is less than 90/60.

2. Antidepressant medications do not have a therapeutic blood level; the effectiveness and side effects of the medication are determined by the client's behavior.

3. **Many antidepressants may cause hepatotoxicity; therefore, the nurse should monitor the client's liver function tests.**

4. **The nurse should ensure the client's safety. Many antidepressants may cause orthostatic hypotension and increase the risk for dizziness, falls, and injuries.**

5. Antidepressant medications take at least 3 weeks to become effective; therefore, when the client is first admitted to the psychiatric department and prescribed an antidepressant, evaluating for the effectiveness of the medication is not an appropriate intervention.

9. 1. Providing phone numbers for the client and family is an intervention that the nurse could implement, but it is not priority over the psychological and physical safety of the client.

2. Follow-up appointments are important for the client after being discharged from a psychiatric facility, but it is not priority over the psychological and physical safety of the client.

3. **Ensuring the psychological and physical safety of the client is priority. As antidepressant medications become more effective, the client is at a higher risk for suicide. Therefore, the nurse should ensure that the client cannot take an overdose of medication.**

4. This is an appropriate intervention, but it is not priority over the psychological and physical safety of the client.

10. 1. The nurse should realize this medication takes at least 3 weeks to work; therefore, this question is not helpful to the client.

2. This is a therapeutic response to encourage the client to ventilate feelings, but the client needs factual information.

3. The nurse should realize this medication takes at least 3 weeks to become effective, and the client does not need to come into the clinic to be told that fact.

4. **The client probably was told this information but may have forgotten it, or the client may not have been told, but the most appropriate response is to provide information so that the client realizes it takes 3 weeks for the medication to work and that he or she may not feel better until that time has elapsed.**

A Client with Bipolar Disorder

11. 1. The lithium level is monitored by a venipuncture serum level, which must be

done by a laboratory; it is not a test to be done at home.

2. **Lithium acts like sodium in the body so dehydration can cause lithium toxicity; therefore, the client should not become dehydrated.**

3. Lithium should not be stopped because bipolar disorder is a chemical imbalance, and the client must continue taking this medication or manic behavior will return.

4. The client should take the medication with food to decrease gastrointestinal upset.

12. 1. **The therapeutic serum level is 0.6 to 1.5 mEq/L. Because the lithium level is within those parameters, the nurse should administer the medication.**

2. This is within the therapeutic range; therefore, the nurse should not hold the medication but should administer it.

3. This is within the therapeutic range; therefore, the nurse should administer the medication.

4. There is no reason to verify the lithium level; therefore, the nurse should administer the medication.

MEDICATION MEMORY JOGGER: The nurse must be knowledgeable about accepted standards of practice for medication administration, including which client assessment data and laboratory data should be monitored prior to administering the medication.

13. 1. The client taking lithium should have adequate sodium intake because a salt-free diet reduces lithium excretion and can lead to lithium toxicity. The nurse would not question administering the medication to this client.

2. Many clients with bipolar disorder are prescribed an antidepressant medication and an antimania drug to treat bipolar disorder; therefore, the nurse would not question administering this medication.

3. **Diuretics increase the excretion of lithium from the kidneys; therefore, the nurse would question administering lithium to this client.**

4. The nurse would not question administering lithium to a client who has an adequate urine output.

14. 1. Depakote may be used to help prevent migraine headaches, but this is not an appropriate question to ask this client.

2. **Depakote is a category D drug, which means it will cause harm to the fetus**

and should not be prescribed to a female of childbearing age who is not taking the birth control pill.

3. Many times a classification of medications can be prescribed for another disease process. The nurse must know what the medication is prescribed for, as stated in the stem of the question.

4. Depakote takes 2–3 weeks to become therapeutic; therefore, this question is not pertinent.

MEDICATION MEMORY JOGGER: Any time a female client of childbearing age is prescribed a routine medication the nurse should think about possible pregnancy.

15. 1. Caffeine has a diuretic effect that can cause lithium sparing by the kidneys, which may cause lithium toxicity. This statement indicates the client understands the medication teaching.

2. **Playing soccer or any sport that includes running can lead to dehydration, and the nurse must make sure the client understands the need to stay well-hydrated during the activity. Therefore, this comment indicates the need for further clarification by the nurse.**

3. The client needs to maintain adequate fluid intake to prevent dehydration. This statement indicates the client understands the medication teaching.

4. Diarrhea is a sign of lithium toxicity, and the client should notify the health-care provider so that a serum lithium level can be evaluated. This statement indicates the client understands the medication teaching.

16. 1. This is an extremely high toxic level that requires immediate treatment. The therapeutic range is 0.6 to 1.5 mEq/L.

2. This is an extremely high toxic level that would require more than intravenous therapy.

3. **Extremely high toxic levels of lithium require hemodialysis and supportive care.**

4. There is no known antidote for lithium toxicity.

17. 1. **Tegretol is an anticonvulsant medication that is prescribed as a mood stabilizer. Mood stabilizers are prescribed because they have the ability to moderate extreme shifts in emotions between mania and depression. Therefore,**

this data indicates the medication is effective.

2. Serum drug levels determine if the medication is at a toxic level, but they do not indicate that the client's mania is controlled. Therefore, this does not indicate the medication is effective.

3. Tegretol is prescribed to treat the mania in bipolar disorder, not the depression. Therefore, a depression scale does not indicate anything about the effectiveness of the medication.

4. A client with bipolar disorder experiences a mood disorder, not a thought disorder such as schizophrenia. Therefore, this data does not indicate the medication is effective in treating the bipolar disorder.

MEDICATION MEMORY JOGGER: The nurse determines the effectiveness of a medication by assessing for the symptoms, or lack thereof, for which the medication was prescribed.

18. 1. This would be an appropriate intervention, but the client's physiological needs are priority.

2. The nurse must assess why the client is not compliant with medication, but in an acute manic state the client cannot answer this question. Therefore, it is not the first intervention.

3. **This is the first intervention because the client is in an acute manic state and the client's physiological need is priority.**

4. Lithium takes 2–3 weeks to become therapeutic; therefore, a stat dose of lithium orally will not help the manic state. Lithium is not available in intramuscular or intravenous route.

19. 1. Recommending use of a soft-bristled toothbrush is specific for clients taking phenytoin (Dilantin), another anticonvulsant medication, but not for Tegretol.

2. Tegretol does not affect visual acuity; therefore, there is no reason to recommend this health promotion activity for this client.

3. Tegretol does not affect the blood pressure; therefore, there is no reason to recommend this health promotion activity for this client.

4. **The client should avoid driving and other hazardous activities until the effects of Tegretol are known because this medication may cause sedation and drowsiness.**

MEDICATION MEMORY JOGGER: The nurse should discuss information with the client that is specific to that medication. There are many health promotion activities that the nurse can discuss with the client, but the nurse should not overload the client with activities that are not specific to the medication prescribed for the client.

20. 1. Lithium has a narrow therapeutic serum level. The level is monitored every 3–5 days initially and every 2–3 months thereafter.

2. Lithium is a salt and may cause dehydration; therefore, the client should maintain an adequate fluid intake of at least 2000 mL or more a day.

3. Insufficient dietary salt intake causes the kidneys to conserve lithium, which increases serum lithium levels; therefore, the client should have sufficient salt intake and not decrease the sodium intake.

4. The radial pulse is not evaluated before taking lithium, and the client should take the medication even if the pulse is less than 60.

5. Lithium does not cause orthostatic hypotension; therefore, the nurse does not need to discuss ways to prevent it.

A Client with Schizophrenia

21. 1. There is no such test as a therapeutic serum level for clozapine.

2. Weekly WBCs are taken because the client is at risk for fatal agranulocytosis. Initially the medication will not be administered if the WBC is not available.

3. The client's RBC count is not affected by clozapine.

4. The respiratory system is not affected by clozapine; therefore, ABGs do not have to be evaluated when taking this medication.

MEDICATION MEMORY JOGGER: Usually if a client is prescribed a new medication and has flulike symptoms within 24 hours of taking the first dose, the client should contact the HCP. These are signs of agranulocytosis, which indicates the medication has caused a sudden drop in the white blood cell count, leaving the body defenseless against bacterial invasion.

22. 1. Atypical antipsychotics do not have any food interactions; a low-tyramine diet is prescribed for clients taking an MAO inhibitor, an antidepressant.
   2. Respirations are not assessed to determine the effectiveness of the medication, nor are they used to determine when to question the medication; therefore, this is not an appropriate intervention for this medication.
   3. **A side effect of all types of antipsychotics is orthostatic hypotension (lightheadedness, dizziness), which can be minimized by moving slowly when assuming an erect posture.**
   4. The client's renal system is not affected by Risperdal; therefore, it does not need to be monitored while taking this medication.

23. 1. Atypical antipsychotic medications have a lower risk of sexual dysfunction than conventional antipsychotic medications; therefore, if the client experiences impotency, he should call his HCP. This statement does not indicate he understands the medication teaching.
   2. Atypical antipsychotic medications do not cause photosensitivity (unlike conventional antipsychotic drugs). This statement does not indicate he understands the medication teaching.
   3. Atypical antipsychotic medications do not cause gynecomastia (unlike conventional antipsychotic drugs). This statement indicates that the client does not understand the medication teaching.
   4. **Geodon is well-tolerated, but the most common side effect is difficulty in sleeping, perhaps because of the histamine antagonist blockade effect of the drug. This comment indicates the client understands the teaching.**

24. 1. **Clozaril can promote significant weight gain; therefore, the client should exercise regularly, monitor weight, and reduce caloric intake.**
   2. Clozaril promotes weight gain, not weight loss.
   3. Clozaril does not cause gastrointestinal distress and can be taken with food or on an empty stomach.
   4. The client should not decrease alcohol intake; the client should avoid alcohol intake completely.

25. 1. Clients with schizophrenia do not have an anxiety disorder, and this medication does not help decrease anxiety.

   2. Abilify affects the receptor sites for dopamine and does not increase the secretion of dopamine.
   3. **Like other antipsychotics, Abilify treats the positive and negative symptoms of schizophrenia—but it does so with fewer side effects than other antipsychotics. This medication does not cause significant weight gain, hypotension, or prolactin release, and it poses no risk of anticholinergic effects or dysrhythmias.**
   4. This medication does not block cholinergic receptors.

26. 1. **Caffeine-containing substances will negate the effects of antipsychotic medication; therefore, the client should drink caffeine-free beverages such as decaffeinated coffee and tea and caffeine-free colas.**
   2. Salt intake does not affect antipsychotic medication, nor does it affect schizophrenia. Therefore, the dietary intake of salt does not need to be decreased.
   3. Small meals and protein do not affect antipsychotic medications, nor will they affect schizophrenia. Therefore, the client does not have to eat high-protein meals.
   4. The client should not drink alcohol at all when taking antipsychotic medication. This will cause an increase in central nervous system depression.

27. 1. The client should be responsible for taking his or her own medication and not rely on the family member to administer it. The nurse should encourage the family member not to make the client dependent on anyone.
   2. There is no reason for the family member to learn CPR because antipsychotic medications do not cause death.
   3. The nurse should encourage the family member to attend a support group for families of people with schizophrenia. If there are any groups available for people with schizophrenia, then the client should attend one. The nurse should encourage the family member to let the client take care of his or her own mental illness.
   4. **Antipsychotic medications lower the seizure threshold, even if the client does not have a seizure disorder. Therefore, the nurse should discuss what to do if the client has a seizure.**

28. 1. Tremors or rigidity indicate the client is having extrapyramidal side effects of antipsychotic medications; such activity

does not indicate the medication is effective.

2. Antipsychotic medications are not prescribed for anxiety; therefore, anxiety cannot be evaluated to determine if the medication is effective.

3. Sleeping all night is a good sign for the client, but it does not determine if the medication is effective.

4. Antipsychotic medications are prescribed to decrease the signs or symptoms of schizophrenia. If the client denies auditory hallucinations, the medication is effective.

MEDICATION MEMORY JOGGER: The nurse determines the effectiveness of a medication by assessing for the symptoms, or lack thereof, for which the medication was prescribed.

29. 1. Rigidity and tremors are signs of extrapyramidal side effects and should be reported to the HCP. The client does not need additional teaching.

2. Haldol has anticholinergic effects, including constipation. Increasing fiber and fluid intake will help prevent constipation. This statement does not indicate that the client needs additional teaching.

3. Haldol causes agranulocytosis, which diminishes the client's ability to fight infection, but the medication (if the client does not develop the adverse effect of agranulocytosis) does not cause the client to have increased susceptibility to colds and the flu. If the client has a fever or sore throat, the HCP should be notified, and if the white blood cell count is elevated, the medication will be discontinued.

4. This statement indicates the client understands why the medication is being taken; this indicates the medication teaching is effective.

MEDICATION MEMORY JOGGER: Usually if a client is prescribed a new medication and has flulike symptoms within 24 hours of taking the first dose, the client should contact the HCP. These are signs of agranulocytosis, which indicates the medication has caused a sudden drop in the white blood cell count, leaving the body defenseless against bacterial invasion.

30. 1. Menstrual irregularity is a common side effect of conventional antipsychotic medications like Thorazine and would not warrant discontinuing the medication.

2. Orthostatic hypotension is a common side effect of conventional antipsychotic medications and would not warrant discontinuing the medication.

3. Anticholinergic effects are common side effects of conventional antipsychotic medications and would not warrant discontinuing the medication.

4. Exhibiting fine, wormlike movements of the tongue is a symptom of tardive dyskinesia, which is an adverse effect that may develop after months or years of continuous therapy with a conventional antipsychotic medication. The medication should be discontinued, and a benzodiazepine should be administered.

A Client with an Anxiety Disorder

31. 1. Xanax has the potential for dependency, but that potential can be minimized by using the lowest effective dosage for the shortest time necessary.

2. Rage, excitement, and heightened anxiety are signs of paradoxical reactions and should be reported to the HCP. The medication will be discontinued.

3. There is no contraindication to eating foods high in vitamin K and taking Xanax.

4. There is no reason for the client to take the medication with 8 ounces of water.

32. 1. The client should inform the obstetrician of the panic attacks and the Ativan therapy, but this is not the nurse's first intervention.

2. The client must quit taking the medication because it has the potential to harm a fetus, but if the client has been on long-term therapy, the medication should be discontinued gradually to prevent withdrawal symptoms.

3. The nurse should first determine how long the client has been taking Ativan and what dosage (or how many pills) to determine if the medication can be discontinued abruptly or if it must be gradually decreased.

4. The nurse should encourage the client to stop taking the Ativan prior to getting pregnant, but the first intervention is to assess the client to determine how long she has been taking the medication.

MEDICATION MEMORY JOGGER: The test taker should question administering any medication to a client who is pregnant or trying to become pregnant. Many medications cross the placental barrier and could affect the fetus.

33. 1. The client's apical pulse would not be monitored prior to the nurse administering the Xanax.
    2. The client's respiratory rate would not be monitored prior to the nurse administering the Xanax.
    3. **The nurse must assess the client's anxiety level on a scale of 1 to 10, with 10 being the most anxious, before administering the Xanax. If the nurse does not do this, there is no way to evaluate the effectiveness of the medication later.**
    4. The client's blood pressure would not be monitored prior to the nurse administering the Xanax.

34. 1. Common side effects of SSRIs include nausea, headache, insomnia, and sexual dysfunction; if these side effects develop, the client would not need to notify the HCP. The client does not understand the medication teaching.
    2. **The beneficial effects of SSRIs develop slowly, taking several months to become maximal when used to treat obsessive–compulsive disorder. The client understands this.**
    3. SSRIs are antidepressants used to treat obsessive–compulsive disorder. They do not have addictive properties. The client does not understand the medication teaching.
    4. The client should continue to go to a counselor or psychologist to determine the cause of the anxiety so that the client can eventually discontinue the SSRI. The client does not understand the medication teaching.

35. 1. This is not an accurate statement. Initial responses can be seen within 2 weeks but may take up to 2–3 months for maximal response.
    2. The nurse should not ask the client "why." It is a confrontational question and does not answer the client's question.
    3. The client should continue with cognitive therapy, but this is a very negative statement and is not the nurse's best response.
    4. SSRIs reduce the three core symptoms of PTSD: re-experiencing, avoidance/

emotional numbing, and hyperarousal. The medication is most effective if taken within 3 months of the traumatic event and may take up to 2 or 3 months for maximal response.

36. 1. This is an appropriate medication for an anxiety attack, but it will take at least 15–30 minutes for the medication to treat the physiological signs or symptoms.
    2. The client is in distress. The nurse should not assess the client; the nurse needs to help the client.
    3. **This is the most appropriate intervention; the nurse should remove the client from the busy day room to help decrease the anxiety attack.**
    4. SSRIs can be used to treat panic attacks, but the medication takes weeks to work; therefore, it would not be helpful in an acute panic attack.

MEDICATION MEMORY JOGGER: Remember that when a client is in distress, medication usually takes too long to work to immediately help the client. The nurse should always treat the client directly.

37. 1. Feeling dizzy and weak when getting out of a chair is indicative of orthostatic hypotension, which is a common side effect of antianxiety medications and is not a reason to quit taking the medication.
    2. Feeling dizzy and weak when getting out of a chair is indicative of orthostatic hypotension, which is a common side effect of antianxiety medications and is not a reason for the client to come to the clinic.
    3. Feeling dizzy and weak when getting out of a chair is indicative of orthostatic hypotension, which is a common side effect of antianxiety medications, and fluid intake would not affect the client's behavior.
    4. **Feeling dizzy and weak when getting out of a chair is indicative of orthostatic hypotension, which is a common side effect of antianxiety medications. The nurse should instruct the client to rise slowly from the sitting to standing position to avoid dizziness.**

38. 1. The first intervention in a case of Xanax overdose is to encourage vomiting—to remove the medication from the stomach before the medication is metabolized and absorbed into the system. Administering an emetic with activated charcoal would induce vomiting.

2. This is an appropriate intervention, but it is not the nurse's first intervention.
3. The antidote is usually not administered if the client is conscious; therefore, this is not the first intervention.
4. This is an appropriate intervention, but it is not the nurse's first intervention.

39. 1. This is subjective and does not best indicate the medication's effectiveness.
2. The pulse rate is elevated in an acute anxiety attack, but pulse rate is not the best assessment data to indicate if the medication is effective.
3. The client hyperventilates in an acute anxiety attack; respiratory rate is not the best assessment data to indicate the medication is effective.
4. **The best indicator of the medication's effectiveness is the client's objective report of his or her anxiety level.**

40. 1. Valium is oil-based and should not be diluted with normal saline.
2. **The nurse should administer the Valium undiluted over 2–3 minutes in the IV port closest to the client's hand so the medication can get to the client's blood stream faster.**
3. The Valium should be administered as an IVP, not as an IV piggyback.
4. Valium can be administered safely via the intravenous route and is recommended for acute, severe anxiety attacks because it will be effective within 1–5 minutes.

A Child with Attention Deficit–Hyperactivity Disorder

41. 1. Weight gain would not warrant intervention; weight loss would be of concern to the nurse.
2. These vital signs are within normal limits for a10-year-old child.
3. **The nurse should further investigate the cause of the bruises because this could be an adverse effect of the medication caused by leukopenia, anemia, or both; it could also be the result of child abuse. Either way it warrants intervention by the nurse.**
4. Sitting quietly in the examination room would indicate the medication is effective and would not warrant intervention by the nurse.

MEDICATION MEMORY JOGGER: If the client verbalizes a complaint, if the nurse

assesses data, or if laboratory data indicates an adverse effect secondary to a medication, the nurse must intervene. The nurse must implement an independent intervention or notify the health-care provider because medications can result in serious or even life-threatening complications.

42. 1. The medication should be taken with food to help decrease gastrointestinal upset and counteract anorexia.
2. The child's weight should be taken weekly and any significant weight loss should be reported.
3. The medication should be administered in the morning, and the last medication should be given no later than 1600 so that the child can sleep. This medication is a central nervous stimulant.
4. **A behavior diary should be kept to chronicle symptoms and response to drug therapy. This diary should be brought to all follow-up visits with the health-care provider.**

43. 1. Ritalin does not affect the glucose level; therefore, the nurse would not need to check this level.
2. The medication should be administered with food to decrease gastrointestinal upset, but it does not need to be given with a full glass of water.
3. **Stimulation of the central nervous system induces the release of catecholamines with a subsequent increase in heart rate and blood pressure. Therefore, the nurse should assess the child's vital signs.**
4. The nurse should assess the child's surgical wound, but it is not pertinent when administering Ritalin. The nurse must administer the Ritalin no matter what the wound looks like.

44. 1. Most schools have a "zero drug tolerance" policy and do not allow students to carry personal medication. The adolescent must keep the medication in the original prescription container. This statement indicates the student does not understand the medication teaching.
2. Ritalin has a high abuse potential and is often sold illegally on the street. This is the reason this medication is not allowed to be carried by students in the school. This statement indicates the adolescent understands the medication teaching—specifically, that

the medication will be kept by the school nurse.

3. Ritalin must be taken daily, usually twice a day. It is not a PRN medication. The student does not understand the medication teaching.

4. The adolescent should not be giving prescription medication to another child. This statement does not support that the adolescent understands the medication teaching.

45. 1. This is a false statement. There are other medications that can be taken for ADHD.

2. The word "why" is considered argumentative, and the nurse should try to provide information to the mother.

3. **Strattera is a medication that has the same efficacy as Ritalin and is not a scheduled drug. Parents who are hesitant to administer stimulants to their child now have a reasonable alternative. The nurse should provide factual information.**

4. The nurse can discuss medications with the mother. The mother would have to obtain a prescription for the medication, but the school nurse must be knowledgeable about medications.

46. 1. **Growth rate may stall in response to nutritional deficiency caused by anorexia. A 4-pound weight loss in 2 weeks is cause for investigation. The child needs to be seen by the HCP.**

2. The medication should not be discontinued abruptly because rebound hyperactivity or withdrawal symptoms can occur.

3. This is not a normal response to Ritalin and the child should be seen by the HCP.

4. This may need to be done, but the child needs to see the HCP to determine why the child has lost 4 pounds in 2 weeks. This is not normal for a 7-year-old child.

47. 1. Inappropriate behavior at school would not indicate the child's medication is effective.

2. Ritalin is not administered to help the child sleep all the time; therefore, this medication is not effective and the child is receiving too much medication.

3. **The child's ability to focus on a specific activity indicates the medication is effective. Inability to focus on one task at a time and jumping from one activity to another are signs of ADHD.**

4. Difficulty in following verbal instruction is a symptom of ADHD; this indicates the medication is not effective.

MEDICATION MEMORY JOGGER: The nurse determines the effectiveness of a medication by assessing for the symptoms, or lack thereof, for which the medication was prescribed.

48. 1. All medication must be kept in a safe place to prevent accidental poisoning of children.

2. Drug holidays may decrease the reduction in growth rate that is associated with this medication. The medication teaching has been effective.

3. Growth rate may be stalled in response to nutritional deficiency caused by anorexia, which often occurs when Ritalin is taken.

4. **Insomnia is an adverse reaction to the medication; central nervous stimulants may disrupt normal sleep patterns. This statement indicates the medication teaching has not been effective.**

49. 1. **Ritalin is metabolized in the liver and excreted by the kidneys. Impaired organ function can increase serum drug levels. The medication may cause leukopenia, anemia, or both. The HCP would order a CBC, differential, and platelet count.**

2. Potassium and sodium levels are not monitored for methylphenidate (Ritalin).

3. The growth rate may stall as a result of nutritional deficiency caused by anorexia, but the child's bone density is not affected; therefore, this diagnostic test is not monitored.

4. There is no serum drug level for methylphenidate (Ritalin).

MEDICATION MEMORY JOGGER: The nurse must be knowledgeable of accepted standards of practice for medication administration, including which client assessment data and laboratory data should be monitored while a client is taking long-term medication.

50. 1. The epiphyseal plate of the bone determines if a person has completed growing, but this would not be assessed in an 8-year-old child. The epiphyseal plate is a thin layer of cartilage between the epiphysis, a secondary bone-forming center, and the bone shaft.

2. **The child's baseline height and weight must be obtained because reduction in**

growth rate is associated with this medication.
3. The HCP would not order an EKG on an 8-year-old child. This medication does not affect the electrical conductivity of the heart.
4. The head circumference would not be measured on an 8-year-old child because the fontanels close at around 2 years old.

A Client with a Sleep Disorder

51. 1. Valium can depress respirations, but this client has already been taking the medication.
2. Valium is administered to clients during a seizure to treat a seizure, but this client has informed the nurse that it is being taken for sleep.
3. The client has already told the nurse that the Valium is used to induce sleep.
4. **Benzodiazepines should be tapered off when the client is trying to stop taking them. The nurse should request an order for the Valium.**

52. 1. **The client is having abdominal surgery so the client will be NPO for a while. Xanax is only manufactured as an oral medication. Therefore, the client will need a similar medication postoperatively. The nurse should discuss this with the HCP.**
2. The client will be NPO after a major abdominal surgery; Xanax only comes in an oral preparation.
3. If the client is going to stop taking Xanax, it should be tapered, but the stem does not indicate a need to discontinue the medication.
4. The Xanax is being taken PRN, not just for sleep but also for anxiety.

53. 1. ACE inhibitors are administered to treat hypertension or for prophylaxis in clients diagnosed with diabetes and would not interfere with a sleep study.
2. **Antihistamines such as diphenhydramine (Benadryl) can cause drowsiness in many clients; the client should not take any medication that would interfere with the test being interpreted correctly.**
3. Loop diuretics are administered early in the day to prevent nocturia, and the effects should have worn off before the

sleep study begins. Sleep studies are conducted during the night.
4. Normal routine doses of thyroid medication would not interfere with a sleep study.

54. 1. **The client should be instructed not to attempt to get pregnant while receiving chemotherapy or taking Ativan. Ativan is a pregnancy category D drug. Ativan is very useful in controlling chemotherapy-induced nausea and vomiting, so the HCP is attempting to achieve a dual use for the medication—improved sleep and relief of chemotherapy-induced nausea.**
2. Ativan can interact with alcohol, increasing central nervous system depression. The client should not consume alcohol at all.
3. Exercise immediately before bedtime can increase the client's inability to sleep. Exercising a few hours prior to bedtime is suggested.
4. Clients taking benzodiazepines may become dependent on the medications, but they do not become addicted to them. The medications are tapered off if they are being discontinued.

55. 1. This situation requires further evaluation by the nurse before notifying the HCP.
2. **Safety is a priority. The client received a sedative medication and an antinausea medication within the last 10 hours. Elderly clients frequently require longer periods of time to clear medications from their systems.**
3. The client is not in a code situation. The client is lethargic, probably from the medications.
4. The nurse should re-evaluate the client in 30–60 minutes, but safety in the mean time is the first intervention.

56. 1. There is only one reason to take Synthroid—thyroid replacement. The nurse should know this.
2. There is no indication that the client is vomiting. Prilosec is frequently taken for gastroesophageal reflux disease (GERD).
3. The blood pressure before beginning Capoten is not important. The current blood pressure and the amount of control the client achieves while taking Capoten are important.
4. **Melatonin is an over-the-counter hormone that many people take to prevent jet lag or induce sleep.**

57. 1. **Ritalin is a stimulant and should be taken early in the day to prevent insomnia at night.**
    2. Taking the medication at bedtime would prevent the client from sleeping.
    3. Most clients do not have a locked cabinet in their home. The medication should be kept out of the reach of children, as should all medications.
    4. This is an expected side effect of Ritalin; the client does not need to notify the HCP.

58. 1. **Caffeine may help the client to achieve some measure of alertness, whereas products containing diphenhydramine can increase the client's problem because this medication is used in over-the-counter sleep aids. The client should be taught about both.**
    2. Flavored water will not have any effect on the narcolepsy, and beta-carotene is a precursor to vitamin A and is often taken to treat degenerative eye diseases.
    3. Milk with vitamin D is useful for clients with osteoporosis, and saw palmetto is used to treat benign prostatic hypertrophy. The question does not state that the client has either of these conditions.
    4. Carbonated drinks should be avoided by clients who have gastroesophageal reflux disease, and black cohosh is used for menstrual irregularities and menopausal symptoms and as an antispasmodic. The question does not state that the client has either of these problems.

59. 1. A mild sedative would increase the child's inability to awaken during the night if needed. There is no medication that is useful to treat sleepwalking.
    2. **This is a safety measure to keep the child from exiting the house during the night.**
    3. It is difficult to arouse a sleepwalker. The child should be guided back to the bed and allowed to remain asleep.
    4. Guided imagery will not stop sleepwalking.
    5. Strattera is administered for attention deficit–hyperactivity disorder (ADHD), not for sleepwalking.

    MEDICATION MEMORY JOGGER: In a "select all that apply" question, only one option may be correct, a few options may be correct, or all options may be correct.

60. 1. This is a situation in which caffeine will not be enough to allow the client to remain awake. NoDoz contains caffeine.

2. An inhaled steroid will not help the client to sleep at night. The client may be placed on a breathing treatment during the night to maintain respirations.
3. **A central nervous system stimulant would be ordered to prevent somnolence.**
4. Elavil can cause drowsiness and should not be administered to a client with a problem of falling asleep at inopportune times.

A Client with Substance Abuse

61. 1. **Librium diminishes anxiety and has anticonvulsant qualities to provide safe withdrawal from alcohol. It may be ordered every 4 hours or PRN to manage adverse effects from withdrawal, after which the dose is tapered to zero.**
    2. Thiamine is a vitamin prescribed for clients with chronic alcoholism; it is prescribed to prevent Wernicke's encephalopathy, not to prevent delirium tremens.
    3. Antabuse is used when a client wishes to quit drinking alcohol. It prevents the breakdown of alcohol and causes the client to vomit when alcohol is consumed.
    4. Antidepressants are not used to prevent delirium tremens.

    MEDICATION MEMORY JOGGER: The nurse must be knowledgeable about accepted standards of practice for disease processes and conditions. If the nurse administers a medication the health-care provider has prescribed and it harms the client, the nurse could be held accountable. Remember that the nurse is a client advocate.

62. 1. Methadone would not help a client addicted to cocaine.
    2. **Methadone blocks the craving for heroin.**
    3. Methadone would not help a client addicted to amphetamines.
    4. Methadone would not help a client addicted to hallucinogens, such as lysergic acid diethylamide (LSD).

63. 1. A smoking cessation support group may be helpful, but nicotine withdrawal is a physical withdrawal, and medication should be used to help with the withdrawal symptoms.

2. Tapering the number of cigarettes daily is not the most successful method to quit smoking cigarettes.
3. **Using a nicotine patch or chewing nicotine gum is the most successful way to help with the nicotine withdrawal symptoms.**
4. Clonidine is used to help prevent delirium tremens in a client with alcohol dependence.

64. 1. Methadone causes gastrointestinal distress, which can be minimized by taking the medication with food.
2. Methadone causes constipation; therefore, the client should increase fiber intake to help prevent constipation.
3. Methadone does not affect the pulse; therefore, the pulse does not need to be monitored before taking the medication.
4. **Methadone causes drowsiness, light-headedness, dizziness, and a transient drop in blood pressure. Therefore, the nurse should discuss how to prevent orthostatic hypotension. Methadone is used to treat heroin withdrawal.**

65. 1. **Nausea, vomiting, and agitation, along with tachycardia, diaphoresis, tremors, and marked insomnia, are adverse effects of central nervous system depressants, such as benzodiazepines.**
2. Yawning, rhinorrhea, and cramps are signs of withdrawal from opiates, such as heroin, meperidine, morphine, and methadone.
3. Disorientation, lethargy, and craving are signs of withdrawal from a stimulant, such as crack cocaine and amphetamines.
4. Ataxia, hyperpyrexia, and respiratory distress are signs of an overdose of a stimulant, such as crack cocaine and amphetamines.

66. 1. The client must want to quit drinking alcohol. Nothing in the question indicates this, so it would not be appropriate to prescribe disulfiram for this client.
2. **Disulfiram is only effective in highly motivated clients because the success of pharmacotherapy is entirely dependent on client compliance. This client is highly motivated to quit drinking alcohol.**
3. Disulfiram inhibits acetaldehyde dehydrogenase, the enzyme that metabolizes alcohol; it is not used for amphetamine abuse.

4. Disulfiram inhibits acetaldehyde dehydrogenase, the enzyme that metabolizes alcohol; it is not used for heroin abuse.

67. 1. The fact that the client has not had any food in 3 days may be a cause for the headache, but the nurse does not need to ask the client the last time he or she had any food because the nurse is aware of this information. The type of diet the client ate prior to being NPO for 3 days would not be an appropriate question in determining the cause of the client's headache.
2. Alcohol withdrawal does not cause a headache.
3. Taking sleeping pills regularly would not cause a headache.
4. **A hallmark symptom of caffeine withdrawal is a headache, along with fatigue, depression, and impaired performance of daily activities. This question would be most appropriate for the nurse to ask the client.**

68. 1. The nurse should implement seizure precautions, but it is not the first intervention.
2. **Immediately on arrival to a hospital the client should be rehydrated with large amounts of intravenous physiological fluids. This is the first intervention.**
3. After treating delirium tremens, it is essential the client go through a course of withdrawal treatment in a therapeutic milieu, but it is not the first intervention in the emergency department.
4. Malnutrition is a serious complication of chronic alcoholism, especially thiamine deficiency, which can result in neurological impairments; therefore, thiamine must be administered intravenously. This is not the first intervention.

69. 1. The nurse would not suspect alcohol overdose with these signs or symptoms.
2. The nurse would not suspect amphetamine overdose with these signs or symptoms.
3. The nurse would not suspect the client inhaling paint thinner with these signs or symptoms.
4. **Respiratory distress, ataxia, hyperpyrexia, convulsions, coma, or stroke are signs and symptoms of cocaine overdose. This question would be most appropriate for the nurse to ask based on the client's signs and symptoms.**

70. 1. Marijuana is psychologically addicting, not physically addicting. There is no

medication that can help the client to quit smoking marijuana.

2. Nicotine replacement therapy is used in clients who are trying to quit smoking cigarettes, not marijuana.

3. Antianxiety medications are not used to treat clients who want to quit smoking marijuana.

4. Marinol is a synthetic derivative of tetrahydrocannabinol (THC), the principal constituent of marijuana. It is prescribed to clients receiving chemotherapy to help treat nausea and vomiting.

1. The nurse is leading a medication group in a psychiatric unit. Which information should the nurse discuss with the clients concerning antipsychotic medications after discharge? Select all that apply.
   1. Chew sugarless gum to help dry mouth.
   2. Teach the client about orthostatic hypotension.
   3. Explain that the medication may cause drowsiness.
   4. Discuss that these medications may cause sexual dysfunction.
   5. Instruct the client to call the HCP if flulike symptoms occur.

2. The female client diagnosed with anorexia nervosa is in the inpatient psychiatric unit receiving amitriptyline (Elavil), an antidepressant, and cyproheptadine (Periactin), an antihistamine. Which data suggests the medications are effective?
   1. The client eats at least 90% of the meal.
   2. The client has a weight gain of 1 kg.
   3. The client has no symptoms of hay fever.
   4. The client states she will eat all her meals.

3. The Asian male client is prescribed fluoxetine (Prozac), a selective serotonin reuptake inhibitor (SSRI), for clinical depression after the death of his wife. Which question should the nurse ask the client when discussing this medication?
   1. "How do you feel about taking this medication?"
   2. "Do you have insurance to pay for the medications?"
   3. "Does your diet include a lot of aged cheese and wine?"
   4. "Are you currently taking any ACE inhibitors?"

4. The clinic nurse is assessing a client 3 weeks after a suicide attempt. The client was prescribed sertraline (Zoloft), an SSRI. Which behavior indicates the medication is effective?
   1. The client sleeps 14–16 hours a day.
   2. The client has lost 3 pounds.
   3. The client regrets the suicide attempt.
   4. The client has started a new job.

5. The client diagnosed with panic disorder is taking a phenelzine (Nardil), an MAO inhibitor. Which statement by the client warrants immediate intervention?
   1. "I am very careful about what I eat."
   2. "I have been taking Robitussin for my cough."
   3. "I took two Tylenol for my headache."
   4. "I only drink one cup of coffee a day."

6. Which task would be most appropriate for the nurse to assign to the licensed practical nurse (LPN) working in the psychiatric department?
   1. Administer alprazolam (Xanax), a benzodiazepine, to a client diagnosed with a panic disorder.
   2. Administer haloperidol (Haldol), an antipsychotic, to a client experiencing tardive dyskinesia.
   3. Administer lithium (Lithobid) to a client diagnosed with bipolar disease who has a lithium level of 2.0 mEq/L.
   4. Administer oral thiamine (B_1), a vitamin, to a client diagnosed with chronic alcoholism who is experiencing delirium tremens.

7. Which statement is the scientific rationale for prescribing atomoxetine (Strattera), a norepinephrine reuptake inhibitor, for a child diagnosed with attention deficit–hyperactivity disorder (ADHD)?
   1. It increases acetylcholine levels and the brain's cholinergic function.
   2. This medication normalizes the reuptake of certain neurotransmitters.
   3. This medication is a nonstimulant, nonnarcotic that regulates impulse control.
   4. It results in mild central nervous stimulation to control the child's behavior.

8. The child diagnosed with ADHD has been taking pemoline (Cylert) for an extended period of time. Which laboratory test should the nurse monitor?
   1. Serum glucose levels.
   2. Amphetamine levels.
   3. Serum melatonin levels.
   4. Liver function tests.

9. The client diagnosed with insomnia asks the nurse, "Why did my HCP prescribe Ambien CR and tell me to quit taking Tylenol PM?" Which response by the nurse would be most appropriate?
   1. "Over-the-counter medications are not as good as prescriptions."
   2. "Tylenol PM is addicting and you should not take it nightly."
   3. "You are concerned your HCP gave you a prescription drug."
   4. "Ambien CR will help you get to sleep and stay asleep through the night."

10. The nurse on the substance abuse unit is administering medications. Which medication would the nurse question administering?
    1. Chlordiazepoxide (Librium), a benzodiazepine, to a client admitted for alcohol detoxification.
    2. Haloperidol (Haldol), an antipsychotic, to a client diagnosed with phencyclidine (PCP) psychosis.
    3. Clonidine (Catapres), an alpha-adrenergic agonist, to client with a blood pressure of 88/60.
    4. Thiamine (B_1), a vitamin, intravenously to a client diagnosed with Wernicke-Korsakoff syndrome.

11. The client is brought to the emergency department by a friend. The client is hyper-vigilant, has not slept in 3 days, has dilated pupils, has an apical pulse of 118, and has a runny nose. Which substance would the nurse suspect the client has been abusing?
    1. Cannabis.
    2. Heroin.
    3. Cocaine.
    4. Alcohol.

12. The client diagnosed with anorexia nervosa is admitted to the medical department for total parenteral nutrition (TPN) because of her emaciated condition. Which task can be delegated to the unlicensed nursing assistant?
    1. Evaluate the client's intake and output.
    2. Obtain the client's daily weight.
    3. Change the TPN tubing during the bath.
    4. Escort the client to the hospital cafeteria.

13. Which statement best supports the scientific rationale for pharmacologic treatment in clients diagnosed with substance abuse?
    1. Medications allow the clients to take a medication legally for their problem.
    2. Medications permit safe withdrawal and help prevent relapse.
    3. Medications will prevent all side effects of substance abuse withdrawal.
    4. Medications allow the client to have a psychological reason to quit the substance abuse.

14. The client diagnosed with bipolar disorder is taking lithium (Lithobid) and has a lithium level of 1.0 mEq/L. Which action should the psychiatric clinic nurse take based on this laboratory result?
    1. Schedule the client's next clinic appointment.
    2. Call the client and have him or her come to the clinic.
    3. Instruct the client to hold the medication for 2 days.
    4. Tell the client to increase daily salt intake.

15. The client wants to quit smoking cigarettes. The client has been to a smoking cessation support group and has used nicotine patches but has not been successful. Which recommendation should the nurse give the client?
    1. "Chew nicotine gum instead of using the patch."
    2. "Try an over-the-counter medication to help quit smoking."
    3. "Take 500 mg of vitamin C twice a day."
    4. "Ask your HCP for a prescription for Wellbutrin, an antidepressant."

16. The client diagnosed with schizophrenia is hallucinating and attacking other clients in the psychiatric unit. The client has a PRN order for 50 mg of chlorpromazine (Thorazine) IM. The medication comes in a vial with 100 mg per mL. How many milliliters should the nurse administer? Designate the spot on the syringe.

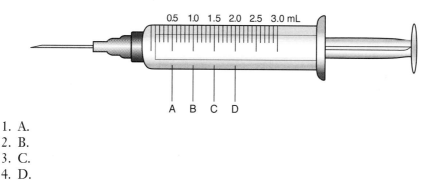

    1. A.
    2. B.
    3. C.
    4. D.

17. The client diagnosed with chronic alcoholism is prescribed multivitamins via intravenous route because of malnutrition. The intravenous solution turns yellow after injecting the multivitamin. Which action should the nurse implement?
    1. Notify the pharmacist about the discoloration of the IV.
    2. Cover the IV bag and tubing with light-resistant material.
    3. Administer the medication as prescribed and take no action.
    4. Discard the intravenous bag and obtain another vial of medication.

18. The client diagnosed with schizophrenia is admitted to the medical department for pneumonia and is exhibiting involuntary movements of the tongue and lips. After reviewing the following MAR, which medication would the nurse question administering?

Client's Name	Account Number: 123456		Allergies: NKDA
Height: 69 inches	Weight: 165 pounds		
Date	Medication	2301–0700	0701–1500	1501–2300
	Chlorpromazine (Thorazine) 50 mg po b.i.d.		0900	1800
	Lorazepam (Ativan) 2 mg po daily			2100
	Cefuroxime (Zinacef) 750 mg IVPB every 6 hours	0600 NN	1200	1800 2400
	Maalox 30 mL PRN		1200	
Signature/Initials	Day Nurse RN/DN		Night Nurse RN/NN

    1. Chlorpromazine (Thorazine).
    2. Lorazepam (Ativan).
    3. Cefuroxime (Zinacef).
    4. The nurse should not question administering any of these medications.

19. The nurse is administering medications on a psychiatric unit. Which client would the nurse discuss with the health-care provider?
1. The 17-year-old client diagnosed with bipolar disorder who is receiving risperidone (Risperdal), an antipsychotic.
2. The client diagnosed with schizophrenia who is receiving cimetidine (Tagamet), a histamine blocker.
3. The client with a heroin dependency who is receiving rifampin (Rifadin), an anti-tuberculin.
4. The 16-year-old client diagnosed with anorexia nervosa who is receiving amitriptyline (Elavil), a tricyclic antidepressant.

20. The 17-year-old adolescent female diagnosed with anorexia is prescribed desipramine (Norpramin), a tricyclic antidepressant. Which data indicates the medication is not effective?
1. The client's mood has improved.
2. The client does not fight with her parents.
3. The client is verbalizing wanting to go college.
4. The client is preoccupied with shape and weight.

1. 1. Antipsychotic drugs produce varying degrees of muscarinic cholinergic blockade, including dry mouth, blurred vision, and photophobia. Chewing sugarless gum may help dry mouth.
   2. Antipsychotic medications promote orthostatic hypotension by blocking alpha–adrenergic receptors on blood vessels. Therefore, the nurse should teach the client about orthostatic hypotension.
   3. The sedative effects of the antipsychotic medications should have subsided by the time the client is discharged. Therefore, this is not an appropriate teaching for discharge. Sedation is common during the early days of treatment, but it subsides within a week or so.
   4. Antipsychotics can cause sexual dysfunction in women and men, so this should be discussed by the nurse.
   5. Flulike symptoms are a sign of agranulocytosis, which is a rare but serious reaction to antipsychotic medications. In agranulocytosis, the body loses its ability to fight infection.

2. 1. The client eating 90% of the meal does not indicate the client has gained weight.
   2. **The medication is effective if the client gains weight, and 2.2 pounds is an excellent weight gain for a client with anorexia.**
   3. The antihistamine would be effective if the client had no signs of hay fever, but this is not why this medication is being administered.
   4. The client can say anything, but weight gain indicates the medication is effective.

MEDICATION MEMORY JOGGER: The nurse determines the effectiveness of a medication by assessing for the symptoms, or lack thereof, for which the medication was prescribed.

3. 1. **The Asian culture does not acknowledge mental illness as a problem, and the client may not believe in taking antidepressant medications. The Asian male may see taking medications as a weakness; therefore, the nurse must determine if the client will take the medications.**
   2. Clients who have difficulty in procuring medications will usually inform the nurse. It is not a question the nurse should ask.

Culturally speaking, an Asian male may find this question offensive.
   3. Aged cheese and wine contain tyramine, which should be avoided when taking an MAO inhibitor, not an SSRI.
   4. Some beta blockers may interact with an SSRI, but ACE inhibitors do not.

4. 1. Sleeping most of the day does not indicate the medication is effective; this may indicate the client is very depressed or is taking too much medication.
   2. Weight loss or gain may indicate the client is depressed.
   3. Verbalizing remorse does not indicate the medication is effective.
   4. **Setting new goals and priorities such as getting a job indicate the client may no longer be depressed and the medication is effective.**

5. 1. Clients taking this medication must not eat foods high in tyramine because it causes a life-threatening complication. This statement does not warrant intervention.
   2. **Dextromethorphan (Robitussin) interacts with MAOIs to produce hypertension, fever, and coma. This statement warrants intervention.**
   3. Tylenol does not interact with MAOIs; therefore, this statement does not warrant intervention.
   4. Caffeine should be limited when taking MAOIs, but it may be consumed in moderation. This statement does not warrant intervention.

MEDICATION MEMORY JOGGER: Some classes of medications are notorious for adverse reactions, and MAO inhibitors, which are prescribed rarely for depression, are among the worst.

6. 1. **This client is stable and has a diagnosis of panic attack; administering Xanax would be an appropriate task to assign to an LCP.**
   2. Tardive dyskinesia is a life-threatening complication of antipsychotic medication, and the nurse should not delegate care of an client who is unstable.
   3. This lithium level is toxic, and the client should not receive any lithium.
   4. The client should receive intravenous, not oral, thiamine medication. The client is not stable and the nurse should not delegate this medication administration.

7. 1. This is the scientific rationale for administering donepezil (Aricept) to a client with Alzheimer's disease.
2. This is the scientific rationale for administering lithium to a client with bipolar disorder.
3. **Strattera is prescribed for ADHD because it is not a CNS stimulant or controlled substance. It acts to increase norepinephrine and regulate impulse control, organizes thoughts, and focuses attention. It does not decrease appetite, and the child does not need to take drug holidays.**
4. This is the scientific rationale for administering methylphenidate (Ritalin) to children with ADHD.

8. 1. The glucose level is not monitored when taking Cylert.
2. The child should test positive for amphetamine because amphetamines are the prototype for Cylert. But this test is not monitored because the drug's effectiveness is determined by the client's behavior.
3. Melatonin is a hormone produced by the body that regulates sleep patterns. Cylert can cause insomnia, but it does not interfere with melatonin levels.
4. **Cylert, as with most medications, is metabolized by the liver and can cause liver dysfunction or liver failure over a long period. Therefore, liver function tests should be monitored.**

MEDICATION MEMORY JOGGER: The kidneys and the liver are responsible for metabolizing and excreting all medications.

9. 1. Some OTC medications are as effective as prescription medications; therefore, this is a false statement.
2. Tylenol PM is a combination of acetaminophen and Benadryl, and it is not addictive.
3. The client did not verbalize this concern. The client needs factual information, not a therapeutic response.
4. **This medication allows the client to fall asleep and stay asleep, which is why it is prescribed for clients with insomnia. Short-term use does not result in an addiction to this medication.**

10. 1. Librium is used to prevent delirium tremens; therefore, the nurse would not question this medication.

2. Haldol is prescribed for psychosis; therefore, the nurse would not question this medication.
3. **Clonidine is administered primarily to treat hypertension, but it is also used to reduce the symptoms of withdrawal from opioids, nicotine, and alcohol. The nurse would question administering this medication because of the client's low blood pressure no matter why it is being prescribed.**
4. Thiamine is used to diminish Wernicke-Korsakoff encephalopathy, which is characterized by confusion, memory loss, and loss of cranial nerve function resulting from chronic alcohol abuse.

11. 1. Cannabis is marijuana and results in a lack of sense of time, apathy, and increased appetite, not the signs and symptoms the client is experiencing.
2. Heroin abuse results in slurred speech, sedated appearance, apathy, and decreased emotional pain, not hypervigilance and insomnia.
3. **Hypervigilance, insomnia, dilated pupils, and a runny nose are the signs or symptoms of cocaine abuse.**
4. Alcohol abuse results in lack of control, hostility, rationalization, grandiosity, confusion, and blackouts, not the signs and symptoms this client has.

MEDICATION MEMORY JOGGER: Many of the illegal substances that are abused by clients may produce the same symptoms, so the test taker must focus on symptoms that are different, such as "runny nose" for cocaine.

12. 1. The nurse cannot delegate evaluation of assessment data. The unlicensed nursing assistant (NA) can obtain the intake and output but not evaluate it.
2. **The NA could obtain the client's weight.**
3. The NA should not be manipulating the IV, the IV pump, or the IV tubing. TPN is a medication, and the nurse cannot delegate the administration of medications.
4. The client is anorexic, and any food intake should be evaluated by the nurse. Having the NA go to the cafeteria removes the employee from the unit for an extended period; therefore, this is not an appropriate task to delegate.

13. 1. Substance abuse, whether involving legal or illegal substances, is still abuse, and the client needs psychological intervention to help with the abuse. The pharmacologic intervention helps with the physiologic withdrawal, with the scientific rationale being to help the client not take any type of medication, legal or illegal.

2. **The two main purposes for prescribing medication for clients who are addicted to alcohol, sedative/hypnotics, and benzodiazepines are to permit safe withdrawal from the substance and to prevent relapse into addiction again.**

3. No medications used in substance abuse detoxification can prevent all side effects.

4. This statement is not true.

14. 1. **This is within the therapeutic range of 0.6 to 1.2 mEq/L. Therefore, the nurse should take no action, except to make sure the client has a follow-up appointment.**

2. This would be appropriate if the client's lithium level was elevated, which it is not.

3. This would be appropriate if the client's lithium level was elevated, which it is not.

4. The lithium level is therapeutic; therefore, the client does not need to adjust his or her salt intake.

MEDICATION MEMORY JOGGER: The nurse must be knowledgeable about accepted standards of practice for medication administration, including which client assessment data and laboratory data should be monitored prior to administering the medication.

15. 1. The nicotine patch and nicotine gum are both nicotine replacement products, and if one doesn't work, neither will the other one.

2. The nicotine patch is an over-the-counter medication, so this recommendation is not helpful to the client.

3. Nicotine lowers vitamin C levels in the body, so it will not help the client with withdrawal symptoms from nicotine.

4. **Bupropion (Wellbutrin) is an antidepressant that has been proved to be an adjunct to smoking cessation.**

16. 1. **This is the correct amount of medication to administer to the client; 100 divided by 50 is 0.5 mL.**

2. This would be a medication error and would be administering 100 mg of medication, or twice the dose prescribed.

3. This would be a medication error and would be administering 150 mg of

medication, or three times the dose prescribed.

4. This would be a medication error and would be administering 200 mg of medication, or four times the dose prescribed.

MEDICATION MEMORY JOGGER: Most pharmaceutical companies package the medication in amounts that are usually prescribed by the HCP. If the nurse uses more than one vial to administer a medication, then the nurse should seek clarification of the prescription.

17. 1. The multivitamins in the IV solution cause the IV solution to be yellow; therefore, there is no reason to notify the HCP.

2. This IV does not need to be protected from light. The yellow color is normal for this IV therapy.

3. **This IV therapy is commonly known as a "banana boat" because of the yellow color of the IV solution. The nurse should administer the medication as prescribed.**

4. This is not cost effective because the yellow color is normal for this medication.

18. 1. **Involuntary movements of the tongue and lips are signs and symptoms of tardive dyskinesia, which is an adverse reaction to first-generation antipsychotic medications such as Thorazine.**

2. Antianxiety medications, such as Ativan, do not cause tardive dyskinesia.

3. Antibiotics, such as Zinacef, do not cause tardive dyskinesia.

4. The client has signs and symptoms of tardive dyskinesia, which is an adverse reaction to a first-generation antipsychotic medication such as Thorazine. The nurse must intervene when assessing these signs and symptoms.

19. 1. Risperdal is the drug of choice for an adolescent diagnosed with bipolar disorder.

2. **Tagamet may reduce the effects of antipsychotic medications and lead to medication failure. The client diagnosed with schizophrenia would be taking an antipsychotic medication, so the nurse should discuss an alternate medication to decrease the client's gastric acidity.**

3. The client receiving antituberculin medications must receive them to prevent resistant strains of TB and protect the community.

4. Elavil has shown efficacy in promoting weight gain in clients with anorexia nervosa. Therefore, the nurse would not need to discuss this medication with the HCP.

20. 1. The antidepressant is administered to improve the mood; therefore, this indicates the medication is effective.
2. Arguing with the parents will not determine the effectiveness of the medication.

3. Verbalizing future goals will not determine the effectiveness of the medication.
4. Being preoccupied with the shape and weight is a symptom of bulimia and indicates the medication is not effective.

MEDICATION MEMORY JOGGER: The nurse determines the effectiveness of a medication by assessing for the symptoms, or lack thereof, for which the medication was prescribed.

13

Sensory Deficits

"Nothing has really happened until it has been recorded."

—Virginia Woolf

PRACTICE QUESTIONS

A Client with an Eye Disorder

1. The client diagnosed with open-angle glaucoma is prescribed pilocarpine (Isopto Carpine), miotic ophthalmic drops. The client is demonstrating instilling the medication. Which action by the client would warrant intervention?
   1. The client washes his or her hands prior to instilling the medication.
   2. The client squeezes the bridge of the nose after administering the medication.
   3. The client keeps the eyes open immediately after administering the medication.
   4. The client does not touch the dropper to the eye when instilling the medication.

2. The client with glaucoma is using an Ocusert system when applying pilocarpine, a miotic ophthalmic medication. Which intervention should the nurse discuss with the client?
   1. Place the Ocusert Pilo system in the lower conjunctival sac.
   2. Apply the Ocusert Pilo system at bedtime.
   3. Replace the system daily the first thing in the morning.
   4. Notify the HCP if increased lacrimation or headache occurs.

3. The client with glaucoma is prescribed epinephrine (Epitrate), mydriatic ophthalmic drops. Which statement indicates the client understands the client teaching?
   1. "I will call my health-care provider if I start experiencing any eye pain."
   2. "This medication does not interfere with any over-the-counter medication."
   3. "I will probably experience anxiety, nervousness, and muscle tremors."
   4. "After putting the medication in my eyes I must lie down for 1 hour."

4. The client is undergoing eye surgery and the nurse is administering a cycloplegic, a ciliary paralytic ophthalmic medication. Which intervention should the nurse implement?
   1. Don sterile gloves prior to administering medication.
   2. Tape the client's eyelids shut with nonadhesive tape.
   3. Place an eye catheter at the outer canthus to insert medication.
   4. Explain that the eyes will be paralyzed for 24 to 48 hours.

5. The client diagnosed with bilateral conjunctivitis is prescribed antibiotic ophthalmic ointment. Which interventions should the nurse implement when discussing the medication with the client? Select all that apply.
   1. Apply a thin line of ointment evenly along inner edge of lower lid margin.
   2. Press the nasolacrimal duct after applying the antibiotic ointment.
   3. Don nonsterile gloves prior to administering the medication.
   4. Apply antibiotic ointment from the outer canthus to the inner canthus.
   5. Instruct the client to sit with head slightly tilted back or lie supine.

6. The client reports having dry and irritated eyes to the clinic nurse. Which intervention should the nurse implement first?
   1. Recommend the client use artificial tears in both eyes.
   2. Assess the eyes for any redness or discharge.
   3. Check the client's eyes using the ophthalmoscope.
   4. Evaluate the client's cardinal fields of vision.

7. The client called the emergency department and told the nurse that bleach had splashed into both eyes. Which action should the nurse tell the client to perform first?
   1. Come to the emergency department immediately.
   2. Determine if the client has normal saline flush.
   3. Apply antibiotic ointment and patch the eyes bilaterally.
   4. Cleanse the eye continuously with tap water.

8. Which client would the nurse question administering the beta-adrenergic blocker betaxolol (Betoptic), ophthalmic drops?
   1. The client diagnosed with open-angle glaucoma.
   2. The client diagnosed with end-stage liver failure.
   3. The client diagnosed with allergies to sulfa.
   4. The client diagnosed with chronic obstructive pulmonary disease (COPD).

9. Which statement best describes the scientific rationale for administering a mydriatic ophthalmic medication to a client diagnosed with glaucoma?
   1. It constricts the pupil, which causes the pupil to dilate in low light.
   2. It dilates the pupil to reduce the production of aqueous humor.
   3. It decreases production of aqueous humor but does not affect the eye.
   4. It is used as adjunctive therapy primarily to reduce intraocular pressure.

10. The nurse is preparing to administer ophthalmic medication to the client. To which area should the nurse administer the medication?

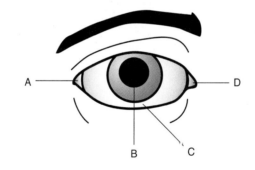

   1. A
   2. B
   3. C
   4. D

A Child with an Ear Infection

11. The nurse is teaching the parents how to instill antibiotic otic drops to the 6-year-old child with otitis media. Which instruction should the nurse discuss with the parents?
    1. After instilling medication gently massage the area immediately anterior to the ear.
    2. Gently pull the pinna downward and straight back when inserting the eardrops.
    3. Allow the child to get up immediately after instilling the ear drops into the affected ear.
    4. Insert the dropper with prescribed medication deep into the ear canal and instill drops.

12. Which statement indicates that the mother understands the procedure for administering otic drops to the child who has otitis media?
    1. "I should clean my child's ear canal very gently with cotton swabs."
    2. "I will warm the drops to room temperature before instilling them."
    3. "I can place a heating pad over my child's ear after putting in drops."
    4. "I need to place the dropper gently into my child's ear canal."

13. The 4-year-old child with otitis media with effusion is not prescribed systemic antibiotics. The mother asks the nurse, "Why didn't the doctor order antibiotics for my child?" Which statement is the nurse's best response?
    1. "Your child is too young to receive antibiotics."
    2. "You should discuss this with your child's health-care provider."
    3. "Because your child did not have a fever the doctor did not order antibiotics."
    4. "Most pediatricians prescribe ear drops instead of antibiotics."

14. The mother of a 5-year-old male child who has had five ear infections in the last 6 months asks the nurse, "What can be done because my child keeps having ear infections?" Which response by the nurse is most appropriate?
    1. "There are many different types of antibiotics, and one will work."
    2. "You are concerned your child keeps having ear infections."
    3. "Does you child dunk his head under water during bath time?"
    4. "Your child may need tubes inserted into both of his ears."

15. The father of a 23-month-old female child with acute otitis media calls the clinic and tells the nurse his daughter is crying and pulling at her ears. Which action should the nurse implement?
    1. Instruct the father to give acetaminophen elixir as prescribed on the bottle.
    2. Determine when the father gave the last dose of prescribed antibiotic.
    3. Tell the father to administer two chewable baby aspirins every 6 hours.
    4. Encourage the father to hold the child and rock her until she falls asleep.

16. The nurse is administering otic drops to a 5-year-old child with acute otitis media. Which interventions should the nurse implement? Rank in order of performance.
    1. Brace the administering hand against the child's head above the ear.
    2. Insert the required number of drops and gently massage the tragus.
    3. Explain the procedure to the child in developmentally appropriate terms.
    4. Gently pull the top of the child's ear up and back.
    5. Keep the child on the unaffected side for several minutes.

17. The 3-year-old female child is diagnosed with acute otitis media. Which statement by the mother indicates the medication teaching has not been effective?
    1. "I will be sure and take my daughter to her follow-up appointment with her doctor."
    2. "My son starting pulling at his ears so I gave him some of my daughter's antibiotics."
    3. "I will give my daughter all of the medication, even if she starts feeling better."
    4. "If my daughter does not get better in 48 hours, I will call her health-care provider."

18. The mother of a 13-year-old child who is diagnosed with external otitis tells the nurse her child spends a lot of time swimming. Which information is most important for the nurse to discuss with the mother?
    1. Insert silicone earplugs prior to entering the water.
    2. Administer a drying agent in the ear canal after swimming.
    3. Wear a tight-fitting swim cap, especially in cold water.
    4. Tilt the head to allow water to drain from the ear.

19. The 2-year-old child has acute otitis media. Which intervention will help increase the mother's compliance with the medical regimen?
    1. Instruct the parent verbally on how to use a calibrated measuring device.
    2. Give the mother a sample of the antibiotic therapy to take home.
    3. Make an appointment for a follow-up visit in 1 week.
    4. Provide written and oral instructions about antibiotic therapy.

20. The primary nurse is administering antibiotic otic drops to a 2-year-old child. Which action by the primary nurse warrants intervention by the charge nurse?
    1. The primary nurse asks the mother if the child has any known allergies.
    2. The primary nurse puts on nonsterile gloves when inserting the otic drops.
    3. The primary nurse washes his or her hands prior to administering medication.
    4. The primary nurse gets assistance to restrain the child when giving otic drops.

A Client with an Eye Disorder

1. 1. The client should wash the hands prior to instilling medication to ensure that bacteria do not fall into the eye. This action does not warrant intervention.
   2. The client should squeeze the bridge of the nose gently after administering the medication to prevent systemic absorption of the medication. This action does not warrant intervention.
   3. **The client should keep the eyes closed for 1–2 minutes after instilling the eye drops to enhance the effectiveness of the medication. This action warrants the nurse correcting the behavior.**
   4. The client should not touch the eye with the dropper to help prevent trauma to the eye. This action does not warrant intervention.

2. 1. The Ocusert Pilo should be placed in the conjunctival sac, preferably under the upper lid. This positioning is different from that for most eye medications.
   2. **The pilocarpine may cause blurred vision; therefore, it should be applied at night. This is a special system that allows medication to be applied to the eye with an ophthalmic device.**
   3. The system should be removed daily and is replaced weekly.
   4. Lacrimation and headache are expected side effects, and the client does not need to call the HCP.

3. 1. **Eye pain may indicate an attack of angle-closure glaucoma and must be reported to the HCP immediately.**
   2. The client should avoid using any over-the-counter sinus and cold medications containing pseudoephedrine and phenylephrine, which may accentuate the side effects of epinephrine.
   3. If the client experiences any central nervous system side effects, such as anxiety, nervousness, or muscle tremors, the client should notify the HCP. Depending on the severity of the side effects, the HCP may or may not discontinue the medication.
   4. There is no reason why the client must lie down for 1 hour after administering this medication.

4. 1. The nurse does not have to don sterile gloves when applying ophthalmic medication; nonsterile gloves can be used.
   2. The client's eyelids should not be shut during surgery. This medication paralyzes the eye during surgery.
   3. There is no such thing as an eye catheter that is inserted into the outer canthus of the eye.
   4. **Cycloplegic medication paralyzes the eye for 1 to 2 days and the client should be aware of this information because most ophthalmic surgery is performed in day surgery. Because the client will be at home, he or she needs to be knowledgeable about the medication.**

5. 1. **The client should instill eye ointment into the lower conjunctival sac, which is the inner edge of the lower lid margin.**
   2. **Applying pressure to the nasolacrimal duct will prevent systemic absorption of the medication.**
   3. The client does not have to wear gloves when applying the ointment to his or her own eyes. The client should be instructed to wash hands prior to and after applying the ointment.
   4. **The antibiotic ointment should be applied from the inner canthus to the outer canthus, from the nose side of the eye to the outer area.**
   5. **The client should sit with the head slightly tilted back or lie supine when applying ophthalmic ointment or drops to better access the lower conjunctival sac.**

MEMORY MEDICATION JOGGER: The nurse must know the correct technique when administering medications. This is considered one of the "six rights" of medication administration.

6. 1. If there is no redness, inflammation, or other signs of an infection, then the nurse could recommend using artificial tears, which is an over-the-counter medication, but this is not the first intervention.
   2. **The nurse should first assess the eyes for redness or inflammation to determine if there is any type of infection, which would need an HCP's prescription for antibiotics.**
   3. The nurse could use the ophthalmoscope to assess the client's eyes, but the first intervention is a visual inspection.
   4. The nurse could evaluate the client's cardinal fields of vision, but the first intervention is a visual inspection.

7. 1. The client should come to the emergency department to determine if permanent damage has occurred and to be seen by an ophthalmologist, but that is not the first intervention.
   2. Normal saline flush would help cleanse the bleach from the eyes, but it is not the first intervention.
   3. Regular antibiotic ointment should not be used in the eye, and bilateral patching is not appropriate for chemical irritation to the eye.
   4. **The nurse should instruct the client to rinse the eye with tap water for at least 5 minutes in each eye and then to come to the emergency department. The bleach must be thoroughly removed from the eyes.**

8. 1. This medication is prescribed for clients with open-angle glaucoma.
   2. There is no contraindication to administering this eye drop to a client in liver failure because the medication should not be absorbed systemically.
   3. There is no contraindication to administering this eye drop to a client who is allergic to sulfa.
   4. **Contraindications to using this medication include clients who may be receiving beta blocker therapy, including clients diagnosed with COPD, asthma, heart block, and heart failure.**

9. 1. Miotic medications, not mydriatic medications, constrict the pupil and block sympathetic nervous system input, which causes the pupil to dilate in low light and contracts the ciliary muscle.
   2. **Mydriatic medications dilate the pupil, reduce the production of aqueous humor, and increase the absorption effectiveness of aqueous humor, thus reducing intraocular pressure in open-angle glaucoma.**
   3. Beta-adrenergic blockers decrease the production of aqueous humor, which reduces intraocular pressure, but they do not affect pupil size and lens accommodation.
   4. Carbonic anhydrase inhibitors are used as adjunctive therapy to reduce intraocular pressure.

10. 1. The medication should not be administered in the inner canthus because it may increase systemic absorption of the medication.
    2. The medication should not be administered on the pupil because the medication will not be retained in the eye.
    3. **The medication should be administered into the lower conjunctival sac. Then the client should close the eye for 1–2 minutes, which will help ensure the medication stays in the eye.**
    4. The medication should not be administered in the outer canthus because it will not be retained in the eye.

A Child with an Ear Infection

11. 1. **Gentle massage of the area immediately anterior to the ear facilitates the entry of drops into the ear canal.**
    2. This should be done with children younger than 3 years of age because it will straighten the ear canal. In children older than age 3 the pinna should be pulled upward and back.
    3. After instillation of ear drops, the child should remain lying on the unaffected side for a few minutes.
    4. The dropper should be held over the ear canal when instilling eardrops. Inserting the dropper deep into the ear could cause injury to the ear.

12. 1. The mother should never attempt to place anything inside the ear to clean the canal because the risk of rupturing the tympanic membrane is high.
    2. **Cold otic drops cause pain when they come in contact with the tympanic membrane. Therefore, otic solutions should be allowed to warm to room temperature before being administered.**
    3. A heating pad could cause the tympanic membrane to rupture. The mother should not put heat or cold over the ear.
    4. The dropper should not be placed in the ear canal; the dropper should be held over the canal when releasing the drops into the canal.

13. 1. Any age child can receive antibiotics.
    2. This is "passing the buck," and the nurse should answer the mother's question.
    3. **Otitis media with effusion differs from acute otitis media in that there are no signs of acute infection. If there are no signs of infection, such as fever or pain, the nurse should explain that, with the emergence of antimicrobial-resistant**

organisms, recent recommendations discourage antibiotic use for otitis media with effusion because 50% of effusions will resolve on their own.

4. Acute otitis media with symptoms is treated with 5–7 days of oral antibiotics.

14. 1. There are only so many antibiotics that treat otitis media, and the HCP will not continue using antibiotics because the child can become resistant to antibiotics.

2. This is a therapeutic response, which is not appropriate because the mother needs factual information. This response is used to help the client ventilate feelings.

3. Dunking the head under water does not cause ear infections.

4. **This is the most appropriate response. A myringotomy with insertion of tympanostomy tubes is performed on children with persistent ear infections despite antibiotic therapy or otitis media with effusion for more than 3 months with associated hearing loss.**

15. 1. **Acetaminophen (Tylenol) is the drug of choice to help relieve discomfort in children.**

2. Determining the last dose of antibiotic will not help relieve the child's pain.

3. Aspirin should not be given to children because of the possibility of their developing Reye's syndrome.

4. This is a good action to take, but the child needs medication to help ease pain.

16. **3, 1, 4, 2, 5**

3. **The nurse should talk to the child and explain the procedure. This will help develop trust with the child. Many nurses talk to the parents and not the child.**

1. **Bracing the hand helps prevent the child from moving the head.**

4. **For children older than 3 years old, the pinna should be pulled up and back to straighten the ear canal so that the drops get to the tympanic membrane.**

2. **After inserting the drops, massaging the tragus (anterior portion) ensures that the drops reach the tympanic membrane.**

5. **This prevents the medication from spilling out of the ear.**

17. 1. This statement indicates the mother understands the medication teaching. Clients should keep all follow-up appointments.

2. Antibiotics are prescribed for a specific condition for a specific client. The mother should not give antibiotics prescribed for her daughter to her son. The mother does not understand the medication teaching.

3. The entire prescription of antibiotics should be taken whether the client is feeling better or not.

4. After 2 days of antibiotic therapy, the child should start feeling better. This statement indicates the mother understands the medication teaching.

18. 1. Silicone earplugs can keep water out of the ear without reducing hearing significantly, but it is not the most important information to discuss with the client.

2. **A 2% acetic acid solution or 2% boric acid in ethyl alcohol is effective in drying the canal and restoring its normal acidic environment. This is the most important information for the nurse to teach because, although suggesting ways to prevent water from entering is helpful, the client must dry the canal to prevent further episodes of external otitis.**

3. A swim cap does not prevent water from entering the ear. It protects the ear from the cold and possibly slows the formation of bony growths in the ears. It also protects the ear from debris in the water.

4. Tilting the head to allow water to drain from the ear is helpful, but it does not ensure the ear will be restored to a normal acidic environment.

19. 1. The nurse should have the mother demonstrate how to use the measuring device to ensure the mother knows how to use the device. Verbal instructions alone do not ensure that the mother knows how to administer medication correctly.

2. Providing the mother with a sample of antibiotics will not ensure compliance.

3. A follow-up visit will not ensure compliance with the medication regimen.

4. **Many times in the HCP's office the mother may be nervous. The child is in the room, and there are many distractions. Therefore, verbal instructions alone may not be thoroughly understood. Written information may increase compliance with the medication regimen.**

20. 1. This indicates the nurse understands the correct procedure for administering otic drops; therefore, this does not warrant intervention by the charge nurse.
    2. **This procedure does not warrant wearing nonsterile gloves because the nurse will not come into contact with any blood or body fluids. The nurse should wash his or her hands and administer medication. This action warrants intervention by the charge nurse.**
    3. This is correct procedure prior to administering medications; therefore, this action does not warrant intervention by the charge nurse.
    4. Assistance in restraining a young child might be necessary; therefore, this would not warrant intervention by the charge nurse.

1. The client diagnosed with glaucoma is prescribed oral acetazolamide (Diamox), a carbonic anhydrase inhibitor. Which information should the client discuss with the client?
   1. Administer the medication in the morning.
   2. Instill medication in the lower conjunctival sac.
   3. Wash hands prior to administering medication.
   4. Hold the eyes shut for 2 minutes after taking medication.

2. The nurse is discussing how to instill artificial tears into the client's eyes. Which information should the nurse discuss with the client? Select all that apply.
   1. Do not allow the artificial tear dropper to touch the eye.
   2. Keep the eyes closed 1–2 minutes after instilling drops.
   3. Apply pressure to the inner canthus after instilling eye drops.
   4. Wash the hands prior to instilling the artificial tears into the eyes.
   5. Lie in the prone position when instilling the eye drops.

3. The client diagnosed with glaucoma is prescribed betaxolol (Betoptic), beta-adrenergic blocker, ophthalmic drops. Which information should the nurse discuss with the client?
   1. Instruct the client to call the HCP if dizziness occurs when getting up too fast.
   2. Discuss that the drops will cause the vision to get worse initially.
   3. Teach the client how to prevent orthostatic hypotension.
   4. Explain the importance of applying pressure at the outer canthus.

4. The client diagnosed with Meniere's disease, also known as endolymphatic hydrops, is prescribed meclizine (Antivert), an antivertigo medication. Which statement best describes the scientific rationale for this medication?
   1. It will help decrease the whirling sensation experienced in Meniere's disease.
   2. It will help prevent an acute episode of nausea and vomiting.
   3. It will help maintain a lower labyrinthine pressure in the ears.
   4. It will help the ear canal vasoconstrict, reducing the pressure in the ears.

5. The client diagnosed with Meniere's disease is admitted with an acute attack and prescribed intravenous diazepam (Valium), a sedative–hypnotic. Which intervention should the nurse implement when administering this medication?
   1. Dilute the Valium to a 10-mL bolus with normal saline.
   2. Administer the diazepam undiluted via a saline lock
   3. Infuse the diazepam via an IV piggyback over 1 hour.
   4. Question the order because diazepam cannot be given IVP.

6. Which interventions should be included when the nurse is teaching the 28-year-old client diagnosed with external otitis how to instill otic drops? Rank in the order of performance.
   1. Loosely place a small piece of cotton in the auditory meatus.
   2. Demonstrate pulling the pinna of the ear up and back when inserting drops.
   3. Warm the medication by holding the container in the hand for 5 minutes.
   4. Tilt the head toward the unaffected side when in the sitting position.
   5. Administer the prescribed number of drops into the ear canal.

7. The client calls the clinic and tells the nurse that a live insect is in the client's right ear. Which action should the clinic nurse take?
   1. Encourage the client to get someone to remove the insect.
   2. Instruct the client to put water into the ear canal.
   3. Have the client put mineral oil into the ear canal.
   4. Tell the client to put a medicated cotton ball in the ear.

8. The client with nasal congestion is prescribed nasal solution. Which information should be included in the medication teaching?
   1. Direct the solution toward the base of the nasal cavity.
   2. Tell the client to blow the nose prior to instilling solution.
   3. Replace remaining nasal solution in the dropper back into the bottle.
   4. Have the client squeeze the nostrils shut after instilling nasal solution.

9. The client is diagnosed with acute bacterial conjunctivitis. The health-care provider prescribed erythromycin ophthalmic ointment. Which information should the nurse discuss with the client?
   1. Apply a thick line of ointment in the upper lid margin of the eye.
   2. Instruct the client to look downward when applying the ointment.
   3. Instruct the client to clean the eye with antibiotic solution prior to applying ointment.
   4. Apply the ophthalmic ointment from the inner to the outer canthus.

10. The client who has undergone eye surgery is complaining of being nauseated. Which intervention should the PACU recovery room nurse implement?
    1. Administer an intravenous antiemetic medication.
    2. Determine if the client had anything to eat preoperatively.
    3. Place a cold washcloth under the chin along the client's throat.
    4. Put the client on the left side and insert a rectal antiemetic medication.

11. The pediatric nurse is administering nasal medication to the 13-month-old child. Which intervention should the nurse implement?
    1. Place the child in a prone position with the head to the side.
    2. Gently place the child's chin on the chest using the nondominant hand.
    3. Turn the child's head slightly from side to side and back to midline.
    4. Allow the child to sit up immediately after the medication is instilled.

12. The 3-year-old child with an eye infection has both an ophthalmic ointment and ophthalmic drops prescribed. Which action by the primary nurse would warrant intervention by the charge nurse?
    1. The primary nurse applies the ophthalmic ointment first.
    2. The primary nurse instills the ophthalmic drops in the lower lid.
    3. The primary nurse does not allow the dropper to touch the eye.
    4. The primary nurse instills the ophthalmic drops first.

13. The nurse is administering silver nitrate 1% (Dey-Drop), an antibiotic, to a 1-hour-old infant. Which statement is the scientific rationale for administering this medication?
    1. It is used to prevent herpes simplex keratitis.
    2. It is used to prevent ophthalmia neonatorum.
    3. It is used to treat bacterial conjunctivitis.
    4. It is used to treat a fungal infection of the eyes.

14. The client with a fungal infection of the eye is prescribed natamycin (Natacyn Ophthalmic) drops. Which medication teaching should the nurse discuss with the client?
    1. Instruct the client to patch both eyes after instilling the medication.
    2. Tell the client to apply cool packs to the eye after instilling medication.
    3. Explain that the medication may cause temporary blurred vision.
    4. Discuss the need to instill drops once a day prior to going to sleep.

15. To which client would the health-care provider recommend Debrox, an over-the-counter ceruminolytic?
    1. The client with "swimmer's ear."
    2. The client with impacted ear wax.
    3. The client with external otitis.
    4. The client with bilateral cataracts.

16. The client with otitis media is prescribed clarithromycin (Biaxin), an antibiotic, 500 mg po every 12 hours for 10 days. Which medication teaching should the nurse discuss with the client?
    1. Discuss the need to take medication with food.
    2. Tell the client to wear sunglasses when going outdoors.
    3. Instruct the client to get cultures after completing medications.
    4. Encourage the client to eat yogurt or buttermilk daily.

17. The client with multiple mouth ulcers is prescribed Nystatin swish and swallow. Which intervention should the nurse implement when administering this medication?
    1. Instruct the client to swish the medication in the mouth and spit it out.
    2. Encourage the client to swish the medication in the mouth for at least 2 minutes.
    3. Tell the client to swish the mouth with normal saline after swallowing the medication.
    4. Apply the Nystatin medication to the mouth ulcers with a sterile cotton swab.

18. The nurse is discussing how to instill nasal drops. Which instructions should the nurse discuss with the client? Rank in order of performance.
    1. Discard any remaining solution that is in the dropper.
    2. Instruct the client to remain in position for 5 minutes.
    3. Instruct the client to open and breathe through the mouth.
    4. Instill the solution laterally toward the nasal septum.
    5. Hold the tip of the dropper just above the nostril without touching the nose.

19. The client just diagnosed with glaucoma is prescribed pilocarpine, a miotic ophthalmic eye drop. Which statement indicates the client needs more teaching concerning the medication?
    1. "I will use nightlights in the halls and in the bathroom."
    2. "I will get my wife or son to drive me around at night."
    3. "I will avoid doing tasks that require sharp vision."
    4. "I will take the eye drops every time I have eye pain."

20. The nurse is administering ophthalmic medication to the client. To which area should the nurse instruct the client to apply pressure for 1–2 minutes after instilling the medication?

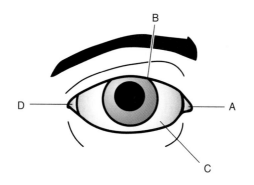

    1. A
    2. B
    3. C
    4. D

1. 1. The oral medication Diamox has a diuretic effect. Therefore, it should be taken in the morning to prevent sleep deprivation because of the need to get up to urinate during the night.
   2. This is an oral medication that is used as adjunctive therapy for clients diagnosed with glaucoma. It is not instilled into the eye.
   3. This is an oral medication that is used as adjunctive therapy for clients diagnosed with glaucoma. The client does not have to wash hands prior to taking an oral medication.
   4. This is an oral medication that is used as adjunctive therapy for clients diagnosed with glaucoma. It is not instilled into the eye, and there is no reason for the client to hold the eyes shut.

2. 1. Not letting the dropper touch the eye ensures that the eye will not be injured during application of the artificial tears.
   2. Keeping the eyes shut for a minute or two after instilling the drops will enhance the effectiveness of the medication.
   3. Applying pressure to the inner canthus is not an appropriate intervention because this prevents systemic absorption of the medication and artificial tears are not a medication that would cause systemic effects.
   4. Washing the hands is an appropriate intervention so that bacteria on the hands will not fall into the eye when instilling eye drops.
   5. Lying on the stomach (prone position) is not an appropriate intervention to discuss with the client. This position would allow the drops to leak out of the eye.

3. 1. Betoptic is a beta blocker that, if absorbed systemically, may cause bradycardia and hypotension. The nurse should discuss orthostatic hypotension with the client, but there is no need for the client to call the HCP.
   2. If the vision gets worse, the client should call the HCP because this is an adverse reaction that warrants intervention.
   3. This is a beta blocker that, if absorbed systemically, may cause bradycardia and hypotension. The nurse should discuss ways to prevent orthostatic hypotension.
   4. The client should apply pressure at the inner canthus (closest to nose) to help prevent systemic absorption of the medication.

4. 1. Antivert helps prevent dizziness and the whirling sensation characteristic of Meniere's disease.
   2. An antiemetic medication, not Antivert, would be prescribed to help prevent nausea and vomiting.
   3. An oral diuretic, not Antivert, is prescribed for clients with Meniere's disease to help maintain a lower labyrinthine pressure.
   4. Vasoconstriction should be avoided in clients with Meniere's disease because it may precipitate an attack. Tobacco products, alcohol, and caffeine should be avoided because they cause vasoconstriction.

5. 1. Diazepam cannot be diluted because it is oil based and will not dissolve with normal saline.
   2. Diazepam cannot be diluted because it is oil based and will not dissolve with normal saline. Diazepam should be administered via a saline lock or at the port closest to the client if administered through an existing intravenous line.
   3. Diazepam is administered via intravenous push over 2–5 minutes, but it is not administered via an intravenous piggyback over 30 minutes.
   4. Diazepam can be administered via intravenous push.

6. Answers 3, 4, 2, 5, 1
   3. Warming the medications promotes comfort when the eardrops are instilled.
   4. Sitting with the head tilted toward the unaffected side allows gravity to assist in moving the medication to the inner portion of the ear canal.
   2. Pulling the pinna up and back straightens the ear canal in adults and allows the medication to travel along the length of the canal.
   5. This ensures the full amount of prescribed medication will be administered to penetrate the length of the canal and achieve full effectiveness.
   1. Leaving a small piece of cotton in the auditory meatus for 15 to 20 minutes helps keep the medication in the canal.

7. 1. A live insect cannot be removed from the ear; the insect must be killed prior to removing the insect.
   2. Water should not be inserted into the ear canal because organic foreign bodies such as an insect or bean will swell when water is

inserted into the ear canal, which makes removal more difficult.
3. Mineral oil or topical lidocaine drops are used to immobilize or kill insects prior to their removal from the ear.
4. There is no such thing as medicated cotton balls available over the counter; therefore, this is not an appropriate action.

8. 1. The solution should be directed laterally toward the midline of the superior concha of the ethmoid bone, not at the base of the nasal cavity because then it will run down the throat and into the eustachian tube.
2. The client should blow his or her nose to clear the nasal passages prior to instilling the nasal solution.
3. The client should discard any solution remaining in the dropper.
4. The client should not squeeze the nostrils but should remain with the head tilted for 5 minutes after instilling the nasal solution.

9. 1. A thin line of ointment should be applied evenly along the inner edge of the lower lid margin of the eye.
2. The client should look upward when applying the ointment.
3. The eye should be cleaned with warm water prior to applying antibiotic ointment. There is no antibiotic solution used prior to using ophthalmic ointment.
4. When applying ointment, a thin line of ointment should be applied evenly along the inner edge of the lower lid margin, from the inner canthus to the outer canthus.

10. 1. The nurse must take action as soon as possible to prevent vomiting because vomiting will increase intraocular pressure.
2. Determining if the client had anything to eat preoperatively should have been done prior to the client having surgery. It is not pertinent information at this time.
3. A cold washcloth will not help prevent the client from vomiting. The client needs an antiemetic medication.
4. The client in the recovery room would have an intravenous route. The nurse should administer the antiemetic via the route that would decrease the nausea as fast as possible; that is the intravenous route.

11. 1. The child should be in the supine position.

2. The nurse should hyperextend the neck slightly by placing a rolled towel or small blanket under the shoulder blades.
3. Turning the head slightly from side to side and back to the midline position will help disperse the medication to the maxillary and frontal sinuses.
4. The child should be kept in the midline position for at least 3 minutes after the medication is instilled into the nose to allow the medication to reach the ethmoid and sphenoid sinuses.

12. 1. The nurse should apply the drops first because if the drops are placed after the ointment, the ophthalmic drops will not be absorbed. This action would warrant intervention by the charge nurse.
2. This is the correct procedure to instill the ophthalmic drops; therefore, this intervention would not warrant intervention by the charge nurse.
3. This is the correct procedure; therefore, this intervention would not warrant intervention by the charge nurse.
4. The ophthalmic drops should be administered first because if the ointment is instilled first, the ophthalmic drops will not be absorbed. This action would not warrant intervention by the charge nurse.

13. 1. Herpes simplex is a virus and is not treated with an antibiotic.
2. This antibiotic ointment is used to prevent an eye infection secondary to the mother having a sexually transmitted disease. It is administered to all newborns within 1 hour of birth.
3. A 1-hour-old infant would not have bacterial conjunctivitis; therefore, this is not the scientific rationale for administering this medication.
4. Antibiotics are not used to treat fungal infections.

14. 1. There is no reason for the client to patch the eyes after administering the medication.
2. There is no reason for the client to apply cool packs after instilling the medication.
3. The nurse should instruct the client that this medication may cause temporary blurring of the vision and may cause transient stinging.
4. The ophthalmic medication is administered one drop every 2 hours for the first 3–4 days; after that, 1 drop should

be administered every 3 hours for 14
to 21 days.

15. 1. The client with swimmer's ear would
need a 2% acetic acid solution or 2%
boric acid in ethyl alcohol to help dry
the ear canal and restore its normal
acidic environment.
2. **A ceruminolytic medication helps to
loosen and remove impacted cerumen
(ear wax) from the ear canal.**
3. This is an inflammation of the external
ear that would not require a ceruminolytic.
4. Cataracts are eye disorders, not ear
disorders.

16. 1. The medication can be taken with or
without food.
2. This medication does not cause photosensitivity.
3. There is no need for the client to get a
culture after antibiotic therapy; otitis
media is not diagnosed with a culture but
with a visual examination of the ear.
4. **Yogurt and buttermilk will help to
maintain the intestinal flora, which may
be destroyed when receiving antibiotic
therapy. The destruction of intestinal
flora will lead to a superinfection,
resulting in diarrhea.**

17. 1. The client should swish the medication in
the mouth for at least 2 minutes and then
swallow the medication.
2. **The client should swish the medication
in the mouth for at least 2 minutes and
then swallow the medication.**
3. The client should not swish the mouth
with normal saline because the medication
should remain in the mouth even after the
medication is swallowed.
4. This is not the correct procedure for
administering this medication.

18.   **3, 5, 4, 2, 1**
3. **The client should first breathe through
the mouth.**
5. **The tip of the dropper should not
touch the nose because this could**

cause contamination of the dropper
when being replaced into the bottle.
4. **The solution should be inserted laterally toward the midline of the superior
concha of the ethmoid bone, not the
base of the nasal cavity where it will
run down the throat and into the
eustachian tube.**
2. **The client should remain lying down
for 5 minutes so that the solution will
not run out of the nose.**
1. **The remaining solution should be
discarded to prevent contamination
of the bottle.**

19. 1. Vision is reduced in dim lights; therefore,
the client should use a nightlight to
prevent falls. This statement indicates the
client understands the teaching.
2. Vision is reduced in dim lights; therefore,
the client should avoid night driving for
the safety of himself and others. This
statement indicates the client understands
the teaching.
3. Visual acuity may be decreased during the
initiation of therapy; therefore, the client
should avoid tasks requiring sharp vision.
This statement indicates the client understands the teaching.
4. **This medication should be taken
routinely every day to reduce intraocular pressure. Glaucoma is painless, so if
the client experiences pain, the client
should call the HCP immediately. This
statement indicates the client needs
more teaching.**

20. 1. Gentle pressure should be applied to
the inner canthus (lacrimal sac) for 1–
2 minutes to increase the local effect
and decrease systemic absorption.
2. Gentle pressure to the eyelid is not helpful
when instilling ophthalmic medication.
3. Gentle pressure to the lower conjunctival
sac is not helpful when instilling
ophthalmic medication.
4. Gentle pressure to the outer canthus is
not helpful when instilling ophthalmic
medication.

14

Emergency Nursing

"Drug interactions that might have trivial consequences in a young adult can have devastating consequences in an older person."

—Mickey Stanley, Kathryn Blair, and Patricia Beare

PRACTICE QUESTIONS

A Client Experiencing Shock

1. The nurse is preparing to administer a nitroglycerin (Tridil) drip to a client in cardiogenic shock. Which intervention should the nurse implement?
   1. Mix the nitroglycerin in 500 mL of lactated Ringer's.
   2. Wrap the intravenous bag and tubing in a foil package.
   3. Use regular intravenous tubing when administering Tridil.
   4. Ensure that the client's nitroglycerin patch is in a nonhairy area.

2. The nurse is preparing to administer dopamine, a beta and alpha agonist, to a client in cardiogenic shock. Which intervention should the nurse implement?
   1. Ensure the client is on a cardiac monitor.
   2. Assess the blood pressure every 4 hours.
   3. Evaluate the intake and output every shift.
   4. Explain that burning at the intravenous site may occur.

3. The client in hypovolemic shock is receiving dextran, a nonblood colloid. Which assessment data would warrant immediate intervention by the nurse?
   1. The client's blood pressure is 102/78.
   2. The client's pulse oximeter reading is 95%.
   3. The client's lung sounds reveal bilateral crackles.
   4. The client's urine output is 120 mL in 3 hours.

4. The nurse is caring for the client in septic shock. The nurse administered the twice-a-day, intravenous, broad-spectrum antibiotic ceftriaxone (Rocephin) at 0900. At 1100 the health-care provider prescribed daily intravenous vancomycin, an aminoglycoside antibiotic. Which action should the nurse implement?
   1. Administer the vancomycin within 2 hours.
   2. Notify the HCP and question the antibiotic order.
   3. Schedule the vancomycin to be administered at 2100.
   4. Assess the client's white blood cell count.

5. The client in cardiogenic shock is receiving norepinephrine (Levophed), a sympathomimetic. Which priority intervention should the nurse implement?
   1. Do not abruptly discontinue the medication.
   2. Administer medication on an infusion pump.
   3. Check the client's creatinine level and BUN.
   4. Monitor the client's blood pressure continuously.

6. The nurse is preparing to administer albumin 5% (Albuminar-5), a colloid solution. Which statement is the scientific rationale for administering this medication?
   1. Albumin acts directly on the smooth muscles to cause vasodilatation.
   2. Albumin mimics the fight-or-flight response of the sympathetic nervous system.
   3. Albumin is a blood volume expander that promotes circulatory volume.
   4. Albumin contains dextrose and increases fluid volume in the interstitial space.

7. During the first 15 minutes of administering blood to a client, the client complains of shortness of breath, low back pain, and itching all over the body. Which action should the nurse implement first?
   1. Administer 0.5 mL of epinephrine, an adrenergic, intravenously.
   2. Assess the client's temperature, pulse, and blood pressure.
   3. Infuse normal saline at 125 mL an hour via a peripheral IV.
   4. Discontinue the blood at the hub of the intravenous catheter.

8. The primary nurse is preparing to administer dobutamine (Dobutrex), a beta$_1$-adrenergic agonist, to a client in cardiogenic shock. Which action by the primary nurse would warrant intervention by the charge nurse?
   1. The primary nurse is administering the dobutamine drip via gravity.
   2. The primary nurse attaches a urometer to the client's Foley catheter.
   3. The primary nurse applies a pulse oximeter to the client's finger.
   4. The primary nurse checks the client for any medication allergies.

9. The client in cardiogenic shock is receiving dopamine, a beta and alpha agonist. The peripheral intravenous site becomes infiltrated. Which action should the nurse implement?
   1. Assess the client's blood pressure and apical pulse.
   2. Elevate the arm and apply ice to the infiltrated area.
   3. Inject phentolamine (Regitine) at the site of infiltration.
   4. Discontinue the IV and take no other action.

10. The nurse is caring for a client diagnosed with cardiogenic shock who is receiving a dopamine drip, a sympathomimetic. Which interventions should the nurse implement? Select all interventions that apply.
   1. Aspirate the injection site to avoid injecting directly into the vein.
   2. Do not administer any alkaline solutions in the same tubing as dopamine.
   3. Assess the client's lung sounds, vital signs, and hemodynamic parameters.
   4. Ask if the client has a living will or durable power of attorney for health care.
   5. Administer the dopamine via a Y-tubing along with normal saline (0.9%).

A Community Facing Bioterrorism

11. The nurse working in an emergency department (ED) receives a call that the ED will be receiving multiple casualties from a chlorine chemical explosion. Which intervention is the most important in preparing for the victims?
   1. Prepare to decontaminate the clients in a decontamination room.
   2. Do not touch any of the clothing the clients are wearing.
   3. Have intravenous supplies ready to start IV lines.
   4. Prepare to administer oxygen immediately to all casualties.

12. The nurse is discussing the bioterrorism threat with a group in the community. Which information regarding smallpox should be included in the discussion?
   1. The incubation period for smallpox is 3–4 days after exposure.
   2. The organism can only live for 5–6 minutes outside the host body.
   3. It can be spread by direct or indirect contact with an infected person.
   4. The rash begins on the lower half of the body and progresses from there.

13. The client is suspected of being exposed to inhaled anthrax. Which nursing intervention has the greatest priority?
    1. Assess the client's lungs.
    2. Start the IVPB antibiotics.
    3. Place the client on respiratory isolation.
    4. Maintain the client's blood pressure.

14. The Homeland Security Office has issued a warning of suspected biological warfare using the *Francisella tularensis* (tularemia) bacteria. Which sign and symptoms would support the initial diagnosis of tularemia?
    1. Fever, chills, headache, and malaise.
    2. Hypotension; red, raised rash; and nasal congestion.
    3. Enlarged cervical lymph nodes and polydipsia.
    4. Metallic taste and disorientation.

15. The client has been diagnosed with botulism. Which isolation procedures should the nurse implement?
    1. Airborne precautions.
    2. Standard precautions.
    3. Contact precautions.
    4. Droplet precautions.

16. The client has been exposed to nitrogen mustard gas. Which solution should be used to decontaminate the client?
    1. Normal saline.
    2. Milk and dairy products.
    3. Soap and water.
    4. Diluted baking soda.

17. The client working in a chemical plant that processes malathion for agricultural use presents to the emergency department with profuse sweating, visual disturbances, gastrointestinal disturbances, and bradycardia. Which medication should the nurse prepare to administer?
    1. Dilantin, an anticonvulsant, IV every 4 hours.
    2. Solu-Medrol, a glucocorticosteroid, IV every 8 hours.
    3. Activated charcoal, an absorbent agent, po every 2 hours.
    4. Atropine, an anticholinergic, IV every 5 minutes.

18. The employee health nurse working in an industrial plant that manufactures cyanide smells the odor of bitter almonds. Which actions should the nurse implement? Select all that apply.
    1. Have the workers evacuate the area.
    2. Close off the area in question.
    3. Notify the Office of Emergency Management.
    4. Call the emergency broadcast system to alert the public.
    5. Assess the workers for respiratory distress.

19. The client is diagnosed with acute radiation syndrome (ARS). Which signs and symptoms would the nurse assess in the acute phase?
    1. Elevated blood pressure and bradycardia.
    2. Fluid and electrolyte imbalance and shock.
    3. Decreased lymphocytes, leukocytes, and erythrocytes.
    4. Nausea, vomiting, diarrhea, and fatigue.

20. The nurse is working as the triage nurse in an emergency department. Five clients have presented to the emergency department within the last 6 hours with complaints of severe abdominal cramping, nausea, vomiting, and diarrhea. Which intervention would be most important for the nurse to implement first?
    1. Notify the public health department of a botulism outbreak.
    2. Check the clients' complete blood count results.
    3. Determine if the clients ate at the same place recently.
    4. Discuss the situation with the house supervisor.

A Client Experiencing a Code

21. A code has been called for the client experiencing ventricular fibrillation. Which medication should the nurse prepare to administer to the client?
    1. Epinephrine, an adrenergic agonist, intravenous push.
    2. Lidocaine, an antidysrhythmic, intravenous push.
    3. Atropine, an antidysrhythmic, intravenous push.
    4. Digoxin, a cardiac glycoside, intravenous push.

22. The client in a code has the following arterial blood gases: pH 7.31, PaO_2 60, $PaCO_2$ 58, and HCO_3 19. Which medication should the nurse prepare to administer to the client?
    1. Dopamine, a vasopressor medication.
    2. Sodium bicarbonate, an alkalinizing agent.
    3. Calcium gluconate, electrolyte replacement.
    4. Adenosine, an antidysrhythmic medication.

23. The nurse is administering epinephrine 0.5 mg intravenous push to a client in a code. The client has a primary intravenous line of D_5W at to keep open (TKO) rate. Which intervention should the nurse implement?
    1. Administer the medication over 5 minutes.
    2. Flush the tubing before and after administering epinephrine.
    3. Elevate the arm after administering the medication.
    4. Dilute the medication with 10 mL normal saline.

24. The HCP orders a lidocaine drip at 3 mg/min for a client who has just converted from ventricular fibrillation to normal sinus rhythm with multiple premature ventricular contractions (PVCs). The intravenous bag has 2 grams of lidocaine in 500 mL normal saline. How would the nurse set the intravenous rate?
    Answer _____

25. The client who is coding is in asystole. Which action should the nurse implement first?
    1. Prepare to defibrillate the client at 200 joules.
    2. Prepare for synchronized cardioversion.
    3. Prepare to administer atropine, intravenous push.
    4. Prepare to administer amiodarone, an antidysrhythmic.

26. The client in a code is in ventricular fibrillation and then is in sinus rhythm with PVCs. After taking vital signs the HCP orders a dopamine, vasopressor, drip at 3 mg/kg per hour. Which intervention should the nurse implement concerning this medication?
    1. Monitor the client's blood pressure every 2 hours.
    2. Assess the client's telemetry reading every 1 hour.
    3. Check the client's urine output every 1 hour.
    4. Evaluate the client's glucometer readings every 4 hours.

27. The client is in a code and is exhibiting ventricular fibrillation. Which medication would the nurse prepare to administer?
    1. Dopamine, a vasopressor, intravenous drip.
    2. Lidocaine, an antidysrhythmic, intravenous push.
    3. Procainamide, an antidysrhythmic, intravenous push.
    4. Dobutamine, an inotropic medication, intravenous drip.

28. The nurse is preparing to hang a dopamine drip on the client who has just been successfully coded. The client is receiving lidocaine 2 mg/min in the existing IV site. Which action should the nurse implement when hanging the dopamine drip?
    1. Initiate another intravenous line to administer the dopamine drip.
    2. Piggyback the dopamine drip in the lidocaine tubing.
    3. Question the order because dopamine cannot be administered with lidocaine.
    4. Prepare to help the HCP insert a subclavian line for the dopamine drip.

29. The client has just been successfully resuscitated and has the following arterial blood gases (ABGs): pH 7.35, PaO₂ 78, PaCO₂ 46, and HCO₃ 22. Which action should the nurse implement?
    1. Prepare to administer sodium bicarbonate IVP.
    2. Administer oxygen 8 L/min via nasal cannula.
    3. Take no action because the ABGs are within normal limits.
    4. Assess the client's pulse oximeter reading.

30. The client in a code is in ventricular fibrillation. Which HCP order would the nurse question?
    1. Administer amiodarone, an antidysrhythmic.
    2. Administer lidocaine, an antidysrhythmic.
    3. Prepare to defibrillate at 360 joules.
    4. Prepare to insert an external pacemaker.

A Child Experiencing Poisoning

31. A 4-year-old child is brought to the emergency department as a suspected poisoning victim. Which interventions should the nurse implement? Select all that apply.
    1. Implement supportive care.
    2. Identify the poison.
    3. Prevent further absorption of the poison.
    4. Promote poison removal.
    5. Administer the antidote.

32. Which statement best describes the scientific rationale for administering activated charcoal to a child who has ingested a poison?
    1. Charcoal neutralizes toxic substances by changing the pH of the poison.
    2. The charcoal binds with the poison, and it is excreted through the bowel.
    3. Charcoal enhances antidotes for better results than antidotes given alone.
    4. The charcoal induces vomiting, and the client eliminates much of the poison.

33. The emergency department is caring for pediatric clients who have ingested poisons. Which client would the nurse question administering a gastric lavage?
    1. The 2-year-old child in a coma who took a bottle of Tylenol.
    2. The 3-year-old child who ate a bottle of unknown tablets.
    3. The hyperactive 6-year-old child who swallowed motor oil.
    4. The 10-year-old child who took a prescription of painkillers.

34. The nurse administered syrup of ipecac to an 18-month-old girl who swallowed her grandparent's prescription of digoxin. Which intervention is most important for the nurse to implement?
    1. Tell the parent to expect vomiting to occur in 20 minutes.
    2. Place the child on telemetry to monitor the cardiac status.
    3. Have the unlicensed assistive personnel monitor the vital signs.
    4. Order a STAT digoxin level to be drawn.

35. The 13-year-old child admitted to the intensive care department diagnosed with an overdose of Ambien CR, a sedative hypnotic, is ordered whole bowel irrigation. Which intervention should the nurse implement?
    1. Administer 0.5 L of GoLYTELY every hour.
    2. Administer 1.0 L of GoLYTELY every hour.
    3. Administer 1.5–2.0 L of GoLYTELY every hour.
    4. Administer 2.5–3.0 L of GoLYTELY every hour.

36. The nurse working in the emergency department receives a child who has ingested a poison. Which referral agency should be contacted for specific information regarding the poison?
    1. The Material Safety Data information line.
    2. The National Poison Control Hotline.
    3. Child Protective Services (CPS).
    4. The local police department.

37. The nurse is admitting a client suspected of poison ingestion to the emergency department. Which method is preferred to aid in the removal of ingested poisons?
    1. Emesis.
    2. Gastric lavage.
    3. Catharsis.
    4. Activated charcoal.

38. The health-care provider has prescribed edetate calcium disodium (Calcium EDTA), a chelating agent, for a child diagnosed with lead poisoning. Which intervention should the nurse implement?
    1. Administer orally with a large glass of water.
    2. Monitor the client's liver function tests.
    3. Check the client's intake and output.
    4. Tell the child to prepare to vomit.

39. The nurse administered the narcotic agonist naloxone (Narcan) to a 7-year-old child who drank a large bottle of narcotic cough syrup. Which intervention should the nurse be prepared to implement?
    1. Administer Narcan again in 30 minutes.
    2. Place the child on a negative pressure ventilator.
    3. Prepare the child for a tracheostomy.
    4. Have the parents discuss the situation with the police.

40. The school-aged child is brought to the emergency department with carbon monoxide poisoning. Which intervention would the nurse implement first?
    1. Place the child on a pulse oximeter.
    2. Have respiratory therapy draw blood gases.
    3. Administer oxygen at 10 L per minute.
    4. Prevent chilling by wrapping the child in blankets.

A Client Experiencing Shock

1. 1. Nitroglycerin should be mixed with D_5W or normal saline (NS) only.
   2. **These drugs must be protected from light. They must be protected in the package that is provided or wrapped in tin foil.**
   3. Regular intravenous tubing can absorb 40%–80% of the nitroglycerin. This medication should be administered in the special tubing that comes with the medication.
   4. Nitroglycerin patches should be removed when administering Tridil to prevent overdosage.

2. 1. **Clients must be connected to a cardiac monitor prior to and during the infusion of cardiotonic drugs. The client in cardiogenic shock will be in the intensive care department.**
   2. Dopamine is administered to increase the blood pressure, and the blood pressure must be monitored every 5 to 15 minutes, not every 4 hours.
   3. The client's urinary output should be monitored hourly to ensure the client has at least 30 mL of urine output an hour.
   4. Extravasation of dopamine causes severe, localized vasoconstriction, resulting in a slough of the tissue and tissue necrosis. The client should report burning at the IV site immediately.

3. 1. A blood pressure of 102/78 is a stable blood pressure reading for a client in hypovolemic shock. A B/P less than 90/60 would warrant intervention by the nurse.
   2. A pulse oximeter reading of greater than 93% indicates the arterial oxygen level is between 80 and 100, which is normal.
   3. **Because of the ability of all colloids, including dextran, to pull fluid into the vascular space, circulatory overload is a serious adverse outcome. Crackles in the lungs reflect pulmonary congestion, a sign of fluid-volume overload.**
   4. A urinary output of 120 mL in 3 hours indicates that the client is urinating 40 mL an hour. If the client has at least 30 mL of urine output an hour, then the kidneys are being perfused adequately.

   MEDICATION MEMORY JOGGER: If the client verbalizes a complaint, if the nurse assesses data, or if laboratory data indicates an adverse effect secondary to a medication, the nurse must intervene. The nurse must implement an independent intervention or notify the health-care provider because medications can result in serious or even life-threatening complications.

4. 1. **Septic shock is secondary to an infection of the blood and a broad-spectrum antibiotic (such as Rocephin) is prescribed until cultures and sensitivity results are obtained. The antibiotic that is specific to the bacteria causing the septic shock—in this case, vancomycin—should be administered as soon as possible.**
   2. There is no reason for the nurse to call the HCP and question this order.
   3. The nurse should not wait 10 hours to administer an antibiotic that will help save the client's life. Septic shock is life threatening and must be treated with the appropriate antibiotic as soon as possible.
   4. The client's white blood cell count does not affect the nurse's responsibility to administer the vancomycin antibiotic as soon as possible.

5. 1. Levophed must be tapered, but this is not the priority nursing intervention when administering this medication. Caring for the client is always priority.
   2. Administering medication on an infusion pump is important, but the priority intervention is caring for the client, not a machine.
   3. The nurse should check the client's renal status, but the priority nursing intervention is assessing the data for which the client is receiving the medication.
   4. **Norepinephrine is a powerful vasoconstrictor; therefore, continuous monitoring of the blood pressure is required to avoid hypertension.**

6. 1. This is the scientific rationale for administering vasodilators such as nitroglycerin (Tridil) or nitroprusside (Nipride), not colloid solutions.
   2. This is the scientific rationale for administering adrenergics (sympathomimetics) such as norepinephrine (Levophed), not colloid solutions.
   3. **This is the scientific rationale for administering a colloid solution. They are blood volume expanders that promote circulatory volume and tissue perfusion.**
   4. Crystalloid solutions, such as isotonic (normal saline 0.9%) or hypotonic (0.45% normal saline) solutions, increase fluid

volume in both the intravascular and the interstitial space.

7. 1. Shortness of breath, low back pain, and itching all over the body are signs of anaphylactic shock and epinephrine is the drug of choice to treat anaphylaxis, but it is not the first intervention.
  2. The client's assessment data indicates an anaphylactic reaction to the blood transfusion, which is life threatening. The nurse should take action and not assess the client.
  3. The nurse should keep an intravenous access so that normal saline and medication can be administered to help prevent anaphylactic shock, but this is not the first intervention when the client is experiencing anaphylactic shock.
  4. **Discontinuing the blood at the hub of the intravenous catheter is the first intervention because the client is exhibiting signs of an anaphylactic reaction, which can lead to anaphylactic shock if the allergen (blood) is not stopped immediately. Many different allergens can cause anaphylactic shock, including medications, blood administration, latex, foods, snake venom, and insect stings.**

MEDICATION MEMORY JOGGER: When answering test questions or when caring for clients at the bedside, the nurse should remember assessing the client may not be the first action to take when the client is in distress. The nurse may need to intervene directly to help the client.

8. 1. An infusion pump should be used when administering dobutamine because an overdose, which could occur if a drip via gravity is used, could cause death in the client. This action by the primary nurse would warrant immediate intervention by the charge nurse.
  2. A urometer is a plastic triangular container that can be attached to a Foley catheter and allows the nurse to obtain hourly urinary outputs. This action would not require intervention by the charge nurse.
  3. Monitoring the client's peripheral oxygen saturation would be appropriate for a client in cardiogenic shock; therefore, this action would not warrant intervention by the charge nurse.
  4. The nurse should always check the client for any types of allergies; therefore, this action would not warrant intervention by the nurse.

9. 1. The nurse should address the infiltrated site because of the toxic effects of the medication in the tissue. The blood pressure reading and apical pulse rate will not help the infiltrated site.
  2. This is not the appropriate action to take when dopamine infiltrates.
  3. **Extravasation of dopamine causes severe, localized vasoconstriction, resulting in a slough of the tissue and tissue necrosis if not reversed with the antidote phentolamine (Regitine) injections at the site of the infiltration.**
  4. The IV should be discontinued, but the nurse must take further action or the IV site may have tissue necrosis.

10. 1. This would be appropriate when injecting medications intramuscularly or subcutaneously, but dopamine can only be administered intravenously.
  2. **Sympathomimetics are incompatible with sodium bicarbonate or alkaline solutions.**
  3. **The client in hypovolemic shock is in critical condition, and a thorough assessment must be completed on the client frequently.**
  4. **This intervention is not specific for the dopamine administration, but a client in cardiogenic shock taking dopamine is in critical condition. An advance directive would be an appropriate intervention for this client.**
  5. Dopamine is not administered via Y-tubing. Blood and blood products are administered via Y-tubing.

A Community Facing Bioterrorism

11. 1. Chlorine is a gas, and, although the clothing may have some chlorine on it, decontamination procedures are not required.
  2. Chlorine is a gas, and, although the clothing may have some chlorine on it, the chlorine in the clothing should not pose a threat to the ED.
  3. Intravenous access is important, but not as important as supplying the clients with oxygen and ventilatory support.
  4. **Chlorine is a gas that when inhaled separates the alveoli from the capillary bed. Oxygenation and ventilatory support are the most important interventions.**

12. 1. The incubation period is about 12 days.
    2. The organism can survive on clothing and blankets in cool temperatures for at least 24 hours.
    3. **Smallpox spreads by direct contact with an infected person, by droplet contact, or by coming into contact with a contaminated item of bedding or clothing. During the French and Indian War (1756–1767), smallpox was used as a weapon when contaminated bedding was sent into Indian villages, resulting in a 50% casualty rate.**
    4. The rash begins on the face, mouth, pharynx, and forearms and then proceeds to the trunk and the rest of the body.

13. 1. Assessing is usually the first intervention, but in this case a delay of any kind in starting the antibiotics could result in death.
    2. **If antibiotics are initiated within 24 hours of the onset of symptoms of inhaled anthrax, death can be prevented. The nurse must keep in mind that the client will have had the symptoms for some hours before seeking medical attention.**
    3. Standard precaution procedures are all that are necessary. However, if the client dies, cremation should be the method of disposal of the body because the body can harbor the spores for decades and pose a threat to mortuary and medical examiner personnel.
    4. The client's blood pressure should remain stable unless sepsis overwhelms the client's body, in which case the treatment is antibiotics.

MEDICATION MEMORY JOGGER: The nurse must remember that if initiation of treatment can prevent a complication (death), then treatment has priority over assessment.

14. 1. Tularemia is extremely contagious and can be contracted by direct contact with infected animals or by breathing aerosolized tularemia bacteria used as a biologic weapon. The initial symptoms are a sudden onset of fever, fatigue, chills, headache, lower backache, malaise, rigor, coryza (profuse discharge from the mucous membranes of the nose), dry cough, sore throat without adenopathy, and nausea and vomiting.
    2. These are not symptoms of tularemia.
    3. These are not symptoms of tularemia.
    4. These are not symptoms of tularemia.

15. 1. Airborne precautions are used for clients suspected of having tuberculosis. Hospital staff must use 0.3-micron filtration masks when caring for these clients. This is not needed for clients diagnosed with botulism.
    2. **Clients diagnosed with botulism were infected by direct contact with the bacteria. It is not transmitted from human to human. Standard precautions are required for all clients.**
    3. Contact precautions are used to prevent contact with bacteria in wounds or infected gastrointestinal secretions. Botulism is not transmitted from human to human.
    4. Droplet precautions are used for respiratory illnesses where transmission can occur when in close contact with the client. Botulism is not transmitted from human to human.

16. 1. The client should wash the chemical off the body with a mild soap and water, not with normal saline.
    2. The client should wash the chemical off the body with a mild soap and water, not with milk products.
    3. **The client should wash the chemical off the body with a mild soap and water.**
    4. The client should wash the chemical off the body with a mild soap and water, not with diluted baking soda.

17. 1. Valium is the drug of choice for the potential convulsions that are associated with nerve-agent toxicity.
    2. Steroid medications would not be administered for excessive nerve stimulation.
    3. Charcoal is administered to prevent absorption of ingested poisons.
    4. Intravenous atropine 2–4 mg, followed by 2 mg every 3–8 minutes for 24 hours, is the drug of choice to reverse the toxic drug effects of malathion, a nerve agent. The ingredients in many pesticides bond with acetylcholinesterase so that acetylcholine cannot be removed from the body. The result is hyperstimulation of the nerve endings.

MEDICATION MEMORY JOGGER: Atropine is the medication administered for symptomatic bradycardia. This might lead the test taker to choose option "4" as the correct answer.

18. 1. The smell of bitter almonds is associated with cyanide gas, a deadly poison. The nurse should evacuate the area.
    2. The smell of bitter almonds is associated with cyanide gas, a deadly poison. The nurse should attempt to contain the gas to the area in question.
    3. The nurse would notify local authorities and the administration of the plant, not federal emergency personnel. Nurses must know and follow emergency procedures and guidelines.
    4. The administration of the plant or the local authorities are responsible for notifying the public. There are procedures designed to limit mass panic.
    5. The signs of cyanide poisoning include respiratory muscle failure, respiratory or cardiac failure, and death.

19. 1. Elevated blood pressure and bradycardia occur in the last phase of radiation sickness and death occurs soon after.
    2. Fluid and electrolyte imbalance and shock occur in the illness phase after 4 or more weeks.
    3. Decreased lymphocytes, leukocytes, and erythrocytes occur in the latent phase and can last for 3 weeks or more.
    4. Nausea, vomiting, diarrhea, and fatigue are the initial presenting symptoms of exposure to radiation and occur within 48–72 hours after exposure.

20. 1. This would not be done until it is determined that all the clients have botulism. Then it is the individual who has the responsibility of working with the public health department who will notify the agency, not the emergency department nurse.
    2. The clients' CBC results will not indicate if the clients have botulism.
    3. Severe abdominal cramping, nausea, vomiting, and diarrhea are the symptoms of botulism, but it has not been determined that this is the diagnosis in the triage area. Determining whether the clients ate in the same place recently is the first step in determining if the client has been exposed to botulism.
    4. The person with the responsibility for the facility should be notified whenever there is a potential situation where the press and the public will be arriving at the facility, but this is not the first intervention.

A Client Experiencing a Code

21. 1. Epinephrine is the first medication administered in a code because it constricts the periphery and shunts the blood to the trunk of the body.
    2. Lidocaine is administered in ventricular fibrillation, but it is not administered first in a code.
    3. Atropine is administered for asystole.
    4. Digoxin is administered for cardiac failure.

22. 1. Dopamine is administered to increase blood pressure.
    2. The ABGs indicate the client is in metabolic acidosis, and the drug of choice is sodium bicarbonate.
    3. Calcium gluconate is administered in clients experiencing hypocalcemia.
    4. Adenosine is the drug of choice for supraventricular tachycardia (SVT).

23. 1. The medication should be pushed as fast as possible in a code situation.
    2. Epinephrine is compatible with the primary intravenous line; therefore, there is no reason to flush the tubing before and after administering the medication.
    3. A client in a code does not have blood circulating in the vascular system. Elevating the client's arm will help the medication get into the central circulation.
    4. The epinephrine in the crash cart is diluted in 10 mL of normal saline in a bristojet and ready for administration; therefore, the nurse should not dilute the medication.

24.   45 mL.
       Drip rates are set per hour. A drip rate of 3 mg/min is 180 mg/hour.
       If 500 mL contains 2000 mg (2 grams) of lidocaine, then each milliliter contains 4 mg of lidocaine (2000 ÷ 500 = 4).
       To determine how many milliliters per hour is needed, divide 180 mg ÷ 4 = 45.
       The nurse should set the intravenous rate at 45 mL.

       MEDICATION MEMORY JOGGER: There is a way to remember this in an emergency situation: 1 mg (15 mL), 2 mg (30 mL), 3 mg (45 mL), 4 mg (60 mL). This is the rate if the medication is 2 g in 500 mL, which is how it comes, prepackaged.

25. 1. The client in asystole would not benefit from defibrillation because there is no heart activity. The client must have some heart activity (ventricular activity) for defibrillation to be successful.
    2. Synchronized cardioversion is used for new-onset atrial fibrillation or unstable ventricular tachycardia.
    3. **Atropine is the drug of choice for asystole because it decreases vagal stimulation and increases heart rate.**
    4. Amiodarone is administered in life-threatening ventricular dysrhythmias, not asystole.

26. 1. This medication increases blood pressure, and the blood pressure should be monitored every 15 minutes, not every 2 hours.
    2. The client's telemetry reading will not indicate the effectiveness of dopamine or identify complications secondary to the dopamine. Therefore, assessing the client's telemetry reading every hour is not a pertinent intervention for the dopamine administration.
    3. **The client's urine output must be assessed every 1 hour to determine the effectiveness of the dopamine administration because dopamine increases the blood pressure. If the client's blood pressure increases, then the urine output increases; if the client's blood pressure decreases, then the urine output decreases. The kidneys will retain water to help increase the blood pressure. The client should have at least 30 mL/hour.**
    4. The glucose level is not used when evaluating the effectiveness of dopamine, nor does it identify complications secondary to the dopamine. Therefore, this is not a pertinent intervention for dopamine administration.

27. 1. Dopamine is used to increase blood pressure.
    2. **Ventricular fibrillation is a very common dysrhythmia in a code situation, and lidocaine is the drug of choice because it suppresses ventricular ectopy.**
    3. Procainamide is an antidysrhythmic (Class 1A) medication that is used for ventricular and atrial dysrhythmias, but it is not the medication the nurse would prepare to administer for this specific dysrhythmia.
    4. This medication is only used for cardiac failure.

28. 1. **Dopamine is incompatible with all other intravenous fluids; therefore, the nurse must initiate another intravenous line to infuse the dopamine in a separate line.**
    2. Dopamine is incompatible with all other intravenous fluids; therefore, it cannot be piggybacked with lidocaine.
    3. The nurse does not need to question the order because the nurse can start another saline lock without talking to the healthcare provider.
    4. The dopamine drip does not have to be administered via a subclavian line as long as it is not piggybacked through any other medication.

29. 1. The ABGs do not indicate metabolic acidosis, so sodium bicarbonate should not be administered.
    2. **The PaO$_2$ is low (normal is 80–100); therefore, the nurse should administer oxygen via a nasal cannula. Oxygen is considered a medication.**
    3. The ABGs are not normal and intervention is needed.
    4. The client's ABGs reveal a low arterial oxygen level and do not need to be verified by a pulse oximeter reading.

30. 1. Amiodarone suppresses ventricular ectopy and is prescribed for life-threatening ventricular dysrhythmias unresponsive to less toxic agents. The nurse would not question this order.
    2. Lidocaine is the drug of choice for ventricular dysrhythmias because it suppresses ventricular ectopy. The nurse would not question this order.
    3. Defibrillation is the treatment of choice for a client in ventricular fibrillation.
    4. **Pacemakers are used for clients in symptomatic sinus bradycardia or asystole. This client is in ventricular fibrillation; therefore, the nurse would question this order.**

A Child Experiencing Poisoning

31. 1. **The child must receive supportive care to maintain life until the poison can be identified and further specific measures can be implemented.**
    2. **Treatment is facilitated by identifying the specific poison and the amount**

ingested. Then specific treatment can be instituted.

3. Limiting the amount of poison absorbed by the body can limit the damage.

4. Measures to eliminate the poison from the body prevent further absorption.

5. An antidote is administered to counter-act the effects of the poison.

32. 1. Charcoal does not change the pH of a substance.

2. **Charcoal binds with the poison to form an inert substance that can be elimi-nated through the bowel because the body is incapable of absorbing char-coal molecules. The charcoal must be administered within 60 minutes of ingesting the poison. The feces will be black.**

3. Charcoal can absorb the antidote. Char-coal should not be administered before, with, or immediately after the antidote.

4. Charcoal does not cause emesis. An emetic such as ipecac would induce vomiting.

33. 1. Gastric lavage would not be contraindi-cated for a 2-year-old child in a coma who ingested the contents of a bottle of Tylenol.

2. Gastric lavage would not be contraindi-cated for a 3-year-old child who ate a bottle of unknown tablets.

3. **Gastric lavage should not be attempted when there has been ingestion of caus-tic agents, convulsions are occurring, high-viscosity petroleum products have been ingested, cardiac dysrhythmias are present, or there is emesis of blood. Antidotes, supportive care, and preventing aspiration are implemented if gastric lavage is not to be performed.**

4. Gastric lavage would not be contraindi-cated for a 10 year old who took painkillers.

34. 1. **Ipecac stimulates vomiting, which can remove the medication from the stom-ach. It takes 20–30 minutes to work.**

2. Telemetry monitoring is not as important as preparing the parent for the child's response to the medication. It is hoped that the medication will be removed from the child's system before significant impact on the heart can occur.

3. The child is unstable, and the nurse cannot delegate a client who is unstable to unlicensed personnel.

4. The digoxin should not remain in the child's body long enough for this to become important.

35. 1. 0.5 L of GoLYTELY every hour is the dose for children younger than 6 years old.

2. 1.0 L GoLYTELY every hour is the dose for children 6–12 years old.

3. **1.5–2.0 L of GoLYTELY is the dose for clients 12 years old or older. Whole bowel irrigation is effective following ingestion of lead, lithium, iron, and sustained-release medications.**

4. This dosage is not recommended for any client.

36. 1. Material Safety Data safety information is required for every chemical in a health-care facility, but it is not an agency to contact regarding specific poisons and the antidotes.

2. **The National Poison Control Hotline (1-800-222-1222) is the equivalent of dialing 911 locally. The hotline can be dialed from anywhere in the United States, and they will connect the nurse with the local poison control agency.**

3. Child Protective Services (CPS) will not be able to help the nurse with information regarding the poison.

4. The police department will not be able to help the nurse with information regarding the poison.

MEDICATION MEMORY JOGGER: In an emergency situation, the client must be cared for first, and then other agencies such as Child Protective Services (CPS) or the police may be notified.

37. 1. Ipecac is not the preferred method for removal of a poison because it should not be given to clients experiencing convul-sions or who have a reduced level of consciousness or otherwise cannot protect their airway.

2. Gastric lavage is not the preferred method of removal of an ingested poison because of the potential for aspiration of stomach contents into the lungs.

3. Catharsis (administration of harsh stimu-lant laxatives) may help to remove the poison, but this method has not been shown to improve clinical outcomes.

4. **Activated charcoal and whole bowel irrigation are the preferred methods of removal of ingested poisons from the body. Activated charcoal binds with the poison and the body cannot absorb**

charcoal so the poison is eliminated in the feces.

38. 1. Calcium EDTA is administered IM or IV because it is poorly absorbed though the gastrointestinal tract.
    2. The drug and lead will be excreted though glomerular filtration. Therefore, kidney function is monitored, not liver function.
    3. **The drug and lead will be excreted through glomerular filtration; the nurse should ensure adequate renal function before administering the medication.**
    4. Calcium EDTA is not an emetic medication.

39. 1. **Narcan has a short half-life and could wear off before the effects of the narcotic cough syrup. The nurse should observe for signs of returning respiratory depression and be ready to intervene.**
    2. Negative pressure ventilators (the old iron lung) are not used anymore. Currently, positive pressure ventilation is preferred.
    3. The child would have an endotracheal tube placed first, not a tracheostomy, for a few days until it is determined if the child needs permanent ventilatory support because of brain damage.
    4. This is not the nurse's responsibility. The nurse would report the case to Child Protective Services (CPS), who could call the police if necessary.

40. 1. A pulse oximeter would give a falsely high reading because the blood is saturated with carbon monoxide.
    2. Arterial blood gases are not priority.
    3. **The client should receive high levels of oxygen. Carbon monoxide binds to the hemoglobin molecule with a greater affinity than oxygen. It is imperative to get oxygen to the client as quickly as possible.**
    4. The child should be prevented from chilling, but oxygen is the priority.

1. The mother of a 2-year-old child calls the emergency department and reports that the child has swallowed a bottle of prenatal vitamins. Which question is most important for the nurse to ask the mother?
   1. "How much does your daughter weigh?"
   2. "Is it prenatal vitamins with or without iron?"
   3. "Have you called the Poison Control Center?"
   4. "When did you purchase the prenatal vitamins?"

2. The client is admitted to the emergency department diagnosed with heatstroke. The client has a temperature of 104°F along with hot, dry skin. Which intervention should the nurse implement?
   1. Start an IV to infuse intravenous fluids.
   2. Administer the antipyretic acetaminophen (Tylenol).
   3. Encourage the client to drink cold water.
   4. Institute seizure precautions per hospital protocol.

3. The emergency department (ED) nurse is notifying the Poison Control Center concerning an accidental poisoning of a 4-year-old child. Which action by the ED nurse warrants intervention by the charge nurse?
   1. The ED nurse tells the center the type of poison ingested.
   2. The ED nurse tells the center the type and estimated time the poison was taken.
   3. The ED nurse informs the center of the client's vital signs.
   4. The ED nurse tells the center the age and weight of the child ingesting the poison.

4. Which document protects the nurse from liability as long as no grossly negligent care or willful misconduct is provided that deliberately harms a person outside the hospital?
   1. The American First Aid Association mission.
   2. The Board of Nurse Examiners First Aid section.
   3. The Good Samaritan Act.
   4. The Lay Rescuer Administration Act.

5. The nurse has just completed administering medication to a client with a cerebrovascular accident (CVA) via a gastrostomy tube. As the nurse is leaving the room, the client starts vomiting. Which action should the nurse implement?
   1. Ask the client if he or she can speak.
   2. Assist the client to sit on the side of the bed.
   3. Place the client in the side-lying position.
   4. Assess the client's bowel sounds.

6. The school nurse is caring for a 14-year-old student who stepped on a rusty nail that punctured the skin. Which interventions should the nurse implement? Rank in the order of performance.
   1. Cleanse the puncture site with soap and water.
   2. Put sterile, nonadhesive dressings on the wound.
   3. Apply an antibiotic ointment to the puncture site.
   4. Determine when the child last had a tetanus shot.
   5. Ask the student if he or she is allergic to any antibiotic.

7. The client with Type 2 diabetes is being discharged from the emergency room after sustaining a head injury. Which statement indicates the client needs more teaching prior to discharge from the emergency room?
   1. "I should not take my insulin if I am unable to eat."
   2. "I should take a couple of Tylenol if I have a headache."
   3. "If I become nauseated or start vomiting, I will call my doctor."
   4. "I will not take any type of sedative medications."

8. The client who has a history of peptic ulcer disease presents to the emergency department with a B/P of 86/42 and an apical pulse of 128. Which intervention should the nurse implement first?
    1. Administer dopamine, a sympathomimetic, by IV constant infusion.
    2. Request a stat CBC, Chem 7, and type and crossmatch.
    3. Prepare to administer intravenous Protonix, a proton-pump inhibitor.
    4. Initiate an IV with lactated Ringer's with an 18-gauge angiocath.

9. Which medication should the nurse administer first to the client experiencing cardiac arrest?
    1. Epinephrine, a sympathomimetic.
    2. Oxygen via Ambu bag.
    3. Lidocaine, an antidysrhythmic.
    4. Atropine, an antidysrhythmic.

10. The client presented to the emergency department (ED) with a rattlesnake bite on the left foot 2 hours ago. Which intervention should the nurse implement during the administration of the antivenin?
    1. Take the client's vital signs every 15 minutes.
    2. Administer diphenhydramine (Benadryl), an H_1 antagonist.
    3. Monitor the circumference of the left leg every 4 hours.
    4. Administer cimetidine (Tagamet), an H_2 histamine blocker.

11. The 22-year-old college student is admitted to the medical department with an overdose of sleeping pills. Which task can be delegated to an unlicensed nursing assistant (NA)?
    1. Ask the NA to assess the stool for color.
    2. Have the NA reset the rate on the IV pump.
    3. Instruct the NA to sit with the client.
    4. Evaluate the client's Glasgow Coma Scale.

12. The client with a chemical burn with lye is brought to the emergency department by the paramedics. Which action by the staff nurse would warrant immediate intervention by the charge nurse?
    1. The nurse is brushing the lye into a biohazard bag.
    2. The nurse wears personal protective equipment.
    3. The nurse starts an IV with a 20-gauge angiocath.
    4. The nurse is washing the lye off the client with water.

13. The client tells the triage nurse in the emergency department (ED) that she has food poisoning like the rest of the people who ate at a local restaurant. The client has been vomiting and has had diarrhea for the last 6 hours and needs help. Which medication should the nurse administer first?
    1. Diphenoxylate (Lomotil), an antidiarrheal.
    2. Ceftriaxone (Rocephin), an antibiotic, intravenous piggyback.
    3. Pantoprazole (Protonix), a proton-pump inhibitor.
    4. Diluted promethazine (Phenergan), an antiemetic, intravenous push.

14. The client who is being discharged from the emergency department (ED) after being raped is offered the medications mifepristone (RU-486), a birth control pill, and misoprostol (Cytotec), a prostaglandin. Which statement best describes the scientific rationale for administering these medications?
    1. These medications will help prevent the client from getting a sexually transmitted disease.
    2. These medications are known as the "morning after pills" and will prevent implantation of an ovum.
    3. These medications will help decrease the anxiety and nervousness of the client.
    4. These medications will promote the healing process of the vaginal tissues.

15. The client has an open fracture of the right forearm. Which interventions should the emergency department nurse implement? Select all that apply.
    1. Administer a prophylactic antibiotic.
    2. Apply a warm pack to the right forearm.
    3. Evaluate the effectiveness of the pain medication.
    4. Prepare to administer the preoperative medication on call.
    5. Explain the surgical procedure to the client and family.

16. The client with Type 1 diabetes is brought to the emergency department (ED) by the family. The client is belligerent, confused, and uncooperative. Which intervention should the nurse implement?
    1. Administer 1 amp of dextrose 50%.
    2. Give the client 2 cups of orange juice.
    3. Inject glucagon subcutaneously in the abdomen.
    4. Request a serum glucose level stat.

17. The HCP is preparing to suture a laceration on the client's right hand. Which question is most important for the nurse to ask the client?
    1. "Are you right- or left-handed?"
    2. "Do you have any allergies?"
    3. "How did you cut yourself?"
    4. "Are you afraid of needles?"

18. The elderly client diagnosed with chronic hypertension is brought to the emergency department by the caregiver. The client has a blood pressure of 198/120, and the nurse notes multiple contusions on the abdomen and forearms. Which question would be most important for the nurse to ask the client?
    1. "How did you get the bruises on your abdomen and forearm?"
    2. "Has anyone forced you to sign papers against your will?"
    3. "When was the last time you took your blood pressure medication?"
    4. "You seem frightened. Are you afraid of anyone in your home?"

19. The Homeland Security Office has issued a warning of suspected biological warfare using the *Francisella tularensis* (tularemia) bacteria. Which intervention should the charge nurse implement?
    1. Initiate the hospital's external emergency disaster plan.
    2. Instruct the staff to prepare the decontamination area.
    3. Prepare to administer the antitoxin intravenously.
    4. Check on the supply of oral doxycycline, an antibiotic.

20. The client with botulism poisoning is prescribed gentamycin, an aminoglycoside antibiotic. The medication is available in 250 mL of normal saline. At which rate should the nurse set the IV pump?
    Answer _____

1. 1. The weight of the child is pertinent information, but it is not the most important question.
   2. **If the prenatal vitamins have iron, this is a life-threatening situation. The child can hemorrhage because of the ulcerogenic effects of unbound iron, causing shock. As few as 10 tablets of ferrous sulfate (3 g) taken at one time can be fatal within 12 to 48 hours. This is the most important question to ask to determine what treatment the child should have for the accidental overdose.**
   3. Because the mother has called the emergency department, it is not priority to know if she called the Poison Control Center.
   4. Determining if the vitamins may have lost potency if they were purchased months ago is not as high a priority as determining if the prenatal vitamins have iron.

2. 1. **The first action the nurse should implement is to start an IV and infuse fluids, which will help rehydrate the client.**
   2. Antipyretic medication will not help decrease the temperature when the hyperpyrexia is secondary to a heatstroke.
   3. The client should be kept NPO to prevent vomiting and possible aspiration.
   4. Seizure precautions are not instituted for a client experiencing a heatstroke.

   MEDICATION MEMORY JOGGER: The stem of the question told the test taker that the situation is a "crisis." The first step in many crises is to make sure that an IV access is available to administer fluids and medications.

3. 1. The Poison Control Center needs to know the type of poison ingested; therefore, this would not warrant intervention by the charge nurse.
   2. The Poison Control Center needs to know the type and estimated time the poison was taken; therefore, this would not warrant intervention by the charge nurse.
   3. **The Poison Control Center does not need to know the client's vital signs; therefore, this would warrant intervention by the charge nurse. The center's responsibility is to inform the nurse of the antidote and treatment to decrease the possibility of life-threatening complications secondary to the poisoning.**
   4. The Poison Control Center needs to know the age and weight of the child to determine the severity of the poisoning; therefore, this would not warrant intervention by the charge nurse.

4. 1. There is no American First Aid Association.
   2. The Board of Nurse Examiners does not have a section addressing emergency care outside the hospital.
   3. **The Good Samaritan Act protects nurses and lay rescuers when they are caring for individuals outside the hospital. Nurses are held to a different standard because the nurse has received teaching on first aid.**
   4. There is no Lay Rescuer Administration Act.

5. 1. Asking the client if he or she can speak is the correct action if the client is choking, not vomiting.
   2. Because the client had a CVA, the client may not be able to sit on the side of the bed.
   3. **The client should be lying on the side to help prevent aspirating vomit contents into the lungs.**
   4. The client is vomiting; therefore, assessing the bowel sounds is not an appropriate nursing intervention.

   MEDICATION MEMORY JOGGER: When answering test questions or when caring for clients at the bedside, the nurse should remember that assessing the client may not be the first action to take when the client is in distress. The nurse may need to intervene directly to help the client.

6. **1, 5, 3, 2, 4**
   1. The nurse must cleanse the area with soap and water to remove any debris.
   5. The nurse should make sure the student is not allergic to any type of antibiotics before applying the ointment. Topical medication can cause allergic reactions.
   3. The nurse should then apply the antibiotic ointment to help prevent a wound infection.
   2. A dressing should be applied over the wound to help prevent infection.
   4. The nurse should then determine when the last tetanus shot was administered to determine if the student needs a booster.

7. 1. **Physiological stress, such as might occur after a head injury, increases the blood glucose level; therefore, the client must take insulin as prescribed but needs glucose (carbohydrates) to prevent**

hypoglycemia. Therefore, the client should drink the amount of carbohydrates in the prescribed ADA diet, which includes popsicles, regular Jell-O, or regular cola. This statement indicates the client needs more teaching prior to discharge.

2. The client can take acetaminophen (Tylenol) for a headache secondary to a head injury. The client does not need more teaching.

3. Nausea and vomiting are signs of increasing intracranial pressure, and the client should call the HCP. This statement indicates the client does not need more teaching.

4. The client should not take any type of sedatives, which may cause further neurological deficit. The client does not need more teaching prior to discharge.

8. 1. Dopamine is administered to increase the client's blood pressure, but the client must have an IV route. Because the client does not have an IV route, this is not the nurse's first intervention.

2. Laboratory tests are important, but not more important than preventing circulatory collapse, which is inevitable in a client in hypovolemic shock, as this client is.

3. Protonix is administered to decrease gastric acid production, but the client must have an IV route; therefore, this is not the first intervention.

4. **The client's vital signs indicate shock, and with the history of PUD, the nurse should suspect hypovolemic shock; however, no matter what type of shock, the nurse must first initiate intravenous therapy because of the low blood pressure and increased heart rate.**

9. 1. Epinephrine is the first medication administered intravenously or intratracheally, but oxygen should be administered when CPR is instituted.

2. **Oxygen is the first medication administered to all clients experiencing cardiac arrest. It will be administered through an Ambu bag via a face mask until the client is incubated.**

3. Lidocaine is the drug of choice for ventricular dysrhythmias, but the client must be monitored by telemetry to determine the specific rhythm.

4. Atropine is the drug of choice for asystole, but the client must be monitored by telemetry to determine the specific rhythm.

10. 1. **The client's vital signs must be monitored every 15 minutes throughout the 6-hour intravenous infusion because of the great potential for a life-threatening reaction to the antivenin.**

2. Benadryl must be administered prior to the initiation of the antivenin infusion to decrease the allergic response to the antivenin. This is an H_1 antihistamine.

3. The leg circumference should be measured every 30–60 minutes for 48 hours after the infusion.

4. Tagamet must be administered prior to the initiation of the antivenin infusion to decrease the allergic response to the antivenin. This is an H_2 antihistamine.

11. 1. The NA can assist the client to the bathroom, but the NA does not have the knowledge to determine if the stool color is normal for this client. If the client received charcoal, the stool should be black.

2. IV fluids are considered medications, and the nurse cannot delegate medication administration to an NA.

3. **An overdose of sleeping pills should be considered a suicide attempt until proved otherwise. The client should be on one-to-one suicide precautions. An NA could sit with the client.**

4. The Glasgow Coma Scale assesses the client's neurological status, and this cannot be delegated to an NA.

12. 1. Lye must be removed by brushing because water can initiate an explosion or deepening of the wound. Using a biohazard bag ensures the lye does not contaminate the environment. This action would not warrant intervention by the charge nurse.

2. Because lye is an alkaline substance and can causing burning of the skin or of the respiratory membranes if inhaled, the nurse should wear PPE. This action would not warrant intervention for the charge nurse.

3. For a burn secondary to lye, the client will be administered blood, which should be infused with an 18-gauge angiocath. The nurse starting the IV with a 20-gauge angiocath would not warrant immediate intervention from the nurse.

4. **Water should not be applied to burns from lye or white phosphorus because**

of the potential for an explosion or deepening of the wound. Lye should be brushed off the client.

13. 1. The client will not be able to tolerate oral medications until the nausea is controlled; therefore, Lomotil will be administered. The client needs to rid the body of the offending substance; therefore, diarrhea is not stopped.
    2. Antibiotics are not administered to clients with food poisoning.
    3. Medications administered to decrease gastric acid may or may not be given to the client, but it is not the first medication administered.
    4. Measures to control nausea and vomiting will prevent further fluid and electrolyte loss; therefore, an antiemetic is the first medication that should be administered.

14. 1. Mifepristone and misoprostol do not prevent STDs.
    2. Mifepristone and misoprostol will cause the client to abort any potential fetus. They must be taken within 3–5 days after the act of sexual intercourse.
    3. Antianxiety medications, not mifepristone and misoprostol, would be prescribed for anxiety and nervousness.
    4. Mifepristone and misoprostol do not promote wound healing.

15. 1. The client with an open fracture will be receiving antibiotics to prevent infection.
    2. The nurse should apply ice, not heat, to an acute injury.
    3. The client with a fracture will have pain; therefore, the nurse should evaluate the effectiveness of the medication given for pain.
    4. The client with an open fracture will have to go to surgery; therefore, preparing to administer the pre-op medication is an appropriate intervention.
    5. The HCP or surgeon is responsible for explaining the surgical procedure; this is not within the realm of the nurse's responsibility.

16. 1. Dextrose 50% is the drug of choice to treat hypoglycemia if the client is in a comatose state or not able to cooperate. This client exhibits signs of hypoglycemia.

2. The client who is uncooperative may refuse fluids or choke when being belligerent. If the client were cooperative, the family could have given the client juice.
3. Glucagon is provided in an emergency kit to be used by significant others at home to treat hypoglycemic reactions. It takes longer to elevate the client's glucose level and is dependent on the client's glycogen stores.
4. The nurse should always treat the client before obtaining laboratory tests.

17. 1. Determining if the client is right- or left-handed really does not matter because the sutures must be placed in the hand with the laceration.
    2. The nurse should determine the client's allergies. The HCP must inject the laceration with lidocaine prior to suturing; therefore, the nurse must determine if the client is allergic to lidocaine. The wound may be cleaned with Betadine (allergy to iodine) and the client may be prescribed antibiotics (allergy to antibiotic); therefore, the nurse must determine any allergies to these substances. In addition, a tetanus injection may be administered.
    3. The history of how the accident occurred is not the most important information.
    4. The statement could possibly initiate an anxiety reaction, and the nurse cannot do anything if the client is afraid of needles.

18. 1. This question is appropriate if the nurse suspects elder abuse, but the client's physiological status is priority at this time.
    2. This question is appropriate if the nurse suspects elder abuse, but the client's physiological status is priority at this time.
    3. The nurse should suspect elder abuse including unfilled medication prescriptions and other forms of neglect. This client's blood pressure is extremely high and could lead to a life-threatening condition if antihypertensive medications are not administered immediately. According to Maslow's Hierarchy of Needs, physiological needs are priority over potential other problems.
    4. This question is appropriate if the nurse suspects elder abuse, but the client's physiological status is priority at this time.

19. 1. This is a warning, not an actual event; therefore, the nurse should not initiate the disaster plan.

2. Tularemia is not contagious from human-to-human contact; it is acquired through direct contact with infected animals or by inhaling aerosolized bacteria. There is no decontamination for this.
3. Antitoxins are available for botulism but not for tularemia.
4. **For persons exposed to this biological bacterium, doxycycline is recommended** for 14 days. The nurse should ensure that a supply of doxycycline is available.

20. **250 mL.** The nurse must know that aminoglycoside antibiotics are very ototoxic and nephrotoxic and must be administered via an infusion pump over a minimum of 1 hour. The IV pump is regulated to infuse mL/hour.

Nonprescribed Medications

15

"The important thing is not to stop questioning. Curiosity has its own reason for existing."

—Albert Einstein

PRACTICE QUESTIONS

A Client Taking Herbs

1. The female client tells the perioperative nurse that she takes dong quai for menstrual cramps. Which action should the nurse implement first?
   1. Assess the client for any abnormal bleeding.
   2. Determine when the client took the last dose.
   3. Document the finding on the front of the client's chart.
   4. Notify the client's surgeon that the client takes this herb.

2. The client asks the nurse, "My grandmother puts aloe vera on her burns when she is cooking. Is that all right?" Which statement would be the nurse's best response?
   1. "Aloe vera juice is safe to use for minor burns but not for deep burns."
   2. "Aloe is approved by the U.S. Food and Drug Administration as a laxative."
   3. "Any type of herbal product or remedy has potential complications."
   4. "Aloe should not be used on any type of burns. Flush the burn with cool water."

3. The client tells the clinic nurse that she is taking St. John's wort for her depression. Which information should the nurse discuss with the client?
   1. Discuss the need to avoid tyramine-rich foods.
   2. Instruct to avoid touching eyes after taking the medication.
   3. Tell the client to apply sunscreen freely when outdoors.
   4. Explain that this medication often causes liver damage.

4. The client admitted to the medical floor for pneumonia tells the nurse that he is taking the herb ephedra. Which intervention should the nurse implement?
   1. Assess the client's blood pressure and pulse.
   2. Check the client's urine for ketones.
   3. Monitor the client for hyperpyrexia.
   4. Avoid giving the client products with caffeine.

5. The client taking valerian root, an herbal product, to decrease anxiety tells the nurse the medication has a pungent odor that smells like "dirty socks" and it makes her drowsy. Which action should the nurse take?
   1. Tell the client to quit taking the medication immediately.
   2. Warn the client that valerian root has addictive potential.
   3. Explain that odor is related to the dried plant and is normal.
   4. Determine if the client has discussed this with the HCP.

6. The nurse is presenting a lecture on herbs to a group in the community. Which guidelines should the nurse discuss with the group? Select all that apply.
   1. Do not take herbs if you are pregnant or attempting to get pregnant.
   2. Administer smaller amounts of herbs to babies and young children.
   3. Store the herbal remedy in a cool, dry, dark place.
   4. Advise against belief in unsubstantiated claims of "miracle cures."
   5. Think of herbs as medicines—more is not necessarily better.

7. The client with atherosclerosis asks the nurse, "I would really like to take herbs instead of medications for my atherosclerosis." Which statement is the nurse's best response?
   1. "You should not take any herbs to treat your atherosclerosis."
   2. "Garlic has been shown to decrease the 'stickiness' of platelets."
   3. "Horehound has sometimes been used to decrease atherosclerosis."
   4. "Taking a baby aspirin daily helps to decrease atherosclerosis."

8. The client is taking *Echinacea purpurea*. Which statement by the client would indicate to the nurse that the herb has been effective?
   1. "It has prevented me from getting diarrhea since I have been taking antibiotics."
   2. "Since I started taking echinacea I do not get nauseated in the morning anymore."
   3. "The fungal infection on my feet is getting better since I started taking echinacea."
   4. "This medication is the reason I have not had a cold the entire winter."

9. With which client would the nurse discuss taking hawthorn, an herb?
   1. The client diagnosed with congestive heart failure.
   2. The client diagnosed with hypertension.
   3. The client diagnosed with Alzheimer's disease.
   4. The client diagnosed with diabetes mellitus.

10. The male client is scheduled for an elective surgical procedure. While in the preoperative waiting area he tells the nurse he is taking ephedra, which he says really helps his asthma. Which action should the preoperative nurse implement?
    1. Document in the chart and take no further action.
    2. Notify the client's nurse anesthetist immediately.
    3. Request a stat electrocardiogram and chest x-ray.
    4. Determine how long the client has been taking the ephedra

A Client Taking Vitamins/Minerals

11. The client is taking vitamin A. Which assessment data would indicate to the nurse that the client is experiencing vitamin A toxicity?
    1. Nausea, vomiting, and diarrhea.
    2. Tingling and numbness of extremities.
    3. Dermatitis, fatigue, and dementia.
    4. Bleeding gums and gingivitis.

12. The client is prescribed folic acid, a vitamin. Which information should the nurse discuss with the client?
    1. Do not use any laxatives that contain mineral oil.
    2. Avoid drinking any type of alcoholic beverages.
    3. See the ophthalmologist periodically.
    4. Increase the intake of milk and milk products.

13. The client diagnosed with anemia is taking an iron tablet, a mineral, daily. Which statement indicates the client understands the medication teaching?
    1. "I will call my HCP if my stools become black or dark green."
    2. "I must take my iron tablet with meals and one glass of milk."
    3. "I will sit upright for 30 minutes after taking my iron tablet."
    4. "I will have to take an iron tablet for the rest of my life."

14. The mother of a newborn African American infant asks the nursery nurse, "Why did you give my baby a vitamin K injection?" Which statement is the nurse's best response?
    1. "It will help protect your child from getting sickle cell anemia."
    2. "Your baby's gut is sterile, and this will help the blood to clot."
    3. "This will help prevent your baby from becoming jaundiced."
    4. "Vitamin K will help your infant's ability to fight off infection."

15. The client diagnosed with pernicious anemia is prescribed cyanocobalamin (Cyanabin), vitamin B_{12}. Which intervention should the nurse implement?
    1. Administer the intramuscular injection via Z-track.
    2. Instruct the client to sip medication through a straw.
    3. Doublecheck the dose with another registered nurse.
    4. Monitor the client's serum potassium level.

16. The female client having her annual physical exam tells the clinic nurse, "I take vitamins daily but I have not had the money to buy any for the last week." Which response would be most appropriate for the nurse?
    1. "I will have the HCP give you a prescription for some vitamins."
    2. "As long as you eat a balanced diet you do not need to take vitamins."
    3. "Daily vitamins are necessary, so please get them as soon as possible."
    4. "This should not hurt you because vitamin deficiencies do not occur for some time."

17. The client asks the clinic nurse, "Vitamin E is a primary antioxidant. What does that mean?" Which statement is the nurse's best response?
    1. "Antioxidants minimize damage and keep your body's cells healthy."
    2. "Vitamin E is essential for general growth and development."
    3. "Antioxidants prevent the formation of free radicals in your muscles and skin."
    4. "The antioxidants are vitamins that help the blood clot."

18. The health-care provider has recommended the client take 100 mg of zinc a day. Which statement best supports the scientific rationale for taking zinc daily?
    1. Zinc is needed for the formation of connective tissue.
    2. Zinc is vital for hemoglobin regeneration in the client's body.
    3. Zinc is thought to help alleviate the common cold.
    4. Zinc aids in the absorption of iron and in the conversion of folic acid.

19. The nurse is discussing vitamins with a group of women at a community center. The nurse is discussing water-soluble vitamins and fat-soluble vitamins. Which vitamins are fat-soluble vitamins? Select all that apply.
    1. Vitamin A.
    2. Vitamin D.
    3. Vitamin E.
    4. Vitamin C.
    5. Folic acid.

20. The nurse is taking the male client's medication history. The client informs the nurse he takes megadoses of vitamin C daily, a daily aspirin, and an iron tablet. Which statement is the nurse's best response?
    1. "I am glad you take megadoses of vitamin C because it prevents the common cold."
    2. "Taking aspirin and megadoses of vitamin C may cause crystals in your urine."
    3. "Megadoses of vitamins and a balanced diet will help prevent you from getting sick."
    4. "You should take megavitamins—not just megadoses of vitamin C alone."

A Client Self-Prescribing Medications

21. The male client tells the clinic nurse that he has been taking the over-the-counter medication Prilosec for heartburn. Which statement would be the nurse's best response?
    1. "You should not take medications without notifying the HCP."
    2. "Have you also had breathing difficulties, especially at night?"
    3. "Be sure to limit taking the medication to less than 1 week."
    4. "OTC Tagamet is cheaper and works better than Prilosec."

22. The adolescent client has been admitted to the intensive care department for an overdose of acetaminophen (Tylenol). Which laboratory data should the nurse monitor for long-term complications from the attempt?
    1. The arterial blood gases.
    2. The liver function tests.
    3. The BUN and creatinine.
    4. The complete blood count.

23. The elderly female client has been diagnosed with compression fractures of the vertebrae and has been taking large doses of ibuprofen for pain. Which nursing intervention should the nurse implement?
    1. Teach the client not to take the medication on an empty stomach.
    2. Have the HCP order PTT/PT and INR laboratory tests.
    3. Ask the HCP to prescribe a narcotic medication for the client.
    4. Determine why the client thinks she needs so much medication.

24. The parent of a 1-year-old child calls the clinic to ask about medications that can be administered to reduce fever. Which medication should the nurse discuss with the parent?
    1. Acetylsalicylic acid (aspirin), an antipyretic.
    2. Diphenhydramine (Benadryl), an antihistamine.
    3. Docosanol (Abreva), an anti-infective.
    4. Docusate sodium (Colace), a gastrointestinal agent.

25. The female client diagnosed with essential hypertension tells the nurse that she has a cold and a runny nose. Which over-the-counter medication should the nurse tell the client to take?
    1. Tylenol Cold and Sinus.
    2. Advil Cold and Sinus.
    3. Nyquil.
    4. Coricidin HBP.

26. The client calls the clinic nurse to discuss problems concerning not being able to sleep at night. Which over-the-counter medications are taken to assist with sleep?
    1. Acetaminophen (Tylenol), an analgesic.
    2. Ibuprofen (Motrin), an NSAID.
    3. Diphenhydramine (Benadryl), an antihistamine.
    4. Zolpidem (Ambien), a sedative–hypnotic.

27. The HCP has instructed the 21-year-old female client diagnosed with allergies to take the over-the-counter medication pseudoephedrine (Sudafed). Which specific information should the nurse tell the client?
    1. An expected side effect is drowsiness, so plan for rest periods.
    2. Plan to use a second method of birth control while taking this medication.
    3. The medication will cause a developing fetus to become deformed.
    4. Take a driver's license to the pharmacy when purchasing this medication.

28. The female client tells the clinic nurse that she has frequent vaginal yeast infections and uses an over-the-counter preparation to cure the infections. Which is the nurse's first response?
    1. "How often do you use the over-the-counter yeast medications?"
    2. "You should tell the HCP about the frequent infections."
    3. "You should take lactic acidophilus when you take antibiotics."
    4. "Have you tried eating yogurt daily to prevent the infections?"

29. The teenaged client asks the nurse about over-the-counter birth control methods. Which intervention or medication should the nurse discuss with the client?
    1. The oral contraceptive medication Ortho Tri-Cyclen.
    2. There are no over-the-counter products that will prevent pregnancy.
    3. Tell her that spermicidal foams used with condoms are the most effective.
    4. Discuss the problems of sexual activity at a young age.

30. The male client diagnosed with cancer tells the oncology clinic nurse that an employee of a health food store suggested that he take 50,000 mg of vitamin C every day to treat the cancer. Which information is most important for the nurse to discuss with the client?
    1. Excessive amounts of water-soluble vitamins are excreted by the body.
    2. Too much acid could result in the client developing mouth ulcers.
    3. This is an alternative treatment to taking chemotherapy or radiation.
    4. The individual at the store wanted to sell the vitamins to the client.

A Client Taking Herbs

1. 1. Dong quai increases the risk of bleeding postoperatively, but the nurse would not need to assess for abnormal bleeding preoperatively.
   2. The American Society of Anesthesiologists recommends that all herbal products be stopped at least 2–3 weeks before surgery to avoid potential complications of herb use. The client should have been NPO since midnight; therefore, determining when the client last took the herb is the nurse's first intervention.
   3. The client's allergies, not the medication the client is currently taking, should be documented on the front of the chart.
   4. The nurse should first determine when she last took the herb before notifying the surgeon.

2. 1. Aloe vera juice is used externally for treatment of minor burns, insect bites, and sunburn. It is a safe herb to use externally and will not hurt the client.
   2. Aloe taken internally is a powerful laxative, but the client is asking about burns, not about using aloe as a laxative.
   3. This is a true statement about many herbal supplements, but topical aloe does not have any known complications that would prevent it from being used for minor burns.
   4. This is a false statement. Aloe can be used externally for treating minor burns. Many lotions have aloe as an ingredient.

3. 1. Users of St. John's wort do not need to avoid tyramine-rich foods. These types of foods should be avoided in clients taking MAO inhibitors for depression.
   2. This would be appropriate when applying capsicum or cayenne pepper lotion. St. John's wort is a pill or can be taken in tea form.
   3. St. John's wort can cause photosensitization dermatitis; therefore, the client should use sunscreen when outside.
   4. Many herbal supplements are hepatotoxic, but St. John's wort is not one that causes liver damage.

4. 1. Ephedra is an herbal stimulant that causes the cardiovascular system to potentially increase the blood pressure and heart rate. It has been implicated in many deaths and serious adverse effects, such as heart attacks and strokes. It may be removed from the U.S. market because of safety concerns. The nurse should assess the client's blood pressure and pulse.
   2. Ketones in the urine may be secondary to weight loss, which may occur when using ephedra, but that information is not included in the stem of the question.
   3. Ephedra does not cause hyperpyrexia, an extremely elevated temperature.
   4. This is an herbal stimulant, but there are no contraindications concerning caffeinated products.

5. 1. There is no reason to quit taking the medication because of the odor.
   2. There have been no reports of habituation or addiction with valerian root.
   3. The "dirty socks" odor is related to the dried plant. Valerian root is known as the "herbal Valium," and it has no hangover effect.
   4. The pungent odor and drowsiness are expected with this medication, and there is no reason to discuss this with the HCP.

6. 1. This is a guideline for prudent use of herbs.
   2. According to guidelines for prudent use of herbs, babies and young children should not be given any types of herbs.
   3. Herbs exposed to sunlight and heat may lose potency.
   4. This is a guideline for prudent use of herbs.
   5. This is a guideline that both consumers and health-care providers must be aware of when using herbal therapy.

7. 1. The nurse should not be judgmental when clients request information about herbal therapy.
   2. Garlic is one of the best-studied herbs. It has been shown to decrease the aggregation of platelets, thus producing an anticoagulant effect that is useful in treating atherosclerosis.
   3. Horehound has been used as an herbal remedy for the treatment of respiratory disorders, including asthma, bronchitis, whooping cough, and tuberculosis, but not atherosclerosis.
   4. This is a true statement, but aspirin is a medical treatment and is not considered an herb.

8. 1. *Lactobacillus acidophilus*, not *Echinacea purpurea*, is used to restore or to maintain the normal flora of the intestine during antibiotic therapy.

2. Ginger is one of the best-studied herbs and is used for treating nausea caused by motion sickness, pregnancy morning sickness, and postoperative procedures.
3. Goldenseal is an herb that when used topically is purported to be of value in treating bacterial and fungal skin infections and oral conditions such as gingivitis and thrush.
4. Some substances in *Echinacea* appear to have antiviral activity. Thus, the herb is sometimes taken to treat or prevent the common cold, a use for which it has received official approval in Germany.

MEDICATION MEMORY JOGGER: The nurse determines the effectiveness of a medication by assessing for the symptoms, or lack thereof, for which the medication was prescribed.

9. 1. Clients taking cardiac glycosides should avoid hawthorn because it has the ability to decrease cardiac output. The client with congestive heart failure would be taking cardiac glycosides.
2. Hawthorn has been purported to lower blood pressure after 4 weeks or longer of therapy; therefore, the nurse would not question the client with hypertension taking this medication.
3. Hawthorn is not recommended for a client diagnosed with Alzheimer's disease. *Ginkgo biloba* is the herb that is recommended for clients with Alzheimer's disease.
4. Hawthorn is not recommended for a client diagnosed with diabetes mellitus. Stevia, an herb indigenous to Paraguay, may be helpful to people with diabetes because it is used as a sweetener.

10. 1. Ephedra can interact with anesthetics; therefore, the nurse should take some action.
2. Ephedra can interact with anesthetics to cause dangerous elevations in blood pressure and heart rate that can lead to arrhythmias, stroke, myocardial infarction, and cardiac arrest. The nurse should notify the nurse anesthetist immediately to make sure he or she is aware of the client taking this herb.
3. These diagnostic tests may be needed prior to the client receiving anesthesia, but the preoperative nurse must notify the anesthetist about the client taking ephedra.

4. It doesn't make a difference if the client has taken ephedra for 1 day, 1 week, or 1 year; the nurse must notify the nurse anesthetist because ephedra use should be a reason to cancel an elective surgical procedure.

A Client Taking Vitamins/Minerals

11. 1. Signs and symptoms of vitamin A overdose include nausea, vomiting, anorexia, dry skin and lips, headache, and loss of hair. The nurse should instruct the client to quit taking the vitamin A immediately.
2. Paresthesia is not a sign of vitamin A toxicity. It may be a sign of thiamine deficiency, along with neuralgia and progressive loss of feeling and reflexes.
3. Dermatitis, fatigue, and dementia are symptoms of advanced niacin deficiency.
4. Bleeding gums and gingivitis are signs of vitamin C deficiency.

12. 1. This is appropriate information for the client who is taking vitamin A. Mineral oil inhibits the absorption of vitamin A.
2. The client should avoid drinking alcohol because it increases folic acid requirements.
3. This is appropriate information for the client who is taking vitamin A. Vitamin A may cause miosis, papilledema, and nystagmus.
4. Milk and milk products are a good source of vitamin D, not folic acid.

MEDICATION MEMORY JOGGER: Alcohol consumption is always discouraged when taking any prescribed or over-the-counter medication because of adverse interactions. The nurse should encourage the client not to drink alcoholic beverages.

13. 1. Iron turns the stool a harmless black or dark green. This statement indicates the client does not understand the medication teaching.
2. The iron tablet should be taken between meals and with 8 ounces of water to promote absorption. The iron tablet should not be taken within 1 hour of ingesting antacid, milk, ice creams, or other milk products such as pudding. This statement indicates the client does not understand the medication teaching.

3. Sitting upright will prevent esophageal corrosion from reflux. This statement indicates the client understands the medication teaching.

4. The drug treatment for anemia is generally less than 6 months. This statement indicates the client does not understand the medication teaching.

14. 1. Sickle cell anemia is a genetically inherited disease, and there is no medication that can prevent a child from getting this disease.

2. **This is the correct scientific rationale for administering vitamin K to newborn infants.**

3. Increasing fluid intake, phototherapy, and exposure to sun will help the infant who is jaundiced.

4. There is no medication that will prophylactically help a newborn fight off an infection.

15. 1. Intramuscular iron, not vitamin B_{12}, must be administered Z-track to prevent staining of the skin.

2. Cyanocobalamin does not stain the teeth and therefore does not need to be administered through a straw. Liquid iron must be administered through a straw.

3. This is required when administering insulin or digoxin intravenous push, but it is not required when administering this medication.

4. **Because conversion to normal blood cell production—the purpose of giving vitamin B_{12}— increases the need for potassium, hypokalemia is a possible side effect of this medication, especially during the first 48 hours medication is administered.**

16. 1. Vitamins are usually over-the-counter medications. If the client does have not money for OTC medications, she would not have money for a prescription.

2. A balanced diet can provide all the vitamins a client needs daily, but if the client was taking a daily vitamin, the nurse should not discourage her from taking the vitamins.

3. Vitamin supplements are not necessary if the person is healthy and receives proper nutrition on a regular basis.

4. **Signs or symptoms of vitamin deficiencies will not occur if the client has not taken the vitamins in more than a week. Vitamin deficiencies may take**
months to occur, and if the client is eating a well-balanced diet, vitamin deficiencies will not occur.

17. 1. Vitamin E is a primary antioxidant that prevents the formation of free radicals that damage cell membranes and cellular structure.

2. This is the role of vitamin A in the body. It is essential for general growth and development.

3. This statement has medical jargon that the client probably would not understand. The nurse needs to explain information in layman's terms.

4. Vitamin K, not the antioxidant vitamin E, is required by the body to help the blood clot.

18. 1. Copper is needed for the formation of red blood cells and connective tissue.

2. Iron is vital for hemoglobin regeneration. More than 60% of the iron in the body is found in hemoglobin.

3. **The use of zinc has greatly increased in the past few years; it is thought by some that zinc can alleviate the symptoms of the common cold.**

4. Vitamin C aids in the absorption of iron and in the conversion of folic acid.

19. 1. Vitamin A is a fat-soluble vitamin that is essential for the maintenance of epithelial tissues, skin, eyes, hair, and bone growth.

2. Vitamin D is a fat-soluble vitamin that has a major role in regulating calcium and phosphorus metabolism and is needed for calcium absorption from the intestines.

3. Vitamin E is a fat-soluble vitamin that has antioxidant properties that protect cellular components from being oxidized and red blood cells from hemolysis.

4. Vitamin C is a water-soluble vitamin that aids in the absorption of iron and conversion of folic acid.

5. Folic acid is a water-soluble vitamin that is essential for body growth; it is needed for DNA synthesis, and without folic acid there is a disruption in cellular division.

20. 1. Most authorities believe that vitamin C does not cure or prevent the common cold. Rather, it is believed that vitamin C has a placebo effect. This would not be appropriate information to share with the client.

2. Megadoses of vitamin C taken with aspirin or sulfonamides may cause crystalluria, crystal formation in the urine.

3. Megadoses of vitamins can cause toxicity and might result in a minimal desired effect.

4. The use of megavitamin therapy, massive doses of vitamins, is questionable at best. The nurse should not recommend this action.

A Client Self-Prescribing Medications

21. 1. Most adult clients self-medicate for minor problems, such as a headache or indigestion, and only seek medical attention if the symptoms are unrelieved. This is not the best response for the nurse to make.

2. **Up to 90% of adult-onset asthma is caused by gastroesophageal reflux disease (GERD). The nurse should assess what other symptoms are occurring.**

3. The medication is taken for up to 2 weeks per package instructions. Many clients have been prescribed Prilosec for many months to years.

4. The histamine$_2$ blockers (Tagamet, Zantac, Pepcid) may or may not be more effective than Prilosec. It depends on the individual's response to the medication. Most clients report better symptom control with the proton-pump inhibitors.

22. 1. The arterial blood gases would give information about the immediate situation, not long-term problems.

2. **Tylenol is toxic to the liver, and the liver function tests should be monitored in the hospital and in the HCP's office afterward to determine if there is permanent liver damage.**

3. BUN and creatinine tests determine kidney functioning. Tylenol does not affect the kidneys.

4. Tylenol does not damage the bone marrow. It is not necessary to monitor the CBC.

23. 1. **NSAIDs interfere with prostaglandin production in the stomach, resulting in the client being susceptible to ulcer formation. To prevent erosion of the stomach lining, the client should not**

take the medication on an empty stomach.

2. NSAIDs will not affect the PTT/PT/INR results.

3. If the NSAIDs are effective, there is no reason for the HCP to prescribe a narcotic.

4. The priority is to prevent complications from the medication; the client is taking the medication because fractures of the bones are painful.

24. 1. **The parent should be taught to never administer aspirin to a child because of the association of aspirin with Reye's syndrome. Tylenol or ibuprofen may be administered to a child for a fever.**

2. Benadryl will make the child drowsy and will help nasal congestion, but it will not treat a fever.

3. Abreva is a topical medication for cold sores, not for fever.

4. Colace is a stool softener, not an antipyretic.

25. 1. Tylenol Cold and Sinus contains ingredients that cause vasoconstriction. The client with hypertension should not take any medication that increases vasoconstriction.

2. Advil Cold and Sinus contains ingredients that cause vasoconstriction. The client with hypertension should not take any medication that increases vasoconstriction.

3. Nyquil contains ingredients that cause vasoconstriction. The client with hypertension should not take any medication that increases vasoconstriction.

4. **Coricidin HBP has been formulated to control symptoms of the cold or flu without causing vasoconstriction. This is the only medication in this list that will not increase the client's blood pressure.**

26. 1. Tylenol is an analgesic. It is not formulated with ingredients that induce sleep. Tylenol PM contains diphenhydramine. This medication can be taken to aid in sleep.

2. Ibuprofen is an analgesic and antipyretic, not a sleeping medication.

3. **Diphenhydramine is an antihistamine that has the side effect of causing drowsiness. This is the main ingredient in over-the-counter sleep aids.**

4. Ambien is not an over-the-counter medication.

27. 1. Pseudoephedrine can cause insomnia, not drowsiness. It is the ability to rev people up that makes it an ingredient of "uppers."
    2. Oral or topical contraceptive hormone products interact with antibiotics, not pseudoephedrine.
    3. This is a class C medication. Its use during pregnancy is questionable, but it is not known to be teratogenic.
    4. The federal government enacted a law limiting the purchase of products containing pseudoephedrine to adults and to no more than two products within a 24-hour time period. The client should be able to prove her age when purchasing the products at the pharmacy.

28. 1. This is an assessment question to determine the extent of the client's problem. This is the first question.
    2. The nurse should assess the problem before making this statement.
    3. This is a true statement, especially for clients diagnosed with chronic illness, but it is not the first statement.
    4. Eating yogurt daily will prevent most yeast infections when the client is taking prescribed antibiotics, but assessing the extent of the problem should be the nurse's first response.

    MEDICATION MEMORY JOGGER: Whenever the question asks for a "first" intervention, even when discussing medications, assessing is usually the correct answer.

29. 1. Ortho Tri-Cyclen is not an over-the-counter medication.
    2. There are several types of over-the-counter birth control methods.
    3. The client should be encouraged to use two forms of over-the-counter products to prevent pregnancy. The condom that is used should be compatible with the spermicidal product. Additionally, condoms provide some protection from acquiring a sexually transmitted disease.
    4. The client is not asking for the nurse's opinion on sexual behavior. The nurse should provide the information requested.

30. 1. This is true, but this is not the most important information to provide the client.
    2. Nutrition is an important consideration for clients diagnosed with cancer and undergoing treatment. Many of the antineoplastic medications can cause stomatitis, and a combination of huge amounts of vitamin C and chemotherapy could result in a serious complication for the client.
    3. There are many alternative treatments that should be encouraged for use by clients with different diseases; this is not one of them.
    4. This is true, but it is not the most important information for the nurse to teach the client.

1. The client diagnosed with anemia is taking an iron tablet. Which assessment data indicates the medication is effective?
   1. The client denies night blindness.
   2. The client has not had a cold this winter.
   3. The client's potassium level is 4.5 mEq/L.
   4. The client's hemoglobin is 12.

2. The 50-year-old female client tells the nurse that she has been having frequent episodes of suddenly feeling hot and flushed and asks the nurse if there is any medication that can help her symptoms. Which statement is the nurse's best response?
   1. "There is really nothing except time that helps these symptoms."
   2. "I would suggest taking a vitamin that has soy in it to help the problem."
   3. "The HCP can prescribe hormone replacement therapy for you."
   4. "Are you concerned about having symptoms of menopause?"

3. The nurse is discussing vitamins with a group of women at a community center. The nurse is discussing water-soluble vitamins and fat-soluble vitamins. Which vitamins are water-soluble vitamins? Select all that apply.
   1. Vitamin C.
   2. Vitamin D.
   3. Folic acid.
   4. Vitamin B_{12}.
   5. Vitamin K.

4. The 60-year-old client who is postmenopausal tells the nurse she is taking the herb chasteberry. Which data indicates the herb is effective?
   1. The client reports decreased pain with sexual intercourse.
   2. The client reports less bleeding and a more regular menstrual cycle.
   3. The client reports an increase in hot flashes and mood swings.
   4. The client reports less bloating and breast fullness.

5. The 27-year-old female client tells the nurse she is taking melatonin, a natural hormone, to help her sleep better at night. Which response is most appropriate by the nurse?
   1. "Melatonin has not shown any efficacy in helping people sleep."
   2. "Is there any chance you may be pregnant or trying to get pregnant?"
   3. "This natural hormone may help you to sleep better at night."
   4. "You should really take a prescription medication to help you sleep."

6. The client tells the nurse, "My grandmother gives me licorice tea to help my stomach ulcers. Is this bad for me?" Which response is most appropriate for the nurse?
   1. "Yes, it is bad for you because it increases gastric acid production."
   2. "Pure licorice root is the best type to take to help heal your ulcer."
   3. "The best thing for a stomach ulcer is an antacid such as Maalox."
   4. "No, it is not bad. It is one of the most effective herbs for stomach protection."

7. The nurse is teaching a class on herbal therapy to a community group. Which information should the nurse share with the group members?
   1. The dandelion herb can be used externally to help heal minor burns.
   2. Peppermint is an herb that exerts a protective effect on the liver.
   3. The herb cascara can be used as a laxative if the client is constipated.
   4. Witch hazel is an herb that is used as a long-term antidepressant.

8. The wife of a client with Alzheimer's disease is requesting information about any herbal therapy that may help with her husband's memory. Which herb should the nurse discuss with the client?
   1. St. John's wort.
   2. Ginkgo biloba.
   3. Psyllium.
   4. Sarsaparilla.

9. The client tells the nurse, "I take garlic every day because my parents did, but I am not sure what it does. Could you tell me?" Which response is most appropriate by the nurse?
   1. "Garlic helps prevent atherosclerosis and helps reduce your cholesterol level."
   2. "This herb has some anti-inflammatory effects and promotes wound healing."
   3. "You take garlic every day just because your parents took this herb every day."
   4. "Garlic is used to help prevent respiratory problems if people smoke cigarettes."

10. The nurse is discussing the importance of antioxidants in the body. Which vitamins and minerals help neutralize the free radical assault and keep the client's body cells healthy? Select all that apply.
    1. Vitamin C.
    2. Vitamin D.
    3. Vitamin E.
    4. Selenium.
    5. Copper.

11. The nurse is preparing to administer the following medications. Which medication would the nurse question administering?
    1. Cyanocobalamin (Cyanabin), vitamin B$_{12}$, to a client diagnosed with end-stage chronic obstructive pulmonary disease.
    2. Ferrous sulfate (Ferralyn), an iron supplement, to a client who is 22 weeks pregnant and is 2 days postoperative appendectomy.
    3. AquaMEPHYTON (vitamin K) to a client who has an International Normalized Ratio of 4.0.
    4. Calcium citrate (Citracal), a mineral, to a client who has a serum calcium level of 4.0 mEq/L.

12. The nurse is discussing nutritional supplements with a client recently diagnosed with cancer. Which supplement should the nurse recommend for the client at this time?
    1. Pulmocare, a supplement formulated for clients with lung diseases.
    2. Glucerna, a supplement formulated for clients with diabetes mellitus.
    3. Boost, a supplement formulated with added fiber.
    4. None. The client should try milkshakes and other foods first.

13. The male client tells the clinic nurse that he purchased over-the-counter Tylenol in Mexico for back pain that worked very well and now he has purchased Tylenol at the local drug store, but now the medication does not work. Which statement would be the nurse's best response?
    1. "Do you still have the container of the Tylenol you purchased in Mexico?"
    2. "The Food and Drug Administration makes the company halve the dose in the United States."
    3. "What makes you think there is a difference in the two bottles of medication?"
    4. "You are still having back pain. Would you like to talk about the pain?"

14. The client who is pregnant tells the clinic nurse that she has been using Preparation H (phenylephrine and cocoa butter), an over-the-counter medication, for hemorrhoids. Which information should the nurse teach the client?
    1. Apply the ointment after a bath but before drying the area.
    2. Do not use the medication because of possible harm to the fetus.
    3. Suppositories may be used up to four times a day for symptom relief.
    4. Tucks (witch hazel) work better than Preparation H for hemorrhoids.

15. The client is diagnosed with mild psoriasis of the scalp. Which shampoo should the nurse recommend to the client? Select all that apply.
    1. Head and Shoulders shampoo.
    2. T-Gel, a tar shampoo.
    3. Scalpicin, an anti-itch shampoo.
    4. Nizoral (ketoconazole), a psoriasis shampoo.
    5. A mild shampoo such as Suave.

16. The female client tells the clinic nurse that she has been having urinary frequency, lower abdominal cramping, and burning on urination. The client has been using an over-the-counter urinary antispasmodic but reports that the burning has not gone away. Which intervention should the nurse implement?
    1. Tell the client to continue taking the antispasmodic.
    2. Encourage the client to decrease the amount of fluid intake.
    3. Make an appointment for the client to see the HCP.
    4. Have the client start drinking cranberry juice daily.

17. Which medications and supplies can be purchased over the counter to treat diabetes mellitus? Select all that apply.
    1. Glargine (Lantus), a steady-state insulin.
    2. Humulin R (regular), a fast-acting insulin.
    3. Glucose tablets.
    4. Glucose monitoring strips.
    5. Humulin N, an intermediate-acting insulin.

18. The school nurse assesses lice and nits (lice eggs) in the hair of a child attending the elementary school. Which instructions should the nurse include when talking with the parent?
    1. Apply Nix (permethrin) topically to the scalp twice a day for 1 week.
    2. Ask the HCP for a prescription for a shampoo to treat the lice.
    3. It is fine to allow the child to continue attending class while being treated.
    4. Shampoo the hair with RID (pyrethrin with piperonyl butoxide) and comb the nits out.

19. Which over-the-counter medication would the nurse caution the use of for a client who is allergic to the numbing medication used in dental offices? Select all that apply.
    1. Benzocaine (Lanacane), a topical preparation for sunburns.
    2. Benzalkonium and lidocaine (Bactine), an antiseptic/pain reliever.
    3. Dibucaine (Nupercainal) for the pain, itching, and burning of hemorrhoids.
    4. Mineral oil, a lubricant laxative used as a preparation for a radiologic exam.
    5. Miconazole (Monistat) Vaginal Cream for a client with a yeast infection.

20. The client diagnosed with macular degeneration asks the nurse why the HCP would prescribe over-the-counter supplements of CoQ10 and flax seed oil. Which statement best describes the scientific rationale for the nurse's response?
    1. This is an unproven folk remedy that the HCP thinks might work.
    2. This is an antioxidant that will support arterial functioning.
    3. This is an omega-3 fatty acid that decreases the risk of heart attack.
    4. This combination of medications has been shown to cure eye problems.

1. 1. This would indicate that vitamin A therapy is effective.
   2. This would indicate zinc therapy is effective.
   3. The potassium level would not indicate that iron therapy was effective.
   4. **The effectiveness of iron therapy can be determined by a normal hemoglobin level and by the client denying fatigue or shortness of breath.**

   MEDICATION MEMORY JOGGER: The nurse determines the effectiveness of a medication by assessing for the symptoms, or lack thereof, for which the medication was prescribed.

2. 1. These symptoms and the client's age suggest that she is having "hot flashes" associated with menopause. There are over-the-counter preparations and hormone replacement that help the symptoms of menopause.
   2. **There are some natural estrogen enhancers such as soy that many women believe help the symptoms of menopause. Soy products come as milk or in some vitamins. This is the best response.**
   3. In some instances the HCP will prescribe HRT for a woman experiencing menopause, but this is rarely done now because current research indicates that, although HRT protects against osteoporosis and treats the symptoms of menopause, it also increases the risk of heart attack, stroke, and breast cancer.
   4. The client is asking for information, not expressing a need to discuss feelings.

3. 1. Vitamin C is a water-soluble vitamin that aids in the absorption of iron and conversion of folic acid.
   2. Vitamin D is a fat-soluble vitamin that has a major role in regulating calcium and phosphorus metabolism and is needed for calcium absorption from the intestines.
   3. Folic acid is a water-soluble vitamin that is essential for body growth. It is needed for DNA synthesis. Without folic acid, there is a disruption in cellular division.
   4. Vitamin B_{12} is a water-soluble vitamin that, like folic acid, is essential for DNA synthesis. It aids in the conversion of folic acid to its active form.
   5. Vitamin K is a fat-soluble vitamin that is needed for synthesis of prothrombin and clotting factors VII, IX, and X.

4. 1. **Chasteberry exerts effects similar to those of progesterone. When used during menopause and postmenopause, it may help reverse vaginal changes and diminished libido.**
   2. The client is postmenopausal; therefore, the client does not have regular menstrual cycles.
   3. The client would have a decrease in hot flashes and mood swings if the herb was helping decrease menopausal discomforts.
   4. This would indicate the herb was helping a client with premenstrual syndrome.

5. 1. Melatonin decreases alertness and decreases the body temperature, both of which make sleep more inviting. Therefore, this is a false statement.
   2. **Melatonin should not be taken by clients who are pregnant because there is a lack of studies that indicate its safety. Large doses of melatonin have been shown to inhibit ovulation, so women trying to conceive should reconsider taking melatonin. This is the most appropriate response for the nurse.**
   3. Melatonin does show efficacy for helping the client sleep, but because the client is 27 years old, the nurse's best response is to discuss pregnancy.
   4. Over-the-counter medications, herbs, and natural hormones have been proved to help clients sleep. Therefore, a prescription medication is not absolutely necessary.

   MEDICATION MEMORY JOGGER: The test taker should question administering any medication to a client who is pregnant or may become pregnant. Many medications cross the placental barrier and could affect the fetus.

6. 1. Licorice does not increase gastric acid production.
   2. Frequent use of pure licorice root can contribute to sodium and water retention, hypertension, and other ill effects; therefore, this is not the nurse's best response.
   3. The client is not asking what the best thing is for a stomach ulcer. The nurse's best response is to answer the client's question.
   4. **Licorice, a weak-tasting herb, contains substances that protect the lining of the stomach. It has been shown in several studies to help heal ulcers. It protects the stomach by increasing mucus production and blood flow through the membranes.**

7. 1. Dandelion, an herb, is used as a digestive aid, laxative, diuretic, and liver and gallbladder protectant, and it prevents iron-deficiency anemia. It is not used to heal minor burns.
   2. Peppermint helps soothe the stomach; it has a direct spasmolytic action on the smooth muscles of the digestive tract.
   3. Cascara is FDA approved as a laxative. It stimulates peristalsis.
   4. Witch hazel is FDA approved as an astringent, not as an antidepressant.

8. 1. St. John's wort is used for its antidepressant effects.
   2. *Ginkgo biloba* has been shown to improve mental functioning and stabilize Alzheimer's disease.
   3. Psyllium is FDA approved as a laxative.
   4. The herb sarsaparilla is best used as a flavoring agent in soft drinks.

9. 1. Garlic appears to provide some protection against atherosclerosis and stroke and may reduce blood cholesterol and blood pressure.
   2. The herb gotu kola has the ability to promote wound healing.
   3. This is a judgmental response, and the nurse should not be judgmental toward alternate therapy. Herbal treatment has shown efficacy.
   4. Eucalyptus has shown some efficacy in treating respiratory disorders.

10. 1. Antioxidants protect the body from damage caused by harmful molecules called free radicals; this damage is a factor in the development of atherosclerosis. Vitamin C captures the free radical and neutralizes it before it causes damage.
    2. Vitamin D is not an antioxidant. It is a fat-soluble vitamin that has a major role in regulating calcium and phosphorus metabolism and is needed for calcium absorption from the intestines.
    3. Vitamin E is a chain-breaking antioxidant. Whenever vitamin E is sitting on a cell membrane, it breaks the chain reaction before the free radicals cause damage.
    4. Selenium is an antioxidant that has shown efficacy in decreasing the risk for lung cancer, prostate cancer, and colorectal cancer.
    5. Copper is a mineral, but it is not an antioxidant. Copper is needed for the formation of red blood cells and connective tissue.

11. 1. Cyanocobalamin is contraindicated in clients with severe pulmonary disease and is used cautiously in clients with heart disease. Clients with these conditions may develop pulmonary edema and heart failure. The nurse should question administering this medication.
    2. Prenatal vitamins with iron are part of a pregnant woman's routine medications. Ferrous sulfate is pregnancy category A, which means it has been proved safe for the fetus. The nurse would not question administering this medication.
    3. The normal INR is 2–3; therefore, the nurse would not question administering this medication because it is the antidote for overdose of Coumadin.
    4. Hypocalcemia occurs when a serum calcium level falls below 4.5 mEq/L; therefore, the nurse would not question administering this medication to the client whose serum calcium level is low.

12. 1. Pulmocare is a supplement recommended for clients diagnosed with chronic lung disease because the supplement does not have as much carbon dioxide as a byproduct of its metabolism as do other supplements; however, the stem did not state the client had lung disease.
    2. Glucerna is the supplement recommended for clients who have diabetes because this supplement has a slower release of carbohydrates and provides more controllable blood glucose, but the stem did not state that the client has diabetes.
    3. Because of the added fiber Boost would be the supplement recommended for clients diagnosed with cancer who have significant pain and are taking narcotic pain medications, but this client is newly diagnosed and pain was not mentioned in the stem of the question.
    4. Newly diagnosed clients should try homemade supplements to support their diets. Supplements are expensive (ranging from $1.75 to more than $2.00 per can), and if the client develops an aversion to the taste, then it is unlikely that anyone else in the family will want to drink the supplement. The nurse should suggest the client try to make milkshakes and use canned soups to supplement the diet first.

13. 1. Many medications that are prescription in the United States are available over the counter in other countries. Antibiotics, narcotics, and steroids are some of the medications that can be purchased over the counter in Mexico. The nurse should investigate to determine if the Tylenol purchased in Mexico was Tylenol #2, #3, or #4. All of these medications have codeine in them.
    2. The Food and Drug Administration is responsible for the safety of medications in the United States, but the agency does not require the manufacturers of Tylenol to halve the dose of each pill.
    3. Pain is what the client says it is and pain relief is what the client says it is. This is not an appropriate question.
    4. This is a therapeutic response; the nurse should assess the situation and provide factual information.

14. 1. The ointment and suppositories should be used after the area is cleaned and patted dry.
    2. The medication will not harm the fetus.
    3. **The labeling directions for Preparation H state four times a day as the safe administration guidelines. The phenylephrine shrinks the size of the hemorrhoids and provides relief from the pain and burning, and the cocoa butter provides some emollient relief for expelling feces.**
    4. Tucks will provide relief from burning and itching but will not shrink the hemorrhoids. Tucks may initially sting when applied to the area.

15. 1. Head and Shoulders is a dandruff shampoo. It is not effective in controlling psoriasis.
    2. **T-Gel is a shampoo formulated with coal tar and is recommended for clients with mild psoriasis.**
    3. **Scalpicin has hydrocortisone and is marketed for mild psoriasis symptoms.**
    4. **Ketoconazole is an antifungal medication that has some efficacy for psoriasis.**
    5. Psoriasis is a painful skin problem accompanied by intense itching. A mild shampoo without some other ingredient will not be effective for this client.

MEDICATION MEMORY JOGGER: Nurses are frequently asked to provide information about over-the-counter medications

and preparations. The test taker could eliminate option "5" in the previous question because of the diagnosis of psoriasis.

16. 1. The over-the-counter antispasmodic is masking some of the client's symptoms. The nurse should recognize the symptoms of a urinary tract infection. The client should see the HCP and have a urine culture performed.
    2. The client should increase the amount of fluids when there is a suspicion of a urinary tract infection.
    3. **The client has symptoms of a urinary tract infection and should see the HCP for a urine culture and prescription for antibiotics.**
    4. Cranberry juice is helpful in preventing urinary tract infections (UTIs), but this client has the symptoms of already having a UTI.

17. 1. Lantus is not available over the counter. A prescription is required.
    2. **Humulin R, N, L, and U are all available over the counter, but they are usually kept behind the counter with the pharmacist. These insulins can be purchased without a prescription. In some states syringes may be purchased without a prescription. A prescription is only required if the client has insurance that is paying for part of the cost.**
    3. **Glucose tablets are recommended for clients to carry with them in case of a hypoglycemic reaction and may be purchased without a prescription.**
    4. **Glucose monitoring devices and strips may be purchased without a prescription. However, if the client has insurance that will pay for the equipment, a prescription is required.**
    5. **Humulin R, N, L, and U are all available over the counter. They are kept behind the counter with the pharmacist but can be purchased without a prescription. In some states syringes may be purchased without a prescription. A prescription is only required if the client has insurance that is paying for part of the cost.**

18. 1. Nix is applied once, and the clean hair is combed to get rid of the nits.
    2. Nix and RID are over-the-counter medications that treat lice.
    3. The child is not allowed to return to school until the nurse determines there are no more lice or nits.

4. This is the correct procedure for treating lice.

19. 1. The most common local anesthetic used in dental procedures is a "-caine" medication, Novocaine. Therefore, a client allergic to Novocaine could be allergic to benzocaine.
    2. The most common local anesthetic used in dental procedures is a "-caine" medication, lidocaine. Therefore, a client allergic to Novocaine could be allergic to lidocaine.
    3. The most common local anesthetic used in dental procedures is a "-caine" medication, dibucaine. Therefore, a client allergic to Novocaine could be allergic to dibucaine.
    4. Mineral oil is not a "-caine"; therefore, the nurse would not caution the client using this medication.
    5. Monistat vaginal cream is not a "-caine"; therefore, the nurse would not caution the client using this medication.

MEDICATION MEMORY JOGGER: If the test taker was not familiar with the local anesthetic Novocaine, the test taker could possibly still get this question correct by reading the ending of the generic names in the first three options.

20. 1. There is evidence that CoQ-10 in combination with fish oil (omega 3 fatty acid) or flax seed oil will reduce damage to blood vessels and may delay degeneration of the macula.
    2. CoQ–10 is a fat-soluble antioxidant found in almost every cell in the body. Flax seed oil (or omega 3 fatty acid) is taken in conjunction with CoQ–10 to help the body utilize the CoQ–10. Antioxidants are supportive of arterial health by decreasing fat deposits in the vessels.
    3. CoQ–10 is not an omega 3 fatty acid.
    4. There is no cure for macular degeneration. An injection has recently been approved by the Food and Drug Administration for use by some clients with macular degeneration. The medication is injected into the eye on a monthly basis.

Administration of Medications

16

"I'm not into working out. My philosophy: No pain, no pain."

—Carol Leifer

PRACTICE QUESTIONS

The Nurse Administering Medications

1. The nurse is teaching the client the correct use of a metered-dose inhaler. Which intervention should the nurse implement?
   1. Instruct the client to push the top of the medication canister while taking a deep breath.
   2. Explain the need to wait 30 seconds before taking a second dose of medication.
   3. Teach to monitor the respiratory rate for 1 full minute after taking medication.
   4. Tell the client to exhale the breath immediately after inhaling the medication.

2. The primary nurse is at the bedside and is preparing to administer 3 mL of medication into the deltoid muscle. Which action should the charge nurse take?
   1. Take no action because this is acceptable standard of practice.
   2. Ask the primary nurse to come to the nurse's station.
   3. Tell the nurse not to inject the medication into the deltoid muscle.
   4. Complete an occurrence report documenting the behavior.

3. The nurse is administering digoxin (Lanoxin) 0.25 mg intravenous push medication to the client. Which intervention should the nurse implement?
   1. Administer the medication undiluted in a 1-mL syringe.
   2. Insert the needle in the port closest to the client's IV site.
   3. Pinch off the intravenous tubing below the port.
   4. Inject the medication quickly and at a steady rate.

4. The nurse is adding a medication to an intravenous bag. Which action indicates the nurse needs more teaching in performing this procedure?
   1. The nurse clamps the roller clamp on the tubing attached to the IV solution.
   2. The nurse inserts the needle into the center of the medication port.
   3. The nurse avoids rotating the solution after administering the medication.
   4. The nurse writes the name and dose of the medication on the medication label.

5. Which intervention should the nurse implement when withdrawing medication from an ampule?
   1. Do not use if the ampule was opened more than 30 days ago.
   2. Ensure that all the medication is in the upper chamber of the ampule.
   3. Snap the neck of the ampule so that it opens toward the nurse.
   4. Insert the needle into the center of the opening of the ampule.

6. Which action by the primary nurse warrants intervention by the charge nurse?
   1. The charge nurse observes the primary nurse carrying a used needle to the medication room.
   2. The charge nurse observes the primary nurse using two methods to identify the client who is receiving medications.
   3. The charge nurse observes the primary nurse injecting air into a vial when preparing an intramuscular injection.
   4. The charge nurse observes the primary nurse documenting the removal of meperidine (Demerol) from the narcotic box.

7. The nurse is administering an unpleasant-tasting liquid medication to a 2-year-old child. Which intervention should the nurse implement?
   1. Prepare the medication in the child's favorite food.
   2. Tell the child the medication will not taste bad.
   3. Put the medication in 4 ounces of apple juice.
   4. Use a dropper to place the medication between the gum and cheek.

8. The nurse administers a medication to a client, and 30 minutes later the client tells the nurse that he/she is starting to itch. The nurse notes a red rash over the client's body. Which action should the nurse implement first?
   1. Have the crash cart brought to the room.
   2. Assess the client's apical pulse and blood pressure.
   3. Notify the health-care provider immediately.
   4. Prepare to administer diphenhydramine (Benadryl), an antihistamine.

9. The nurse is preparing to administer 15 mL of the antacid Maalox from a bottle to a client. Which intervention should the nurse implement?
   1. Determine the correct amount at the sides of the cup.
   2. Measure the medication at the base of the meniscus.
   3. Avoid shaking the bottle of Maalox.
   4. Draw the medication into a 20-mL syringe.

10. The nurse is preparing to administer 0.1 mL of medication intradermally to the client. How much medication would the nurse draw up in the tuberculin (1.0-mL) syringe?

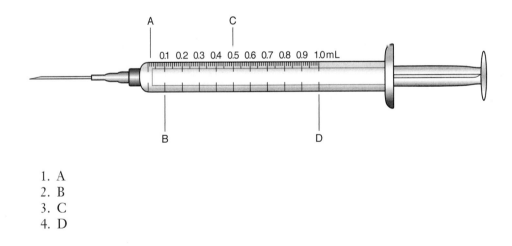

   1. A
   2. B
   3. C
   4. D

The Nurse Computing Math to Administer Medications

11. The client who has had abdominal surgery has an IV of Ringer's lactate infusing at 150 mL/hour. The nurse is hanging a new bag of fluid. The IV administration set delivers 10 gtts/mL. At what rate would the nurse set the infusion?

    Answer _____

12. The nurse is preparing to administer vancomycin, an aminoglycoside antibiotic, IVPB via an infusion pump. The IVPB is delivered in 250 mL of normal saline. At which rate should the nurse set the pump?

    Answer _____

13. The order is penicillin 2.0 millions units IM. The medication comes in a powder form of 5 million units per vial with directions to reconstitute with 3.2 mL of sterile diluent to produce 3.5 mL of solution. How many milliliters will the nurse administer?

    Answer _____

14. The order reads administer acetaminophen 15 mg/kg PRN every 6 hours to an infant weighing 33 pounds. How many milligrams of acetaminophen could the infant receive in a 24-hour time period?

    Answer _____

15. The client's MAR reads:

Client Name:	Account Number: 0 1234 56		Allergies: NKDA	
Date of Birth: 01 01	Weight: 165 lbs		Height: 70 inches	
Date	Medication	2301–0700	0701–1500	1501–2300
	Heparin 40,000 units in 500 mL D₅W infuse per protocol	2400 @ 15 mL/hour NN		
	For PTT Results : <50 increase rate by 4 mL/hour and redraw PTT in 4 hours			
	For PTT Results : <60 increase rate by 2 mL/hour and redraw PTT in 4 hours			
	For PTT Results : 60–90 maintain rate and redraw PTT in 4 hours × 2	0400 PTT 69 NN		
	For PTT Results : >90 decrease rate by 2 mL/hour and redraw PTT in 4 hours			
Sig: Night Nurse RN/NN	**Sig: Day Nurse RN/DN**			

   At 0800 the client's PTT result is 58. How many units per hour will the client receive for the next 6 hours?

    Answer _____

16. The client is receiving a heparin infusion at 24 mL/hour via an infusion pump. The medication comes 25,000 units in 500 mL of D₅W. How much heparin is the client receiving during a 12-hour shift?

    Answer _____

17. The client is to receive a preoperative medication of morphine 10 mg and Phenergan 25 mg IM on call to the operating room. The medication comes as morphine 15 mg/mL and Phenergan 25 mg/mL. How many milliliters of medication will the nurse administer?

    Answer _____

18. The nurse is preparing to administer an IVPB of 40 mEq of potassium in 200 mL of IV solution over 4 hours. At what rate would the nurse set the pump?

    Answer _____

19. The client is to receive 1.5 grams of a medication every morning. The medication comes 1000 mg per tablet. How many tablets would the nurse administer?

    Answer _____

20. The HCP has ordered 3 mcg/kg per minute of dopamine 2 G/500 mL of D_5W to be administered to a client in the intensive care unit. The client weighs 165 pounds. At which rate would the nurse set the IV pump in mL/hour?

    Answer _____

The Nurse Administering Medications

1. 1. This is the correct way to administer a metered-dose inhaler.
   2. The client should wait 2 minutes before taking a second dose of medication.
   3. The client should monitor the pulse rate, not the respiratory rate, because this medication causes tachycardia.
   4. The breath should be held as long as possible and then exhaled through pursed lips.

2. 1. This is not the acceptable standard of practice. The ventrogluteal muscle (on the side of the hip between the trochanter and ischium) is the injection site of choice because it is a large muscle mass that is free of major nerves and adipose tissue to ensure the medication goes in the muscle.
   2. **This is the correct action to take because the charge nurse should not correct the primary nurse in front of the client. The deltoid muscle (in the upper arm) should not be used to administer 3 mL of medication intramuscularly because the muscle is small and can only accommodate small doses of medications, no more than 1–2 mL of medication.**
   3. The charge nurse should not correct the primary nurse at the bedside in front of the client. This embarrasses the primary nurse and will make the client lose confidence in the primary nurse.
   4. An occurrence report should not be completed because the charge nurse stopped the action before the client received the injection in the incorrect muscle. The charge nurse would want to discuss the correct site for administering intramuscular medication with the primary nurse.

3. 1. The medication should be diluted with normal saline to increase the longevity of the vein for intravenous medication and fluids. Diluting decreases the client's pain secondary to the IV push. A 5-mL or 10-mL amount allows the nurse to inject the medication over a 5-minute time frame better than a 0.5-mL amount.
   2. **Using the closest port ensures the least resistance to the flow of medication into the client and helps to control the rate at which the medication reaches the client's bloodstream.**
   3. The nurse should pinch off the tubing above the port, not below, to ensure that the medication flows into the client's vein and not upward into the IV tubing.
   4. The medication should be injected slowly over 5 minutes (2 minutes for most IV medications) and at a steady rate because a rapid injection could cause speed shock. Speed shock is a sudden adverse physiological reaction secondary to an IVP medication where the client develops a flushed face, headache, a tight feeling in the chest, irregular pulse, loss of consciousness, and possible cardiac arrest.

4. 1. The roller clamp should be closed on the tubing to prevent fluid loss from the IV bag. The nurse does not need more teaching.
   2. The medication should be inserted into the center of the port to prevent accidental puncture of the sides of the port or the IV bag. The nurse does not need more teaching.
   3. **This indicates the nurse needs more teaching because the IV bag should be gently rotated to distribute the medication evenly throughout the IV solution.**
   4. The label must clearly identify what the nurse added to the IV solution. The nurse does not need more teaching.

5. 1. This is appropriate when withdrawing medication from a vial. An ampule is a one-time use container.
   2. All the medication should be in the lower chamber of the ampule; the nurse should tap the upper chamber to make sure all the medication is in the lower chamber.
   3. The ampule should be snapped away from the nurse so that any glass fragments are directed away from the nurse, not toward the nurse.
   4. **The nurse should not allow the needle to touch the rim of the ampule because the rim is considered contaminated. The correct procedure is to insert the needle in the center of the opening of the ampule.**

6. 1. **The primary nurse must discard the used needle in the sharps container in the client's room and, according to OSHA, cannot remove a used or "dirty" needle from the client's room. This action would require intervention from the charge nurse.**
   2. The Joint Commission mandates that the nurse use two forms of identification when administering medications to a client to ensure that the correct client is given the

prescribed medication. This action would not warrant intervention by the charge nurse.

3. Air should be injected into a vial to create a positive pressure inside the vial to ease the medication withdrawal and prevent a vacuum when withdrawing the medication. This action would not warrant intervention by the charge nurse.

4. Narcotics must be documented and accounted for when removed from the narcotics box or container. This action would not warrant intervention by the charge nurse.

7. 1. Do not use a favorite food or essential dietary item when administering a medication because the child may refuse the food in the future. The medication will cause the favorite food to taste bad or "funny."

2. The nurse should be honest with the child and the parent or guardian and tell the truth. Not telling the truth will damage the parent's trust in the nurse. Even if a 2-year-old does not understand, the child gagging or spitting out the medication indicates it is unpleasant tasting, and the parent will know the nurse lied about the medication.

3. The nurse should not use large volumes of fluid because if the child does not drink the entire amount, then the nurse cannot determine if the entire dose has been taken.

4. **This action promotes swallowing and prevents the medication from being aspirated or spit out.**

8. 1. The client appears to be having an anaphylactic reaction and bringing the crash cart to the bedside is an appropriate intervention, but it is not the first intervention.

2. The client is in distress, and taking the vital signs will not help an allergic reaction.

3. **The HCP should be notified so that the order for a medication to counteract the anaphylactic reaction can be obtained. Therefore, this is the first intervention.**

4. The nurse can prepare to administer the medication, but the HCP determines if in fact the client is having an allergic reaction and then orders the appropriate medication. Very few clients have a PRN order in place from the HCP for a possi-

ble allergic reaction, so this is not the first intervention.

9. 1. This is not the correct way to determine the prescribed amount when using a calibrated measuring cup.

2. **The liquid Maalox must be poured into a calibrated measuring cup and measured at the base of the meniscus to ensure the correct dose.**

3. The Maalox bottle must be shaken vigorously to ensure the medication is well-dispersed in the bottle.

4. A syringe is primarily used to give liquid medications to children to ensure accurate dosing. It is not used to administer antacids to an adult.

10. 1. If the nurse drew up this much medication, then the dose would be 10 times less than the prescribed dose.

2. **This is the correct amount of medication to administer to the client intradermally. This is the prescribed dose when administering a PPD intradermal injection to a client who is being tested for possible exposure to tuberculosis.**

3. This is five times the prescribed dose of medication.

4. If the nurse drew up this much medication, then the dose would be 10 times too much medication. This much medication intradermally would cause damage to the intradermal layer of the skin.

The Nurse Computing Math to Administer Medications

11.   **25 gtts/minutes**
The nurse should divide 150 mL/hour by 60 minutes to get 2.5 mL/minute.

Then multiply 2.5 mL/minute by 10 gtts/mL to get 25 gtts/minutes as the rate to set the infusion set.

12.   **250 mL/hour**
Vancomycin is administered over a minimum of 1 hour. Pumps deliver fluids at an hourly rate. The nurse should set the pump to deliver the 250 mL of fluid over 1 hour.

13.   **1.4 mL will be administered intramuscularly**
To set up this equation the nurse would write the equation:

5,000,000 units : 3.5 mL = 2,000,000 units : X mL

Cross-multiply to get:

7,000,000 = 5,000,000 X

To solve for X, divide both sides of the equation by 5,000,000

X = 1.4 mL

14. **900 mg/24-hour time period**
The nurse must first determine the infant's weight in kilograms. To do this, divide 33 pounds by 2.2 conversion factor = 15 kg of body weight.

Then multiply 15 kg times 15 mg per kg to equal 225 mg per dose.

The medication can be administered every 6 hours. The question asks how many milligrams could be administered within 24 hours. To find out the number of potential dosing times, divide 24 by 6, which equals 4.

Multiply 225 mg per dose times 4 doses to obtain 900 mg of Tylenol administered in a 24-hour time period.

15. **1360 units of heparin per hour**
The heparin mixture is 40,000 per 500 mL of fluid. The first step in solving this problem is to find out how many units of heparin are in each mL of fluid. Divide 40,000 by 500 = 80 units of heparin per milliliter of IV fluid.

The current rate is 15 mL per hour, but the client should have the IV infusion rate increased by 2 mL per hour per the protocol = 17 units per hour.

Multiply 80 units per mL times 17 = 1360 units of heparin per hour for the next 6 hours.

16. **14,400 units of heparin per 12-hour shift**
The first step in solving this problem is to find out how many units are in each milliliter of IV fluid. To do this divide 25,000 units by 500 mL of IV fluid = 50 units per milliliter of IV fluid.

The next step is to multiply the number of units per milliliter times the number of milliliters per hour the client is receiving: 15 × 24 = 1200 units of heparin infusing per hour.

Many math problems will ask for the number of units per hour. If this is the question, then 1200 units is the answer, but this question is asking the cumulative shift total of medication. Multiply 1200 times 12 = 14,400 units per 12-hour shift.

17. **1.67 mL**
To find out how many milliliters of morphine should be administered:

15 : 1 = 10 : X

Then cross-multiply:

10 = 15 X

To solve for X, divide both sides of the equation by 15

$$\frac{10}{15} = \frac{15\,X}{15}$$

10 divided by 15 = 0.666 or 0.67 mL of morphine

For Phenergan, the dose is 25 mg. Phenergan comes as 25 mg/mL, so 1 mL contains the dose prescribed.

Then add the two: 1 mL + 0.67 mL = 1.67 mL

18. **50 mL per hour**
The nurse would divide the amount of fluid—200 mL—by the number of hours—4— to infuse the medication. 200÷4 = 50 mL per hour. Pumps are always set at the rate per hour to infuse.

19. **1 1/2 tablets**
To set up this problem convert grams to milligrams. There are 1000 mg in 1 g, so 1.5 g equals 1500 mg.

The set up the problem:

1000 : 1 = 1500 : X

Then cross-multiply

1000 X = 1500

To solve for X divide each side of the equation by 1000

$$\frac{1000\,X}{1000} = \frac{1500}{1000}$$

X = 1.5

20. **3.4 mL per hour**
This is a multistep problem. The first step is to find out how many kg the client weighs. Divide 165 pounds by 2.2 conversion factor to equal 75 kg of body weight.

Then multiply 3 times 75 = 225 mcg/minute infusion rate.

Multiply 225 times 60 equals 13,500 mcg per hour to infuse. Pumps are set at an hourly rate in mL/hour.

Next convert the mg of medication to mcg: multiply 2 g times 1000 = 2000 mg, and then multiply 2000 times 1000 = 2,000,000 μg (or 2 g times 1,000,000)

$$13500 : X = 2{,}000{,}000 : 500$$

$$2{,}000{,}000\,X = 6{,}750{,}000$$

$$\frac{2{,}000{,}000\,X}{2{,}000{,}000} = \frac{6{,}750{,}000}{2{,}000{,}000}$$

3.375 or 3.4 mL per hour. Most pumps in an intensive care unit can be set in increments of tenths of a milliliter.

1. Which intervention should the nurse implement when administering sublingual medication?
   1. Place the medication between the gumline and the cheek.
   2. Assess the client's ability to swallow the medication.
   3. Instruct the client to allow the tablet to dissolve completely.
   4. Wear gloves when administering sublingual medication.

2. The nurse is preparing to administer medication via a nasogastric tube. Which intervention should the nurse implement first?
   1. Assess and verify tube placement.
   2. Check the residual volume.
   3. Elevate the foot of the client's bed.
   4. Pour medication into the syringe barrel.

3. Which interventions should the nurse implement when administering a tablet to the client? List in the specific order.
   1. Offer a glass of water to facilitate swallowing the medication.
   2. Assess that the client is alert and has the ability to swallow.
   3. Open the medication and place in the medication cup.
   4. Check the client's identification band and date of birth.
   5. Remain with the client until all medication is swallowed.

4. The charge nurse is making rounds on the clients and notices that the primary nurse left a medication cup with three tablets at the client's bedside. Which action should the charge nurse implement?
   1. Administer the client's medications.
   2. Remove the medication cup from the room.
   3. Request the primary nurse come to the room.
   4. Leave the cup at the bedside and talk to the primary nurse.

5. The nurse is preparing to administer a rectal suppository to a client. Which interventions should the nurse implement? Select all that apply.
   1. Insert the suppository beyond the anal–rectal ridge.
   2. Instruct the client to lie in the supine position.
   3. Lubricate the suppository with a water-soluble lubricant.
   4. Apply a sterile glove on the dominant hand.
   5. Encourage the client to retain the suppository for 30 minutes.

6. Which action indicates the nurse needs more teaching when administering a transdermal medication to a client?
   1. The nurse rotates the site when administering the transdermal patch.
   2. The nurse removes the previous transdermal patch and cleans the area.
   3. The nurse applies the transdermal patch using nonsterile gloves.
   4. The nurse applies the transdermal patch to a dry, hairy area.

7. The nurse is administering heparin via the subcutaneous route. Which intervention should the nurse implement?
   1. Prepare the medication using a 20-gauge, 1.5-inch needle.
   2. After injecting the needle, aspirate and observe for blood.
   3. After removing the needle, massage the area gently.
   4. Check previous injection sites and administer in another area.

8. Which intervention should the nurse implement when administering a medication via the intradermal route?
   1. Insert the needle with the bevel up at a 10-degree angle in the skin.
   2. Prepare the medication in a 3-mL syringe using a 23-gauge 1-inch needle.
   3. Bunch the skin between the thumb and index finger of the nondominant hand.
   4. Quickly inject the medication as to not form a wheal or bleb.

9. The nurse is administering ophthalmic drops to the client. Which intervention should the nurse implement?
   1. Firmly press the lacrimal duct for 5 minutes after instilling drops.
   2. Do not remove any discharge from the eye prior to instilling drops.
   3. Apply nonsterile gloves prior to administering ophthalmic drops.
   4. Administer the ophthalmic drops in the lower conjunctival sac.

10. The charge nurse is observing the primary nurse administering otic drops to a 2-year-old child by pulling down and back on the auricle. Which action should the charge nurse take?
    1. Stop the primary nurse and ask the nurse to step out of the room.
    2. Demonstrate inserting the otic drops by pulling up and back on the auricle.
    3. Take no action because this is the correct way to administer the eye drops.
    4. Allow the nurse to administer the otic drops and then discuss the technique with the nurse.

11. Which action indicates the nurse needs more teaching when administering nasal drops to the client?
    1. Instruct the client to blow the nose prior to administering the nasal drops.
    2. Have the client keep the head tilted back for 5 minutes after instilling drops.
    3. During the administration have the client tilt the head back and to the affected side.
    4. Place a sterile cotton ball into the nostril where the nasal spray was administered.

12. The nurse prepared 2 mg of morphine with 9 mL normal saline for a client who is complaining of pain. When the nurse enters the room the client tells the nurse, "I don't want to take a shot. I would like to have a pain pill." Which action should the nurse take?
    1. Explain that the medication must be administered because it has been drawn up.
    2. Ask another nurse to watch the medication being wasted into the sink.
    3. Place the syringe in the sharps container in the client's room.
    4. Notify the pharmacy that a narcotic was not administered to the client.

13. The nurse is preparing to administer the morning medications to a group of clients in a medical department. Which intervention should the nurse implement first?
    1. Compare the medication with the Medication Administration Record.
    2. Take the medication and the Medication Administration Record to the bedside.
    3. Check the client's identification band with the Medication Administration Record.
    4. Wash the hands with soap and warm water for at least 30 seconds.

14. The nurse is administering medications through a gastrostomy tube (GT). Which intervention should the nurse implement first?
    1. Place the crushed pills in the gastrostomy tube.
    2. Flush the gastrostomy with at least 30 mL of tap water.
    3. Use the plunger to push the medication into the GT.
    4. Clamp the gastrostomy tube closed.

15. The nurse is preparing to administer intravenous fluids to a 2-year-old child. Which intervention is most important for the nurse to implement?
    1. Use a volume-controlled chamber to administer the intravenous fluids.
    2. Ensure that the intravenous catheter is securely taped to the child's skin.
    3. Request that an adult hold the child's hand when hanging the IV fluid.
    4. Check the intravenous solution type with another nurse before administering.

16. The nurse is preparing to administer 3 mL of a medication intramuscularly. Which muscle is the best site to administer the medication?
    1. The deltoid muscle.
    2. The dorsogluteal muscle.
    3. The ventrogluteal muscle.
    4. The vastus lateralis muscle.

17. The client is prescribed vaginal cream. Which information should the nurse discuss with the client?
   1. Instruct the client to lie down for 10 to 15 minutes after inserting medication.
   2. Tell the client not to use a perineal pad after administering the medication.
   3. Teach the client not to insert the vaginal applicator very far into the vagina.
   4. Discuss the need to douche 30 minutes prior to inserting the vaginal cream.

18. The nurse is preparing to administer a liquid-form oral medication. Which intervention should the nurse implement?
   1. Place the lid of the bottle right side up so the outer surface is up.
   2. Do not shake the medication before pouring it into the medication cup.
   3. Hold the medication cup at chest level when reading the proper dose.
   4. Pour the liquid into the bottle with the label against the hand.

19. The nurse on a medical unit is providing discharge instructions to a client who is prescribed fluticasone (AeroBid), a glucocorticoid, and a metered-dose inhaler. Which statement by the client would warrant intervention?
   1. "I will use a spacer when using my inhaler."
   2. "I will hold the medication in my mouth for 10 seconds."
   3. "I will wait a few minutes between puffs."
   4. "I will notify my HCP if I get mouth sores."

20. The nurse is preparing to administer 14 units of regular insulin and 28 units of intermediate insulin. How much insulin would the nurse draw up on the insulin syringe?

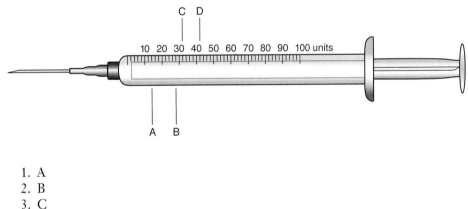

   1. A
   2. B
   3. C
   4. D

ADMINISTRATION OF MEDICATIONS
COMPREHENSIVE EXAMINATION ANSWERS AND RATIONALES

1. 1. The medication should be placed under the tongue, not between the gumline and the cheek (buccal).
   2. The medication should be placed under the tongue, not swallowed.
   3. Sublingual medication is placed under the tongue and should be kept there until the tablet is totally dissolved before swallowing the saliva.
   4. The nurse does not need to don gloves when administering this medication. It will not absorb into the nurse's skin.

2. 1. Assessment is the first intervention, and verifying that the tube is in the stomach is priority when administering medications via the nasogastric tube.
   2. If the residual is greater than 100 mL for an adult, the medication should not be administered because this indicates the client is not digesting the feedings.
   3. The head of the client's bed should be elevated to prevent aspiration. The foot of the bed should not be elevated.
   4. The medication should not be poured into the syringe until the placement of the tube is verified, the residual is checked, and the head of the bed is elevated.

3. 4, 2, 3, 1, 5
   4. The nurse must first check to make sure the right client is getting the right medication.
   2. The nurse should determine if the client can swallow the medication.
   3. The nurse should check the medication against the Medication Administration Record, open the medication package, and place it in the medication cup at the bedside. If the client cannot swallow or refuses the medication, the package can be sent back to the pharmacy if it has not been opened, preventing an unnecessary charge to the client.
   1. The nurse should offer water so that the client can swallow the medication.
   5. The nurse should remain with the client until the medication is swallowed.

4. 1. The charge nurse cannot administer these medications without verifying the medications against the Medication Administration Record.

2. The nurse should take the medication cup back to the medication room and discuss this situation with the primary nurse. Medications should never be left at the bedside.
3. The charge nurse should not correct the primary nurse in front of the client; therefore, this would not be an appropriate intervention.
4. The charge nurse should not leave the medications at the bedside. Medication should never be left at the bedside.

5. 1. Inserting the suppository beyond the anal–rectal ridge will ensure the suppository is retained.
   2. The client should lie on the left side (Sims' position).
   3. A water-soluble lubricant will ensure the suppository is inserted without trauma to the rectal area and will allow the suppository to dissolve.
   4. The nurse should wear nonsterile gloves on both hands, not just on the dominant hand.
   5. Thirty minutes will allow absorption of the medication.

6. 1. Rotating the sites prevents skin irritation. The nurse understands the correct way to apply a transdermal patch and does not need more teaching.
   2. The old patch must be removed and the area must be cleansed to prevent further medication absorption. The nurse does not need more teaching.
   3. The nurse should use nonsterile gloves to prevent absorption of the medication through the nurse's hands. The nurse does not need more teaching.
   4. The patch should be applied to a clean, dry, hairless area to ensure adherence and proper absorption of the medication. Because the nurse is applying the medication to a hairy area, the nurse needs more teaching.

7. 1. The nurse should prepare the medication using a 25-gauge, 3/8- to 5/8-inch needle.
   2. For heparin, do not aspirate for blood because this can damage surrounding tissue and cause bruising.
   3. Do not massage after injecting heparin because this may cause bruising or bleeding.

4. The nurse should not administer the heparin in the same site because this may cause tissue necrosis or other damage to the tissue.

8. 1. This is the correct way to administer an intradermal medication.
2. The medication should be administered in a tuberculin or 1-mL syringe using a 25–27-gauge, 3/8- to 5/8-inch needle.
3. The nurse should use the thumb and index finger of the nondominant hand to spread the skin taut, not bunch the skin.
4. The medication should be injected slowly to form a small wheal or bleb.

9. 1. The nurse should gently press on the lacrimal duct for 1–2 minutes to prevent systemic absorption through the lacrimal canal.
2. The nurse should remove any discharge by gently wiping out from the inner canthus, using a separate cloth for each eye.
3. The nurse should wash hands prior to administering eye drops, but the nurse does not need to wear gloves when administering ophthalmic drops.
4. Medication placed directly on the cornea can cause discomfort or damage, which is why the medication is placed in the lower conjunctival sac.

10. 1. The nurse is administering the eardrops correctly so there is no reason to stop the nurse from administering the eardrops.
2. This is the correct way to administer eardrops to an adult, but not to a young child.
3. The nurse should administer eardrops to a child younger than age 3 in this manner. This is done because of the short eustachian tube of a child. The charge nurse need take no action.
4. This is the correct way to administer the eardrops to a 2-year-old child. Therefore, the charge nurse does not need to discuss the administration technique with the primary nurse.

11. 1. The nurse should have the client blow the nose prior to instilling nasal drops to clear the nasal passage. Instructing the client to blow the nose indicates the nurse does not need more teaching.

2. This action allows the drops to have time to work effectively. The nurse does not need more teaching.
3. The client should tilt the head back for the drops to reach the frontal sinus and tilt the head to the affected side to reach the ethmoid sinus. This action indicates the nurse knows the correct administration of nasal drops and does not need more teaching.
4. Some nasal drops require the client to close one nostril and tilt the head to the closed side or to hold the breath or breathe through the nose for 1 minute. None of the nasal drops require a sterile cotton ball to be inserted into the nostril. The nurse needs more teaching.

12. 1. The client has the right to refuse medication; therefore; the nurse cannot force the client to take the medication.
2. This nurse must have a witness when wasting a narcotic.
3. Legally the nurse must have someone witness the narcotic being wasted.
4. The pharmacy does not need to be notified that a narcotic was wasted; it must be witnessed and documented on the narcotics log.

13. 1. The nurse must compare the medication with the MAR to make sure it is the right medication, but this is not the nurse's first intervention.
2. The nurse must take the MAR to the bedside with the medication to make sure the medication is being administered to the correct client, but this is not the nurse's first intervention.
3. The nurse must check the MAR with at least two forms of identification, one of which can be the client's identification band, but this is not the nurse's first intervention.
4. Washing the hands is essential to avoid contaminating the medication. Although it seems like an obvious step, it is often neglected by the nurse as a result of being busy and in a hurry.

14. 1. Only crushed or liquid medication should be administered through the GT tube, but this is not the first intervention the nurse should implement.

2. The nurse should first flush the GT with tap water to ensure that it is patent before putting any medication into the gastrostomy tube.

3. The medication can be administered via gravity or a plunger can be used, if needed, but this is not the nurse's first intervention.

4. After the medication is administered, the nurse should flush the GT with tap water to make sure all the medication is in the stomach and not in the tubing.

15. 1. A volume-controlled chamber (Buretrol) along with an intravenous administration pump should be used when administering intravenous fluids to children to ensure that the child does not experience fluid-volume overload. Fluid-volume overload in a child could cause death.

2. The IV catheter should be secured, but this is not the most important intervention because even if it is not secured the child would not experience fluid-volume overload, which is a potentially life-threatening complication of IV fluid therapy.

3. Having the mother or father at the bedside is an appropriate intervention because the child will be frightened, but it is not the most important intervention.

4. Double-checking a routine intravenous fluid is not necessary, but the nurse should double-check medication according to the child's weight.

16. 1. The deltoid muscle (in the upper arm) should not be used to administer 3 mL of medication intramuscularly because the muscle is small and can only accommodate small doses, no more than 1 to 2 mL, of medications.

2. The dorsogluteal (the buttocks) is not recommended for intramuscular injections because the sciatic nerve may be injured if the nurse fails to identify the proper landmarks to ensure missing it.

3. The ventrogluteal muscle on the side of the hip between the trochanter and ischium is the injection site of choice because it is a large muscle mass that is free of major nerves and adipose tissue to ensure the medication goes in the muscle.

4. The vastus lateralis muscle (lateral side of the thigh) can be used for administering intramuscular injections, but the client often complains that this is more painful than other areas.

17. 1. The client should lie down for 10 to 15 minutes so that all the medication can melt and coat the vaginal walls.

2. The client may need to use a perineal pad to catch any drainage or prevent staining of the undergarments.

3. The filled vaginal applicator should be inserted as far into the vaginal canal as possible, and then the client should push the plunger, depositing the medication in the vagina.

4. The client should not douche prior to administering vaginal cream because douching removes the normal flora of the vagina.

18. 1. The lid should be placed with the lid upside down so that the outer surface is down. This protects the inside of the lid from dirt or contamination.

2. Many liquids or medications in a solution must be shaken before they are poured. Make sure the lid is tightly closed before shaking.

3. The medication should be held at eye level when reading the proper dose. Often the medication in the cup is not level—it is higher on the sides than in the middle. Read the level at the lowest point in the medication cup.

4. Holding the medication label against the hand prevents the medicine from running down onto the label so that it cannot be read.

19. 1. The use of a spacing device increases the amount of medication reaching the lungs with less of the medication being deposited in the mouth and throat. This is the correct procedure, and the nurse would not have to correct the information.

2. The site of action for inhalers is the lungs. The client should not hold the medication in the mouth because this will increase the likelihood of the client developing a fungal infection of the mouth. The client should inhale deeply and hold the breath after the medication is in the lung. The nurse should correct this misinformation.

3. Pausing between puffs allows the lungs to absorb more of the medication. This is correct information.

4. Mouth sores may indicate a fungal mouth infection as a result of the medication and the HCP should be notified. This is correct information

20. 1. This point indicates the amount of regular insulin only—14 units.

2. This point indicates the amount of intermediate insulin only—28 units.

3. This point is 32 units, which is the incorrect dosage.

4. **The nurse would first draw up 14 units of regular-acting insulin and have** another RN check the dosage. Then the nurse should draw up 28 units of intermediate-acting insulin to total 42 units of insulin and verify the dosage with another RN. Drawing up regular insulin first ensures that the intermediate-acting insulin does not accidentally get inserted into the regular insulin, thereby altering the peak time of the regular insulin.

MEDICATION MEMORY JOGGER: Remember clear to cloudy when combining regular-acting and intermediate-acting insulin.

Comprehensive Examination

17

1. The client with cardiac disease is prescribed amiodarone (Cordarone), an antidys-rhythmic, orally. Which teaching intervention should the nurse implement?
   1. Notify the health-care provider of dyspnea, fatigue, and cough.
   2. Instruct the client to take the medication prior to going to bed.
   3. Tell the client not to take the medication if the apical pulse is less than 60.
   4. Explain that this medication may cause the stool to turn black.

2. The nurse is administering 0900 medications to the following clients. To which client would the nurse question administering the medication?
   1. The client receiving a calcium channel blocker who drank a full glass of water.
   2. The client receiving a beta blocker who has a blood pressure of 96/70.
   3. The client receiving a nitroglycerin patch who is complaining of a headache.
   4. The client receiving an antiplatelet medication who has a platelet count of 33,000.

3. The client with a head injury is ordered a CT scan of the head with contrast dye. Which intervention should the nurse include when discussing this procedure?
   1. Instruct the client to not take any of the routine medications.
   2. Inform the client an intravenous line will be started prior to the procedure.
   3. Ask about any allergies to nonsteroidal anti-inflammatory medication.
   4. Explain that the client will be given sedatives prior to the procedure.

4. The obstetric clinic nurse is discussing folic acid, a vitamin, with a client who is trying to conceive. Which information should the nurse discuss with the client when taking this medication?
   1. Do not use any laxatives containing mineral oil when taking folic acid.
   2. The client should drink one glass of red wine daily to potentiate the medication.
   3. This medication will help prevent spina bifida in the unborn child.
   4. Notify the health-care provider if the client's vision becomes blurry.

5. Which statement best describes the scientific rationale for prescribing the thiazo-lidinedione pioglitazone (Actos)?
   1. This medication increases glucose uptake in the skeletal muscles and adipose tissue.
   2. This medication allows the carbohydrates to pass slowly through the large intestine.
   3. This medication will decrease the hepatic production of glucose from stored glycogen.
   4. This medication stimulates the beta cells to release more insulin into the blood-stream.

6. The client is experiencing ventricular tachycardia and has a weak, thready apical pulse. Which medication should the nurse prepare to administer to the client?
   1. Epinephrine, an adrenergic agonist, intravenous push.
   2. Lidocaine, an antidysrhythmic, intravenous push.
   3. Atropine, an antidysrhythmic, intravenous push.
   4. Digoxin, a cardiac glycoside, intravenous push.

7. The client with major depressive disorder is prescribed the selective serotonin reuptake inhibitor (SSRI) fluoxetine (Prozac). Which intervention should the nurse teach the client concerning this medication?
   1. Instruct the client not to eat any type of tyramine-containing foods such as wines or cheeses.
   2. Notify the health-care provider if the client becomes anxious or has an elevated temperature.
   3. Encourage the client to take the medication with grapefruit juice.
   4. Explain that tremors and sweating are initial expected side effects.

8. The client who has had abdominal surgery has an IV of Ringer's lactate infusing at 100 mL/hour. The nurse is hanging a new bag of fluid. At which rate should the nurse set the pump to infuse the Ringer's lactate?

   Answer _____

9. The client admitted for an acute exacerbation of reactive airway disease is receiving intravenous aminophylline. The client's serum theophylline level is 18 μg/mL. Which action should the nurse implement first?
   1. Continue to monitor the aminophylline drip.
   2. Assess the client for nausea and restlessness.
   3. Discontinue the aminophylline drip.
   4. Notify the health-care provider immediately.

10. The nurse is administering 0800 medications. Which medication would the nurse question?
    1. Misoprostol (Cytotec), a prostaglandin analog, to a 29-year-old male with an NSAID-produced ulcer.
    2. Omeprazole (Prilosec), a proton-pump inhibitor, to a 68-year-old male with a duodenal ulcer.
    3. Furosemide (Lasix), a loop diuretic, to a 56-year-old male with a potassium level of 3.0 mEq/L.
    4. Acetaminophen (Tylenol), a nonnarcotic analgesic, to an 84 year old with a frontal headache.

11. The elderly client calls the clinic and is complaining of being constipated and having abdominal discomfort. Which interventions should the nurse implement? Select all that apply.
    1. Instruct the client to take an OTC laxative as recommended on the label.
    2. Recommend the client drink clear liquids only, such as tea or broth.
    3. Determine when the client last had a bowel movement.
    4. Tell the client to go to the emergency department as soon as possible.
    5. Ask the client what other medications are currently being taken.

12. The nurse is administering morning medications on a medical floor. Which medication should the nurse administer first?
    1. Regular insulin sliding scale to an elderly client diagnosed with Type 1 diabetes mellitus.
    2. Methylprednisolone, a glucocorticoid, to a client diagnosed with lupus erythematosus.
    3. Morphine, a narcotic analgesic, to a client diagnosed with Guillain-Barré syndrome.
    4. Etanercept, a biologic response modifier, to a client diagnosed with rheumatoid arthritis.

13. The nurse is caring for clients diagnosed with acquired immunodeficiency syndrome (AIDS). Which action by the unlicensed assistive personnel (UAP) warrants immediate action by the nurse?
    1. The UAP uses nonsterile gloves to empty a client's urinal.
    2. The UAP is helping a client take OTC herbs brought from home.
    3. The UAP provides a tube of moisture barrier cream to a client.
    4. The UAP fills a client's water pitcher with ice and water.

14. Which intervention should the nurse implement when administering the biologic response modifier filgrastim (Neupogen) subcutaneously?
    1. Shake the vial well prior to preparing the injection.
    2. Apply a warm washcloth after administering the medication.
    3. Discard any unused portion of the vial after withdrawing the correct dose.
    4. Keep the medication vials in the freezer until preparing to administer.

15. The elderly client diagnosed with coronary artery disease has been taking aspirin daily for more than a year. Which data would warrant notifying the health-care provider?
    1. The client has lost 5 pounds in the last month.
    2. The client has trouble hearing low tones.
    3. The client reports having a funny taste in the mouth.
    4. The client is complaining of bleeding gums.

16. The nurse is reviewing the laboratory data of a male client receiving chemotherapy. Based on the laboratory results, which action should the nurse implement?

Client Name	Account Number: 1 234 56	Date: Today
Laboratory Data	Client Values	Normal Values
WBC	7.4	4.5–11.0 (10^3)
RBC	2.0	M: 4.7–6.1 (10^6) F: 4.2–5.4 (10^6)
Hemoglobin	6.6	M: 13.5–17.5 g/dL F: 11.5–15.5 g/dL
Hematocrit	19.2	M: 40%–52% F: 36%–48%
MCV	83	81–96 μg/m^3
MCHC	31	33–36 g/dL
RDW	12	11%–14.5%
Reticulocyte	1.4	0.5%–1.5%
Platelets	110	150–400 (10^3)
Differential		
Neutrophils	40	40%–75% (2500–7500/mm^3)
Lymphocytes	50	20%–50% (1500–5500/mm^3)
Monocytes	2	1%–10% (100–800/mm^3)
Eosinophils	6	0%–6% (0–440/mm^3)
Basophils	2	0%–2% (0–200/mm^3)

1. Assess for an infection.
2. Assess for petechiae.
3. Assess for shortness of breath.
4. Assess for rubor.

17. The client experienced a full-thickness burn to 45% of the body including the chest area. The HCP ordered fluid resuscitation. Which data indicates the fluid resuscitation has been effective?
    1. The client's urine output is less than 30 mL/hour.
    2. The client's has a productive cough and clear lungs.
    3. The client's blood pressure is 110/70.
    4. The client's urine contains sediment.

18. Which statement best describes the scientific rationale for administering a miotic ophthalmic medication to a client diagnosed with glaucoma?
    1. It constricts the pupil, which causes the pupil to dilate in low light.
    2. It dilates the pupil to reduce the production of aqueous humor.
    3. It decreases production of aqueous humor but does not affect the eye.
    4. It is used as adjunctive therapy primarily to reduce intraocular pressure.

19. The charge nurse on an orthopedic unit is transcribing orders for a client diagnosed with back pain. Which HCP order should the charge nurse question?
    1. Morphine sulfate, a narcotic analgesic, Q 4 hours ATC.
    2. CBC and CMP (complete metabolic panel).
    3. Hydrocodone (Vicodin), an opioid analgesic, Q 4 hours PRN.
    4. Carisoprodol (Soma), a muscle relaxant, po, B.I.D.

20. The nurse is administering medications to clients on an orthopedic unit. Which medication should the nurse question?
    1. Ibuprofen (Motrin), an NSAID, to a client diagnosed with back pain.
    2. Morphine, an opioid analgesic, to a client with a "2" back pain on the pain scale.
    3. Methocarbamol (Robaxin), a muscle relaxant, to a client with chronic back pain.
    4. Propoxyphene (Darvon N), a narcotic, to a client with mild back pain.

21. Which is the scientific rationale for prescribing decongestants for a client with a cold?
    1. Decongestants vasoconstrict the blood vessels, reducing nasal inflammation.
    2. Decongestants decrease the immune system's response to a virus.
    3. Decongestants activate viral receptors in the body's immune system.
    4. Decongestants block the virus from binding to the epithelial cells of the nose.

22. The nurse is caring for clients on the telemetry unit. Which medication should the nurse administer first?
    1. The cardiotonic digoxin to the client diagnosed with CHF whose digoxin level is 1.9 mg/dL.
    2. The narcotic morphine IVP to the client who has pleuritic chest pain that is a "7" on a 1–10 pain scale.
    3. The sodium channel blocker lidocaine to the client exhibiting two unifocal PVCs per minute.
    4. The ACE inhibitor lisinopril (Vasotec) to the client diagnosed with HTN who has a B/P of 130/68.

23. The nurse is preparing to administer medications to the following clients. Which medication would the nurse question administering?
    1. The loop diuretic furosemide (Lasix) to the client with a serum potassium level of 4.2 mEq/L.
    2. The osmotic diuretic mannitol (Osmitrol) to the client with a serum osmolality of 280 mOsm/kg.
    3. The cardiac glycoside digoxin (Lanoxin) to the client with a digoxin level of 1.2 mg/dL.
    4. The anticonvulsant phenytoin (Dilantin) to the client with a Dilantin level of 24 µg/mL.

24. The nurse is administering digoxin (Lanoxin) 0.25 mg intravenous push medication to the client. Which intervention should the nurse implement?
    1. Administer the medication undiluted in a 1-mL syringe.
    2. Check the client's potassium level.
    3. Pinch off the intravenous tubing below the port.
    4. Inject the medication quickly and at a steady rate.

25. To which client would the nurse expect the health-care provider to prescribe chlordiazepoxide (Librium), a benzodiazepine?
    1. A client addicted to cocaine.
    2. A client addicted to heroin.
    3. A client addicted to amphetamines.
    4. A client addicted to alcohol.

26. The client is discussing wanting to quit smoking cigarettes with the clinic nurse. Which intervention is most successful in helping the client to quit smoking cigarettes?
    1. Encourage the client to attend a smoking cessation support group.
    2. Discuss tapering the number of cigarettes smoked daily.
    3. Instruct the client to use varenicline (Chantix), a smoking cessation medication.
    4. Explain that clonidine can be taken daily to help decrease withdrawal symptoms.

27. Each of the following clients has a head injury. To which client would the nurse question administering the osmotic diuretic mannitol (Osmitrol)?
    1. The 34-year-old client who is HIV positive.
    2. The 84-year-old client who has glaucoma.
    3. The 68-year-old client who has congestive heart failure.
    4. The 16-year-old client who has cystic fibrosis.

28. The nurse is administering 1.0 inch of Nitropaste, a coronary vasodilator. How much paste should the nurse apply to the application paper?

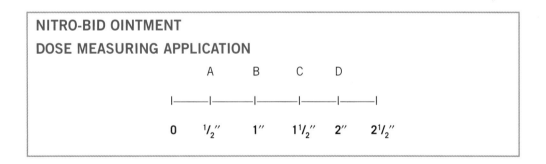

    1. A
    2. B
    3. C
    4. D

29. The client receiving telemetry is exhibiting supraventricular tachycardia. Which antidysrhythmic medication should the nurse administer?
    1. Lidocaine.
    2. Atropine.
    3. Adenosine.
    4. Epinephrine.

30. The client diagnosed with coronary artery disease is prescribed atorvastatin (Lipitor), an HMG-CoA reductase inhibitor. Which statement by the client indicates the medication is effective?
    1. "I really haven't changed my diet, but I am taking my medication every day."
    2. "I am feeling good since my doctor told me my cholesterol level came down."
    3. "I am swimming at the local pool about three times a week for 30 minutes."
    4. "Since I have been taking this medication the swelling in my legs is better."

31. The nurse is preparing to administer medications on a pulmonary unit. Which medication should the nurse administer first?
    1. Prednisone, a glucocorticoid, for a client diagnosed with chronic bronchitis.
    2. Ceftriaxone (Rocephin), an intravenous antibiotic, an initial dose (ID).
    3. Lactic acidophilus (Lactinex) to a client receiving IVPB antibiotics.
    4. Cephalexin (Keflex) po, an antibiotic, to a client being discharged.

32. The client diagnosed with chronic obstructive pulmonary disease is prescribed methylprednisolone (Solu-Medrol), a glucocorticoid, IVP. Which laboratory data would warrant immediate intervention by the nurse?
    1. The white blood cell (WBC) count is 15,000.
    2. The hemoglobin and hematocrit levels are 13 g/dL and 39%.
    3. The blood glucose level is 138 mg/dL.
    4. The creatinine level is 1.2 mg/dL.

33. The client's arterial blood gas results are pH 7.35, PaO_2 75, PCO_2 35, and HCO_3 24. Which action would be most appropriate for this client?
    1. Administer oxygen 10 L/min via nasal cannula.
    2. Administer an antianxiety medication.
    3. Administer 1 amp of sodium bicarbonate IVP.
    4. Administer 30 mL of an antacid.

34. Which data would indicate that the antibiotic therapy has been successful for a client diagnosed with a bacterial pneumonia?
    1. The client's hematocrit is 45%.
    2. The client is expectorating thick green sputum.
    3. The client's lung sounds are clear to auscultation.
    4. The client has complaints of pleuritic chest pain.

35. Which statement is the scientific rationale for administering an antacid to a client diagnosed with gastrointestinal reflux disease (GERD)?
    1. Antacids neutralize the gastric secretions
    2. Antacids block H_2 receptors on the parietal cells.
    3. Antacids inhibit the enzyme that generates gastric acid.
    4. Antacids form a protective barrier against acid and pepsin.

36. The client with a severe acute exacerbation of Crohn's disease is prescribed total parenteral nutrition (TPN). Which interventions should the nurse implement when administering TPN? Select all that apply.
    1. Monitor the client's glucose level daily.
    2. Administer the TPN via an intravenous pump.
    3. Assess the subclavian line insertion site.
    4. Check the TPN according to the five rights prior to administering.
    5. Encourage the client to eat all of the food offered at meals.

37. The client is prescribed a stool softener. Which statement best describes the scientific rationale for administering this medication?
    1. The medication acts by lubricating the stool and the colon mucosa.
    2. Stool softeners irritate the bowel to increase peristalsis.
    3. The medication causes more water and fat to be absorbed into the stool.
    4. Stool softeners absorb water, which adds size to the fecal mass.

38. The nurse is preparing to administer medications to the following clients. To which client would the nurse question administering the medication?
1. Lactulose (Cephulac), a laxative, to a client who has an ammonia level of 10 μg/dL.
2. Furosemide (Lasix), a loop diuretic, to a client who has a potassium level of 3.7 mEq/L.
3. Spironolactone (Aldactone), a potassium-sparing diuretic, to a client with a potassium level of 3.5 mEq/L.
4. Vasopressin (Pitressin) to a client with a serum sodium level of 137 mEq/L.

39. The nurse administered 25 units of Humulin N to a client with Type 1 diabetes at 0700. Which intervention should the nurse implement?
1. Assess the client for hypoglycemia around 1800.
2. Ensure the client eats the nighttime snack.
3. Check the client's serum blood glucose level.
4. Serve the client the lunch tray.

40. The nurse is administering Humalog, a fast-acting insulin, at 0730 to a client diagnosed with Type 1 diabetes. Which intervention should the nurse implement?
1. Ensure the client eats at least 90% of the lunch tray.
2. Do not administer unless the breakfast tray is in the client's room.
3. Check the client's blood glucose level 1 hour after receiving insulin.
4. Have 50% dextrose in water at the bedside for emergency use.

41. The client diagnosed with hypothyroidism is prescribed levothyroxine (Synthroid). Which assessment data would support that the client is taking too much medication?
1. The client has a 2-kg weight gain.
2. The client complains of being too cold.
3. The client's radial pulse rate is 110 bpm.
4. The client complains of being constipated.

42. The client diagnosed with chronic pancreatitis is complaining of steatorrhea. Which medication should the nurse prepare to administer?
1. Humalog, a fast-acting insulin, intravenously, then monitor glucose levels.
2. Pancrelipase (Cotazym) sprinkled on the client's food with meals.
3. Humulin R subcutaneously after assessing the blood glucose level.
4. Ranitidine (Zantac), a histamine$_2$ receptor blocker, orally.

43. The client in end-stage renal disease is receiving oral Kayexalate, a cation exchange resin. Which assessment data indicates the medication is not effective?
1. The client's serum potassium level is 5.8 mEq/L.
2. The client's serum sodium level is 135 mEq/L.
3. The client's serum potassium level is 4.2 mEq/L.
4. The client's serum sodium level is 147 mEq/L.

44. The nurse observes the unlicensed assistive personnel (UAP) performing nursing tasks. Which action by the UAP requires immediate intervention?
1. The UAP increases the rate of the saline irrigation for a client who had a transurethral resection of the prostate.
2. The UAP tells the nurse that a client who is on strict bed rest has green, funny-looking urine in the bedpan.
3. The UAP encourages the client to drink a glass of water after the nurse administered the oral antibiotic.
4. The UAP assists the client diagnosed with a urinary tract infection to the bedside commode every 2 hours.

45. The male client is diagnosed with herpes simplex 2 viral infection and is prescribed Valacyclovir (Valtrex). Which information should the nurse teach?
    1. The medication will dry the lesions within a day or two.
    2. Valtrex is taken once a day to control outbreaks.
    3. The use of condoms will increase the spread of the herpes.
    4. After the lesions are gone, the client will not transmit the virus.

46. The client who is 38 weeks pregnant and diagnosed with preeclampsia is admitted to the labor and delivery area. The HCP has prescribed intravenous magnesium sulfate, an anticonvulsant. Which data indicates the medication is not effective?
    1. The client's deep tendon reflexes are 4+.
    2. The client's blood pressure is 148/90.
    3. The client's deep tendon reflexes are 2 to 3+.
    4. The client's deep tendon reflexes are 0.

47. The client who is postmenopausal is prescribed alendronate (Fosamax), a bisphosphonate, to help prevent osteoporosis. Which information should the nurse discuss with the client?
    1. Chew the tablet thoroughly before swallowing.
    2. Eat a meal prior to taking the medication.
    3. Take the medication at night before going to sleep.
    4. Remain upright for 30 minutes after taking medication.

48. The client with low back pain syndrome is prescribed chlorzoxazone (Parafon Forte), a skeletal muscle relaxant. Which statement by the client would warrant intervention by the nurse?
    1. "I have not had the flu since I started the medication."
    2. "I am always drowsy after taking this medication."
    3. "I find driving my car difficult when I take my back pain medicine."
    4. "If I miss a dose I wait until the next dose time to take a pill."

49. The client is prescribed methotrexate (Rheumatrex), an antineoplastic agent, for psoriasis. Which intervention should the nurse teach the client?
    1. Teach the client that the urine may turn a red–orange color.
    2. Have the client drink Ensure to increase nutritional status.
    3. Tell the client to notify the HCP if a fever develops.
    4. Encourage the client to increase green, leafy vegetables in the diet.

50. With which client would the nurse use caution when applying mafenide acetate (Sulfamylon), a topical antimicrobial agent, to a burned area?
    1. A client with a creatinine level of 2.8 mg/dL.
    2. A client with congestive heart failure.
    3. A client with a pulse oximeter reading of 95%.
    4. A client with diabetes Type 2 taking insulin.

51. The long term care nurse is administering botulinum toxin Type A (Botox), an antispasmodic, to a client diagnosed with a brain attack. Which statement best describes the scientific rationale for administering this medication?
    1. This medication is administered for the cosmetic effect to reduce wrinkles.
    2. This medication reduces muscle spasticity associated with strokes.
    3. This medication will improve the client's residual limb strength.
    4. This medication will decrease the pain associated with neuropathy.

52. The client has second- and third-degree burns to 40% of the body. The HCP writes an order for 8000 mL of fluid to be infused over the next 24 hours. The order reads that half of the total amount should be administered in the first 8 hours with the other half being infused over the remaining 16 hours. At what rate would the nurse set the intravenous pump for the first 8 hours?
    Answer _____

53. The client has a severe anaphylactic reaction to insect bites. Which priority discharge intervention should the nurse discuss with the client?
    1. Wear an insect repellent on exposed skin.
    2. Keep prescribed antihistamines on their person.
    3. Keep an EpiPen in the refrigerator at all times.
    4. Wear a MedicAlert identification bracelet.

54. Which statement is the scientific rationale for prescribing the regimen known as highly active antiretroviral therapy (HAART) to clients diagnosed with HIV infection?
    1. HAART will cure clients diagnosed with HIV infection.
    2. HAART poses less risk of toxicity than other regimens.
    3. HAART can decrease HIV to undetectable levels.
    4. HAART is less costly than other medication regimens.

55. The client with rheumatoid arthritis is prescribed hydroxychloroquine sulfate (Plaquenil), a disease-modifying antirheumatic drug (DMARD). Which statement indicates the client understands the medication teaching?
    1. "I will get my eyes checked yearly."
    2. "I can only have two beers a week."
    3. "It is important to take this medication with milk."
    4. "I will call my HCP if the pain is not relieved in 2 weeks."

56. The nurse is preparing to administer morning medications on an oncology floor. Which medication should the nurse administer first?
    1. An analgesic to a female client with a headache of "3" on the pain scale.
    2. An anxiolytic to a female client who thinks she might get anxious.
    3. A mucosal barrier agent to a male client who has peptic ulcer disease.
    4. A biologic response modifier to a male client with low red blood cell counts.

57. The client calls the nursing station and requests pain medication. When the nurse enters the room with the narcotic medication, the nurse finds the client laughing and talking with visitors. Which action should the nurse implement first?
    1. Administer the client's prescribed pain medication.
    2. Assess the client's perception of pain on a 1–10 scale.
    3. Wait until the visitors leave to administer any medication.
    4. Check the MAR to see if there is a nonnarcotic medication ordered.

58. The nurse administered a narcotic pain medication 30 minutes ago to a client diagnosed with cancer. Which data indicates the medication was effective?
    1. The client keeps his or her eyes closed and the drapes drawn.
    2. The client uses guided imagery to help with pain control.
    3. The client is snoring lightly when the nurse enters the room.
    4. The client is lying as still as possible in the bed.

59. The client has received chemotherapy 2 days a week every 3 weeks for the last 8 months. The client's current lab values are Hgb and Hct 10.3 and 31, WBC 2000, neutrophils 50, and platelets 189,000. Based on the laboratory results which information should the nurse teach the client?
    1. Avoid individuals with colds or other infections.
    2. Maintain nutritional status with supplements.
    3. Plan for periods of rest to prevent fatigue.
    4. Use a soft-bristled toothbrush and electric razor.

60. The nurse is preparing to administer lithium (Eskalith), an antimania medication, to a client diagnosed with bipolar disorder. The lithium level is 3.5 mEq/L. Which action should the nurse implement first?
    1. Administer the medication.
    2. Hold the medication.
    3. Notify the health-care provider.
    4. Verify the lithium level.

61. The 8-year-old child newly diagnosed with attention deficit–hyperactivity disorder (ADHD) is prescribed methylphenidate (Ritalin), a central nervous stimulant. Which statement by the mother indicates the medication teaching is effective?
    1. "I will keep the medication in a safe place."
    2. "I will give my child this medication every 12 hours."
    3. "It may cause my child to have growth spurts."
    4. "My child will probably experience insomnia."

62. The client diagnosed with bilateral conjunctivitis is prescribed antibiotic ophthalmic ointment. Which medication teaching should the nurse discuss with the client? Select all that apply.
    1. Apply a thin line of ointment evenly along the inner edge of the lower lid margin.
    2. Press the nasolacrimal duct after applying the antibiotic ointment.
    3. Don nonsterile gloves prior to administering the medication.
    4. Apply antibiotic ointment from the outer canthus to the inner canthus.
    5. Instruct the client to sit with the head slightly tilted back or lie supine.

63. The nurse has administered an ophthalmic medication to the client. To which area should the nurse hold pressure to prevent systemic absorption?

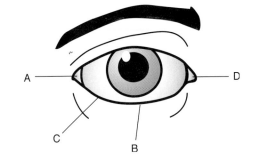

    1. A
    2. B
    3. C
    4. D

64. The client in hypovolemic shock is receiving normal saline by rapid intravenous infusion. Which assessment data would warrant immediate intervention by the nurse?
    1. The client's blood pressure is 89/48.
    2. The client's pulse oximeter reading is 95%.
    3. The client's lung sounds are clear bilaterally.
    4. The client's urine output is 120 mL in 3 hours.

65. The client who is coding is in asystole. Which action should the nurse implement first?
    1. Prepare to defibrillate the client at 360 joules.
    2. Prepare for synchronized cardioversion.
    3. Prepare to administer atropine, intravenous push.
    4. Prepare to administer amiodarone, an antidysrhythmic.

66. Which statement best describes the scientific rationale for administering acetylcysteine (Mucomyst), an antidote, to a child who was brought to the emergency room?
    1. Mucomyst neutralizes toxic substances by changing the pH of the poison.
    2. Mucomyst binds with bleach, and it is excreted through the bowel.
    3. Mucomyst is the antidote for acute acetaminophen (Tylenol) poisoning.
    4. Mucomyst induces vomiting, and the client eliminates much of the narcotics.

67. The mother of a 2-year-old child calls the emergency department and reports that the child drank some dishwashing detergent. Which question is most important for the nurse to ask the mother?
    1. "How much does your child weigh?"
    2. "Is your child complaining of a stomachache?"
    3. "Have you called the Poison Control Center?"
    4. "Where did you keep the dishwashing soap?"

68. The client admitted to the medical floor for pneumonia informs the nurse of taking an aspirin every day. Which intervention should the nurse implement?
    1. Assess the client's blood pressure and pulse.
    2. Check the client's urine for ketones.
    3. Monitor for an elevated temperature.
    4. Document the information in the chart.

69. The client diagnosed with anemia is taking an iron tablet, a mineral, daily. Which statement indicates the client needs more medication teaching?
    1. "I will not call my HCP if my stools become black or dark green."
    2. "I must take my iron tablet with meals and one glass of milk."
    3. "I will sit upright for 30 minutes after taking my iron tablet."
    4. "I will have to take an iron tablet for about 6 months."

70. Which statement best explains the scientific rationale for a client taking antioxidants?
    1. Antioxidants will increase the availability of oxygen to the heart muscle.
    2. Antioxidants will help prevent platelet aggregation in the arteries.
    3. Antioxidants decrease the buildup of atherosclerotic plaque in the arteries.
    4. Antioxidants decrease the oxygen demands of the peripheral tissues.

71. The nurse is presenting a lecture on herbs to a group in the community. Which guideline should the nurse discuss with the group?
    1. Administer smaller amounts of herbs to babies and young children.
    2. Store the herbal remedy in a sunny, warm, moist area.
    3. Encourage clients to use herbs as an alternative to other medications.
    4. Consumers need to think of herbs as medicines; more is not necessarily better.

72. Which intervention should the nurse implement first when administering a tablet to the client?
    1. Offer a glass of water to facilitate swallowing the medication.
    2. Assess that the client is alert and has the ability to swallow.
    3. Open the medication and place it in the medication cup.
    4. Remain with the client until all medication is swallowed.

73. The unlicensed assistive personnel (UAP) is making rounds on the clients and notices that the primary nurse left a medication cup with three tablets at the client's bedside. Which action should the UAP implement?
    1. Administer the client's medications.
    2. Remove the medication cup from the room.
    3. Request the primary nurse come to the room.
    4. Leave the cup at the bedside and do nothing.

74. The nurse is administering heparin via the subcutaneous route. Which intervention should the nurse implement?
    1. Prepare the medication using a 25-gauge, $1/_2$-inch needle.
    2. After injecting the needle, aspirate and observe for blood.
    3. After removing the needle, massage the area gently.
    4. Administer the medication in the client's "love handles."

75. The nurse is administering therapeutic heparin, an anticoagulant, for a client diagnosed with deep vein thrombosis. Which laboratory value should the nurse monitor?
    1. International Normalized Ratio (INR).
    2. Prothrombin time (PT).
    3. Partial thromboplastin time (PTT).
    4. Platelet count.

76. Which discharge instruction should the emergency department (ED) nurse discuss with the client who sustained a concussion and is being discharged home?
    1. Instruct the client to not take any acetaminophen (Tylenol) for at least 48 hours.
    2. Tell the client to stay on a clear liquid diet for the next 24 hours.
    3. Instruct the client to take one hydrocodone (Vicodin) if experiencing a headache.
    4. Tell the client to return to the ED if experiencing nausea and vomiting.

77. The nurse is preparing to administer the following anticonvulsant medications. Which medication would the nurse question administering?
    1. Carbamazepine (Tegretol) to the client who has a Tegretol serum level of 22 μg/mL.
    2. Clonazepam (Klonopin) to the client who has a Klonopin serum level of 60 ng/mL.
    3. Phenytoin (Dilantin) to the client who has a Dilantin serum level of 19 μg/mL.
    4. Ethosuximide (Zarontin) to the client who has a Zarontin serum level of 45 μg/mL.

78. Which information should the nurse teach the client and family of a client prescribed donepezil (Aricept), a cholinesterase inhibitor?
    1. Aricept may delay the progression of Alzheimer's for 6 months to a year.
    2. Aricept will repair the brain damage in clients with Alzheimer's.
    3. Aricept is still experimental as far as how it works to treat Alzheimer's.
    4. Aricept is difficult for clients to tolerate because of the many side effects.

79. Which statement is the scientific rationale for prescribing dexamethasone (Decadron), a glucocorticoid, to a client diagnosed with a primary brain tumor?
    1. Decadron will prevent metastasis to other parts of the body.
    2. Decadron is a potent anticonvulsant and will prevent seizures.
    3. Decadron increases the uptake of serotonin in the brain tissues.
    4. Decadron decreases intracranial pressure by decreasing inflammation.

80. The HCP in the emergency department has prescribed alteplase (Activase) for a client with complaints of new onset of slurred speech, difficulty swallowing, and paralysis of the left arm. Which situation would cause the nurse to question administering the medication?
    1. The client has the comorbid condition of congestive heart failure.
    2. The client has not had a computerized axial tomography scan done.
    3. The client's insurance will not cover this medication.
    4. The client has a history of deep vein thrombosis with pulmonary embolism.

81. The emergency department nurse received a client on warfarin (Coumadin) who has an International Normalized Ratio (INR) of 1.5. Which intervention should the nurse implement?
    1. Prepare to administer protamine sulfate, an antidote.
    2. Document the laboratory result and take no action.
    3. Prepare to administer AquaMEPHYTON (vitamin K).
    4. Notify the client's health-care provider.

82. The nurse is preparing to administer a nitroglycerin patch to a client diagnosed with coronary artery disease. Which interventions should the nurse implement first?
    1. Date and time the nitroglycerin patch.
    2. Remove the old patch.
    3. Apply the nitroglycerin patch.
    4. Check the patch against the MAR.

83. The client with congestive heart failure is taking digoxin (Lanoxin), a cardiac glycoside. Which data indicates the medication is ineffective?
    1. The client's blood pressure is 110/68.
    2. The client's apical pulse rate is 68.
    3. The client's potassium level is 4.2 mEq/L.
    4. The client's lungs have crackles bilaterally.

84. The client receiving telemetry is showing ventricular fibrillation and has no pulse. Which medication should the nurse administer first?
    1. Lidocaine.
    2. Atropine.
    3. Adenosine.
    4. Epinephrine.

85. The nurse is preparing to administer medications to the following clients. To which client would the nurse question administering the medication?
    1. The client receiving the angiotensin receptor blocker losartan (Cozaar) who has a B/P of 168/94.
    2. The client receiving the calcium channel blocker diltiazem (Cardizem) who has 2+ pitting edema.
    3. The client receiving the alpha blocker terazosin (Hytrin) who has a regular apical pulse of 56.
    4. The client receiving the thiazide diuretic hydrochlorothiazide (HCTZ), who is complaining of a headache.

86. The nurse is discharging a client diagnosed with chronic obstructive pulmonary disease (COPD). Which discharge instructions should the nurse provide regarding the client's prednisone, a glucocorticoid?
    1. Take the prednisone as directed and do not discontinue.
    2. Take the prednisone on an empty stomach with a glass of water.
    3. Stop taking the prednisone if a noticeable weight gain occurs.
    4. The medication will decrease the risk of developing an infection.

87. Which assessment data best indicates the client with reactive airway disease has not achieved "good" control with the medication regimen?
    1. The client's peak expiratory flow rate (PEFR) is greater than 80% of his or her personal best.
    2. The client's lung sounds are clear bilaterally both anteriorly and posteriorly.
    3. The client has only had three acute exacerbations of asthma in the last month.
    4. The client's monthly serum theophylline level is 18 μg/mL.

88. The nurse is preparing to administer the following medications. To which client would the nurse question administering the medication?
    1. The client receiving prednisone, a glucocorticoid, who has a glucose level of 140 mg/dL.
    2. The client receiving ceftriaxone (Rocephin), an antibiotic, who has a white blood cell count of 15,000.
    3. The client receiving heparin, an anticoagulant, who has a PTT of 108 seconds with a control of 39.
    4. The client receiving theophylline (Theo-Dur) who has a theophylline level of 12 mg/dL.

89. The nurse is preparing to administer warfarin (Coumadin), an anticoagulant. The client's current laboratory values are as follows:

    PT 48   PTT 40
    Control 12.9   Control 36
    INR 4.2

    Which action should the nurse implement?
    1. Question administering the medication.
    2. Prepare to administer protamine sulfate.
    3. Notify the health-care provider to increase the dose.
    4. Administer the medication as ordered.

90. The nurse is caring for a client diagnosed with pneumonia. Which data indicate that antibiotic therapy has been effective?
    1. The white blood cell count is 7.2 (10^3) mg/dL.
    2. The C&S shows gram-negative rods.
    3. The client completed taking all the prescribed antibiotics.
    4. The client complains of pleurisy.

91. The nurse is administering 0800 medications. Which medication should the nurse question?
    1. Ibuprofen (Motrin), a nonsteroidal anti-inflammatory drug, to a 49-year-old female with a peptic ulcer.
    2. Omeprazole (Prilosec), a proton-pump inhibitor, to an 18-year-old male with a duodenal ulcer.
    3. Digoxin (Lanoxin), a cardiotonic, to a 76-year-old male with a potassium level of 4.2 mEq/L.
    4. Riopan, an antacid, to a 67-year-old client diagnosed with congestive heart failure who is complaining of indigestion.

92. The client diagnosed with inflammatory bowel disease is prescribed mesalamine (Asacol) suppository, an aspirin product. Which statement indicates the client does not understand the medication teaching?
    1. "I should retain the suppository for at least 15 minutes."
    2. "The suppository may stain my underwear or clothing."
    3. "I should store my medication in my medication cabinet."
    4. "I should have an empty rectum when applying the suppository."

93. The client postgastrectomy has a patient-controlled analgesia (PCA) pump. Which data indicates the client and family understand the instructions regarding the PCA pump?
    1. The family pushes the PCA button whenever the time limit has expired.
    2. The client uses the PCA before turning, coughing, and deep breathing.
    3. The family discourages the client from using the PCA pump.
    4. The client pushes the PCA button when the pain is an 8 or 9 on the pain scale.

94. The client who is obese is prescribed sibutramine (Meridia), a selective serotonin reuptake inhibitor, therapy to aid in weight reduction. Which information should the nurse teach the client?
    1. While taking the medications the client does not need to limit the caloric intake.
    2. The medications cannot be taken with antihypertensive medications.
    3. Report a sustained increase of heart rate and blood pressure immediately.
    4. The client will be taking the medications for 2 or 3 weeks at a time.

95. The elderly male client diagnosed with diverticulosis tells the nurse he takes bisacodyl (Dulcolax), a stimulant laxative, daily. Which teaching would be most important for the nurse to provide the client?
    1. "It is not necessary for you to have a bowel movement every day."
    2. "You need to increase fluids to prevent dehydration when taking this medication."
    3. "You should use a bulk laxative when taking laxatives daily."
    4. "You will need to increase the dose of laxative if you do not get good results."

96. The unlicensed assistive personnel (UAP) notified the primary nurse that the client is complaining of being jittery and nervous and is diaphoretic. The client is diagnosed with diabetes mellitus. Which interventions should the primary nurse implement first?
    1. Have the UAP check the client's glucose level.
    2. Tell the UAP to get the client some orange juice.
    3. Check the client's Medication Administration Record.
    4. Immediately go to the room and assess the client.

97. The nurse is administering medications to a client diagnosed with Type 1 diabetes. The client's 1100 glucometer reading is 299. Which action should the nurse implement?

Client's Name:		Account Number: 123456		Allergies: NKDA
Height: 69 inches		Weight: 165 pounds		
Date	Medication	2301–0700	0701–1500	1501–2300
	Regular insulin by bedside glucose subcu ac & hs			
	<60 notify HCP <150 0 units 151–200 2 units		0730 DN BG 142 0 units	
	201–250 4 units 251–300 6 units			
	301–350 8 units 351–400 10 units >400 notify HCP			
Signature/Initials		Day Nurse RN/DN		

    1. Have the laboratory verify the glucose results.
    2. Notify the health-care provider of the results.
    3. Administer 6 units of regular insulin subcutaneously.
    4. Recheck the client's glucometer reading at 1130.

98. The client diagnosed with chronic pancreatitis is prescribed the pancreatic enzyme Pancrease. Which data indicate that the medication is effective?
    1. No bowel movement for 3 days.
    2. Fatty, frothy, foul-smelling stools.
    3. Brown, soft, formed stools.
    4. Normal bowel sounds in four quadrants.

99. The client diagnosed with diabetes insipidus (DI) is receiving desmopressin (DDAVP), a pituitary hormone, intranasally. Which assessment data would warrant the client notifying the health-care provider?
    1. The client complains of being thirsty all the time.
    2. The client is able to sleep through the night.
    3. The client has lost 1 pound in the last 24 hours.
    4. The client has to urinate at least five times daily.

100. The client diagnosed with Addison's disease is being discharged. Which statement indicates the client understands the medication discharge teaching?
    1. "I will be sure to keep my dose of steroid constant and not vary."
    2. "I may have to take two forms of steroids to remain healthy."
    3. "It is normal to get weak and dizzy when taking this medication."
    4. "I must take prophylactic antibiotics prior to getting my teeth cleaned."

1. 1. These are adverse affects that would cause the HCP to discontinue this medication. This medication can cause pulmonary toxicity, which is progressive dyspnea, cough, fatigue, and pleuritic pain.
   2. The medication can be taken at the client's convenience; the medication should be taken at the same time each day.
   3. The client checks the radial pulse at home, not the apical pulse, which requires a stethoscope.
   4. This medication does not cause the stool to turn black. Iron supplements make the client's stool turn black.

2. 1. The client receiving a calcium channel blocker (CCB) can take the medication with water; therefore, the nurse would not question administering this medication.
   2. This blood pressure is above 90/60; therefore, the nurse would not question administering this medication.
   3. Headache is a side effect of nitroglycerin; therefore, the nurse would not question administering this medication but could administer Tylenol or a nonnarcotic analgesic.
   4. **The client's platelet count is not monitored when administering antiplatelet medication, but if the nurse is aware that the client has a low platelet count the nurse would question administering any medication that would inactivate the platelets.**

3. 1. Antihypertensive medications do not interfere with the contrast dye that is used when performing a CT scan. Glucophage may be held prior to or following the procedure until a normal creatinine level can be established.
   2. **The client will have an intravenous line to administer the contrast dye.**
   3. The contrast dye is iodine based so an allergy to shellfish would be important, but there is no contraindication to taking an NSAID.
   4. Sedatives are not administered for this procedure, but if the client is anxious about the machine sometimes an antianxiety medication is administered.

4. 1. Mineral oil will not affect folic acid, but it will inhibit the absorption of vitamin A.
   2. The client should avoid drinking alcohol products because they increase folic acid requirements.
   3. Research has proved that decreased stores of folic acid in the maternal body directly affect the development of spina bifida in the fetus.
   4. This would be significant if a client is at risk for developing pregnancy-induced hypertension but not when taking folic acid.

5. 1. This is scientific rationale for administering thiazolidinediones, pioglitazone (Actos), or rosiglitazone (Avandia).
   2. This is the scientific rationale for administering an alpha-glucosidase inhibitor, acarbose (Precose), or miglitol (Glyset).
   3. This is the scientific rationale for administering metformin (Glucophage). It diminishes the increase in serum glucose following a meal and blunts the degree of postprandial hyperglycemia.
   4. This is the scientific rationale for administering meglitinides, repaglinide (Prandin), sulfonylureas, or nateglinide (Starlix).

6. 1. Epinephrine is the first medication administered in a code because it constricts the periphery and shunts the blood to the trunk of the body.
   2. **Lidocaine, an antidysrhythmic, is a drug of choice for treating ventricular dysrhythmias.**
   3. Atropine is administered for asystole.
   4. Digoxin is administered for cardiac failure.

7. 1. This would be appropriate for monoamine oxidase inhibitors (MAOIs).
   2. **Serotonin syndrome (SES) is a serious complication of SSRIs that produces mental changes (confusion, anxiety, and restlessness), hypertension, tremors, sweating, hyperpyrexia (elevated temperature), and ataxia. Conservative treatment includes stopping the SSRI and using supportive treatment. If untreated it can lead to death.**
   3. Grapefruit juice does not specifically affect SSRIs, but the nurse should be aware that many medications interact negatively with grapefruit juice and its consumption should not be encouraged.
   4. These are additional signs of serotonin syndrome and should be reported to the health-care provider.

8. **100 mL.** The pump is set at the rate to be administered per hour; therefore, the nurse should set the rate at 100.

9. 1. The therapeutic level for theophylline is 10–20 μg/mL; therefore, the nurse should continue to monitor the medication because this is within therapeutic range.
   2. If the serum theophylline level rises above 20 μg/mL, the client will experience nausea, vomiting, diarrhea, insomnia, and restlessness. This theophylline level may result in serious effects such as convulsion and ventricular fibrillation; therefore, the client should not be assessed first.
   3. The nurse should not discontinue the medication because the client's blood level is within therapeutic range.
   4. There is no reason to notify the HCP because the theophylline level is within the therapeutic range.

10. 1. The client with an ulcer would be prescribed a medication that decreases gastric acid secretion; therefore, the nurse would not question administering this medication. Females of childbearing age should not receive this medication because it can cause an abortion.
    2. Prilosec is prescribed to treat duodenal and gastric ulcers; the nurse would not question this medication.
    3. **The potassium level is low (3.5–5.5 mEq/L); therefore, the nurse should question this medication and request a potassium supplement or possibly telemetry.**
    4. Tylenol is frequently administered for headaches; the nurse would not question this medication.

11. 1. **The nurse can recommend the client take over-the-counter (OTC) medication to help relieve the constipation.**
    2. The client should be encouraged to eat high-fiber foods and increase fluid intake, preferably water.
    3. **The nurse should determine when the last bowel movement was so that appropriate action can be taken to resolve the constipation.**
    4. The client does not need to go to the emergency department because the constipation should resolve with medication, but the client may need to be seen in the clinic if there is still no bowel movement within several days.
    5. **The nurse should determine what other medications the client is taking because constipation can be a side**

effect of many prescribed and OTC medications.

12. 1. Regular insulin sliding scale is administered prior to meals; therefore, this medication should be administered first.
    2. This medication can be administered within the 30-minute acceptable time frame.
    3. A pain medication is a priority, but it can be administered after the sliding scale.
    4. Etanercept (Enbrel) can be administered within the 30-minute acceptable time frame.

13. 1. This is standard precaution and does not require intervention by the nurse.
    2. **Herbs are considered medications, and the UAP cannot administer medications to the client even if they are from home. Many herbs will interact with prescribed medications, and the nurse must be aware of what the client is taking.**
    3. The client can apply his or her own moisture barrier protection cream. This does not warrant immediate intervention by the nurse.
    4. This is a comfort measure and does not warrant intervention by the nurse.

14. 1. Do not shake the vial because shaking may denature the glycoprotein, rendering it biologically inactive.
    2. The nurse should apply ice to numb the injection site, not a warm washcloth.
    3. **The nurse should only use the vial for one dose. The nurse should not reenter the vial and should discard any unused portion because the vial contains no preservatives.**
    4. The medication should be stored in the refrigerator, not the freezer, and should be warmed to room temperature prior to administering the medication.

15. 1. A 5-pound weight loss in 1 month would not make the nurse suspect the client is experiencing any long-term complications from taking daily aspirin.
    2. Elderly clients often have a loss of hearing, but it is not a complication of long-term aspirin use.
    3. Elderly clients often lose taste buds, which may cause a funny taste in their mouth, but it is not a complication of taking daily aspirin.

4. A complication of long-term aspirin use is gastric bleeding, which could also result in bleeding gums; this data would warrant further intervention.

16. 1. The WBC count is within normal range; therefore, the nurse would not need to assess for infection.
    2. The client's platelet count is less than normal of 150,000 but still greater than 100,000. Less than 100,000 is thrombocytopenia. Critical values begin at 50,000, which would cause the client to have petechiae.
    3. The client's hemoglobin is critically low; therefore, the client might fatigue easily because of oxygen demands on the body and have shortness of breath.
    4. The client would not have rubor (redness); the client would be pale.

17. 1. This would not indicate the fluid resuscitation is effective.
    2. This would indicate the respiratory system is functioning but does not indicate fluid resuscitation is effective.
    3. The client's blood pressure indicates that the fluid resuscitation is effective and able to maintain an adequate blood pressure to perfuse the vital organs.
    4. This would indicate that the fluid resuscitation is not effective because this is a sign of decreased urine output.

18. 1. This is the scientific rationale for miotic medications, which constrict the pupil and block sympathetic nervous system input, causing the pupil to dilate in low light and contract the ciliary muscle.
    2. This is the scientific rationale for mydriatic medications, which dilate the pupil, reduce the production of aqueous humor, and increase the absorption effectiveness, reducing intraocular pressure in open-angle glaucoma.
    3. This is the scientific rationale for beta-adrenergic blockers, which reduce intraocular pressure but do not affect pupil size and lens accommodation.
    4. This is the scientific rationale for carbonic anhydrase inhibitors, which reduce intraocular pressure.

19. 1. Morphine is a potent analgesic with addictive properties, and the nurse should question a routine administration of this medication. The HCP may

have failed to write PRN after the order.
    2. Many medications can affect the kidneys or the liver and the blood counts. Baseline data should be obtained. There is no reason to question this order.
    3. This medication order is an appropriate order. The nurse would not question this order.
    4. Soma comes in one strength so this order is complete. There is no reason to question this order.

20. 1. NSAIDs are appropriate interventions for clients diagnosed with back pain. They decrease pain and inflammation.
    2. Opioid analgesics are administered for pain. The client is in the mild pain range. The nurse would question administering this medication because of its addictive properties. A less potent analgesic should be administered.
    3. Muscle relaxant medications are administered to clients with back pain to relax the muscles and decrease the pain. The nurse would administer this medication.
    4. Darvon N is a pain medication. The nurse would administer this medication.

21. 1. Decongestants vasoconstrict the blood vessels, resulting in decreased inflammation in the nasal passages. This vasoconstriction is the reason that OTC cold medications are labeled not to be used by clients diagnosed with hypertension and diabetes.
    2. Decongestants do not decrease the immune system's response to the virus.
    3. Activating viral receptors would increase the symptoms of a cold.
    4. This is the rationale for zinc. Theoretically, zinc blocks the virus from binding to nasal epithelium. Research has shown that increased amounts of zinc can prevent the binding and development of rhinovirus.

22. 1. The digoxin level is within therapeutic range; therefore, the nurse could administer this medication, but it is a routine medication and can be administered at any time.
    2. Pleuritic pain is pain involving the thoracic pleura, and pain of a "7" should be addressed before routine medications.
    3. A client with two unifocal PVCs in a minute would be considered normal,

and no intervention would be needed at this time.

4. This blood pressure is within normal limits, and this medication could be given within the 30-minute time frame.

23. 1. The normal serum potassium level is 3.5–4.5 mEq/L; therefore, the nurse would administer this medication.

2. The normal serum osmolality is 275–300 mOsm/kg; therefore, the nurse would administer this medication.

3. The normal digoxin level is 0.8–2.0 mg/dL; a digoxin level of 1.2 mg/dL is within therapeutic range. The nurse would administer this medication.

4. **The therapeutic serum level of Dilantin is 10–20 μg/mL; therefore, the nurse should question administering this medication.**

24. 1. The medication should be diluted with normal saline to increase the longevity of the vein for intravenous medication and fluids. Diluting decreases the client's pain secondary to the IV push. A 5-mL or 10-mL amount allows the nurse to inject the medication over a 5-minute time frame with better control than a 0.5-mL amount.

2. **Hypokalemia may potentiate digoxin toxicity; therefore, the nurse should check the client's potassium level.**

3. The nurse should pinch off the tubing above the port, not below, to ensure that the medication flows into the client's vein and not upward into the IV tubing.

4. The medication should be injected slowly over 5 minutes (2 minutes for most IV medications, except for medications that act directly on the cardiovascular system and narcotics) and at a steady rate because a rapid injection could cause speed shock. Speed shock is a sudden adverse physiological reaction secondary to an IVP medication where the client develops a flushed face, a headache, a tight feeling in the chest, an irregular pulse, loss of consciousness, and possible cardiac arrest.

25. 1. Librium would not help a client addicted to cocaine.

2. Methadone, not Librium, blocks the craving for heroin.

3. Librium would not help a client addicted to amphetamines.

4. **Librium is the drug of choice for preventing neurological complications**

and delirium tremens, which is a life-threatening complication of alcohol withdrawal.

26. 1. A smoking cessation support group may be helpful, but nicotine is a physical withdrawal and medication should be used to help with the withdrawal symptoms.

2. Tapering the number of cigarettes daily is not the most successful method to quit smoking cigarettes.

3. **Research has shown that 44% of smokers were able to quit smoking at the end of 12 weeks with Chantix as compared to other smoking cessation medications, which have a 30% chance of success. It reduces the urge to smoke.**

4. Clonidine is used to help prevent delirium tremens in clients with a alcohol dependence.

27. 1. Mannitol would not be contraindicated in a client who is HIV positive.

2. Mannitol, an osmotic diuretic, would not be contraindicated in a client who has glaucoma. The osmotic diuretic medication Diamox is administered to clients with glaucoma.

3. **Because mannitol will pull fluid off the brain by osmosis into the circulatory system it can lead to a circulatory overload, which the heart could not handle because the client already has CHF. This client would need an order for a loop diuretic to prevent serious cardiac complications.**

4. The client is 16 years old, and even with CF the client's heart should be able to handle the fluid-volume overload.

28. 1. A. This would be half the dose prescribed.

2. **B. The line is in increments of 0.5 (1/2 inch) and the order is 1 inch.**

3. C. This would be 1 1/2 inches, which is not the correct dose.

4. D. This would be 2 inches, which is not the correct dose.

29. 1. Lidocaine suppresses ventricular ectopy and is a first-line drug for the treatment of ventricular dysrhythmias.

2. Atropine decreases vagal stimulation, which increases the heart rate, and is the drug of choice for asystole, complete heart block, and symptomatic bradycardia.

3. Adenosine is the drug of choice for terminating paroxysmal supraventricular

tachycardia by decreasing the automaticity of the SA node and slowing conduction through the AV node.

4. Epinephrine constricts the periphery and shunts the blood to the central trunk and is the first medication administered in a client who is coding.

30. 1. The client should adhere to a low-fat, low-cholesterol diet, but this does not indicate the medication is effective.

2. **This medication is prescribed to help decrease the client's cholesterol level; therefore, this statement indicates it is effective.**

3. A sedentary lifestyle is a risk factor for developing atherosclerosis; therefore, exercising should be praised but it does not indicate the medication is effective.

4. The medication is not administered to decrease edema; therefore, this statement does not indicate the medication is effective.

31. 1. This is an oral preparation and one that can be given daily; this is not the first medication to be administered.

2. **An initial dose of intravenous antibiotic is priority because the client must be started on the medication as soon as possible to prevent the client from becoming septic.**

3. Lactinex is administered to replace the good bacteria in the body destroyed by the antibiotic, but it does not need to be administered first.

4. Keflex is an oral antibiotic, but this client is being discharged, indicating the client's condition has improved. This client could wait until the initial dose of an IV antibiotic is administered.

32. 1. **White blood cells are monitored to detect the presence of an infection, and an elevated WBC is a sign of infection that would warrant intervention. Steroids mask infection.**

2. The hemoglobin and hematocrit are monitored to detect blood loss, not for steroid therapy.

3. Steroid therapy interferes with glucose metabolism and increases insulin resistance. The blood glucose levels should be monitored to determine if an intervention is needed, but a glucose level of 138 would not warrant immediate intervention and would be expected.

4. The creatinine is monitored to determine renal status. The adrenal glands produce cortisol.

33. 1. **This client has normal ABGs, but the oxygen level is below normal (80–100); therefore, the nurse should administer oxygen.**

2. The client has normal ABGs; therefore, an antianxiety medication does not need to be administered. The client needs oxygen.

3. Sodium bicarbonate is the drug of choice for metabolic acidosis and this client has normal ABGs except for hypoxia.

4. The client has normal ABGs with hypoxia.

34. 1. This hematocrit is normal but does not indicate that the client is responding to the antibiotics.

2. Thick-green sputum is a symptom of pneumonia, which indicates the antibiotic therapy is not effective. If the sputum were changing from a thick-green sputum to a thinner, lighter-colored sputum, it would indicate an improvement in the condition.

3. **The symptoms of pneumonia include crackles and wheezing in the lung fields. Clear lung sounds indicate an improvement in the pneumonia and that the medication is effective.**

4. Pleuritic chest is a symptom of pneumonia and does not indicate the medication is effective. Lack of symptoms indicates the medication is effective.

35. 1. **This is the mechanism of action for antacids.**

2. This is the mechanism of action for histamine$_2$ blockers.

3. This is the mechanism of action for proton-pump inhibitors.

4. This is the mechanism of action for mucosal barrier agents.

36. 1. The TPN is 50% dextrose; therefore, the client's blood glucose level should be checked every 6 hours and sliding scale insulin coverage should be ordered.

2. **TPN should always be administered using an intravenous pump and not to gravity; fluid volume and increased glucose resulting from an overload of TPN could cause a life-threatening fluid-volume or hyperglycemic crisis.**

3. **TPN must be administered via a subclavian line, and any infection may lead to endocarditis; therefore, the nurse should assess the site.**

4. **TPN is considered a medication and should be administered as any other medication.**

5. The client with severe acute exacerbation of Crohn's is NPO to rest the bowel; when a client is on TPN they are usually NPO because the TPN provides all necessary nutrients; therefore, the nurse would not encourage the client to eat food.

37. 1. This is the rationale for administering mineral oil.

2. This is the rationale for administering stimulants.

3. **Stool softeners or surfactants have a detergent action to reduce surface tension, permitting water and fats to penetrate and soften the stool.**

4. This is the rationale for bulk-forming agents.

38. 1. **The normal plasma ammonia level is 15–45 μg/dL (varies with method); this is below the normal level. The client with end-stage liver failure would be receiving this medication, and the client does not need to receive a laxative that will cause diarrhea**

2. The normal serum potassium level is 3.5–5.5 mEq/L; therefore, the nurse should administer this medication because the potassium level is within normal limits.

3. The normal serum potassium level is 3.5–5.5 mEq/L; therefore, the nurse should not question administering this medication because the potassium level is within normal limits.

4. Hyponatremia (normal sodium 135–145 mEq/L) may occur when the client is taking vasopressin therapy. This sodium level is within normal limits; therefore, the nurse would not question administering this medication.

39. 1. Humulin N is an intermediate-acting insulin that will peak 6–8 hours after administration; therefore, the client would experience signs of hypoglycemia around 1300–1500.

2. The nurse needs to ensure the client eats the nighttime (HS) snack to help prevent nighttime hypoglycemia if the Humulin N is administered at 1600. This insulin has been administered at 0700, so the nurse should ensure that the client eats lunch and/or a mid-afternoon snack for this administration time.

3. A serum blood glucose level would have to be done with a venipuncture and the blood sample must be taken to the laboratory; if the client needed the blood glucose checked, it should be done with a glucometer at the bedside.

4. **Eating the food from the lunch tray will help prevent a hypoglycemic reaction because the Humulin N is an intermediate-acting insulin that peaks in 6–8 hours.**

40. 1. The insulin will not be working 4–5 hours after being administered.

2. **This insulin peaks in 15–20 minutes after being administered; therefore, the meal should be at the bedside prior to administering this medication.**

3. The glucose level should be checked prior to meals, not after meals.

4. This medication is administered when a client is unconscious secondary to hypoglycemia and should not be kept at the bedside. Orange juice or some type of simple glucose should be kept at the bedside.

41. 1. Weight gain indicates the client is not taking enough medication.

2. Intolerance to cold indicates the client is not taking enough medication.

3. **Tachycardia, heart rate greater than 100, is a sign of hyperthyroidism and indicates the client is taking too much medication.**

4. Decreased metabolism, constipation, indicates the client is not taking enough thyroid hormone.

42. 1. Humalog is not administered intravenously, and glucose levels should be monitored prior to insulin administration.

2. **Steatorrhea is fatty, frothy stools that indicate the pancreatic enzymes are not sufficient for digestive purposes. The nurse should be prepared to administer pancreatic enzymes.**

3. Humulin R insulin is administered by sliding scale to decrease blood glucose levels. Clients with pancreatitis should be monitored for the development of diabetes mellitus.

4. Zantac would not treat the client's symptoms.

43. 1. **Kayexalate is a medication that is administered to decrease an elevated serum potassium level; therefore, an**

elevated serum potassium (5.5 mEq/L) would indicate the medication is not effective.

2. Kayexalate is not used to alter the serum sodium level.

3. Kayexalate is a medication that is administered to decrease an elevated serum potassium level; therefore, a potassium level within the normal range of 3.5–5.5 mEq/L indicates the medication is effective.

4. Kayexalate is not used to alter the serum sodium level.

44. 1. **The saline irrigation is being instilled into the bladder and requires nursing judgment; therefore, this nursing task requires immediate intervention.**

2. The UAP reporting abnormal data is appropriate. A green–blue color indicates the client is taking bethanechol (Urecholine), a urinary stimulant used for clients with a neurogenic bladder. This is an expected color.

3. The client should be encouraged to drink fluids. The nurse would not intervene to stop this action.

4. This action encourages bowel and urine continence and is part of a falls prevention protocol. The nurse would not intervene to stop this action.

45. 1. The time period for the lesions to heal depends on several factors, including the immune status of the individual who is infected and the amount of stress the individual is experiencing at the time. It usually requires several days to more than a week for an outbreak to be healed.

2. **Suppressive therapy with Valtrex is once daily, every day. This is an advantage of Valtrex over other antiretroviral medications, which require twice-a-day dosing.**

3. The use of condoms may prevent the spread of herpes infections; it does not increase the spread of the virus.

4. It is possible to transmit the virus to a sexual partner with no visible signs of a lesion being present. Valtrex will not absolutely prevent the spread of the virus. It will treat an outbreak and decrease the risk of transmission.

46. 1. **If the client's deep tendon reflexes are 4+, this indicates the client may have a seizure at any time, which indicates the medication is not effective.**

2. Magnesium sulfate is not administered to treat the client's blood pressure; therefore, this data cannot be used to evaluate the effectiveness of the medication.

3. Magnesium sulfate is administered to prevent seizure activity and is determined to be effective and in the therapeutic range when the client's deep tendon reflexes are normal, which is 2+ to 3+ on a 0–4+ scale.

4. A "0" deep tendon reflex indicates the client has received too much magnesium sulfate but the client would not have seizure activity; therefore, it is effective. The client is at risk for respiratory depression.

47. 1. The client should swallow the medication. The client should not crush, chew, or suck the medication.

2. The medication should be taken on an empty stomach at least 30 minutes before eating or drinking any liquid. Foods and beverages greatly decrease the effect of Fosamax.

3. The medication will irritate the stomach and esophagus if the client lies down; therefore, the medication should be taken when the client can remain upright at least 30 minutes.

4. **Fosamax can be taken daily or weekly, but because of the high risk of esophageal complications if the client does not take Fosamax exactly as prescribed, most HCPs prescribe the medication to be taken once a week. The client must take the medication on an empty stomach and remain in an upright position for a minimum of 30 minutes.**

48. 1. Parafon Forte would not have an effect on whether or not the client has had the flu.

2. This medication can make the client drowsy; this is why the nurse teaches the client not to drive or operate heavy machinery when taking a muscle relaxant.

3. **The client should not be driving at all when the medication makes them less than alert. The nurse should address this with the client.**

4. This would keep the client from overdosing on the medication.

49. 1. The urine does not change color when the client takes methotrexate.
    2. The client should be encouraged to eat a balanced diet; drinking a supplement is not necessary.
    3. **Methotrexate suppresses the bone marrow, resulting in decreased numbers of white blood cells; the client should notify the HCP if a fever develops because this could indicate an infection.**
    4. There is no reason to increase the amount of green, leafy vegetables consumed when taking this medication.

50. 1. **This medication affects the acid–base balance in the body and should not be administered to clients with renal disease. A 2.8 mg/dL serum creatinine level indicates renal insufficiency; therefore, the nurse would use caution with this client.**
    2. Clients with congestive heart failure would not be affected by this medication.
    3. This client has adequate respiratory status; therefore, the nurse would not need to use caution with this client.
    4. There is no reason a client with diabetes could not be prescribed mafenide acetate.

51. 1. Botox will reduce wrinkles, but that is not why it is administered to a client with a cerebrovascular accident, a brain attack. The paralysis of the facial muscles lasts from 3–6 months.
    2. **Botox produces partial chemical denervation of the muscle, resulting in localized reduction in muscle activity and spasticity.**
    3. This medication will not improve limb weakness.
    4. This medication does not help with pain secondary to neuropathy.

52. **500 mL/hour.** The nurse should divide 8000 mL by 2, which equals 4000 mL. The 4000 must be divided by 8, which equals 500 mL/hour. There are formulas that are used to determine the client's fluid-volume resuscitation. The formulas specify that the total amount of fluid must be infused in 24 hours, 50% in the first 8 hours followed by the other 50% over the other 16 hours. This is a large amount of fluid, but it is not uncommon in clients with full-thickness burns over greater than 20% total body surface area burned.

53. 1. Wearing insect repellent is an appropriate intervention, but if the client has an insect bite, the repellent will not help prevent anaphylaxis; therefore, this is not the priority intervention.
    2. Antihistamines are used in clients with anaphylaxis, but it takes at least 30 minutes for the medication to work, and if the client has an insect bite, it is not the priority medication.
    3. Clients with documented severe anaphylaxis should carry an EpiPen, which is a prescribed epinephrine injectable device that the client can administer to themselves in case of an insect bite. Keeping the medication in the refrigerator does not allow it to be available to the client at all times.
    4. **The client should wear an identification bracelet because even if the client uses insect repellent, a sting could occur. The bracelet indicates the client is at risk for an anaphylactic reaction; therefore, this is the priority intervention.**

54. 1. There is not a cure for the HIV infection; HIV is a retrovirus that never dies as long as the host is alive.
    2. HAART is complex and expensive and poses a risk of toxicity and serious drug interactions.
    3. **Because of HAART plasma levels of HIV can be reduced to undetectable levels with current technology.**
    4. HAART medications are very expensive.

55. 1. Plaquenil can cause pigmentary retinitis and vision loss, so the client should have a thorough vision examination every 6 months; therefore, the client does not understand the medication teaching.
    2. Plaquenil may increase the risk of liver toxicity when administered with hepatotoxic drugs, so alcohol use should be eliminated during therapy; therefore, the client does not understand the medication teaching.
    3. **The medication should be taken with milk to decrease gastrointestinal upset. This statement indicates the client understands the medication teaching.**
    4. The medication takes 3–6 months to achieve the desired response; therefore, the client needs more medication teaching.

56. 1. A "3" is considered mild pain and could wait until the client whose needs are more emergent is medicated.
    2. An antianxiety medication is not priority over a client who must take the medication on an empty stomach. This is a potential anxiety attack over a physiological problem.
    3. **The medication must be administered prior to a meal. Administering a mucosal barrier agent after a meal places medication in the stomach that will coat the food, not the stomach lining. This medication should be administered first.**
    4. This medication stimulates the bone marrow to produce red blood cells; the full effect of the medication will not be seen for 30–90 days. It could be administered after the antianxiety medication and the analgesic.

57. 1. The nurse should not administer pain medication until after assessing the client's pain.
    2. **The first action is to always assess the client in pain to determine if the client is having a complication that requires medical intervention rather than PRN pain medication.**
    3. The nurse should assess the client, then administer the pain medication whether the client has visitors or not.
    4. The nurse should first assess the client's pain.

58. 1. Keeping the eyes closed and drapes drawn would not indicate the pain medication is effective. These actions may be the client's way of dealing with the pain.
    2. Using guided imagery is an excellent method to assist with the control of pain, but its use does not indicate effectiveness of the medication.
    3. **Light snoring indicates the client is asleep, which would indicate the medication is effective.**
    4. This action may be the client's way of dealing with the pain, but it does not indicate the medication is effective.

59. 1. **The client's WBC is low and the absolute neutrophil count is 1100, which indicates the client is immunosuppressed; therefore, the client should not be exposed to people with active infections.**

2. This is good information to teach, but it is not based on the laboratory values. The client may develop mouth ulcers as a result of chemotherapy administration and the nurse should discuss methods of maintaining nutrition for this reason, not the laboratory values.
    3. This is good information to teach, but it is not based on the laboratory values. Cancer and treatment-related fatigue are real and should be addressed; an Hgb and Hct of around 8 and 24 could cause fatigue, but at the current level this is not indicated.
    4. A platelet count of less than 100,000 is the definition of thrombocytopenia; therefore, this client is not at risk for bleeding.

60. 1. This level is above therapeutic range; therefore, the nurse should not administer the medication.
    2. **The therapeutic serum level is 0.6 to 1.5 mEq/L; therefore, the first intervention is to hold the medication.**
    3. After holding the medication, the nurse should notify the health-care provider.
    4. The nurse should first hold the medication and then can verify the level at a later time.

61. 1. **All medication must be kept in a safe place to prevent accidental poisoning of children.**
    2. The last medication should be administered no later than 1400 in the afternoon or the child will not be able to sleep at night. Ritalin is a stimulant. This statement indicates the mother does not understand the medication teaching.
    3. Growth rate may be stalled in response to nutritional deficiency caused by anorexia; it does not cause growth spurts. This statement indicates the mother does not understand the medication teaching.
    4. Insomnia is an adverse reaction to the medication; central nervous stimulants may disrupt normal sleep patterns. This statement indicates the medication teaching has not been effective.

62. 1. **The client should instill eye ointment into the lower conjunctival sac, which is the inner edge of the lower lid margin.**
    2. **This pressure will prevent systemic absorption of the medication.**
    3. The client does not have to wear gloves when applying the ointment to his or her

own eyes; the client should be instructed to wash hands prior to and after applying the ointment.

4. The antibiotic ointment should be applied from the inner canthus to the outer canthus, from the nose side of the eye to the outer area.

5. **The client should be in this position when applying ophthalmic ointment or drops to better access the lower conjunctival sac.**

63. 1. The outer canthus does not have access to the systemic system; therefore, the nurse would not hold pressure in this area.
    2. The nurse should not hold pressure under the eyelid because the medication will not be retained in the eye.
    3. The nurse cannot hold pressure in the lower conjunctival sac because this would be painful for the client and would not prevent systemic absorption of the medication.
    4. **The lacrimal duct is located in the inner canthus area, and systemic absorption of the medication can occur if the nurse does not apply light pressure to the area.**

64. 1. **This is a low blood pressure reading for a client in hypovolemic shock. A B/P less than 90/60 warrants intervention by the nurse and indicates the fluid resuscitation is not effective.**
    2. A pulse oximeter reading of greater than 93% indicates the arterial oxygen level is between 80 and 100, which is normal.
    3. The client's lungs are clear, which indicates the client is not in fluid-volume overload; therefore, this does not warrant immediate intervention.
    4. If the client has at least 30 mL of urine output an hour, then the kidneys are being perfused adequately. This indicates the client is urinating 40 mL an hour.

65. 1. The client in asystole would not benefit from defibrillation because there is no heart activity; the client must have some heart activity (ventricular activity) for defibrillation to be successful.
    2. Synchronized cardioversion is used for new-onset atrial fibrillation or unstable ventricular tachycardia.
    3. **Atropine is the drug of choice for asystole because it decreases vagal stimulation and increases heart rate.**

4. Amiodarone is administered in life-threatening ventricular dysrhythmias, not asystole.

66. 1. Mucomyst does not neutralize substances by changing their pH.
    2. Mucomyst is not used to treat bleach poisonings. Charcoal binds with poisons to form an inert substance that can be eliminated through the bowel because the body is incapable of absorbing charcoal molecules.
    3. **This is the scientific rationale for administering Mucomyst.**
    4. Mucomyst does not cause emesis. An emetic such as ipecac would induce vomiting.

67. 1. The weight of the child is pertinent information, but it is not the most important question.
    2. **Most dishwashing liquids are vegetable-based products and will produce osmotic diarrhea when ingested; therefore, the nurse should ask about abdominal cramping. The soap is not poisonous, but the child may become dehydrated and be uncomfortable.**
    3. Because the mother has called the emergency department it is not priority to know if she called the Poison Control Center.
    4. Determining where the soap was is not going to help the child.

68. 1. Aspirin does not affect the blood pressure and pulse; therefore, the nurse would not need to implement this intervention.
    2. Aspirin will not cause a breakdown of fat, which results in increased ketone production.
    3. Daily aspirin is taken as an antiplatelet medication, not as an antipyretic.
    4. **This information should be documented in the chart, and no further action should be taken.**

69. 1. Iron turns the stool a harmless black or dark green. This statement indicates the client does understand the medication teaching.
    2. **The iron tablet should be taken between meals and with 8 ounces of water to promote absorption. The iron tablet should not be taken within 1 hour of ingesting antacid, milk, ice cream, or other milk products such as pudding. This statement indicates the**

client does not understand the medication teaching.

3. Sitting upright will prevent esophageal corrosion from reflux. This statement indicates the client understands the medication teaching.

4. The drug treatment for anemia generally lasts less than 6 months. This statement indicates the client understands the medication teaching.

70. 1. This is the scientific rationale of a coronary vasodilator.
2. This is the scientific rationale for antiplatelet medications.
3. **Antioxidants are being prescribed to help prevent cardiovascular diseases.**
4. Rest is the only action that will help decrease the oxygen demands of the peripheral tissues.

71. 1. According to guidelines for prudent use of herbs, babies and young children should not be given any types of herbs.
2. Herbs exposed to sunlight and heat may lose their potency.
3. When presenting information as a nurse, the nurse must encourage a discussion with a health-care provider when substituting herbs for prescribed medications.
4. **This is a guideline that both consumers and health-care providers must be aware of when using herbal therapy.**

72. 1. The nurse should offer water so that the client can swallow the medication, but it is not the first intervention.
2. **The nurse should determine if the client can swallow the medication; this is the first intervention.**
3. The nurse should check the medication against the Medication Administration Record, open the medication package, and place it in the medication cup at the bedside, but this is not the first intervention. If the client cannot swallow or refuses the medication, the medication can be sent back to the pharmacy if it has not been taken out of the package.
4. The nurse should remain with the client until the medication is swallowed.

73. 1. The UAP cannot administer medications, and the medications should not be left at the bedside. Medication aides are permitted in some states to practice in long term care facilities. This was not stated in the stem. Regardless, no one should adminis-

ter a medication dispensed by another person.
2. **The UAP should take the medication cup back to the medication room and tell the primary nurse. Medications should never be left at the bedside.**
3. The UAP nurse should not correct the primary nurse in front of the client; therefore, this would not be an appropriate intervention. This is not in the realm of a UAP's duties. The person over the nurse is the one to confront the nurse.
4. The UAP is a vital part of the health-care team and is expected to maintain safety for the client.

74. 1. **The nurse should prepare the medication using a 25-gauge, $^1/_2$- to $^5/_8$-inch needle.**
2. The nurse should not aspirate for blood when administering heparin because this can damage surrounding tissue and cause bruising.
3. The nurse should not massage after injecting heparin because this may cause bruising or bleeding.
4. Heparin is administered in the lower abdominal area at least 2 inches from the umbilicus. Lovenox is administered in the "love handles," located anterolateral to the upper abdomen.

75. 1. INR is monitored for oral anticoagulant therapy, warfarin (Coumadin).
2. PT is not directly monitored for oral anticoagulant therapy but will be elevated in clients receiving oral anticoagulants.
3. **The PTT should be 1.5 to 2.0 times the normal PTT or a control to determine if intravenous heparin is therapeutic.**
4. The platelet count is not monitored during heparin therapy.

76. 1. The client can take nonnarcotic analgesics if experiencing a headache, and Tylenol would be appropriate to take for a headache.
2. The client can eat anything after experiencing a concussion.
3. Narcotic analgesics should not be taken after a head injury because of further depression of the neurological status.
4. **Any nausea, vomiting (especially projectile), or blurred vision could be increasing ICP; therefore, the client should return to the ED for further evaluation.**

77. 1. **The therapeutic serum level of Tegretol is 5–12 µg/mL; therefore, the nurse should question administering this medication.**
    2. The therapeutic serum level of Klonopin is 20–80 ng/mL; therefore, the nurse should administer this medication.
    3. The therapeutic serum level of Dilantin is 10–20 µg/mL; therefore, the nurse should administer this medication.
    4. The therapeutic serum level of Zarontin is 40–100 µg/mL; therefore, the nurse should administer this medication.

78. 1. **Aricept and other cholinesterase inhibitors have shown the potential to delay the progression of Alzheimer's disease. The client and family should be told that, although it offers them hope, it only lasts for a time.**
    2. Aricept does not repair the brain tissue; there is no medication that repairs lost brain tissue.
    3. Aricept is not an experimental medication. Aricept works by preventing the breakdown of acetylcholine (Ach) by acetylcholinesterase and thereby increases the availability of Ach at the cholinergic synapses.
    4. Aricept is the best tolerated of the cholinesterase inhibitors because it has fewer side effects.

79. 1. Primary brain tumors rarely metastasize outside of the cranium because they kill by occupying space and increasing intracranial pressure.
    2. Decadron is not an anticonvulsant; it may decrease the chance of seizures by decreasing intracranial pressure, but the client may still have a seizure while taking Decadron.
    3. Decadron does not affect the uptake of serotonin,
    4. **Decadron decreases the inflammatory response of tissues. It is particularly used for edema (swelling) of the brain tissues.**

80. 1. Administration of Activase is not contraindicated in clients who are diagnosed with congestive heart failure.
    2. **A CT scan must be done before administering Activase to make sure that the cerebrovascular accident (CVA) is not being caused by an intracranial hemorrhage. There are three types of stroke: thrombotic,** embolic, and hemorrhagic. If the client is experiencing a hemorrhagic stroke, then administering a medication that dissolves clots could initiate more bleeding and cause death.
    3. The medication is very expensive, but in an emergency situation the nurse does not question administering a medication based on cost or insurance coverage.
    4. This history would indicate the client has experienced an embolic stroke and would be helped by the Activase, and it is not a reason to question administering the medication.

81. 1. Protamine sulfate is the antidote for heparin toxicity.
    2. **The therapeutic range for INR is 2–3; therefore, the nurse should document the results and take no action.**
    3. AquaMEPHYTON, vitamin K, is the antidote for Coumadin toxicity, which is supported by an elevated INR greater than 3.
    4. The nurse does not need to notify the HCP for a normal laboratory value.

82. 1. After opening the medication the nurse should date and time the patch prior to putting it on the client so that the nurse is not pressing on the client when writing on the patch.
    2. The old patch should be removed but not before checking the MAR.
    3. The nurse should administer the patch in a clean, dry, nonhairy place while wearing gloves.
    4. **The nurse should implement the five rights of medication administration, and the first ones are to make sure it is the right medication and the right client.**

83. 1. Digoxin does not affect the client's blood pressure; therefore, it cannot be used to determine the effectiveness of the medication.
    2. The client's apical pulse must be assessed prior to administering the medication, but it is not used to determine the effectiveness of the medication.
    3. The client's potassium level must be assessed prior to administering the medication, but it is not used to determine the effectiveness of the medication.
    4. **Signs or symptoms of CHF are crackles in the lungs, jugular vein distention,**

and pitting edema; therefore, the medication is not effective.

84. 1. Lidocaine suppresses ventricular ectopy and is a first-line drug for the treatment of ventricular dysrhythmias, but it is not the first medication to be administered in a code.
   2. Atropine decreases vagal stimulation, which increases the heart rate and is the drug of choice for asystole, complete heart block, and symptomatic bradycardia.
   3. Adenosine is the drug of choice for terminating paroxysmal supraventricular tachycardia by decreasing the automaticity of the SA node and slows conduction through the AV node.
   4. **Epinephrine constricts the periphery, shunts the blood to the central trunk, and is the first medication administered in a client who is coding. The client does not have a pulse; therefore, the nurse must call a code.**

85. 1. The nurse would want to give this antihypertensive medication to a client with an elevated blood pressure; the nurse would question the medication if the B/P was low.
   2. The client with 2+ pitting edema would not be affected by a calcium channel blocker.
   3. **The nurse should question this medication if the apical rate is less than 60.**
   4. A headache is not an adverse effect of HCTZ; therefore, the nurse would not question administering this medication.

86. 1. **Steroids (glucocorticoids) cannot be abruptly discontinued because the adrenal glands stop producing cortisol (a steroid) when the client is taking them exogenously and the client could experience a hypotensive crisis.**
   2. Prednisone can produce gastric distress; it is given with food to minimize the gastric discomfort.
   3. Weight gain is a side effect of steroid therapy; the client should not stop taking the medication. This medication must be tapered off if the client is able to discontinue the medication at all.
   4. Prednisone, a steroid, suppresses the immune system response of the body, increasing the risk of developing an infection.

87. 1. The PEFR is defined as the maximal rate of air flow during expiration; it can be measured with a relatively inexpensive, handheld device. If the peak flow is less than 80% of the client's personal best, more frequent monitoring should be done. The PEFR should be measured every morning.
   2. A normal respiratory assessment does not indicate that the medication regimen is effective and has "good" or "bad" control.
   3. **Three asthma attacks in the last month would not indicate the client has "good" control of the reactive airway disease.**
   4. A serum theophylline level between 10 and 20 μg/mL indicates the medication is within the therapeutic range, but it is not the best indicator of the client's control of the signs or symptoms.

88. 1. Steroids increase insulin resistance; this would be an expected effect of the prednisone. The nurse would not question administering this medication.
   2. This WBC is elevated and indicates an infection. Antibiotics are administered for bacterial infections. The nurse would not question administering this medication.
   3. **The therapeutic range for this control would be 59–78 seconds. This is an extremely high PTT level, and the client is at risk for bleeding. The heparin should be discontinued immediately. The nurse would question this medication.**
   4. This theophylline level is in therapeutic range (10–20 mg/dL); the nurse would not question administering this medication.

89. 1. **The INR is outside of therapeutic range; therefore, the nurse should question administering this medication.**
   2. Vitamin K is the antidote for Coumadin toxicity. Protamine sulfate is the antidote for heparin toxicity.
   3. There is no reason to notify the HCP to request an increase in the dose; the dose should be discontinued. The HCP should be notified of this abnormal lab data.
   4. When the nurse is administering Coumadin the International Normalized Ratio (INR) must be monitored to determine therapeutic level, which is 2–3. Because the INR is 4.2, the nurse should not administer this medication.

90. 1. **The client's WBC count indicates a normal value, which would indicate the medication is effective.**
    2. This culture indicates there is still infection; therefore, the medication is not effective.
    3. This indicates medication compliance, not effectiveness of the medications.
    4. Pleurisy is noncardiac chest pain, which indicates that the medication is not effective.

91. 1. **NSAIDs decrease prostaglandin and increase the client's risk for ulcer disease. They are contraindicated for use in clients diagnosed with ulcer disease. The nurse should question this medication.**
    2. Prilosec is prescribed to treat duodenal and gastric ulcers; the nurse would not question this medication.
    3. Hypokalemia can increase digoxin toxicity. This potassium level is within normal range (3.5–5.5 mEq/L); the nurse would not question this medication.
    4. Riopan is a low sodium antacid and is the antacid of choice for clients diagnosed with CHF. The nurse would not question this medication.

92. 1. **The suppository should be retained for 1–3 hours if possible to get the maximum benefit of the medication. This statement indicates the client does not understand the medication teaching.**
    2. The client should use caution when using the suppository because it may stain clothing, flooring, painted surfaces, vinyl, enamel, marble, granite, and other surfaces. This statement indicates the client understands the teaching.
    3. The medication should be stored at room temperature away from moisture and heat. This indicates the client understands the teaching.
    4. The client should empty the bowel just before inserting the rectal suppository. This statement indicates the client understands the teaching.

93. 1. No one but the client should push the PCA button. If the client has pain, the client should push the button. Family members administering doses "whenever" could overdose the client. This statement indicates the client and family do not understand the correct use of the PCA.
    2. **The client should premedicate himself or herself with the PCA so that effective coughing, deep breathing, and turning can be performed with some degree of comfort. This indicates the client understands the teaching.**
    3. The family should let the client decide when he or she is in pain and the client should use the PCA at that time. This statement indicates the family does not understand the correct use of the PCA.
    4. The client should use the PCA before the pain level reaches this high. This statement indicates the client does not understand the correct use of the PCA.

94. 1. Medications alone will not guarantee weight loss. The client should exercise regularly and limit calories to lose an appreciable amount of weight.
    2. Some of the medications have drug interactions with selective serotonin reuptake inhibitors, MAO inhibitors, triptans, and some opioids but not with antihypertensive medications.
    3. **These symptoms indicate serotonin syndrome and can be life threatening. The nurse should teach the client to monitor the pulse and blood pressure and report significant changes.**
    4. The medications are prescribed for up to a year at a time.

95. 1. This is true, but the client is using stimulant laxatives on a daily basis. This is not the most important teaching.
    2. Fluids are increased when taking bulk laxatives to have fluid available to increase the volume of stool.
    3. **If the client insists on taking a laxative daily, it should be a bulk-forming laxative such as Metamucil. This type of laxative encourages the bowel to perform its normal job and will not harm the integrity of the bowel. Stimulant laxative use over time causes a narrowing of the lumen of the bowel and will increase the likelihood of obstipation and bowel obstruction.**
    4. Increasing the amount of stimulant laxative will increase the potential for serious complications related to laxative abuse.

96. 1. The nurse cannot delegate care of an client who is unstable, and hypoglycemia is a complication of treatment for diabetes mellitus.
2. The treatment of choice for a client who is conscious and experiencing a hypoglycemic reaction is to administer food or a source of glucose, but it is not the first intervention. Orange juice is a source of glucose and the UAP can get it.
3. The nurse should check the MAR to determine when the last dose of insulin or oral hypoglycemic medication was administered, but it is not the first intervention.
4. **These are symptoms of a hypoglycemic reaction and the nurse should assess the client immediately; therefore, this is the first intervention.**

97. 1. According to the sliding scale, blood glucose results should be verified when less than 60 or greater than 400.
2. The HCP does not need to be notified unless the blood glucose is greater than 400.
3. **The client's reading is 299; therefore, the nurse should administer 6 units of regular insulin as per the HCP's order.**
4. There is no reason for the nurse to recheck the results.

98. 1. Constipation does not determine the effectiveness of the medication.
2. Steatorrhea (fatty, frothy, foul-smelling stools) or diarrhea indicates a lack of pancreatic enzymes in the small intestines. This would indicate the dosage is too small and needs to be increased.
3. **Normal bowel movements indicate the medication is effective in preventing steatorrhea.**
4. Normal bowel sounds would not indicate the medication is effective.

99. 1. **The major symptom with DI is polyuria resulting in polydipsia (extreme thirst); therefore, the client being thirsty indicates the medication is not effective and would warrant notifying the health-care provider.**
2. If the client is able to sleep throughout the night, this indicates the client is not up urinating as a result of polyuria; therefore, the medication is effective.
3. A weight loss of 1 pound would not warrant notifying the health-care provider.
4. The client only urinating five times a day indicates the medication is effective; therefore, the client would not have to notify the HCP.

100. 1. The dose of corticosteroids may have to be increased during the stress of an infection or surgery; therefore, this statement indicates the client does not understand the discharge teaching.
2. **This statement indicates the client understands the discharge teaching. The client may be prescribed both mineral and glucocorticoid medications.**
3. If the client gets weak or dizzy, it may indicate an underdosage of medication; therefore, this indicates the client does not understand the discharge teaching.
4. The client does not have to take prophylactic antibiotics prior to invasive procedures.

Index

A

Abilify (*see* Aripiprazole)
Accidents (*see* Injuries)
Accutane, 235, 238
Acetaminophen, 124, 211, 381
  Tylenol, 31, 372
    and arthritis, 255
    and children, 240, 333, 364
    and the liver, 369
    and neurological conditions, 12, 17
Acetazolamide (Diamox), 335, 338
Acetylcysteine (Mucomyst), 77, 85–86, 403
Acetylsalicylic acid (aspirin), 50, 186
  as an antiplatelet, 73, 211
  and arthritis
    osteoarthritis, 205
    rheumatoid, 246, 255
  and coronary artery disease, 39–40, 45, 47, 397
  and gastric irritation, 55, 62
    gastric ulcers, 30, 33
Acidophilus, 110, 127
Acne, 228, 234
  SMART, 235, 238
Acquired immunodeficiency syndrome (AIDS), 242–244, 250–252, 258, 269, 396
  see also HIV
Acromegaly, 12
Actisorb Silver, 226
Activase (*see* Alteplase)
Actonel (*see* Risedronate)
Actos (*see* Pioglitazone)
Acyclovir
  Cytogenesis, 258
  Zovirax, 176, 236–237, 239
Addison's disease, 145, 162–163, 409
  crisis, 146, 156, 167
Adenosine (Adenocard), 43, 413
Adolescents, 175–176, 187–189
Adrenal disorders, 145–146, 155–158
  insufficiency, 146, 162
Adrenalectomy, 145
Adrenaline (*see* Epinephrine)
Adrenocorticotropic hormone (ACTH), 146, 157, 166
  Acthar, 162
Adriamycin (*see* Doxorubicin)
Adult respiratory distress syndrome (ARDS), 79
AeroBid (*see* Fluticasone)
African Americans, 73, 363
Afrin (*see* Oxymetazoline)
Agranulocytosis, 221
Albumin (Albuminar-5), 342
Albuterol (Ventolin), 80
Alcohol, 35, 304–305, 321
  interaction with medications, 137, 188, 367
Aldactone (*see* Spironolactone)
Aldosterone agonists, 162
Alendronate (Fosamax), 145, 206–207, 402, 416
Alkaloid, vinca, 147, 159
Allegra (*see* Fexofenadine)
Allergies, 244–245, 252–254, 373
  latex, 196, 260, 263

medications
    oxymetazoline (Afrin), 78
    pseudoephedrine (Sudafed), 77, 364, 370
  sulfa, 261
  see also Antihistamines
Allopurinol (Zyloprim), 173, 242
Aloe, 121, 234, 361, 366
Alopecia, 289
Alpha-adrenergic agonists, 172
Alpha-beta blockers, 69
5-alpha-reductase inhibitors
  dutasteride (AVODART), 172–173, 185
  finasteride (Proscar), 172, 184, 236
Alprazolam (Xanax), 299–300, 302, 305, 311–312, 315
  and neurological conditions, 10, 12
Alteplase (Activase), 10, 83
Aluminum hydroxide (Amphojel), 169–170
Alupent (*see* Metaproterenol)
Alzheimer's disease (AD), 14–15, 25–26, 371, 421
Amantadine (Symmetrel), 13, 24, 29, 32
Ambien CR, 320, 345
Aminophylline, 80, 396
Amiodarone (Cordarone), 395
Amitriptyline (Elavil), 296, 319
Ammonia, 106, 121
Amoxicillin (Augmentin), 77
Amphetamines, 301–302, 304, 313–314, 316, 403
Amphotericin B (Fungizone), 243
Amputation (*see* Surgery)
Anakinra (Kineret), 269
Analgesics
  acetaminophen, 124, 211, 381
    and arthritis, 255
    and children, 240, 333, 364
    and the liver, 369
    and neurological conditions, 12, 17
    Tylenol, 31, 372
  acetylsalicylic acid (aspirin), 50
    and arthritis, 246, 255
    and coronary artery disease, 397
    and gastric irritation, 30, 33, 55, 62
  capsaicin cream
    Capsin, 205
    Zostrix, 246
  narcotics, 12, 50
    see also Opioids
  patient-controlled (PCA), 131, 215
    and cancer, 273
    and narcotics, 174, 186, 208
    postsurgery, 114, 408
Anastrozole (Arimidex), 269
Ancef (*see* Cephalosporin)
Anemia, 51–52, 66–68, 269, 362, 371
  aplastic, 51
  and cancer, 290
  folic acid deficiency, 52, 67
  immunohemolytic, 52, 68
  iron-deficiency, 51, 71, 404
  pernicious, 363
  sickle cell, 51

Anesthesia
  bupivacaine (Marcaine), 219
  epidural, 174, 187
    catheter, 177
  general, 113–114, 131–132
  post-care unit (PACU), 114
  pramoxine (Proctofoam), 177
  spinal, 172–173, 184–186, 196, 200, 273
Angelica sinensis (*see* Dong quai)
Angina, 37–38, 40, 53–54
Angioedema, 57
Angiotensin converting enzyme (ACE) inhibitors,
    42, 56
  and African Americans, 73
  captopril (Capoten), 48
  enalapril (Vasotec), 10, 41
  lisinopril (Zestril), 38
Anorexia nervosa, 319–320, 322
Anorexiants, 32
Antabuse (*see* Disulfiram)
Antacids, 101, 104, 400
  aluminum hydroxide (Amphojel), 169–170
  Maalox, 134, 380, 384
  magnesium hydroxide (Milk of Magnesia),
    104, 119
  and pancreatitis, 144
  Riopan, 118
Anthrax, 343, 349
Antibacterial agents, 226
Antibiotics, 47, 61, 86, 120
  aminoglycoside
    gentamycin, 46, 356
    vancomycin, 171, 183, 218, 341, 381
  amoxicillin (Augmentin), 77
  ceftriaxone (Rocephin), 105, 175, 188, 341, 347
  cephalosporin (Ancef), 95, 208
  clarithromycin (Biaxin), 337
  clavulanate, 77
  mupirocin (Bactroban), 236
  natamycin (Natacyn), 336
  reaction to, 245
  resistant organisms, 79, 86–87
  silver nitrate (Dey-Drop), 336
  sulfa, 109
  sulfasalazine (Azulfidine), 102–103, 117, 255
  topical, 220
    Neosporin, 17
    ophthalmic ointment, 327, 339
Anticholinergics, 24
  benztropine (Cogentin), 13
  scopolamine (Transderm Scop), 136
  tolterodine (Detrol-LA), 195
Anticoagulants
  heparin, 220, 381
    administration of, 385, 387, 404–405
    and CVA, 21
    and DVT, 49–50, 65–66
    and pulmonary embolism, 83–84, 91–92
  warfarin (Coumadin), 405, 408
    and DVT, 49, 65, 71
    interaction with medications, 138
    and pulmonary embolism, 83, 91
Anticonvulsants, 9–10, 19
  carbamazepine (Tegretol), 8, 18, 297, 308–309
  fosphenytoin (Cerebyx), 9, 19
  magnesium sulfate, 195
  phenytoin (Dilantin), 8, 12, 19, 23, 29–30, 413
  valproic acid (Depakote), 297, 308
Antidepressants, 296, 307
  bupropion (Wellbutrin), 325
  nefazodone (Serzone), 296
  tricyclic
    amitriptyline (Elavil), 296, 319
    desipramine (Norpramin), 322
    imipramine (Tofranil), 296
  Zyban, 128

Antidiabetic medications
  exenatide (BYETTA), 164, 168
  glyburide (Glucovance), 143
  metformin, 143
    Glucophage, 111, 166
Antidiarrheals, 113, 134
Antidysrhythmics, 399
  adenosine (Adenocard), 43, 413
  amiodarone, 395
  atropine sulfate, 43
  lidocaine, 44, 59, 73, 205, 344
Antiemetics, 114, 131
  prochlorperazine (Compazine), 110, 286
  promethazine (Phenergan), 133, 135, 138, 382
Antiepileptic drugs (AED), 33
Antifungals
  amphotericin B (Fungizone), 243
  ketoconazole, 157, 292, 376
Antihistamines, 123, 245, 252–253, 315
  cyproheptadine (Periactin), 319
  diphenhydramine (Benadryl), 244, 263, 315, 369
  meclizine (Antivert), 31, 335
  see also Allergies
Antihyperlipidemics, 39, 55
Antimania medications, 296–298, 308–309, 320, 403
Antimicrobials
  hydrocolloid, 227
  topical
    mafenide acetate (Sulfamylon), 225–226, 230, 402
    silver nitrate, 225
Antineoplastic agents, 287
  doxorubicin (Adriamycin), 289
  megestrol (Megace), 269, 280
  methotrexate (Rheumatrex), 228, 233, 402, 417
  vesicant, 289
  vinca alkaloid, 265
Antiobesity medication, 110–111, 127–129
Antioxidants, 372, 375, 404, 420
Antiplatelets, 62
  acetylsalicylic acid (aspirin), 73, 186, 211
    and coronary artery disease, 39–40, 45, 47
  clopidogrel bisulfate (Plavix), 40, 47, 293
Antipruritics, 136, 233
Antipsychotics, 298–299, 310–311, 319, 323
  atypical
    clozapine (Clozaril), 298, 310
    quetiapine (Seroquel), 299
    risperidone (Risperdal), 298
    ziprasidone (Geodon), 298, 310
  chlorpromazine (Thorazine), 242, 299, 321
  haloperidol (Haldol), 33, 299, 311
  sedative effects, 25, 33
Antirejection medications, 197, 200
Antiretrovirals
  acyclovir (Zovirax), 176, 237, 239
  HAART, 251
Antirheumatics
  disease-modifying drugs (DMARD)
    hydroxychloroquine sulfate (Plaquenil), 245, 259,
      262, 403
    leflunomide (Arava), 245
    methotrexate (Rheumatrex), 246, 254, 259, 262
    sulfasalazine (Azulfidine), 246
Antispasmotics, 373
  baclofen (Lioresal), 204, 210, 242
  botulinum toxin (Botox), 402
  propantheline (Pro-Banthine), 134
Antithyroid medications, 161
  propylthiouracil (PTU), 148–149, 160
Antituberculars, 94
Antitussives, 95, 97–98
  dextromethorphan, 77
    Robitussin, 323
  hydrocodone
    Hycodan, 94
    Vicodin, 31, 35, 78, 86

Antivirals
  acyclovir
    Cytogenesis, 258
    Zovirax, 236
  amantadine (Symmetrel), 13, 24, 29, 32
  ganciclovir (Cytovene), 243, 261
  interferon alfacon (Infergen), 108
  ribavirin (Virazole), 108, 124
Anxiety disorders, 299–300, 311–313
Anxiolytics
  alprazolam (Xanax), 300, 311–312, 315
  diazepam (Valium), 300
Appendectomy, 301
Appetite suppressants (*see* Anorexiants)
AquaMEPHYTON, 64–65, 74, 195
Aranesp (*see* Darbepoetin)
Arava (*see* Leflunomide)
Aricept (*see* Donepezil)
Arimidex (*see* Anastrozole)
Aripiprazole (Abilify), 298, 310
Aromatase inhibitors, 280
  anastrozole (Arimidex), 269
Arterial occlusive disease, 46–47, 61–63
  hypertension, 47–49, 63–64
Arthritis
  osteoarthritis, 204–206, 210–212
  rheumatoid, 245–246, 254–255, 259, 271, 403
Arthrocentesis, 217, 220
Asacol (*see* Mesalamine)
Ascites, 107
Asian Americans, 323
Aspirin (*see* Acetylsalicylic acid)
Asthma, 81–82, 362, 422
  acute exacerbation, 94–95
  and GERD, 102, 369
  intermittent, 81, 90
  zone system, 82, 90–91
Asystole, 344, 351, 403
Atarax (*see* Hydroxyzine)
Atenolol (Tenormin), 10, 49
Atherosclerosis, 362
Athlete's foot (*see* Tinea pedis)
Ativan (*see* Lorazepam)
Atomoxetine (Strattera), 314, 319, 324
Atopic dermatitis (eczema), 228
Atorvastatin (Lipitor), 39, 56, 400
Atrial fibrillation, 59
Atropine, 29, 34, 58, 419
  and asystole, 59, 351
  and glaucoma, 32
  sulfate, 43
Attention deficit-hyperactivity disorder (ADHD), 301–302, 313–315, 319–320, 403
Augmentin (*see* Amoxicillin)
Autoimmune disease, 241–242, 249–250
Autolytic medications, 226
Autotransfusion drainage system (cell saver), 208
AVODART (*see* Dutasteride)
Avonex (*see* Interferon)
Azathioprine (Imuran), 102, 116, 259, 262
AZT, 251
Aztreonam (Azactam), 171
Azulfidine (*see* Sulfasalazine)

B

Bacid, 129
Back pain (*see* Pain)
Baclofen (Lioresal), 204, 210, 242, 249
Bactrim (*see* Trimethoprim sulfa)
Bactroban (*see* Mupirocin)
Baldness, male pattern, 236
Balneotherapy, 233
Belladonna and opiate (B & O), 172, 185
Benadryl (*see* Diphenhydramine)
Benzodiazepines, 315
  alprazolam (Xanax), 10, 12, 299–300, 302, 305

chlordiazepoxide (Librium), 399
  diazepam (Valium), 302, 313, 335, 338
  lorazepam (Ativan), 299, 302, 311, 315
Benztropine (Cogentin), 13
Beta-adrenergics
  betaxolol (Betoptic), 328, 335
  terbutaline (Brethine), 176, 190
Beta blockers, 48–49, 63, 338
  atenolol (Tenormin), 10
  metoprolol (Lopressor), 47
  propranolol (Inderal), 16
Beta$_1$-adrenergic agonists, 56, 342
Betadine, 209
Betaxolol (Betoptic), 328, 335
Bethanechol (Urecholine), 29, 183
Betoptic (*see* Betaxolol)
Biaxin (*see* Clarithromycin)
Bigeminy, 59, 74
Biguanides, 142, 152, 163
Bilberry, 109, 125
Bile-acid sequestrants, 39
Biologic response modifiers, 268–269, 277–279
  erythropoietin, 278
    Epogen, 169, 181, 278–279
  filgrastim (Neupogen), 397
  interferon
    alfa (Roferon), 134
    beta-1a (Avonex), 259
    Intron A, 268, 278
Bioterrorism, 342–343, 348–350
Bipolar disorder, 296–298, 307–309, 320, 403
Birth control, 179–180, 192–194, 365
  condoms, 179, 193
  contraceptives (oral), 179–180, 193, 198, 235, 239
  depot medroxyprogesterone (Depo-Provera), 180
  mifepristone (RU-486), 355, 359
  spermicide, 179, 192
  vaginal rings, 180, 193
Bis in die (b.i.d.), 5
Bisacodyl (Dulcolax), 262, 408
Bismuth subcarbonate, 136, 139
Bisphosphonate regulators, 145, 206–207, 402, 416
Bladder
  infections, 171
  spasms, 172
Bleeding, esophageal, 107
Blood, packed red cells (PRBC), 208, 290
Bone deformities, 147
Bone resorption inhibitors, 218
Botox injections, 228, 402, 417
Botulism, 343, 349–350, 356
Bowels, inflammatory disease (IBD), 102–103, 116–118
Brain
  natriuretic peptide (BNP), 41
  tumors, 11–12, 21–23, 31, 270, 273, 405
Brethine (*see* Terbutaline)
Bromocriptine (Parlodel), 178
Bronchodilators, 80
Bronkodyl (*see* Theophylline)
Bruising (*see* Ecchymosis)
Bulimia, 326
Bulk-forming agents, 106, 121
Bumetanide (Bumex), 48
Bundle branch block (BBB), 58
Bunionectomy, 219
Bupivacaine (Marcaine), 219
Bupropion (Wellbutrin), 325
Burns, 225–226, 230–231, 236, 361, 398
  and antimicrobials, 402
  chemical, 355, 358–359
  electrical, 230
  and Zantac, 104
Butazolidin (*see* Phenylbutazone)
Buttermilk, 340
BYETTA (*see* Exenatide)

C

Caffeine, 88, 99, 310, 316–317
Caladryl, 263
Calcibind (*see* Cellulose sodium phosphate)
Calcitonin (Calcimar), 206, 212–213
Calcitriol (Rocaltrol), 169, 181
Calcium alginate, 47
Calcium channel blockers (CCB), 42, 49, 53
Calcium EDTA (*see* Edetate calcium disodium)
Calcium gluconate (Kalcinate), 206
Cancer, 136, 365
    breast, 267, 269–270, 280, 289
    colon, 272
    lung, 267, 273
    osteosarcoma, 275
    ovarian, 273
    pancreatic, 272–273
    prostate, 269, 273
    skin, 229
    surgery, 272–273, 282–284, 290
    terminal, 273
    treatments, 265–294
    see also Chemotherapy
Cannabinoids, 139
    dronabinol (Marinol), 136
Capsaicin cream
    Capsin, 205
    Zostrix, 246
Captopril (Capoten), 48
Carafate (*see* Sucralfate)
Carbamazepine (Tegretol), 8, 18, 297, 308–309
Carbidopa (Sinemet), 12–13, 23
Carbon monoxide, 346, 353
Carbonic anhydrase inhibitors, 335, 338
Cardiac disorders, 45–46, 59–61
Cardiac glycosides
    and CHF, 41–42, 70
    digoxin, 18, 57, 72, 345
        Lanoxin, 2–3, 69, 379, 399, 407
Cardiovascular system, 37–75
Cascara, 106, 121, 375
Castor oil, 129
Catapres, 73
Catechol-O-methyltransferase (COMT) inhibitors, 13, 24
Catheterization
    cardiac, 71
    epidural, 177
    indwelling, 170, 172, 181
    urinary (Foley), 196, 199
Cation exchange resins, 170, 181, 401, 415
Ceftriaxone (Rocephin), 105, 175, 188, 341, 347
Celecoxib (Celebrex), 204, 206, 218, 222
Cellulitis, 236
Cellulose sodium phosphate (Calcibind), 174, 187
Cephalosporin, 175
    Ancef, 95, 208
Cephulac (*see* Lactulose)
Cerebrovascular accidents (CVA), 10–11, 20–21, 31, 354
Cerebyx (*see* Fosphenytoin)
Ceruminolytics, 336, 340
Cervidil, 190
Charcoal, activated, 345, 352
Chasteberry, 371, 374
Chelating agents, 346
Chemotherapy, 265–268, 276–277, 397, 403
Chickenpox, 247
Childbearing (*see* Pregnancy; Women's issues)
Children
    gastroenteritis, 109–110, 125–127
    immunizations, 247–248, 255–257
    oral replacement therapy (ORT), 126
    poisons, 345–346, 351–353
    reactive airway disease, 81–82, 90–91
Chlamydia trachomatis, 175, 196, 199

Chlordiazepoxide (Librium), 144, 154, 316, 399, 413
Chlorine gas, 342, 348
Chlorothiazide (Diuril), 48
Chlorpromazine (Thorazine), 242, 299, 321
Chlorpropamide (Diabinese), 147, 158
Chlorzoxazone (Parafon Forte), 218, 402
Cholecystectomy, 78, 113–114
Cholesterol, 39, 55
Cholestyramine, 125
Cholinesterase inhibitors, 25
    donepezil (Aricept), 14–15, 26, 405, 421
    edrophonium (Tensilon), 242
    galantamine (Reminyl), 14–15, 25–26
    rivastigmine (Exelon), 14, 25
Chondroitin, 218
Chorionic gonadotrophin (Chorigon), 147
Chronic obstructive pulmonary disease (COPD) (*see* Pulmonary disease)
Chronulac (*see* Lactulose)
Cimetidine (Tagamet), 101, 115, 325
Citrucel (*see* Methylcellulose)
Clarithromycin (Biaxin), 337
Clavulanate, 77
Clemastine (Tavist), 244
Clomiphene (Clomid), 178, 191
Clonidine, 324
Clopidogrel bisulfate (Plavix), 21, 40, 47, 293
Clorthalidone, 49
Clostridium
    difficile, 109
    tetani, 230
Clozapine (Clozaril), 298, 310
Code, 344–345, 350–351
Codeine, 376
Cogentin (*see* Benztropine)
Colace (*see* Docusate sodium)
Colitis, ulcerative, 102
Colloids, 347
    albumin (Albuminar-5), 342
    dextran, 341
Colonoscopy, 106
CombiDerm (*see* Hydrocolloids)
Compazine (*see* Prochlorperazine)
Computed tomography (CT) scan, 7–8, 17, 163, 300, 395
Computing math (medications), 380–382, 384–386
Comtan (*see* Entacapone)
Concussions, 7, 17, 405
Condoms, 179, 193
Conduction problems, 42–44, 57–59
Congestive heart failure (CHF), 41–42, 56–57
Conjunctivitis
    acute bacterial, 336
    bilateral, 327, 403
Constipation, 22, 112–113, 129–131, 396
Contin (*see* Morphine)
Contraceptives (oral), 20, 179–180, 193, 198, 235, 239
    emergency, 200
    see also Birth control
Contrast dye, 8, 17, 395, 410
CoQ10, 373, 377
Cordarone (*see* Amiodarone)
Coricidin HBP, 369
Cornstarch, 133, 137
Coronary artery disease (CAD), 39–40, 54–56, 397, 400
    and aspirin, 70
    and nitroglycerin, 71, 405
Corticosteroids, 155, 191
    anti-inflammatory, 18
    intraarticular, 205
    mineral, 156–157
        fludrocortisone (Florinef), 146
    prednisolone, 81
    therapy, 177
Cough suppressants (*see* Antitussives)

Coumadin (*see* Warfarin)
COX-2 inhibitors, 204, 206, 218, 222
Crabs (*see* Pediculosis)
Cranberry juice, 182
Crohn's disease, 52, 67, 103, 400
Cromolyn (Intal), 81–82, 90
Cryotherapy, 176
Crystalluria, 116
Curling's ulcer, 119, 231
Cushing's disease, 145–146, 157
    iatrogenic, 146
Cyanide, 343, 350
Cyanocobalamin (Cyanabin), 363, 375
Cyclobenzaprine (Flexeril), 203
Cycloplegics, 327, 331
Cyclosporine, 197, 200, 263
    Gengraf, 260
Cylert (*see* Pemoline)
Cyproheptadine (Periactin), 319
Cystic fibrosis (CF), 94–95, 162
Cytogenesis (*see* Acyclovir)
Cytomel (*see* Liothyronine)
Cytotec (*see* Misoprostol)
Cytovene (*see* Ganciclovir)

D

Darbepoetin (Aranesp), 268, 290, 293
DDAVP (*see* Vasopressin)
DDS (*see* Dopamine)
Debriding agents, 232
    Accuzyme papain-urea, 227
    dextranomer (Debrisan), 47
    enzymatic, 235, 238
Debrisan (*see* Dextranomer)
Debrox, 336
Decadron (*see* Dexamethasone)
Decongestants, 398, 412
Deep vein thrombosis (DVT), 49–50, 64–66, 71,
    82, 405
Deltasone (*see* Prednisone)
Demerol (*see* Meperidine)
Depakote (*see* Valproate; Valproic acid)
Depot medroxyprogesterone (Depo-Provera), 180, 194
Depressive disorder, 29, 108, 295–296, 306–307, 396
DermaDress, 227, 233
DermaKlenz, 232
Dermatitis
    allergic, 245
    seborrheic, 235
DES (*see* Diethylstilbestrol)
Desipramine (Norpramin), 322
Desmopressin (DDAVP), 146, 159, 162, 409
Detrol-LA (*see* Tolterodine)
DEXA, 221
Dexamethasone, 22
    Decadron, 270, 280, 405, 421
Dexedrine, 111
Dextran, 341
Dextranomer (Debrisan), 47
Dextromethorphan (Robitussin), 77, 85, 323
Dextrose, 359
Dey-Drop (*see* Silver nitrate)
Diabetes
    gestational, 195
    insipidus (DI), 146–147, 158, 162, 409, 424
        nephrogenic, 147
    mellitus, 163, 373, 409
        education, 143, 153
        and immunizations, 247
        type 1, 141–142, 150–151, 163–164, 356, 401
        type 2, 111, 142–144, 151–154, 164, 354
Diabetic ketoacidosis (DKA), 150, 163
Diabinese (*see* Chlorpropamide)
Diamox (*see* Acetazolamide)

Diarrhea, 111–113, 129–131
    and chemotherapy, 267, 277
    and gastroenteritis, 109, 125
    and peptic ulcers, 104
Diazepam (Valium), 9, 19, 300, 302, 313
    and endolymphatic hydrops, 335, 338
Diethylstilbestrol (DES), 270, 280
Digestive enzymes, 136
Digoxin, 18, 57, 72, 345
    and CHF, 41–42, 70
    Lanoxin, 2–3, 69, 379, 399, 407
    sample card, 4
Dilantin (*see* Phenytoin)
Dilaudid (*see* Hydromorphone)
Dimenhydrinate (Dramamine), 34
Diphenhydramine (Benadryl), 244, 263, 315, 369
Diphenoxylate (Lomotil), 113, 134, 137
Disulfiram (Antabuse), 305, 317
Diuretics, 123
    loop, 48–49, 56
        bumetanide (Bumex), 48
        furosemide (Lasix), 2–3, 10, 14, 41, 147, 173
    osmotic, 7–8
        mannitol (Osmitrol), 11, 17–18, 22, 30–31, 399, 413
    potassium-sparing, 72
        spironolactone (Aldactone), 69, 107, 123, 162
    thiazide, 49, 56, 173, 186
        chlorothiazide (Diuril), 48
        hydrochlorothiazide, 41, 170
Diuril (*see* Chlorothiazide; Hydrochlorothiazide)
Diverticulitis/diverticulosis, 105–106, 120–121, 408
DMARD (*see* Antirheumatics)
Dobutamine (Dobutrex), 56, 342
Docusate calcium (Surfak), 106
Docusate sodium (Colace), 105–106, 120–121
Donepezil (Aricept), 14–15, 26, 405, 421
Dong quai (*Angelica sinensis*), 195, 199, 361
Dopamine, 341–342, 344, 348, 351, 382
    agonists, 24
    system stabilizers (DDS), 298, 310
Doxorubicin (Adriamycin), 289
Dramamine (*see* Dimenhydrinate)
Dronabinol (Marinol), 136
Drug cards (samples), 3–5
Dulcolax (*see* Bisacodyl)
Dutasteride (AVODART), 172–173, 185
Dyspnea, 82
Dysrhythmias, 42–44, 57–59

E

E Mycin (*see* Erythromycin)
Ear infections, 328–330, 332–334
Ecchymosis, 217, 220
Echinacea purpurea, 362, 367
Ectoparasiticides, 176
Eczema (*see* Atopic dermatitis)
Edetate calcium disodium (Calcium EDTA), 346
Edrophonium (Tensilon), 242
Elavil (*see* Amitriptyline)
Eldepryl (*see* Selegiline)
Elderly clients, 5
Electroconvulsive therapy (ECT), 29
Electrolytes, 170, 182
Embolus, pulmonary, 82–84, 91–93
Emergency department (ED), 342–343, 354
Emphysema, 78
Enalapril (Vasotec), 10, 41
Endocarditis, subacute bacterial (SBE), 45–46
Endocrine system, 141–168
Endolymphatic hydrops (Meniere's disease), 335,
    338
Endometriosis, 178
Endoscopic examination, 110
Entacapone (Comtan), 13, 24

Ephedra, 361–362, 366–367
Epiglottitis, 96
Epilepsy, 9, 19, 29–30
  remission, spontaneous, 30
Epinephrine, 344, 350, 422
  adrenaline, 94
  Epitrate, 327
  racemic, 95
EpiPen, 252
Episiotomy, 177
Epogen (*see* Erythropoietin)
Erectile dysfunction, 20, 38, 48
Ergot alkaloids, 177
Erythromycin
  E Mycin, 175
  ophthalmic ointment, 336
Erythropoietin, 278
  Epogen, 169, 181, 268, 278–279
  Procrit, 66, 268–269
Escherichia coli, 110, 127, 129
Eskalith (*see* Lithium)
Esomeprazole (Nexium), 102
Estar (*see* Tar preparation)
Estrogen, 192, 194, 235
  clomiphene (Clomid), 178, 191
  diethylstilbestrol (DES), 270, 280
  SERM, 206
  tamoxifen (Nolvadex), 270, 279, 281
Ethambutol, 252
Etodolac (Lodine), 246
Evista (*see* Raloxifene)
Exelon (*see* Rivastigmine)
Exenatide (BYETTA), 164, 168
Exercise, 128, 130
Exubera (*see* Insulin)
Eye disorders, 327–328, 331–332
Ezetimibe (Zetia), 39, 55

F

Face peel, chemical, 236
Famotidine (Pepcid), 226
Ferrous sulfate (Feosol), 176
Fertilization, in vitro (IVF), 178
Feverfew, 15, 27
Fexofenadine (Allegra), 244, 253
Fibrillation, ventricular, 344–345, 351, 407
Filgrastim (Neupogen), 397
Finasteride (Proscar), 172, 184, 236
Flagyl (*see* Metronidazole)
Flax seed oil, 373
Fleets Phospho-Soda (*see* Sodium biphosphate)
Flexeril (*see* Cyclobenzaprine)
Flomax (*see* Tamsulosin)
Florinef (*see* Fludrocortisone)
Fludrocortisone (Florinef), 146
Fluoride, 213
Fluoxetine (Prozac), 295, 319, 396
Fluticasone
  AeroBid, 389
  Flonase, 244
Folic acid, 362, 367, 374, 395, 410
  deficiency, 52, 67
Fosamax (*see* Alendronate)
Fosphenytoin (Cerebyx), 9, 19
Fosrenol (*see* Lanthanum)
Francisella tularensis (tularemia), 343, 349, 356, 360
Fungizone (*see* Amphotericin B)
Furosemide (Lasix), 2–3, 10, 14, 41, 48, 147, 173
  sample card, 4

G

Galantamine (Reminyl), 14–15, 25–26
Gallbladder, 78, 113–114
Gamma globulin, 261

Ganciclovir (Cytovene), 243, 261
Gardasil, 260
Garlic, 85, 366, 372, 375
Gastrectomy, 114
Gastric bleeding, 55
Gastritis, 40
Gastroenteritis, 109–110, 125–127, 133
Gastrointestinal agents, 134, 138
Gastrointestinal reflux disease (GERD), 101–102, 115–116, 369, 400
Gastrointestinal system, 101–139
Gengraf (*see* Cyclosporine)
Genitourinary system, 169–201
Gentamycin, 46, 356
Geodon (*see* Ziprasidone)
Gingival hyperplasia, 18
Ginkgo biloba, 62, 205, 211
  and Alzheimer's disease, 15, 29, 33, 375
Ginseng, 143, 153
Glasgow Coma Scale, 34
Glaucoma, 24, 328, 335, 337, 340
  and atropine, 32
  open-angle, 327
  and ophthalmic medications, 398
Glipizide (Glucotrol), 142
Glomerulonephritis, 171
Glucocorticoids, 156, 241, 245, 422
  dexamethasone, 22
    Decadron, 270, 280, 405, 421
  fluticasone
    AeroBid, 389
    Flonase, 389
  hydrocortisone, 219, 245
    Solu-Cortef, 241
    topical, 237
  inhalers, 80
  methylprednisolone sodium succinate (Solu-Medrol), 45, 79, 400
  prednisolone, 261
    Pediapred, 258
  prednisone, 103, 133, 163, 167
    and arthritis, 246, 255
    and COPD, 407
    Deltasone, 145
Glucocorticosteroids, 244
Glucophage (*see* Metformin)
Glucosamine, 218
Glucose, blood levels, 152–153
Glucotrol (*see* Glipizide)
Glyburide (Glucovance), 143
GnRH medications, 178, 191, 269
Gold salts, 259, 262
GoLYTELY, 135, 138, 352
Gonadotrophin, human chorionic (HCG), 178
Gonorrhea, 175, 188
Good Samaritan Act, 357
Gout, 242
Grapefruit juice, 32, 53, 198
Growth hormone (GH), 12, 23, 166
Guillain-Barré (GB) syndrome, 258, 261

H

H_1 receptor antagonists
  clemastine (Tavist), 244
  fexofenadine (Allegra), 244, 253
H_2 receptor blockers, 115
  ranitidine (Zantac), 104
HAART (*see* Therapies)
Hallux valgus, 219, 222
Haloperidol (Haldol), 33, 299, 311
Hawthorn extract, 41, 56, 362, 367
Head lice, 238, 373
Headaches, 143
  brain tumor, 12

cluster, 28
medication overuse (MOH), 27
migraine, 15–16, 26–28
rebound, 27
and substance abuse, 305
tension, 16
Heart failure, congestive (CHF), 41–42, 56–57, 73, 104, 173, 407
Heartburn (*see* Pyrosis)
Heatstroke, 354
Helicobacter pylori, 104–105, 118
Hematocrit, 104, 119
Hematomas, 71
Hematopoietic growth factors, 268
    darbepoetin (Aranesp), 268, 290, 293
    erythropoietin
        Epogen, 169, 181, 268
        Procrit, 66, 268–269
    oprelvekin (Neumega), 268, 277
Hematuria, 181
Hemodialysis, 170
Hemoglobin, 104, 119
    glycosylated (A1C), 151
Hemorrhage, postpartum, 177
Hemorrheologic agents, 46
Hemorrhoids, 372
Heparin, 220, 381
    administration of, 385, 387, 404–405
    and CVA, 21
    and DVT, 49–50, 65–66
    Lovenox, 65, 208, 215, 217
    and pulmonary embolus, 83–84, 91–92
Hepatitis, 108–109, 123–125, 134
    A, 108, 123–124
    B, 108–109, 247, 256, 258
        immune globulin (HBIG), 124
    C, 108, 124, 268
Herbs (*see* Natural remedies)
Hernia
    disc, 204
    hiatal, 102, 116
    inguinal, 113
Herpes, 237
    simplex 2, 176, 188, 402
    zoster, 236
Histamine$_2$ antagonists, 226
Histamine$_2$ blockers, 101, 115, 325
HMG-CoA reductase inhibitors
    atorvastatin (Lipitor), 39, 56, 400
    simvastatin (Zocor), 39
Hodgkin's disease, 147
Hormones
    adrenocorticotropic (ACTH), 146, 157, 162, 166
    antiestrogen, 270, 279, 281
    estrogen, 192, 235
        antagonists, 178, 191
        diethylstilbestrol (DES), 270, 280
        excess, 194
    gonadotrophin
        human chorionic (HCG), 178
        releasing (GnRH), 178
    growth (GH), 12, 23, 166
        somatropin (Humatrope), 162
    leptin, 111
    melatonin, 315, 371, 374
    pituitary
        desmopressin (DDAVP), 162, 409
        vasopressin, 11, 22, 107, 122
    replacement, 162
    replacement therapy (HRT), 206, 213
    SIADH, 147, 159
    stimulatory, 145
    substitutes, 147
    suppressants, 12, 23, 145, 155, 158
    therapy, 26, 269–270, 279–281
    thyroid

levothyroxine (Synthroid), 148–149, 160, 162, 401
    liothyronine (Cytomel), 148
Hospice, 273
HPV (*see* Papillomavirus)
Humalog, 142, 151
Human immunodeficiency virus (HIV), 188, 243, 251, 403
    see also AIDS
Humatrope (*see* Somatropin)
Humulin, 141, 155, 376, 401, 415
Hyalgan (*see* Sodium hyaluronate)
Hydrochlorothiazide
    Diuril, 41
    HydroDIURIL, 170
Hydrocodone, 273, 284
    Hycodan, 94
    Vicodin, 31, 35, 78, 86, 219
Hydrocolloids, 227, 232
    CombiDerm, 227
Hydrocortisone, 219, 245
    Solu-Cortef, 241, 249
    topical, 237
Hydrogels, 227, 232
Hydromorphone (Dilaudid), 219
Hydroxychloroquine sulfate (Plaquenil), 245, 259, 262, 403
Hydroxyzine (Atarax), 136, 233
Hyperaldosteronism, 162, 165
Hyperalimentation, 103
Hypercalcemia, 213
Hyperglycemia, 23
Hypermagnesemia, 139
Hyperphosphatemia, 181
Hypertension (HTN), 10, 20–21, 85, 356
    arterial, 47–49, 63–64
    essential, 48, 106, 364
    and herbs, 78
Hyperthyroidism, 148–149, 163
Hyperuricemia, 250
Hypoglycemia, 152–153, 167–168, 359, 424
    medications, 143–144
Hypokalemia, 64, 72, 165, 413
Hyponatremia, 159
Hypotension, 53, 185
    orthostatic, 54, 63
Hypothyroidism, 148–149, 162, 167, 401
Hysterectomy, 162
Hytrin, 185

I

Ibuprofen, 364
    Motrin, 45, 104, 241
Ileostomy, 136, 139
Imferon (*see* Iron dextran)
Imipramine (Tofranil), 296
Imitrex (*see* Sumatriptan)
Immune inflammatory system, 241–263
Immunizations (children), 247–248, 255–257
Immunomodulators, 269
Immunosuppressants
    azathioprine (Imuran), 102, 116, 259, 262
    cyclosporine (Gengraf), 260
Impetigo, 236
Imuran (*see* Azathioprine)
Incontinence, 195
Inderal (*see* Propranolol)
Indigestion, 104
Indomethacin (Indocin), 174
Infections
    anthrax, 343, 349
    bladder, 171
    botulism, 343, 349–350, 356
    Chlamydia trachomatis, 175, 196, 199
    Clostridium
        difficile, 109
        tetani, 230

Infections (*Continued*)
  cytomegalovirus, 243
  ear, 328–330, 332–334
  Escherichia coli, 110, 127, 129
  eye, 336
  Francisella tularensis (tularemia), 343, 349, 356, 360
  Helicobacter pylori, 104–105, 118
  human papillomavirus, 260
  kidney, 109
  Pneumocystis carinii, 244, 251
  respiratory
    lower, 78–79, 86–88
    upper, 77–78, 85–86
  rotavirus, 110
  Shigella, 110
  smallpox, 342, 349
  Staphylococcus aureus, 171
  urinary tract (UTI), 170–172, 182–184, 195
  yeast, 89, 365
Infergen (*see* Interferon)
Infertility, 177–179, 191–192
Inflammatory bowel disease (IBD), 102–103, 116–118, 133, 408
Inflammatory cardiac disorders, 45–46, 59–61
Influenza, 77–78
Injuries, head, 7–8, 17–18, 354, 395, 399
Insect bites, 244, 403
Insomnia, 302, 314, 320, 364
Insulin, 142, 163, 167
  human origin (Exubera), 164
  pen injector, 141, 150
  pump, 142, 150
  rapid-acting (Humalog), 142, 151
  sliding-scale, 143
  therapy, 141, 150
  vial storage, 142, 151
Intal (*see* Cromolyn)
Integumentary system, 225–240
Interferon, 137
  alfa (Roferon), 134
  alfacon (Infergen), 108
  beta-1a (Avonex), 259
  Intron A, 268, 278
International Normalized Ratio (INR), 65, 71, 91–92, 405, 422
Intron A (*see* Interferon)
Investigational protocols, 270–272, 281–282
Iodine, 74, 131
  radioactive (I^{131}), 148–149
Iodosorb gel, 227, 232
Ipecac, 345, 352
Iron dextran (Imferon), 51
Iron preparation, 189, 362, 371, 374, 404, 419
  and anemia, 71
  ferrous sulfate (Feosol), 176
  iron dextran (Imferon), 51
Irritable bowel syndrome (IBS), 134, 138
Isoniazid (INH), 95, 99
Isopto Carpine (*see* Pilocarpine)
Isoxsuprine (Vasodilan), 46

K

Kalcinate (*see* Calcium gluconate)
Kayexalate, 170, 181, 401, 415
Ketoconazole, 157, 292, 376
Kidney disease
  chronic, 197, 268
    renal failure, 169–170, 181–182
  infections, 109
  renal calculi (stones), 173–175, 186–187
  transplant, 197
Kineret (*see* Anakinra)
Kwell (*see* Lindane)

L

L-dopa (*see* Levodopa)

Labetalol (Normodyne), 69
Lacerations, 7
Lactase (Lactaid), 136, 139
Lactose intolerance, 136
Lactulose, 138
  Cephulac, 106–107
  Chronulac, 135
Lanoxin (*see* Digoxin)
Lanthanum (Fosrenol), 170, 182
Laparotomy, 113
Laryngotracheobronchitis (LTB), 95
Lasix (*see* Furosemide)
Laxatives, 22, 129, 136
  bulk, 120, 139, 423
    methylcellulose (Citrucel), 105
    psyllium mucilloid (Metamucil), 14, 105
  cascara, 375
  castor oil, 129
  lactulose
    Cephulac, 106–107
    Chronulac, 135
  osmotic, 106, 121
  stimulant, 129, 139
    bisacodyl (Dulcolax), 262, 408
    GoLYTELY, 135, 138, 352
    senna (Senokot), 113, 121, 130
Lead, 346
Leflunomide (Arava), 245
Leptin, 111, 127
Leucovorin, 252
Leukocytes, 183
Leukopenia, 226, 230
Leukotriene receptor inhibitors, 80–81
Leuprolide (Lupron), 178, 191, 269, 279
Levodopa (L-dopa), 13–14, 23–24
Levophed (*see* Norepinephrine)
Levothyroxine (Synthroid), 148–149, 160, 162, 401
Librium (*see* Chlordiazepoxide)
Licensed practical nurse (LPN), 319
Licorice, 162, 165, 371, 374
Lidocaine, 44, 59, 73, 205, 344, 410
Lindane (Kwell), 228, 235
Lioresal (*see* Baclofen)
Liothyronine (Cytomel), 148
Lipase inhibitors, 110–111, 127–128
Lipitor (*see* Atorvastatin)
Lisinopril (Zestril), 38
Lithium (Eskalith), 296–298, 308–309, 320, 403
Livedo reticularis, 32
Liver failure, 106–107, 121–123
Lodine (*see* Etodolac)
Lomotil (*see* Diphenoxylate)
Lopressor (*see* Metoprolol)
Lorazepam (Ativan), 31, 290, 299, 302, 311, 315
Lovenox, 65, 208, 215, 217
Lower respiratory infections, 78–79, 86–88
Lupron (*see* Leuprolide)
Lupus, systemic erythematosus (SLE), 241, 250, 259
Lye, 355
Lymphoma, 292
  non-Hodgkin's, 289

M

Maalox, 134, 139, 380, 384
Macrodantin (*see* Nitrofurantoin)
Macular degeneration, 373
Mafenide acetate (Sulfamylon), 225–226, 230, 402
Magnesium hydroxide (Milk of Magnesia), 104, 119
Magnesium sulfate, 195
Malathion, 343
Mannitol (Osmitrol), 7–8, 17–18, 22, 30–31, 399, 413
Marcaine (*see* Bupivacaine)
Marijuana (*see* Cannabinoids)
Marinol (*see* Dronabinol)

Measles, 237, 247, 256
Meclizine (Antivert), 31, 335
Medical administration, 1–6
MedicAlert bracelets, 19, 156
Medication Administration Record (MAR), 135
  angina, 40
  cancer treatments, 267, 275, 287
    brain tumor, 31
  gastroenteritis, 133
  mental health disorders, 303
  petechiae, 50
Medications, 21
  administration of, 11, 379–393
    computing math, 380–382, 384–386
    by nurses, 379–380, 383–384
  "drug holiday," 13
  nonprescribed, 361–377
  polypharmacy, 70
  self-prescribing, 364–365, 369–370
Megestrol (Megace), 269, 280
Melatonin, 315, 371, 374
Meniere's disease (see Endolymphatic hydrops)
Menopause, 206
  hormone replacement therapy (HRT), 270
Menotropin (Pergonal), 178
Men's issues
  erectile dysfunction, 20, 38, 48
  prostate cancer, 269–270, 273
  prostatic hypertrophy, benign (BPH), 172–173, 184–186
Menstruation (irregular), 180, 194
Mental health disorders, 295–326
Meperidine (Demerol), 114, 145, 208
  and children, 22
  and headaches, 28
  toxicity, 33
  withdrawal, 155
Meridia (see Sibutramine)
Mesalamine (Asacol), 102–103, 408
Mestinon, 249
Metamucil (see Psyllium mucilloid)
Metaproterenol (Alupent), 80
Metformin (Glucophage), 111, 142–143, 152, 163, 166
Methadone, 304–305, 316–317
Methergine (see Methylergonovine)
Methocarbamol (Robaxin), 204
Methotrexate (Rheumatrex), 262, 402, 417
  and arthritis, 246, 254, 259
  and skin disorders, 228, 233
Methylcellulose (Citrucel), 105
Methylergonovine (Methergine), 177
Methylphenidate (Ritalin), 301–302, 304, 313–314, 316, 403
Methylprednisolone sodium succinate (Solu-Medrol), 45, 79, 400
Metoprolol (Lopressor), 47
Metronidazole (Flagyl), 175, 188
Mifepristone (RU-486), 355, 359
Migraines, 15–16, 26–28
  see also Headaches
Milk of Magnesia (see Magnesium hydroxide)
Milrinone lactate (Primacor), 69, 72
Minerals, 362–363, 367–369
  iron, 67, 362, 374, 404, 419
    deficiency, 51
  selenium, 375
  sodium fluoride, 207
  zinc, 78, 86, 363, 368
  see also Natural remedies; Vitamins
Mirapex (see Pramipexole)
Misoprostol (Cytotec), 355
Mitotane, 157
Monoamine oxidase (MAO) inhibitors, 295, 306, 319, 323
Montelukast sodium (Singulair), 80–81
Moon face, 157
Morphine, 31, 87, 185
  and burns, 226
  epidural, 195

  and immunocompromised systems, 258
  and orthopedic surgery, 207
  with pancreatitis, 154
  preoperatively, 382
  and renal calculi, 174, 197
  sulfate, 37, 53, 203
    Contin, 79, 286
    Roxanol, 12, 275
Morton's neuroma, 219, 223
Motion sickness, 31, 34, 136
Motrin (see Ibuprofen)
MRSA (see Staphylococcus aureus)
Mucolytics, 77, 85–86, 403
Mucomyst (see Acetylcysteine)
Mucosal barrier agents, 119
Multiple sclerosis (MS), 241–242, 259
Mumps, 247, 256
Mupirocin (Bactroban), 236
Muscarinic agonists
  atropine, 29, 419
  bethanechol (Urecholine), 29, 183
Muscle relaxants
  baclofen (Lioresal), 204, 249
  chlorzoxazone (Parafon Forte), 218, 402
  cyclobenzaprine (Flexeril), 203
  methocarbamol (Robaxin), 204
Musculoskeletal system, 203–223
Mushrooms, 34
Mustard gas, 343
Myasthenia gravis (MG), 242, 249
Mylanta, 197
Myocardial infarction (MI), 37–38, 53–54, 69
Myringotomy, 333

N

Naloxone (Narcan), 346, 353
Narcolepsy, 304
Narcotic agonists, 346, 353
Narcotics (see Analgesics; Opioids)
Nardil (see Phenelzine)
Nasal congestion, 336
Natamycin (Natacyn), 336
National Childhood Vaccine Act of 1986, 255
National Poison Control Hotline, 352
Natural remedies, 361–362, 366–367
  aloe, 121, 234, 361, 366
  bilberry, 109, 125
  buttermilk, 340
  cascara, 106, 121
  chasteberry, 371, 374
  CoQ10, 373, 377
  cranberry juice, 182
  dong quai (Angelica sinensis), 195, 199, 361
  Echinacea purpurea, 362, 367
  ephedra, 361–362, 366–367
  feverfew, 15, 27
  flax seed oil, 373
  folic acid, 367
  garlic, 85, 366, 372, 375
  Ginkgo biloba, 62, 205, 211
    and Alzheimer's disease, 15, 29, 33, 375
  ginseng, 143, 153
  hawthorn extract, 41, 56, 362, 367
  herbal therapy, 371
  and hypertension, 78
  licorice, 162, 165, 371, 374
  primrose oil, 8, 18
  rhubarb, 121
  saw palmetto, 172, 184
  senna, 121
  St. John's wort, 108, 124, 177, 191, 361, 366
  valerian root, 361, 366
  yogurt, 340
NCLEX-RN exam, 5–6

Nebulizers, 80–81, 89–90
Nefazodone (Serzone), 296
Neomycin sulfate, 106, 122
Neosporin, 17
Nervousness, 143, 160, 163
Neulasta (*see* Pegfilgrastim)
Neumega (*see* Oprelvekin)
Neupogen, 278, 290
Neurological system, 7–35
Neuromuscular blockers, 29
Neutrexin (*see* Trimetrexate)
Nexium (*see* Esomeprazole)
Nicotine, 61, 317
Nicotinic acid (Niacin), 39
Nitrofurantoin (Macrodantin), 171, 183
Nitroglycerin (NTG), 53, 58
    Nitrobid, 38
    patch, 71, 405
    sublingual, 37, 54
    Tridil, 341
Nitropaste, 38, 399
Nix (*see* Permethrin)
Nocturia, 172
Nolvadex (*see* Tamoxifen)
Nonsteroidal anti-inflammatory drugs (NSAIDs), 27
    and Alzheimer's disease, 26
    and autoimmune disease, 249
    and cardiac disorders, 57, 60
    celecoxib (Celebrex), 206, 218, 222
    etodolac (Lodine), 246
    and gastric irritation, 118, 209–210, 212
    ibuprofen, 364
        Motrin, 45, 104, 241
    indomethacin (Indocin), 174
    and pituitary disorders, 159
    pyrazoline, 246
    side effects, 369, 423
Norepinephrine, 347
    Levophed, 341
    reuptake inhibitors, 314, 319, 324
Normodyne (*see* Labetalol)
Norpramin (*see* Desipramine)
Nursing
    administering medications, 379–380, 383–384
        computing math, 380–382, 384–386
    assistants, 324
    emergency, 341–360
Nutrition, 370
    and cancer, 283, 372, 375
    total parenteral (TPN), 273, 320, 400, 414
        and Crohn's disease, 103
        and IBD, 116–117
        and pancreatitis, 144, 155
Nystatin, 337

O

Obesity, 29, 110–111, 127–129, 408
    and diabetes, 143
Obsessive-compulsive disorder (OCD), 300
Octreotide (Sandostatin), 12, 23, 145, 155, 158
Ocusert system, 327
Oncovin (*see* Vincristine)
Ophthalmic medications, 328, 388
    antibiotic ointment, 327, 336, 403
    ciliary paralytic, 327
    miotic, 398, 412
        pilocarpine (Isopto Carpine), 327, 331, 337
    mydriatic, 328, 332
        epinephrine (Epitrate), 327
Opioids, 412
    belladonna and opiate (B & O), 172, 185
    codeine, 376
    hydrocodone, 284
        Vicodin, 35, 219, 273
    hydromorphone (Dilaudid), 219

meperidine (Demerol), 114, 145, 208
    and children, 22
    and headaches, 28
    toxicity, 33
    withdrawal, 155
methadone, 304–305
morphine, 31, 87, 185
    and burns, 226
    Contin, 79, 286
    epidural, 195
    and immunocompromised systems, 258
    and orthopedic surgery, 207
    with pancreatitis, 154
    preoperatively, 382
    and renal calculi, 197
    Roxanol, 12, 275
    sulfate, 37, 53, 203
    see also Analgesics
Oprelvekin (Neumega), 268, 277
Organ failure, 106–107, 121–123
Orlistat (Xenical), 110–111, 127–128
Orthopedic surgery, 207–208, 214–216
Osmitrol (*see* Mannitol)
Osteoarthritis, 204–206, 210–212
Osteomalacia, 218, 221
Osteomyelitis, 218
Osteoporosis, 206–207, 212–214, 218, 402
    prevention, 145
Osteosarcoma, 275
Otic medications, 328–330, 332–333, 335, 388
Otitis media, 328–330, 332, 335, 337
Ovaries
    cancer, 273
    hyperstimulation syndrome, 178, 192
    stimulants, 178
Ovulation, 158
Oxygen, 87, 90, 98, 358
Oxymetazoline (Afrin), 78, 86, 245
Oxytocin (Pitocin), 177

P

Pain, 174
    abdominal, 144, 173
    chronic, 273–275, 284–286
    leg cramps, 64, 72
    lower back, 104, 203–204, 209–210, 398
    stomach, 47
Pancrease, 163
Pancreatic enzymes, 163, 409
Pancreatitis, 144–145, 154–155, 163, 401, 409
Pancreatoduodenectomy, 272–273, 283
Panic attack disorder, 300, 319
Pantoprazole (Protonix), 105, 146, 157
Papillomavirus, human (HPV), 260, 263
Parafon Forte (*see* Chlorzoxazone)
Parkinson's disease (PD), 12–14, 23–25, 29
Parlodel (*see* Bromocriptine)
Paroxetine (Paxil), 300
Peak expiratory flow rate (PEFR), 89
Pediapred (*see* Prednisolone)
Pediatric clients, 5
Pediculocides, 228, 235
Pediculosis
    capitis, 235
    pubis (crabs), 176, 189
Pegfilgrastim (Neulasta), 268
Pemoline (Cylert), 320, 324
Penicillin, 183, 188, 381
Pentoxifylline (Trental), 46
Pepcid (*see* Famotidine)
Peptic ulcer disease, 104–105, 118–120
Pergonal (*see* Menotropin)
Periactin (*see* Cyproheptadine)
Pericarditis, 45, 60
Permethrin (Nix), 176

Pharmacology tests, 1–3
Phenazopyridine (Pyridium), 171, 183
Phenelzine (Nardil), 295, 319
Phenergan (*see* Promethazine)
Phenylbutazone (Butazolidin), 246
Phenylephrine (Preparation H), 372, 376
Phenytoin (Dilantin), 8–10, 12, 19, 23, 29–30, 413
Phosphodiesterase inhibitors, 69, 72
Photosensitivity, 238
Pickwickian syndrome, 304
Pilocarpine (Isopto Carpine), 327, 331, 337
Pioglitazone (Actos), 395, 410
Pitocin (*see* Oxytocin)
Pitressin (*see* Vasopressin)
Pituitary disorders, 146–148, 158–159
    tumors, 11–12, 147
Placebos, 271
Plaquenil (*see* Hydroxychloroquine sulfate)
Plavix (*see* Clopidogrel bisulfate)
Pneumocystis carinii, 244, 251
Pneumonia, 14, 78, 88, 404, 408
    and alcoholism, 304
    and antidepressants, 295
    bacterial, 79
    with kidney disease, 197
    Pneumocystis carinii (PCP), 244, 251
    and respiratory infections, 96, 98
Poison Control Center, 354, 357
Poison ivy, 163, 235, 260
Poisons
    carbon monoxide, 346
    children, 345–346, 351–354
    cyanide, 343, 350
    food poisoning, 355
    household products, 404, 419
    lead, 346
    malathion, 343
    muscarinic, 34
    overdose, 355, 358
Polio, inactivated poliovirus vaccine (IPV), 248, 257
Polycythemia vera, 51, 67
Polydipsia, 145
Polyuria, 145
Positive protein derivative (PPD) skin test, 96
Posttraumatic stress disorder (PTSD), 300
Potassium, 57, 63, 122, 382, 411
    channel blockers, 58
Pramipexole (Mirapex), 13, 24
Pramoxine (Proctofoam), 177
Prednisolone, 81, 258, 261
Prednisone, 87, 103, 133, 163, 167
    and arthritis, 246, 255
    and COPD, 407
    Deltasone, 145
    and poison ivy, 235
Preeclampsia, 177, 195, 402
Pregnancy, 176–177, 189–191
    and epilepsy, 9, 19
    and HIV, 243, 251
    labor and delivery, 176, 190
        cesarean section, 195
        preeclampsia, 177, 195, 402
Premarin, 162
Premature ventricular contractions (PVC), 44, 70, 344
Preparation H (*see* Phenylephrine)
Pressure ulcers, 226–227, 231–233
Prilosec, 138, 364
Primacor (*see* Milrinone lactate)
Primrose oil, 8, 18
Pro re nata (PRN), 5, 31
Prochlorperazine (Compazine), 110, 286
Procrit (*see* Erythropoietin)
Proctofoam (*see* Pramoxine)
Progesterone, 192
Promethazine (Phenergan), 133, 135, 138, 382
Propantheline (Pro-Banthine), 134

Propranolol (Inderal), 16
Propylthiouracil (PTU), 148
Proscar (*see* Finasteride)
Prostaglandin, 60, 355, 423
Prostate
    cancer, 269–270, 273
    prostatic hypertrophy, benign (BPH), 10, 172–173, 184–186
    resection, transurethral (TURP), 172–173, 185
Protocols, investigational, 270–272, 281–282
Protonix (*see* Pantoprazole)
Proton-pump inhibitors (PPI), 101, 115
    esomeprazole (Nexium), 102
    pantoprazole (Protonix), 105, 146, 157
    ranitidine (Zantac), 119
Protopic (*see* Tacrolimus ointment)
Prozac (*see* Fluoxetine)
Pruritus, 233, 236–237
    and liver failure, 107, 123, 139
    and poison ivy, 260
Pseudoephedrine (Sudafed), 77, 364, 370
Psoriasis, 228, 236, 372, 376, 402
Psychiatric unit, medical, 14
Psyllium mucilloid (Metamucil), 14, 105
Pulmonary disease
    chronic obstructive (COPD), 17, 77–79, 94–95, 302, 407
    embolus (PE), 82–84, 91–93
Pulmonary system, 77–100
Pyelogram, intravenous dye (IVP), 174–175
Pyelonephritis, 170
Pyridium (*see* Phenazopyridine)
Pyrosis, 133, 137, 364

Q

Quetiapine (Seroquel), 299

R

Radiation, 350
    acute syndrome (ARS), 343
    therapy, 12, 23
Raloxifene (Evista), 206
Ranitidine (Zantac), 104, 119
Rape, 196, 200
Raynaud's disease, 46, 61
Reactive airway disease, 79–81, 88–90, 396, 407
    children, 81–82, 90–91
Recombivax HB, 123
Reflux, gastroesophageal, 101–102, 115–116
Religious conflicts, 197, 269
Reminyl (*see* Galantamine)
Renal calculi, 173–175, 186–187
    calcium/oxalate, 173
Renal failure
    chronic, 169–170, 181–182
    end-stage renal disease (ESRD), 169–170
Reproductive issues
    birth control, 179–180, 192–194
        mifepristone (RU-486), 355
    contraceptives (oral), 20
    fertilization, in vitro (IVF), 178
    infertility, 177–179, 191–192
    pregnancy, 176–177, 189–191
        endometriosis, 178
        episiotomy, 177
        and HIV, 243, 251
        labor and delivery, 176, 190, 195
        preeclampsia, 177, 195, 402
    see also Birth control; Infertility; Pregnancy
Respiratory alkalosis, 99
Respiratory infections
    adult respiratory distress syndrome (ARDS), 79
    lower, 78–79, 86–88
    upper, 77–78, 85–86
Retinitis, 243
Reye's syndrome, 369
Rh factor, 197

Rheumatoid arthritis, 245–246, 254–255
Rheumatrex (*see* Methotrexate)
Rhinitis, 212, 244
RhoGAM, 197, 201
Rhubarb, 121
Ribavirin (Virazole), 108, 124
Rifampin (Rifadin), 94
Ringer's lactate, 225, 380, 396
Riopan, 118
Risedronate (Actonel), 218
Risperidone (Risperdal), 298
Ritalin (*see* Methylphenidate)
Rivastigmine (Exelon), 14, 25
Robaxin (*see* Methocarbamol)
Robitussin (*see* Dextromethorphan)
Rocaltrol (*see* Calcitriol)
Rocephin (*see* Ceftriaxone)
Roferon (*see* Interferon)
Rotavirus, 110, 127
Roxanol (*see* Morphine)
RU-486 (*see* Mifepristone)
Rubella, 247, 256

S

Sandostatin (*see* Octreotide)
Saw palmetto, 172, 184
Scabies, 228
Schizophrenia, 242, 298–299, 309–311, 321
Sclerotherapy, 107
Scopolamine (Transderm Scop), 136
Secretin, 145
Sedatives
    Ambien CR, 320, 345
    chlordiazepoxide (Librium), 144, 316, 399, 413
    lorazepam (Ativan), 31, 290
Seizures, 8–9, 18–20
Selective estrogen receptor modulator (SERM), 206
Selegiline (Eldepryl), 30, 33
Selenium, 375
Senna (Senokot), 113, 121, 130
Sensory deficits, 327–340
Seroquel (*see* Quetiapine)
Serotonin
    receptor agonists, 16, 30
    selective reuptake inhibitors (SSRI), 306, 312
        fluoxetine (Prozac), 295, 319, 396
        paroxetine (Paxil), 300
        sertraline (Zoloft), 300, 319
        sibutramine (Meridia), 408
    syndrome (SES), 410, 423
Sertraline (Zoloft), 300, 319
Serzone (*see* Nefazodone)
Sexually transmitted diseases (STD)
    acquired immunodeficiency syndrome (AIDS), 242–244,
        250–252, 396
    adolescents, 175–176, 187–189
    Chlamydia trachomatis, 175, 196, 199
    education, 175
    genital warts, 176, 189
    gonorrhea, 175, 188
    pediculosis pubis (crabs), 176, 189
    syphilis, 175, 188
    see also Hepatitis
Shigella, 110
Shock, 341–342, 347–348
    cardiogenic, 341–342
    hypovolemic, 341, 348, 403
    septic, 341, 347
Sibutramine (Meridia), 110–111, 127–129, 408
Sickle cell disease (SCD), 51, 66
Sildenafil (Viagra), 38, 53, 195, 198
Silver nitrate, 225, 230, 336
Silver sulfadiazine (Silvadene), 226
Simvastatin (Zocor), 39

Sinemet (*see* Carbidopa)
Singulair (*see* Montelukast)
Skin disorders, 228–229, 233–234
Sleep disorders, 302–304, 315–316
Sleepwalking, 304
Slo-Phyllin (*see* Theophylline)
Smallpox, 342, 349
Smoking, 61, 304, 321
    cessation, 111, 128, 399, 413
Snake bites, 355
Sodium biphosphate (Fleets Phospho-Soda), 106, 121
Sodium fluoride, 207
Sodium hyaluronate (Hyalgan), 205, 210
Solu-Cortef (*see* Hydrocortisone)
Somatropin (Humatrope), 162
Spermicide, 179, 192
Spironolactone (Aldactone), 69, 107, 123, 162
St. John's wort, 108, 124, 177, 191, 361, 366
Staphylococcus aureus (MRSA), 171
Statins, 54
Status epilepticus, 9
Steatorrhea, 166, 415
Steroids, 118, 204, 238
    anabolic, 197, 200
    hydrocortisone, 219, 245
    and lupus, 259
    prednisone, 87, 103, 133, 163, 167
        and poison ivy, 235
    and pulmonary disorders, 97, 99
    therapy, 87–88, 146
    topical, 240
    see also Cushing's disease
Stomatitis, 290, 294
Stool softeners, 400, 415
    docusate calcium (Surfak), 106
    docusate sodium (Colace), 105, 120–121
Strattera (*see* Atomoxetine)
Strep throat, 70, 74
Streptase (*see* Streptokinase)
Streptokinase (Streptase), 83, 91–92
Stroke, 10–11
    hemorrhagic, 11, 20
Study of Tamoxifen and Raloxifene (STAR), 279
Substance abuse, 85, 109, 304–305, 316–318, 320
    see also Alcohol; Smoking
Sucralfate (Carafate), 119
Sudafed (*see* Pseudoephedrine)
Suicide, 296, 306, 319
Sulfamylon (*see* Mafenide acetate)
Sulfasalazine (Azulfidine), 102–103, 117, 246, 255
Sulfonylureas, 152, 166
    chlorpropamide (Diabinese), 147, 158
    glipizide (Glucotrol), 142
Sumatriptan (Imitrex), 16, 30
Sunburn, 229, 234
Surfactants, 196
Surfak (*see* Docusate calcium)
Surgery
    abdominal, 113–114, 131–132, 380, 396
    amputation, 217
    cancer, 272–273, 282–284, 290
    eye, 327, 336
    gastric bypass, 51, 135
    open-heart, 44
        valve replacement, 71, 74
    open reduction and internal fixation (ORIF), 208
    orthopedic, 30, 207–208, 214–216
        hip replacement, 50, 217
        knee replacement, 260
Symmetrel (*see* Amantadine)
Sympathomimetics, 253, 348
    norepinephrine (Levophed), 341
    oxymetazoline (Afrin), 78, 86, 245
Syndrome of inappropriate antidiuretic hormone (SIADH),
    147, 159

Synthroid (*see* Levothyroxine)
Syphilis, 175, 188
System to Manage Accutane-Related Teratogenicity (SMART), 235, 238

T

Tachycardia, 59, 395, 415
  supraventricular (SVT), 43, 58, 399
Tacrolimus ointment (Protopic), 228, 234
Tagamet (*see* Cimetidine)
Tamoxifen (Nolvadex), 270, 279, 281
Tamsulosin (Flomax), 172
Tar preparation (Estar), 236, 240
Tavist (*see* Clemastine)
Tegaserod (Zelnorm), 134, 138
Tegretol (*see* Carbamazepine)
Telemetry, 42–44, 58, 70–71, 398, 407
Tenoretic, 49
Tenormin (*see* Atenolol)
Tensilon (*see* Edrophonium)
Terbutaline (Brethine), 176, 190
Tetracycline, 235, 238
Theophylline, 97, 411
  Bronkodyl, 82
  Slo-Phyllin, 79
  Theo-Dur, 96
  toxicity, 91
Therapies
  acid, 238
  antibiotic, 45–46, 79, 239, 400
  electroconvulsive (ECT), 29
  herbal, 371
  highly active antiretroviral (HAART), 251, 403, 417
  hormone, 12, 269–270, 279–281
    replacement (HRT), 206, 213, 270, 280
  insulin, 141, 150
  oral replacement (ORT), 109, 126
  pharmacological, 218
  radiation, 12
    I^{131}, 161
  steroid, 87–88, 146
    corticosteroid, 177
  thrombolytic, 38
Thiazolidinediones, 395, 410
Thioamides, propylthiouracil (PTU), 148–149, 160
Thorazine (*see* Chlorpromazine)
Thrombocytopenia, 254, 276, 292
Thrombolytics
  alteplase (Activase), 83
  streptokinase (Streptase), 83, 91–92
  urokinase, 282
Thyroid disorders, 148–149, 160–161
Thyroidectomy, 163
Tinea pedis, 228, 233
Tocolytic agents, 177
Tofranil (*see* Imipramine)
Tolterodine (Detrol-LA), 195
Transderm Scop (*see* Scopolamine)
Transient ischemic attacks (TIA), 30
Trauma, 196
  bleach in the eyes, 328
  chemical explosions, 342
  foreign objects in ear, 335
  fractures, 356, 364
  lacerations, 354, 356, 359
Trental (*see* Pentoxifylline)
Tridil (*see* Nitroglycerin)
Trimethoprim sulfa (Bactrim), 109, 171, 201, 243
Trimetrexate (Neutrexin), 244
Tuberculosis (TB), 59, 94–95, 98, 244, 252
Tubocurarine, 29, 32
Tularemia, 343, 349, 356, 360

Tumors
  brain, 11–12, 21–23, 31, 270, 273, 405
  bronchogenic, 146
  pituitary, 11–12, 147
Twinrix, 125
Tylenol (*see* Acetaminophen)

U

Ulcers
  arterial, 47
  Curling's, 119, 231
  gastric, 30, 33
  mouth, 287, 337
  peptic, 104–105, 118–120
    disease (PUD), 104–105, 355
  pressure, 217, 226–227, 231–233, 235
    tunneling, 227
  stomach, 371
  ulcerative colitis, 102
  venous stasis, 46
Unlicensed assistive personnel (UAP), 171, 198, 401
  and AIDS patients, 243, 396
  and cancer patients, 290
  and childbirth, 195
  and COPD, 95
  and diabetes patients, 163, 409
  and kidney disorders, 175, 187
  and leftover medications, 404, 420
  and orthopedic patients, 208, 216
  and skin issues, 236, 240
Upper respiratory infections, 77–78, 85–86
Urecholine (*see* Bethanechol)
Uric acid stone calculi, 173
  see also Renal calculi
Urinary retention, 29
Urinary tract infections (UTI), 170–172, 182–184, 195

V

Vaccines, 247
  hepatitis
    A, 108
    B, 108–109, 125, 247, 256, 258
    Twinrix, 125
    yeast-recombinant (Recombivax HB), 123
  human papillomavirus (HPV), 260, 263
  inactivated poliovirus (IPV), 248, 257
Vaginal cream, 389
Valacyclovir (Valtrex), 176, 189, 237, 402, 416
Valerian root, 361, 366
Valium (*see* Diazepam)
Valproate (Depakote), 8, 18
Valproic acid (Depakote), 297, 308
Vancomycin, 171, 183, 218, 341, 381
Varicella, 247, 256
Varices, esophageal, 107
Vasodilan (*see* Isoxsuprine)
Vasodilators
  coronary
    Nitropaste, 38, 399
    sublingual nitroglycerin (NTG), 37
  peripheral, 46
Vasopressin, 122
  DDAVP, 11, 22, 158
  Pitressin, 107
  tannate, 147
Vasotec (*see* Enalapril)
Venous insufficiency, 46
Ventolin (*see* Albuterol)
Vertigo, 31
Viagra (*see* Sildenafil)
Vicodin (*see* Hydrocodone)
Vinca alkaloid, 147,159, 265
Vincristine (Oncovin), 147, 159
Virazole (*see* Ribavirin)

Viscera, enlarged, 147
Vistaril, 220
Vitamins, 362–363, 367–369
   A, 362, 367–368
   B$_{12}$, 51, 66–67, 363, 368, 374
   C, 363, 365, 369, 374
   D, 169, 368
   deficiency, 368
   E, 15, 363, 368, 375
   fat-soluble, 363, 371
   folic acid, 52, 67, 362, 374, 395, 410
   K, 199, 220, 363, 368
     AquaMEPHYTON, 64–65, 74, 195
     and liver failure, 107, 122
   prenatal, 354, 357
   see also Minerals; Natural remedies

W

Warfarin (Coumadin), 405, 408
   and DVT, 49, 65, 71
   interaction with medications, 138
   and pulmonary embolus, 83, 91
   toxicity, 64–65, 74
Warts
   genital, 176, 189
   verruca vulgaris, 235
Wellbutrin (*see* Bupropion)
Wheals, 57, 100
Whipple procedure (*see* Pancreatoduodenectomy)
Women's issues
   cancer
     breast, 267, 269–270, 289
     ovarian, 273
   hysterectomy, 162

   menopause, 206
   menstruation (irregular), 180, 194
   ovulation, 158
   pregnancy, 5, 175–177, 189–191
     endometriosis, 178
     episiotomy, 177
     and HIV, 243, 251
     labor and delivery, 176, 190, 195
     preeclampsia, 177, 195, 402
   yeast infections, 365

X

Xanax (*see* Alprazolam)
Xanthine bronchodilators, 79
Xenical (*see* Orlistat)

Y

Yogurt, 340

Z

Zantac (*see* Ranitidine)
Zelnorm (*see* Tegaserod)
Zestril (*see* Lisinopril)
Zetia (*see* Ezetimibe)
Zinc preparations, 78, 86, 363, 368
Ziprasidone (Geodon), 298, 310
Zithromax, 197
Zocor (*see* Simvastatin)
Zoloft (*see* Sertraline)
Zostrix (*see* Capsaicin creme)
Zovirax (*see* Acyclovir)
Zyban, 128
Zyloprim (*see* Allopurinol)